Principles and Practice

For further volumes:
http://www.springer.com/series/3580

Michał Witt · Małgorzata Dawidowska
Tomasz Szczepański
Editors

Molecular Aspects of Hematologic Malignancies

Diagnostic Tools and Clinical Applications

Springer

Editors
Michał Witt
International Institute of Molecular and Cell Biology
Warsaw
Poland

and

Department of Molecular and Clinical Genetics
Institute of Human Genetics
Polish Academy of Sciences
Poznań
Poland

Małgorzata Dawidowska
Department of Molecular and Clinical Genetics
Institute of Human Genetics
Polish Academy of Sciences
Poznań
Poland

Tomasz Szczepański
Department of Pediatric Hematology and Oncology
Medical University of Silesia
Zabrze
Poland

ISSN 1866-914X ISSN 1866-9158 (electronic)
ISBN 978-3-642-29466-2 ISBN 978-3-642-29467-9 (eBook)
DOI 10.1007/978-3-642-29467-9
Springer Heidelberg New York Dordrecht London

Library of Congress Control Number: 2012940269

Based in part on the Polish language edition: Hematologia Molekularna: patogeneza, patomechanizmy i metody badawcze (ISBN 978-83-7314-119-3)

Printed on acid-free paper

Springer is part of Springer Science+Business Media (www.springer.com)

Preface

In recent years, there has been rapid development in molecular techniques, allowing for precise and highly sensitive support of existing traditional methods used in hemato-oncology. The most frequent applications of molecular techniques in hematology include the identification of fusion genes resulting from chromosomal translocations, the detection of minimal residual disease, and the analysis of chimerism following allogeneic hematopoietic stem cell transplantation. They provide a methodological basis for the widening of horizons in hematology toward molecular problems, significantly modernizing basic research and allowing fundamental questions to be tackled relating to hematopoietic stem cell biology, the process of leukemogenesis, the response to therapy, etc. These methods are also quickly becoming an essential component of modern diagnostic and therapeutic programs, revolutionizing clinical hemato-oncology toward more targeted treatment. At the moment it is hard to imagine effective care for patients subjected to transplantation or to other forms of therapy consistent with modern criteria, without the systematic monitoring of molecular markers of disease, giving usually the most precise insight into the prognostic dilemma. This results in the widespread creation of molecular hematology laboratories performing analyses exclusively for the needs of relevant clinical units and creates the necessity for collaboration between hematology clinical units and existing molecular genetic labs. This entails understanding and collaboration between specialists from these two quite different fields.

This monograph is neither another handbook of clinical hemato-oncology nor an exclusive practical laboratory guide. Descriptions of selected hematological malignancies (Part I), diagnostic procedures (Part II), and various aspects of hematopoietic stem cell transplantation (Part III) focus on their molecular aspects and in most of the cases correspond to a set of relevant laboratory protocols as their counterparts (Part IV), giving, together with appropriate references to a clinical realm, a bigger picture of the problem. Such a layout of the text proved appropriate in our previous publications on the topic, while the smooth blend of clinical and molecular problems perfectly matches the realities of medicine today.

M. Witt
M. Dawidowska
T. Szczepański

Contents

Part I Molecular Biology of Selected Hemato-oncologic Diseases

1 **Molecular Biology of Acute Lymphoblastic Leukemia** 3
Małgorzata Dawidowska, Monika D. Kraszewska, Katarzyna Derwich and Tomasz Szczepański

2 **Genetic Mechanisms and Molecular Markers of Neoplastic Transformation in Acute Myeloid Leukemia** 29
Agata A. Filip, Marta Libura, Sebastian Giebel and Olga Haus

3 **Molecular Pathogenesis of Aggressive B-cell Lymphomas** 55
Przemysław Juszczyński and Krzysztof Warzocha

4 **Molecular Biology and Classification of Multiple Myeloma** 71
Anna Dmoszyńska and Norbert Grząśko

5 **Chronic Lymphocytic Leukemia** 85
Anton W. Langerak and Yorick Sandberg

6 **Molecular Biology of Chronic Myeloid Leukemia** 103
Tomasz Sacha, Kajetana Foryciarz and Aleksander B. Skotnicki

7 **Molecular Biology of Myelodysplastic Syndromes** 117
Francesc Solé

8 **Myeloproliferative Neoplasms** 129
Andrzej Hellmann, Maria Bieniaszewska, Witold Prejzner and Aleksandra Leszczyńska

Part II Diagnostics and Monitoring of Therapy of Hemato-oncologic Diseases

9 **Flow Cytometric Immunophenotyping as Diagnostic Tool of Hematopoietic Malignancies** 143
Łukasz Sędek, Juan Flores-Montero, Joanna Bulsa, Susana Barrena, Julia Almeida, Alberto Orfao and Tomasz Szczepański

10 **Cytogenetics in Hematology** 161
Olga Haus, Anna Poluha and Katarzyna Skonieczka

11 **Monitoring of Minimal Residual Disease in Acute Lymphoblastic Leukemia** 183
Tomasz Szczepański, Małgorzata Dawidowska and Katarzyna Derwich

12 **Gene Expression Profiling in Hematologic Malignancies** 199
Przemysław Juszczyński, Bjoern Chapuy, Małgorzata Szczepaniak and Krzysztof Warzocha

Part III Molecular Procedures Involved in Hematopoietic Stem Cell Transplantation

13 **Allogeneic Transplantation of Hematopoietic Stem Cells** 217
Jacek Wachowiak

14 **Genetic Basis of Donor–Recipient Matching in Allogeneic Transplantation of Hematopoietic Stem Cells** 237
Jacek Nowak and Jacek Wachowiak

15 **Chimerism Following Allogeneic Transplantation of Hematopoietic Stem Cells** 255
Małgorzata Dawidowska, Katarzyna Guz, Ewa Brojer, Jacek Wachowiak and Michał Witt

16 **Peritransplantation Monitoring of Minimal Residual Disease in Acute Lymphoblastic Leukemia** 275
Małgorzata Dawidowska, Katarzyna Derwich and Tomasz Szczepański

17 **Biobanks of Cellular Material** 285
Wiesław Wiktor-Jędrzejczak and Elżbieta Urbanowska

Part IV Molecular Diagnostic Protocols

18 Biobanking of Cellular Material 299
Anna Poluha and Elżbieta Urbanowska

19 Isolation of Mononuclear Cells from Human Blood and Bone Marrow by Density Gradient Centrifugation 305
Małgorzata Dawidowska

20 Molecular Techniques Commonly Used in Hemato-oncology 309
Monika D. Kraszewska and Ewa Ziętkiewicz

21 Genetic Methods of HLA Typing 325
Jacek Nowak, Renata Mika-Witkowska and Elżbieta Graczyk-Pol

22 Post-Transplant Chimerism Analysis Through STR-PCR and RQ-PCR 341
Małgorzata Dawidowska, Katarzyna Guz, Agnieszka Orzińska, Justyna Smolarczyk-Wodzyńska, Monika D. Kraszewska and Michał Witt

23 Analysis of Minimal Residual Disease with the Use of Rearrangements of Ig/TCR Genes Through RQ-PCR 363
Małgorzata Dawidowska, Vincent H. J. van der Velden, Michał Witt and Tomasz Szczepański

24 Molecular Diagnostics of Acute Myeloblastic Leukemia 387
Marta Libura, Agata A. Filip and Olga Haus

25 Assessment of the Presence and the Level of *BCR-ABL* Fusion Gene Expression and Mutational Status in *ABL* Kinase Domain 411
Sylwia Czekalska, Magdalena Zawada and Izabela Florek

26 Studies of Rearrangements and Somatic Hypermutation of IGHV Genes in Chronic Lymphocytic Leukemia 429
Anton W. Langerak, Richard Rosenquist, Paolo Ghia, Chrysoula Belessi, Kostas Stamatopoulos and Frederic Davi

27 Molecular Biology Methods in the Diagnosis of Multiple Myeloma 443
Anna Dmoszyńska and Sylwia Chocholska

28 Molecular Methods in Myeloproliferative Neoplasms 451
Aleksandra Leszczyńska, Witold Prejzner, Maria Bieniaszewska and Andrzej Hellmann

29 Informed Consent for Participation in Research Project 463
Małgorzata Dawidowska and Michał Witt

Index 473

Part I
Molecular Biology of Selected Hemato-oncologic Diseases

Chapter 1
Molecular Biology of Acute Lymphoblastic Leukemia

Małgorzata Dawidowska, Monika D. Kraszewska, Katarzyna Derwich and Tomasz Szczepański

Abstract Acute lymphoblastic leukemia (ALL) is the most common but also the most successfully treated malignancy in children. Current cure rates of approximately 85 % have been reached through multi-agent therapeutic regimens and particularly through risk-stratification enabling therapy individualization. Nevertheless, relapse is still the main cause of treatment failure. Therefore, the main effort is now focused on improving the outcome of high risk ALL subtypes, i.e., Ph + ALL, infant ALL, ALL with *MLL* gene rearrangements, hypodiploid ALL, some T-ALL subsets, recurrent and refractory leukemia. Recent research using advanced molecular techniques, in particular microarray-based genomic gene expression profiling (GEP) and high resolution single nucleotide polymorphism (SNP) microarray approaches, resulted in the identification of novel genetic factors with a potential impact on ALL classification and treatment. The main goal is now

M. Dawidowska (✉) · M. D. Kraszewska
Department of Molecular and Clinical Genetics, Institute of Human Genetics,
Polish Academy of Sciences, Strzeszyńska 32, 60-479 Poznań, Poland
e-mail: ma.dawidowska@wp.pl

M. D. Kraszewska
e-mail: m.kraszewska@gmail.com

K. Derwich
Department of Pediatric Oncology, Hematology and Transplantology,
Poznań University of Medical Sciences, Szpitalna 27/33, 60-572 Poznań, Poland
e-mail: kderwich@poczta.onet.pl

T. Szczepański
Department of Pediatric Hematology and Oncology,
Medical University of Silesia, 3 Maja 13/15, 41-800 Zabrze, Poland
e-mail: szczep57@poczta.onet.pl

M. Witt et al. (eds.), *Molecular Aspects of Hematologic Malignancies*,
Principles and Practice, DOI: 10.1007/978-3-642-29467-9_1,

to translate these findings on ALL blast biology and those on pharmacogenetics of patient response to therapy into improved diagnostics, prognostic classification, and treatment of this malignancy.

1.1 Introduction

Acute lymphoblastic leukemia (ALL) is the most common malignancy in children accounting for approximately 30 % of all childhood neoplasms, with peak incidence at the age of 3–4 years (Kaatsch 2010). In adults ALL is less common, accounting for approximately 20 % of adults leukemias, with two incidence peaks—before the age of 30 and after the age of 70 (Piccaluga et al. 2007).

According to the revised World Health Organization (WHO) classification, two major ALL subtypes are distinguished: B lymphoblastic leukemia/lymphoma, traditionally termed B-cell precursor ALL (BCP-ALL) and T lymphoblastic leukemia/lymphoma (T-ALL). These subtypes are characterized by neoplastic outgrowth of lymphoid progenitor cells, within B or T lineage, respectively, which may occur at any stage of lymphoid differentiation, and results in a substantial heterogeneity of the disease (Vardiman et al. 2009).

With current protocols, based on a multi-agent chemotherapy, approximately 80 % of patients reach long-term remission; however, relapse still remains the main cause of treatment failure. Rapid development of molecular technologies in the recent years has enabled significant advances in the understanding of ALL biology. It is now evident that several disease subtypes can be distinguished within BCP-ALL and T-ALL, characterized by specific genetic abnormalities, distinct biology of leukemic blasts, and thus different prognosis (Pui et al. 2011). Therefore, the current challenge is to implement the recent findings on the biology of ALL cells, in combination with those on host-related pharmacogenetics of treatment response, to further improve prognostic classification, treatment individualization, and enable development of novel more targeted therapeutic strategies.

1.2 Etiopathogenesis

ALL is perceived as a complex disease, caused by a combination of genetic and environmental factors, although its etiology is still not fully elucidated. It is known that conditions characterized by chromosomal instability (ataxia-telangiectasia, Fanconi anemia, Nijmegen breakage syndrome), and those related to constitutional chromosomal abnormalities (Down syndrome) are associated with higher ALL prevalence. However, these syndromes are the cause of leukemia in only up to 5 % of ALL patients (Schrappe 2003; Houlston 2010).

The commonly accepted hypothesis states that at least two genetic aberrations (two hits) must take place for neoplastic transformation of a single cell, followed by uncontrolled proliferation of the leukemic clone (Knudson 1971). In most children, the first hit presumably takes place in their prenatal life, the second, is most probably caused by environmental exposition to toxins, ionizing radiation, or viral infections and triggers the disease onset (Greaves 1999). The suspected infectious etiology of ALL has been addressed by two hypotheses; one suggesting existence of a virus directly involved in pathogenesis of ALL and another implying that ALL might be the consequence of an abnormal immune response to infection. Of these two, the latter seems more plausible (Greaves 2006).

Since most environmental factors studied so far failed to provide strong epidemiological evidence for their causative role in ALL, it is probable that susceptibility to ALL upon exposure to these factors might be determined by genetic polymorphism. A candidate gene approach, focused on a limited number of ALL functionally related genes, revealed a positive association of increased risk of ALL with polymorphism in several genes (e.g., *MTHFR*, methylenetetrahydrofolate reductase or *GSTM1*, glutathione S-transferase mu-1); however, these results have not been consistent (Houlston 2010). The more recent research, based on genome-wide association study (GWAS) approach, enabling analysis of hundreds of thousands of SNPs (single nucleotide polymorphisms), with no prior knowledge on their possible involvement in pathogenesis, revealed that polymorphic variants of three genes contribute to higher leukemia prevalence in children: *IKZF1* (IKAROS; early lymphoid development transcription factor), *ARID5B* (AT-rich interactive domain 5B; B-lineage commitment transcription factor), and *CEBPE* (CAAT/enhancer-binding protein, epsilon; T-cell differentiation transcription factor) (Houlston 2010; Mullighan 2010; Prasad et al. 2010). It is noteworthy that, ALL risk alleles identified through the candidate gene strategy have not been confirmed by GWAS.

Results of GWAS analyses indicate that common genetic variants of multiple genes, most probably involved in regulation of lymphocyte differentiation, contribute to increased risk of ALL development. The impact of a single loci is low, and individual susceptibility to ALL likely depends on the cumulative effect of variation in multiple genes (low-penetrance susceptibility alleles) (Houlston 2010). Some genetic variants are specifically associated with increased ALL risk in particular populations, e.g., 657del5 *NBN* (nibrin; encoding a component of a protein complex crucial for response to DNA damage) gene mutation in Polish population (Pastorczak et al. 2011).

1.3 Classification of ALL and Risk Factors

1.3.1 Morphological Versus Immunophenotypic Classification of ALL

Diagnosis of ALL is based on the presence of at least 25 % of lymphoblasts in bone marrow along with clinical symptoms suggestive of leukemic infiltrations. Based on lymphoblast morphology, according to the guidelines of French–American–British (FAB) classification, three types of lymphoblasts were distinguished:

Table 1.1 Immunophenotypic classification of BCP-ALL (Bene et al. 1995)

Leukemia subtype	CD10	cyIgμ	smIg[a]
B–I (pro-B) ALL	–	–	–
B-II (common) ALL	+	–	–
B-III (pre-B) ALL	±	+	–

cyIg cytoplasmic immunoglobulin, μ heavy chain protein, *sIg* surface immunoglobulin
[a] In a small subset of BCP-ALL, expression of surface membrane Ig is observed together with the surrogate light chains. Such subset is called transitional pre-B-ALL and is associated with favorable outcome

Table 1.2 Immunophenotypic classification of T-ALL (Bene et al. 1995)

Leukemia subtype	cy CD3	sm CD3	CD7	CD2	CD5	CD4	CD8	CD1a	TCR$\alpha\beta$	TCR$\gamma\delta$
T-I (pro-T) ALL	+	–	+	–	–	–	–	–	–	–
T-II (pre-T) ALL	+	–	+	+	+	–	–	–	–	–
T-III (cortical-T) ALL	+	±	+	+	+	+	+	+	–	–
T-IVa (α/β + mature-T) ALL	+	+	+	+	+	±	±	–	+	–
T-IVb (γ/δ + mature-T) ALL	+	+	+	+	+	±	±	–	–	+

TCR$\alpha\beta$ $\alpha\beta$ T cell receptor, *TCR$\gamma\delta$* $\gamma\delta$ T cell receptor

L1—observed in 85 % of cases,
L2—observed in 10–15 % of cases,
L3—observed in 1–3 % of cases.

The L3 cell morphology is typically associated with surface expression of immunoglobulins (Ig) (normally observed only in mature B cells) and translocations typical for Burkitt Lymphoma: t(8;14), t(2;8) or t(8;22). Historically, this type of leukemia was classified as B-ALL. Currently, according to recent WHO recommendations, it is included as a subtype of Burkitt Lymphoma/Leukemia. It should be noted that FAB classification is no longer advocated as the sole basis for ALL diagnosis due to its limited clinical and prognostic value.

Based on flow cytometric immunophenotypic assessment of bone marrow two basic ALL types are distinguished: BCP-ALL (80–85 % of cases) and T-ALL (15–20 %), which are further divided, according to current recommendations of the European Group for the Immunological Characterization of Leukemias (EGIL), into several subtypes listed in Tables 1.1 and 1.2. The immunophenotype of blast cells reflects the differentiation stage, at which the neoplastic transformation occurred (maturation arrest), which might be complemented by the analysis of rearranged immunoglobulin (Ig) and T-cell receptor (TCR) genes, further discussed in Sect. 1.5.1.

Table 1.3 Prognostic factors in ALL (Pui and Jeha 2007)

Prognostic factor	Favorable	Unfavorable
FAB classification	L_1	L_2, L_3
Immunophenotype		
pro-B-ALL	No	Yes
T-ALL	No	Yes
Leukocyte count (G/L)	<20	≥20
Age at diagnosis	1–10 years old	Infants, and ≥10 years old
Response to initial 7 day prednisone therapy	Blast count $<10^9$/L	Blast count $>10^9$/L
DNA index	>1,16	<1,16
Ploidy	>50 chromosomes	<44 chromosomes
Translocations		
t(12;21)/*ETV6–RUNX1*	Yes	No
t(9;22)/*BCR–ABL1*	No	Yes
t(4;11)/*MLL–AF4*	No	Yes
MRD levels at the end of induction therapy	$<10^{-3}$ or below detection levels	$\geq 10^{-3}$
Remission on day 33	Yes	No

1.3.2 Conventional Versus Molecular-Based Prognostic Factors in ALL

In the 'pre-molecular' era prognostic factors were based on clinical observations and laboratory findings such as sex, race, age, and leukocyte count at diagnosis, blast morphology, and response to initial steroid therapy. With current ALL therapy regimens only some of these factors proved to be useful for risk stratification. This indicates their relevance to biological features of leukemic blasts (e.g., chromosomal translocations) or those of leukemic blasts in combination with host genetic features (e.g., prednisone response, now complemented by assessment of minimal residual disease; MRD) (Pui 2010). Prognostic factors currently applied in the vast majority of ALL therapeutic protocols are listed in Table 1.3.

Rapid development of molecular techniques (e.g., molecular cytogenetics, real-time polymerase chain reaction) provided a new basis for the prognostic classification of ALL. More advanced techniques like genome-wide profiling of copy number alterations (CNAs) or gene expression enable the identification of novel factors that might influence prognosis and potentially be incorporated into ALL therapy protocols for risk stratification.

1.3.2.1 Chromosomal Abnormalities in BCP-ALL

In approximately 80 % of pediatric ALL cases, aberrations of the number and the structure of chromosomes are observed. High hyperdiploidy with >50 chromosomes (25–30 % ALL cases), particularly in combination with trisomies of chromosomes 4, 10, and 17 have been associated with favorable prognosis, while hypodiploidy with <44 chromosomes (5–6 %) have been reported to correlate with poor outcome (Sutcliffe et al. 2005; Nachman et al. 2007). The most frequent chromosomal aberrations in pediatric ALL are listed in Table 1.4, those of recognized prognostic significance, widely used for risk group stratification are presented in Table 1.3 and discussed below.

TEL–AML1 (ETV6–RUNX1) Fusion Gene
The *TEL–AML1* (*TEL*, translocation-Ets-leukemia; *AML1*, acute myeloid leukemia-1) fusion gene, resulting from t(12;21)(p13;q22) translocation (approximately 25 % of pediatric ALL) is generally related to favorable prognosis (Gandemer et al. 2007). Since clonally related late relapses occur in some patients even 5–20 years after diagnosis, it is believed that the actual prognostic significance of this aberration is dependent on the therapeutic protocol (Ford et al. 2001). *TEL–AML1* is regarded as a very early or even ALL initiating (pre-leukemic) event, though alone it is not sufficient for the overt leukemia to occur (Greaves and Wiemels 2003). Its frequency in healthy children (found in Guthrie spots) is 100-fold higher than that observed in ALL patients. One of the proposed second hits is the deletion of the nonrearranged *TEL* allele (Konrad et al. 2003).

Transcription factors, encoded by wild-type *TEL* and *AML1* genes, are crucial for regulation of expression of many genes, including these involved in hematopoiesis. TEL–AML1 fusion protein acts as an aberrant transcription factor impairing different pathways of hematopoiesis, including cell differentiation, proliferation, apoptosis, and motility, which has been recently confirmed in gene expression profiling experiments (Gandemer et al. 2007). Moreover, it interferes in a negative dominant manner with a wild-type TEL and AML1, and inactivates the tumor suppressor function of the TEL.

BCR–ABL1 Fusion Gene
The *BCR–ABL1* fusion gene (*BCR*, breakpoint cluster region; *ABL1*, Abelson murine leukemia viral oncogene) and occurrence of Philadelphia (Ph) chromosome (truncated chromosome 22) resulting from t(9;22)(q34;q11) is detected in 5–10 % and 20–30 % of pediatric and adult ALL cases, respectively. It defines a subtype of ALL termed Ph + ALL, related to poor prognosis (Piccaluga et al. 2007). This fusion gene encodes for an constitutively active tyrosine kinase impairing various signal transduction pathways, causing uncontrolled cell proliferation, reduced apoptosis, and altered cell adhesion (Piccaluga et al. 2007; De Braekeleer et al. 2011). The use of tyrosine kinase inhibitors, mostly imatinib, in combination with chemotherapy and/or HSCT, has improved the outcome of childhood Ph + ALL patients (Schultz et al. 2009). Nevertheless, Ph + still

Table 1.4 Typical chromosomal aberration found in pediatric ALL (Szczepanski et al. 2010)

Aberration	Involved genes (detection level)	Frequency in pediatric ALL (%)
BCP-ALL		
t(9;22)(q34;q11)	*BCR–ABL1* (mRNA)	2–3
t(1;19)(q23;p13)	*TCF–PBX1* (mRNA)	5–6
t(4;11)(q21;q23)	*MLL–AF4* (mRNA)	3–5
11q23 aberrations	*MLL* rearrangements (mRNA)	5–8
t(12;21)(p13;q22)	*ETV6–RUNX1* (mRNA)	20–25
T-ALL		
Translocations to TCRD/A or TCRB		40–50
t(11;14)(p15;q11)	*LMO1–TCRD* (DNA)	9
t(11;14)(p13;q11)	*LMO2–TCRD* (DNA)	4–5
t(1;14)(p34;q11)	*TAL1–TCRD* (DNA)	3
t(10;14)(q24;q11) t(7;10)(q35;q24)	*HOX11–TCRD* or *TCRB* (mRNA)	~10
inv(7)(p15q34)	*HOXA–TCRB* (mRNA)	5
Aberrations resulting in fusion genes		
del(1)(p32)	*SIL–TAL1* (DNA/mRNA)	20–30
t(10;11)(p13-14;q14-21)	*CALM–AF10* (mRNA)	8
t(10;11)(p12;q14)	*PICALM–MLLT10* (mRNA)	10
t(5;14)(q35;q32)	*HOX11L2–BCL11B* (mRNA)	20
MLL rearrangements	*MLL–ENL/AF10* and other (mRNA)	5–10
t(9;22)(q34;q11)	*BCR–ABL1* (mRNA)	very rare
Episomal amplification 9p34	*NUP214–ABL1* (mRNA)	5–6
Gene deletions		
del(9)(p21)	*CDKN2A, CDKN2B* (DNA/mRNA)	65–80
del(9)(q34.11q34.13)	*SET–NUP214* (mRNA)	Not established so far

TCF (transcription factor 3); *PBX1* (pre-B-cell leukemia homeobox 1, encodes a transcriptional activator); *LMO1* (LIM domain only 1, probably involved in transcriptional regulation); *LMO2* (LIM domain only 2, encoding a transcription factor involved in erythropoiesis); *TAL1* (T-cell acute lymphocytic leukemia protein 1, encoding a transcription factor involved in erythropoiesis); *HOX11* (T-cell leukemia, homeobox 1, encoding a transcription factor); *HOXA* cluster (homeobox A cluster of genes involved in embryonic development and cell differentiation); *SIL* (*SCL/TAL1* interrupting locus, involved in embryonic development and cellular growth and proliferation); *CALM* (clathrin assembly lymphoid-myeloid leukemia gene) also termed *PICALM* (phosphatidylinositol binding clathrin assembly); *MLLT10* (gene from chromosome 10 involved in translocation to *MLL*, encoding a protein probably involved in transcriptional regulation); *HOX11L2* (homeobox 11-like 2, encoding a transcription factor); *BCL11B* (B-cell lymphoma/leukemia 11B, probably a key regulator of differentiation and survival during thymocyte development); *NUP214* (nucleoporin 214 kDa, involved in receptor-mediated transport across the nuclear pore complex); *SET* (*SET* nuclear oncogene, encoding for a protein involved in apoptosis, transcription, nucleosome assembly and histone binding); the names and functions of the remaining genes are included in the text

remains an adverse prognostic factor in ALL. For more details on BCR–ABL1 inhibitors, including agents with improved tolerability and efficacy (dasatinib, nilotinib) see also Chap. 6.

MLL Abnormalities

Alterations of the *MLL* gene (mixed-lineage leukemia; also named *ALL-1*, *HRX* or *HTRX-1*), mostly chromosomal translocations, but also deletions, inversions, insertions, and complex recombinations involving 11q23 occur in 3–8 % of ALL (Meyer et al. 2009; Tamai and Inokuchi 2010). Rearrangements of the *MLL* gene are particularly regarded as the hallmarks of infant ALL (diagnosed in children <1 year of age, presenting pro-B immunophenotype and *MLL* rearrangements in approximately 80 % of cases), which is a rare ALL subtype characterized by very poor prognosis (5-year disease free survival around 40 %) (Pieters et al. 2007). Early onset of the disease and high concordance between monozygotic twins presenting with *MLL*-r infant ALL, provide evidence for the *MLL* alteration to be the first oncogenic hit, leading to in utero malignant transformation (Ford et al. 1993).

The most frequent aberrations of the *MLL* gene in ALL include: t(4;11), t(11;19), t(9;11), t(10;11), and t(6;11) resulting in *MLL–AF4*, *MLL–ENL*, *MLL–AF9*, *MLL–AF10*, and *MLL–AF6* fusion proteins. All these genes: *ENL* (eleven-nineteen leukemia gene), *AF4*, *AF9*, *AF10*, and *AF6* (*ALL-1* fused genes from chromosomes 4, 9, 10, and 6, respectively) encode for transcriptional transactivation factors. However, the transforming activity of the fusion genes is attributed to a disruption of the *MLL* gene and not to the biological function of the translocation partner genes (TPGs) (Meyer et al. 2009).

Rearrangements of the *MLL* gene result in a fusion of the N-terminal portion of the MLL and the C-terminal part of the protein encoded by a TPG. The resulting fusion proteins retain the DNA binding capacities and putative DNA methyltransferase activity of wild-type MLL (transcriptional repression domain of the *MLL* exhibits homology to DNA methyltransferase 1, DNMT1) but lack histone methyltransferase functions (conveyed by SET domain, SU(var)3-9, enhancer-of-zeste, trithorax) (Liedtke 2010). Therefore, they act through disruption of transcriptional but most possibly also—epigenetic regulation of downstream MLL target genes, including HOX genes (homeobox genes, crucial for differentiation of cells, including embryogenesis and hematopoiesis (Tamai and Inokuchi 2010). *MLL* gene rearrangements are related to poor outcome in infant ALL (Pieters et al. 2007). In older children only t(4;11) is associated with poor outcome and qualifies patients into high risk group. The prognostic significance of other *MLL* rearrangements in children >1 year of age is intermediate (Pui et al. 2002; Szczepanski et al. 2010).

Aberrations Resulting in CRLF2 Overexpression

Recently, overexpression of *CRLF2* gene (cytokine receptor-like factor 2, encoding a receptor for thymic stromal lymphopoietin) in leukemic cells has been identified as adverse prognostic factor. In most patients (including 60 % of children with Down Syndrome associated ALL) *CRLF2* overexpression is caused by fusion of this gene with *IGH* locus on 14q32. Overexpression of *CRLF2* might also be caused by a fusion with *P2RY8* (P2Y purinoceptor 8 gene, located on X chromosome, encoding for a receptor for purines coupled to G-proteins) due to an intrachromosomal deletion centromeric to *CRLF2*. The treatment outcome is particularly dismal for patients with *P2RY8–CRLF2* fusion (6-year EFS of 28 %;

cumulative incidence of relapse 67 %) (Cario et al. 2010) This chromosome aberration might become a novel independent prognostic factor, since most of these patients show non-high risk MRD profile.

1.3.2.2 Chromosomal Abnormalities in T-ALL

The most common aberrations observed in T-ALL are translocations of various oncogenes to loci encoding T-cell receptors *TCRD/A* (delta/alpha) or *TCRB* (beta), detected in about 35 % of all T-ALL cases (Cauwelier et al. 2006). Other recurrent changes involve translocation of transcription factor genes to strong promoter regions of highly active genes, which lead to the formation of fusion genes (Aifantis et al. 2008). The last type of chromosomal aberrations in T-ALL are deletions of tumor suppressor genes. All of these changes cause deregulation of cell proliferation/differentiation, and apoptosis. The most common aberrations found in T-ALL are listed in Table 1.4.

1.3.2.3 Minimal Residual Disease

The level of residual leukemic cells, detected at standard time points during ALL treatment with the use of molecular or flow cytometric approaches, is currently the most significant prognostic factor in ALL. Detailed information about MRD monitoring and its clinical significance in hematological malignancies is presented in Chaps. 11, 16 and 23.

The exceptional prognostic value of MRD, stems from the fact that the reduction of the tumor load reflects the resistance to therapy of the leukemic clone as well as host-related features associated with therapy response, both influencing the risk of relapse. Therefore, recent research, using mainly GWAS approach, has been focused on pharmacogenetics of MRD and identification of germline genetic polymorphisms influencing individual differences in response to treatment, as measured by MRD reduction (Yang et al. 2009).

1.4 Implications of Recent Findings on Molecular Biology of ALL

Due to high prevalence of ALL in children, particularly BCP-ALL, it has been one of the most intensively studied and thus well-characterized malignancies. Despite identification of a wide range of genetic lesions related to ALL, translation of this data into improved prognostic classification and treatment has always been challenging. The advent of novel molecular approaches, particularly (i) microarray-based genomic gene expression profiling (GEP) and (ii) high resolution SNP microarrays enabling GWAS, detection of copy number alterations (CNAs) and loss of heterozygosity (LOH) analysis, but also tools for (iii) second generation sequencing and (iv) analysis of epigenetic changes, provide new insights into molecular biology of ALL. Recent research with the use of these advanced technologies, focused particularly on ALL subtypes related to the most unfavorable prognosis, resulted in the identification of novel genetic factors with a potential impact on classification and treatment. Moreover, complex interactions between previously recognized prognostic factors and newly identified genetic features have been revealed.

1.4.1 Copy Number Alterations

According to the two-hit hypothesis, most of the recurrent chromosomal translocations found in ALL act as the first oncogenic hit, and alone are not sufficient to cause leukemia. Implementation of SNP microarrays into the study of copy number alterations (CNAs) enabled a genome-wide search for cooperating mutations, with a much greater efficiency than the traditionally used candidate gene approach or low resolution approaches for loss of heterozygosity analysis. The use of SNP microarrays revealed that ALL is characterized by an average of 6.46 CNAs/case, mainly affecting genes of crucial importance for lymphoid differentiation and development. It is also noteworthy that the number of lesions is ALL- subtype specific, e.g., *BCR–ABL1*-positive and *ETV6–RUNX1*-positive ALL cases present with relatively high number of CNAs in contrast to *MLL*-r ALL (a mean CNAs/case >6 and <1, respectively) (Mullighan and Downing 2009a, b). These results are consistent with the hypothesis that additional cooperating mutations are needed in *BCR–ABL1* or *ETV6-RUNX1* ALL cases, while the *MLL* rearrangements are regarded early (in utero) leukemia initiating events, with little or no contribution of other genetic lesions (Bardini et al. 2010).

Further analysis of the CNA-involved regions resulted in the identification of numerous genes, including those engaged in normal lymphoid developmental pathways, to be recurrently deleted in ALL (Mullighan 2009; Mullighan and Downing 2009b). These include:

- genes of lymphoid transcription factors involved in B-lymphoid commitment: *PAX5* (paired box gene 5), *IKZF1*, *IKZF2*, *IKZF3* (IKAROS family of transcription factors), *EBF1* (early B-cell factor);
- recombination activating genes: *RAG1* and *RAG2*;
- suppressor genes: *CDKN2A/B* (cyclin-dependent kinase inhibitors 2A/2B), *PTEN* (phosphatase and tensin homolog), *RB1* (retinoblastoma);
- genes presumably involved in the regulation of apoptosis like *BTG1* (B-cell translocation gene 1);
- genes involved in lymphoid signaling like *TOX* (thymus high mobility group box protein);

- genes involved in drug response: *NR3C1* (glucocorticoid receptor), *NR3C2* (mineralocorticoid receptor).

The questions on the actual biological role of CNAs in ALL pathogenesis, whether these lesions are so-called 'driver mutations' or 'passenger mutations' (genetic background noise), as well as on their clinical prognostic significance and involvement in therapy response, remain to be elucidated. Of the above genes, the *IKZF1* and *PAX5* have been most extensively studied so far.

1.4.1.1 *IKZF1*

The *IKZF1* gene encoding for IKAROS, a transcription factor regulating early lymphoid development, appears to be a key player in high risk ALL. Deletions or mutations of this gene are frequent in *BCR–ABL1*- positive ALL (approximately 80 % of cases) and often accompanied by deletions of *CDKN2A/B* and alterations of *PAX5* gene (Mullighan 2009; Mullighan and Downing 2009b; Hunger et al. 2011). Gene expression profiling revealed significant convergence of expression signatures between high risk *BCR–ABL1*-positive leukemia and high risk *BCR–ABL1*-negative ALL subtype with *IKZF1* alterations, which suggests a similar mechanism of leukemogenesis (Mullighan et al. 2009a). Characterization of the latter subtype resulted in the identification of constitutively active tyrosine kinases, other than BCR–ABL1, in approximately 10 % of patients (due to mutations of Janus kinases genes *JAK1*, *JAK2* and *JAK3*) (Mullighan et al. 2009b). These results have significant clinical implications, since altered JAK signaling might be a promising therapeutic target in *BCR–ABL1*-negative ALL, analogous to a tyrosine kinase inhibitor-based therapeutic strategy used in *BCR–ABL1*-positive ALL and CML. Moreover, alterations of *IKZF1* have been related to high levels of minimal residual disease (MRD) and significantly increased risk of ALL relapse in both *BCR–ABL1*-positive and *BCR–ABL1*-negative patients (Waanders et al. 2011; Martinelli et al. 2009; Mullighan et al. 2009a).

1.4.1.2 *PAX5*

In contrast to *IKZF1* alterations, abnormalities regarding the *PAX5* gene serve as an example of genetic lesions of high prevalence in both childhood and adult ALL (approximately 39 % and 35 %, respectively), but with no proved prognostic utility, as revealed to date (Familiades et al. 2009; Iacobucci et al. 2010). The *PAX5* is a member of a highly conserved family of genes, paired-box domain of transcription factors, and encodes for the B-cell lineage specific activator protein (BSAP), involved in early stages of B-cell differentiation. In normal hematopoiesis *PAX5* acts as both transcriptional activator and repressor. *PAX5* is disrupted through partial or complete deletions, but also through partial or complete amplification, point mutations, or rearrangements, resulting in underexpression of

PAX5 or expression of *PAX5* products with impaired DNA-binding affinity. Alterations of *PAX5* gene have been frequently found in *BCR-ABL1*-positive ALL patients with *IKZF1* deletions; however, in contrast to the latter, have not been associated with clinical outcome. This might be attributed to different biological roles of *IKZF1* and *PAX5* genes (Mullighan et al. 2009a; Iacobucci et al. 2010).

1.4.2 Gene Expression Profiling

1.4.2.1 Gene Expression Profiling for Improved Prognostic Classification of ALL

Microarray-based gene GEP has proven that distinct BCP-ALL subtypes: characterized by hyperdiploidy >50 chromosomes, *BCR–ABL1*, *TEL–AML1*, *E2A–PBX*, and *MLL* rearrangements, as well as T-ALL are characterized by unique expression signatures, reflecting differences in molecular biology of these subtypes and hence prognosis (Yeoh et al. 2002; Ross et al. 2003).

Specific expression profiles, highly predictive of relapse within individual leukemia subtypes, have been identified, although it was not possible to point a single relapse-predicting expression profile, common to all leukemia subclasses. These results suggest the existence of multiple mechanisms of therapy resistance and disease recurrence (Yeoh et al. 2002; Ross et al. 2003). Therefore, GEP research has been subsequently focused on expression profiles specific for therapy resistant and therapy sensitive ALL, as measured by MRD levels, and on the development of expression classifiers, based on a limited number of selected genes that best predict outcome (Flotho et al. 2007; Cario et al. 2005). The use of such an approach in pediatric high risk ALL resulted recently in the development of 38-gene and 21-gene expression classifiers that were highly predictive of relapse-free survival (RFS) and end-induction MRD level, respectively. The use of these classifiers, independently and in combination with *IKZF1* deletions, *JAK* mutations and kinase expression profiles, resulted in improved outcome prediction (Kang et al. 2010).

Moreover, results of GEP studies has enabled further prognostic classification of patients within previously defined ALL subtypes. It has been recently shown that *MLL*-r and *MLL*-germline infant ALL cases present with unique gene expression profiles, and are characterized by event-free survival rates of 20–50 % and 75–95 %, respectively (Stam et al. 2010). For more information about GEP in ALL, see Chap. 12.

1.4.2.2 Gene Expression Profiling of T-ALL

Results of GEP analyses has also greatly improved our understanding of molecular heterogeneity and prognostic classification of T-ALL. It has been shown that some of the aberrantly expressed genes can be used for improved T-ALL prognostic classification. Based on the altered expression of only five oncogenes: *LYL1* (lymphoblastic leukemia-derived sequence 1, encoding for a transcription factor), *HOX11* (*TLX1*), *TAL1* and *LMO2*, and *HOX11L2* (*TLX3*), it is possible to classify T-ALL patients into four major T-ALL subtypes of differential prognosis (Ferrando et al. 2002) (for the names and functions of the genes see Table 1.4). *HOXA* cluster overexpression was further proposed as a fifth T-ALL subclass delineating GEP classifier (Dik et al. 2005). These overexpressed genes, regarded as hallmarks of T-ALL subtypes, are associated with specific expression signatures and different therapy response. Hence, the *HOX11* and *HOXA* groups are characterized by a favorable prognosis, in contrast to *LYL1*, *TAL1/LMO2* and *HOX11L2* subtypes, which are related to poor outcome.

The limited number of T-ALL subtypes delineated based on gene overexpression is surprising, considering the abundance of different cytogenetic aberrations observed in this disease. This can be explained by the fact that various molecular aberrations can lead to overexpression of the same oncogene (e.g., *MLL*, *HOXA–TCRB*, *SET–NUP214* and *CALM–AF10* lead to *HOXA* up-regulation (see also Table 1.4).

Recently, gene expression profiling, complemented by immunophenotyping and SNP analysis, resulted in the identification of a novel subtype of T-ALL, termed early T-cell precursor leukemia (ETP-ALL), related to very inferior prognosis due to poor response to therapy targeting lymphoid cells (Coustan-Smith et al. 2009). This subtype originates from stem-cell-like precursors of thymocytes, characterized by a specific gene expression profile, particular cell surface antigens and genomic instability reflected by increased number and size of genetic alterations (CNAs) as compared to typical T-ALL blast cells. These findings explain low responsiveness to current T-ALL therapeutic protocols and opens possibilities for development of novel, ETP-specific therapy options.

1.4.3 Epigenetics

The role of aberrant DNA methylation in leukemogenesis is still not fully understood. However, it is now evident that both hypermethylation of promoter regions of tumor suppressor genes (resulting in their inactivation) and hypomethylation of large areas of repetitive genome sequences (leading to general genome instability) is present in tumor cells. Since the aberrant methylation occurs at very early stages of leukemogenesis and the levels of CpG island methylation density increase with malignancy progression, it can be regarded as one of the leukemia initiating processes, but also possibly could be used for improved risk assessment and outcome prediction, as illustrated by example of *MLL*-r ALL and T-ALL (Stumpel et al. 2009; Roman-Gomez et al. 2005). It is also worth noting that DNA hypermethylation is reversible and might serve as a therapy target. Demethylating agents have been shown to reverse aberrant hypermethylation, inducing apoptosis in *MLL*-r cells (Stumpel et al. 2011).

1.4.3.1 CpG Island Methylation in Infant MLL-r ALL

The identification of expression signature characteristic of *MLL*-r infant ALL, the most aggressive type of childhood ALL, inspired the search for the epigenetic basis of this specific expression profile. It has been demonstrated that *MLL*-r ALL is characterized by global genomic hypermethylation, as compared to other ALL types and controls. Moreover, distinct subtypes of *MLL*-r infant ALL present with differential patterns of CpG island methylation, i.e., aberrantly high levels of hypermethylation in patients with t(4;11) and t(11;19), while methylation levels resembling those found in control bone marrow in cases with t(9;11) and *MLL*-germline infant ALL cases. The risk of ALL relapse have been reported to increase with the increasing degree of hypermethylation of promoter regions (Stumpel et al. 2009; Schafer et al. 2010). Recent findings show that *MLL*-r infant ALL specific expression profiles should be attributed not only to CpG hypermethylation of promoter regions of protein-coding genes, but also to those of miRNA-coding genes, and to aberrant histone modifications (Stumpel et al. 2011; Benedikt et al. 2011).

1.4.3.2 CpG Island Methylation in T-ALL

T-ALL remains the most heterogeneous subtype of ALL (Kraszewska et al. 2012b). In contrast to BCP-ALL, patient outcome cannot be simply correlated with cytogenetic or molecular aberrations. CpG island hypermethylation in T-ALL concerns genes from many functional groups, namely genes encoding for tyrosine kinases, adhesion molecules, proteins belonging to p53 network, to WNT signaling pathway, those involved in apoptosis, cell cycle control, and tumor suppression. Many of these genes are observed to be hypermethylated in different neoplasms, while others seem to be unique for T-ALL (Roman-Gomez et al. 2004; Roman-Gomez et al. 2005). As reported by Roman-Gomez et al. (2005), and recently confirmed by Kraszewska et al. (Kraszewska et al. 2011), T-ALL patients can be divided into two distinct groups based on the number of hypermethylated genes. This is referred to as CpG methylator phenotype (CIMP). The CIMP + patients, with many simultaneously hypermethylated genes, seem to have poorer prognosis and higher relapse rate as compared to those characterized as CIMP- (Roman-Gomez et al. 2005). It still needs to be elucidated, whether DNA hypermethylation analyses can be turned into diagnostics and improve patient stratification.

1.4.4 Point Mutations in T-ALL

Since only about half of T-ALL patients present with an aberrant karyotype, the attention has been drawn to smaller, not cytogenetically detectable aberrations, such as point mutations of genes responsible for normal thymocyte development and lineage determination. Among those, two appear to be of crucial importance for T-ALL pathogenesis and potentially for prognostic classification: *NOTCH1* and *FBXW7* (Kraszewska et al. 2012b).

1.4.4.1 *NOTCH1*

The *NOTCH1* gene (*TAN1*; translocation-associated Notch homolog) is located in 9q34.3. About half of T-ALL patients carry *NOTCH1* activating mutations, only detectable with molecular methods, which makes it the most frequently mutated gene in this disease (Weng et al. 2004). *NOTCH1* encodes for a signal transduction cell membrane receptor, taking part in the control of hematopoietic cell proliferation, maturation, adhesion, and apoptosis (Demarest et al. 2008). In T-cells, it plays a key role in lineage determination: as early as B versus T commitment and then at the $\alpha\beta$ versus $\gamma\delta$ determination stage of T-cell maturation. Both its inactivation and constitutive activation lead to dramatic abruption in T-cell development (Varnum-Finney et al. 2000; Wilson et al. 2001). The receptor is encoded as a pre-protein, which is proteolytically cleaved to give two NOTCH1 subunits, the extracellular receptor unit and the intracellular (ICN) transcription factor interacting unit, in two cleavage steps, the second processed by γ secretase. Understanding the molecular biology of aberrant *NOTCH1* activation triggered the introduction of γ-secretase inhibitors (GSI) as therapeutic agents. Unfortunately, the first attempts to use them in T-ALL therapy failed due to low cytotoxicity and severe gastrointestinal side effects (Milano et al. 2004). Nevertheless, the γ-secretase inhibitors still remain promising therapeutic agents (Real et al. 2009).

1.4.4.2 *FBXW7*

The *FBXW7* gene (*FBW7;* F-box and WD40 domain protein 7) located in 4q31.3 codes for a component of the ubiquitin ligase complex, which plays a role in degradation of various proteins including c-MYC (a homolog of v-myc myelocytomatosis viral oncogene encoding a transcription factor) and NOTCH1 (O'Neil et al. 2007). Mutant FBXW7 protein fails to bind its targets (NOTCH1) or binds, but fails to tag them for degradation (c-MYC), in both cases prolonging their half-life. For NOTCH1 and c-MYC (which is a NOTCH1 downstream target and becomes overexpressed due to high activity of NOTCH1), this leads to a significant increase in the protein activity that contributes to the malignant proliferation of thymocytes. *NOTCH1* and *FBXW7* mutations result in elevated intracellular NOTCH1 activity and overexpression of its downstream targets, impairing cell cycle control and leading to tumor development.

Frequency of *FBXW7* mutations in T-ALL reported by different authors varies between 8.6 (O'Neil et al. 2007) and 19 % (Matsuoka et al. 2008). *FBXW7* and *NOTCH1* mutations are also frequently observed in the same patient, suggesting cooperation between these two mutational events leading to the development of T-ALL.

Many authors indicate that *NOTCH1* and *FBXW7* mutations delineate a low relapse risk T-ALL (Malyukova et al. 2007; Asnafi et al. 2009), but contradictory reports have also been published (Clappier et al. 2010; Zuurbier et al. 2010). *FBXW7* mutations have been observed in cell lines resistant to NOTCH1 inhibitors. These findings improved our understanding of γ-secretase inhibitor treatment resistance, pointing to a necessity of incorporation of additional downstream NOTCH1 target inhibitors into T-ALL therapeutic approaches.

1.5 Immunoglobulin and T-Cell Receptor Gene Rearrangements

1.5.1 Immunoglobulin/T-Cell Receptor Gene Rearrangements in Normal Cells: Implications for ALL Study

Immunoglobulin and T-Cell Receptor (Ig/TCR) diversity is achieved by rearrangements between multiple V (variable), D (diversity) and J (joining) gene segments within Ig and TCR loci. This process, occurring at the early stages of lymphocyte development, is mediated by recombinase enzyme complex, which nearly randomly joins unique V, D, and J fragments (*combinatorial diversity*). Additionally, small deletions of nucleotides as well as random insertions of nucleotides (N) at V, D, and J segment borders occur, mediated by exonucleases and terminal deoxynucleotidyl transferase (TdT), respectively (*junctional diversity*). This results in the generation of almost unlimited number of Ig/TCR gene rearrangements, unique for each lymphocyte/lymphocyte clone, including leukemic clones, therefore used as patient-specific markers of residual leukemic blasts and clonality markers in the diagnosis of suspected lymphoproliferations (van Dongen et al. 2003).

During B lymphocyte development, the *IGH* (Ig heavy chain genes) locus is first rearranged, and, if functional, blocks further changes within this locus, enabling rearrangements within *IGK* (Ig kappa light chain genes) locus. If these turn out to be non-functional, *IGL* (Ig lambda light chain genes) rearrange. In T lymphocytes, *TCRD* (T-cell receptor delta chain genes), followed by *TCRG* (gamma) rearrangements occur, potentially leading to TCR$\gamma\delta$ expression, while *TCRB* (beta) and *TCRA* (alpha) rearrangements (the latter resulting in *TCRD* deletions) potentially lead to TCR$\alpha\beta$ expression. Within each locus containing D genes (*IGH*, *TCRB*, *TCRD*) first the D and J segments rearrange to form incomplete rearrangements, then the D-J segments are joined to V segments to form complete rearrangements. In loci lacking the D segments (*IGK*, *IGL*, *TCRA*, *TCRG*), the V and the J genes are joined directly (van Dongen et al. 2003). The sequential manner of this process is attributed to chromatin accessibility for the recombinase complex, changing for different DNA regions along with lymphocyte maturation (Schlissel 2003).

Although the general chronological order of the rearrangements occurring during normal lymphocytes development is largely reflected in leukemic blasts, the patterns of the rearrangements (defined as frequencies of the rearrangements in each Ig/TCR locus) in ALL differ from those found in normal lymphoid counterparts. In normal lymphocytes usually only lineage-specific rearrangements occur (Ig genes in B cells and TCR genes in T cells), while in 90 % of BCP-ALL and 20 % of T-ALL *cross-lineage* rearrangements take place. This can be explained by a high activity of the recombinase complex and an abnormal Ig/TCR locus accessibility in leukemic cells. This phenomenon limits the usefulness of Ig/TCR gene rearrangements as leukemia lineage markers, but increases the repertoire of markers for MRD analysis.

Since malignant transformation may take place at any stage of lymphocyte development, the study of the rearrangement pattern enables assessment of the maturation arrest of blast cells (a consequence of malignant transformation), and thus immunogenotype-based classification of leukemia. It has been shown that selected subtypes of ALL are characterized by a specific pattern of Ig/TCR gene rearrangements, e.g., *MLL*-r ALL, including infant ALL, both regarded as leukemia originating in utero, are characterized by an immature pattern of Ig/TCR gene rearrangements as compared to that of overall BCP-ALL group (Jansen et al. 2007). The pattern of the rearrangements has also been documented to be influenced by age and the presence of ALL-specific chromosomal translocations (van der Velden et al. 2003).

It should be noted, however, that the frequencies of the rearrangements depend on the methodology chosen for the study of the rearrangement pattern. The Southern blot approach, exploits digestion of genomic DNA with restriction enzymes and hybridization with radiolabeled probes specific for Ig and TCR genes. It allows for detection of a broad spectrum of not only rearranged but also deleted Ig/TCR genes, based on the number and sizes of restriction fragments obtained for rearranged genes and those in germ-line configuration (differing patterns of rearranged and germ-line bands). It also enables discrimination between monoclonal, biclonal, oligoclonal and polyclonal rearrangements. This approach was mainly used in the past for extensive study of the patterns of Ig/TCR gene rearrangements in ALL, which provided insights into the biology of the disease and the basis for diagnostic application of Ig/TCR gene rearrangements (Szczepanski et al. 1998). The more recent approach, focused particularly on detection of the rearrangements as markers of MRD, is based on polymerase chain reaction (PCR) with the use of oligonucleotide primers, complementary to selected Ig and TCR genes and heteroduplex (HD) analysis for assessment of clonality of the rearrangements (See also Chaps. 11 and 23). This method aims at detection of the rearrangements that are most frequent in ALL (van Dongen et al. 2003; Pongers-Willemse et al. 1999; Dawidowska et al. 2006; Kraszewska et al. 2012a; Dawidowska et al. 2008).

1.5.2 Ig/TCR Gene Rearrangements in BCP-ALL

Frequencies of Ig/TCR gene rearrangements in BCP-ALL are presented in Table 23.1. Briefly, the most predominant rearrangements in BCP-ALL are those in *IGH* locus, detected in as many as 95 % of patients. Rearrangements of Ig light chain genes are detected in 60–75 % (*IGK*) and 15–20 % (*IGL*) of patients. Cross-lineage *TCR* gene rearrangements are found in a vast majority of BCP-ALL patients: *TCRB* gene rearrangements in 30–40 %, *TCRG* rearrangements in approximately 50–60 % and *TCRD* rearrangements in as many as 55 % of patients (van der Velden and van Dongen 2009; Dawidowska et al. 2008; Flohr et al. 2008).

Although ALL in principle originates from a clonal proliferation of a single malignantly transformed cell, the presence of subclones (oligoclonality) is observed in a substantial proportion of patients. In BCP-ALL it concerns 30–40 % of *IGH* and 5–10 % of *IGK* rearrangements detected at diagnosis (Szczepański et al. 2001). Oligoclonality should be considered while designing MRD diagnostics. Preferably all clones, the major clone and the subclones, should be quantified during follow-up since it is difficult to predict which of them might emerge in ALL relapse. Comparative analysis of BCP-ALL samples collected at diagnosis and during relapse indicates that the Ig/TCR gene rearrangement pattern can be different at these two time points, particularly in cases showing significant level of oligoclonality at diagnosis (Szczepański et al. 2002). The multiple rearrangements resulting from oligoclonality and relatively high instability of rearrangements during the disease course can be explained by occurrence of ongoing and secondary rearrangements due to high activity of recombinase complex and abnormal accessibility of Ig/TCR gene loci due to maturation arrest (Szczepański et al. 1999b).

1.5.3 Ig/TCR Gene Rearrangements in T-ALL

Frequencies of Ig/TCR gene rearrangements in T-ALL are presented in Table 23.1. The most frequent rearrangements in T-ALL are those in *TCRG* locus, detected in 85–95 % of patients followed by *TCRB* rearrangements found in approximately 70–90 % of patients, and *TCRD* rearrangements in 40–50 % of patients (Flohr et al. 2008; Kraszewska et al. 2012a; van der Velden and van Dongen 2009).

However, it should be noted that immunophenotypic T-ALL subtypes, distinguished, dependent on the presence of CD3 cell surface antigen and the type of TCR receptor ($CD3^-$, $TCR\gamma\delta^+$ and $TCR\alpha\beta^+$) are each characterized by a different pattern of Ig/TCR gene rearrangements. In $CD3^-$ T-ALL, *TCRD* genes are rearranged in a vast majority of cases (80 %), while in approximately 10 % of cases are subject to biallelic deletion (van Dongen et al. 1990; Breit et al. 1993). In all of $TCR\gamma\delta^+$ T-ALL cases *TCRG* and *TCRD* rearrangements are detected; *TCRB* rearrangements are observed in up to 95 % of patients (Breit et al. 1993; Langerak et al. 1999). In all TCR$\alpha\beta^+$ T-ALL cases rearrangements of *TCRB* and *TCRG* genes and deletions of at least one *TCRD* allele, which usually corresponds to the rearrangement of *TCRA* genes, are detected. Despite the generally high frequency of TCR gene rearrangements in T-ALL, approximately 10 % of CD3$^-$ patients have all TCR genes in germline configuration (van Dongen et al. 1990; van Dongen and Wolvers-Tettero 1991). This applies in particular to cases of leukemia originating from very early T-cell precursors (CD1$^-$).

Cross-lineage Ig gene rearrangements are present in T-ALL with low frequency of approximately 20 %. In most cases they are limited to *IGH* locus, in which incomplete DH–JH gene rearrangements significantly predominate over complete VH–JH. *IGH* gene rearrangements occur more frequently in the CD3$^-$ T-ALL (19 %) and TCR$\gamma\delta^+$ T-ALL (50 %) than in the TCR$\alpha\beta^+$ T-ALL (<5 %) (Szczepański et al. 1999b). Oligoclonality is rarely observed in T-ALL; if it occurs, it most often concerns *IGH* locus and is observed in approximately 30 % of all *IGH* rearrangements detected in T-ALL (Szczepański et al. 1999a).

Comparative analysis of T-ALL samples collected at diagnosis and relapse, indicates that as many as 40–50 % of patients show some changes in rearrangement pattern at these two time points. This is most likely caused, as in BCP-ALL, by high recombinase activity and occurrence of secondary rearrangements (van der Velden et al. 2004). However, the stability of TCR gene rearrangement patterns between diagnosis and relapse in T-ALL is significantly higher than in BCP-ALL (Szczepański et al. 2003).

1.6 Conclusions

Acute lymphoblastic lukemia is regarded as a success story of pediatric oncology treatment. With contemporary multi-agent therapy protocols the overall survival rate for childhood ALL reaches approximately 85 %. The challenge is now to find effective treatment regimens for ALL subtypes characterized by the worst prognosis, i.e., ETP-ALL, *MLL*-r ALL, including ALL in infants, hypodiploid ALL, recurrent and refractory leukemia, but also ALL in adolescents and adults. Further intensification of therapy regimens is limited by short-term and long-term side effects. Therefore, the main goal is currently to translate recent findings on molecular biology of ALL into refined prognostic classification and design of new therapy options, directed toward newly identified target molecules. Further advance in development and application of molecular and bioinformatic tools will hopefully significantly improve our understanding and the outcome of this malignancy in the near future.

Acknowledgments This chapter was partly supported by the Ministry of Science and Higher Education, grant N N407 311 839.

References

Aifantis I, Raetz E, Buonamici S (2008) Molecular pathogenesis of T-cell leukaemia and lymphoma. Nat Rev Immunol 8(5):380–390. doi:10.1038/nri2304

Asnafi V, Buzyn A, Le Noir S, Baleydier F, Simon A, Beldjord K, Reman O, Witz F, Fagot T, Tavernier E, Turlure P, Leguay T, Huguet F, Vernant JP, Daniel F, Bene MC, Ifrah N, Thomas X, Dombret H, Macintyre E (2009) NOTCH1/FBXW7 mutation identifies a large subgroup with favorable outcome in adult T-cell acute lymphoblastic leukemia (T-ALL): a Group for research on adult acute lymphoblastic leukemia (GRAALL) study. Blood 113(17):3918–3924. doi:10.1182/blood-2008-10-184069

Bardini M, Spinelli R, Bungaro S, Mangano E, Corral L, Cifola I, Fazio G, Giordan M, Basso G, De Rossi G, Biondi A, Battaglia C, Cazzaniga G (2010) DNA copy-number abnormalities do not occur in infant ALL with t(4;11)/MLL-AF4. Leukemia 24(1):169–176. doi:10.1038/leu.2009.203

Bene MC, Castoldi G, Knapp W, Ludwig WD, Matutes E, Orfao A, van't Veer MB (1995) Proposals for the immunological classification of acute leukemias. European Group for the Immunological Characterization of Leukemias (EGIL). Leuk: Off J Leuk Soc Am Leuk Res Fund UK 9(10):1783–1786

Benedikt A, Baltruschat S, Scholz B, Bursen A, Arrey TN, Meyer B, Varagnolo L, Muller AM, Karas M, Dingermann T, Marschalek R (2011) The leukemogenic AF4-MLL fusion protein causes P-TEFb kinase activation and altered epigenetic signatures. Leukemia 25(1):135–144. doi:10.1038/leu.2010.249

Breit TM, Wolvers-Tettero IL, Beishuizen A, Verhoeven MA, van Wering ER, van Dongen JJ (1993) Southern blot patterns, frequencies, and junctional diversity of T-cell receptor-delta gene rearrangements in acute lymphoblastic leukemia. Blood 82(10):3063–3074

Cario G, Stanulla M, Fine BM, Teuffel O, Neuhoff NV, Schrauder A, Flohr T, Schafer BW, Bartram CR, Welte K, Schlegelberger B, Schrappe M (2005) Distinct gene expression profiles determine molecular treatment response in childhood acute lymphoblastic leukemia. Blood 105(2):821–826. doi:10.1182/blood-2004-04-1552

Cario G, Zimmermann M, Romey R, Gesk S, Vater I, Harbott J, Schrauder A, Moericke A, Izraeli S, Akasaka T, Dyer MJ, Siebert R, Schrappe M, Stanulla M (2010) Presence of the P2RY8-CRLF2 rearrangement is associated with a poor prognosis in non-high-risk precursor B-cell acute lymphoblastic leukemia in children treated according to the ALL-BFM 2000 protocol. Blood 115(26):5393–5397. doi:10.1182/blood-2009-11-256131

Cauwelier B, Dastugue N, Cools J, Poppe B, Herens C, De Paepe A, Hagemeijer A, Speleman F (2006) Molecular cytogenetic study of 126 unselected T-ALL cases reveals high incidence of TCRbeta locus rearrangements and putative new T-cell oncogenes. Leukemia 20(7):1238–1244. doi:10.1038/sj.leu.2404243

Clappier E, Collette S, Grardel N, Girard S, Suarez L, Brunie G, Kaltenbach S, Yakouben K, Mazingue F, Robert A, Boutard P, Plantaz D, Rohrlich P, van Vlierberghe P, Preudhomme C, Otten J, Speleman F, Dastugue N, Suciu S, Benoit Y, Bertrand Y, Cave H (2010) NOTCH1 and FBXW7 mutations have a favorable impact on early response to treatment, but not on outcome, in children with T-cell acute lymphoblastic leukemia (T-ALL) treated on EORTC trials 58881 and 58951. Leukemia. doi:10.1038/leu.2010.205

Coustan-Smith E, Mullighan CG, Onciu M, Behm FG, Raimondi SC, Pei D, Cheng C, Su X, Rubnitz JE, Basso G, Biondi A, Pui CH, Downing JR, Campana D (2009) Early T-cell precursor leukaemia: a subtype of very high-risk acute lymphoblastic leukaemia. Lancet Oncol 10(2):147–156. doi:10.1016/S1470-2045(08)70314-0

Dawidowska M, Derwich K, Szczepanski T, Jolkowska J, van der Velden VH, Wachowiak J, Witt M (2006) Pattern of immunoglobulin and T-cell receptor (Ig/TCR) gene rearrangements in Polish pediatric acute lymphoblastic leukemia patients–implications for RQ-PCR-based assessment of minimal residual disease. Leuk Res 30(9):1119–1125

Dawidowska M, Jolkowska J, Szczepanski T, Derwich K, Wachowiak J, Witt M (2008) Implementation of the standard strategy for identification of Ig/TCR targets for minimal residual disease diagnostics in B-cell precursor ALL pediatric patients: Polish experience. Arch Immunol Ther Exp (Warsz) 56(6):409–418. doi:10.1007/s00005-008-0045-y

De Braekeleer E, Douet-Guilbert N, Rowe D, Bown N, Morel F, Berthou C, Ferec C, De Braekeleer M (2011) ABL1 fusion genes in hematological malignancies: a review. Eur J Haematol 86(5):361–371. doi:10.1111/j.1600-0609.2011.01586.x

Demarest RM, Ratti F, Capobianco AJ (2008) It's T-ALL about Notch. Oncogene 27(38): 5082–5091. doi:10.1038/onc.2008.222

Dik WA, Brahim W, Braun C, Asnafi V, Dastugue N, Bernard OA, van Dongen JJ, Langerak AW, Macintyre EA, Delabesse E (2005) CALM-AF10 + T-ALL expression profiles are characterized by overexpression of HOXA and BMI1 oncogenes. Leukemia 19(11):1948–1957. doi:10.1038/sj.leu.2403891

Familiades J, Bousquet M, Lafage-Pochitaloff M, Bene MC, Beldjord K, De Vos J, Dastugue N, Coyaud E, Struski S, Quelen C, Prade-Houdellier N, Dobbelstein S, Cayuela JM, Soulier J, Grardel N, Preudhomme C, Cave H, Blanchet O, Lheritier V, Delannoy A, Chalandon Y, Ifrah N, Pigneux A, Brousset P, Macintyre EA, Huguet F, Dombret H, Broccardo C, Delabesse E (2009) PAX5 mutations occur frequently in adult B-cell progenitor acute lymphoblastic leukemia and PAX5 haploinsufficiency is associated with BCR-ABL1 and TCF3-PBX1 fusion genes: a GRAALL study. Leukemia 23(11):1989–1998. doi:10.1038/leu.2009.135

Ferrando AA, Neuberg DS, Staunton J, Loh ML, Huard C, Raimondi SC, Behm FG, Pui CH, Downing JR, Gilliland DG, Lander ES, Golub TR, Look AT (2002) Gene expression signatures define novel oncogenic pathways in T cell acute lymphoblastic leukemia. Cancer Cell 1(1):75–87 S1535610802000181 [pii]

Flohr T, Schrauder A, Cazzaniga G, Panzer-Grumayer R, van der Velden V, Fischer S, Stanulla M, Basso G, Niggli FK, Schafer BW, Sutton R, Koehler R, Zimmermann M, Valsecchi MG, Gadner H, Masera G, Schrappe M, van Dongen JJ, Biondi A, Bartram CR (2008) Minimal residual disease-directed risk stratification using real-time quantitative PCR analysis of immunoglobulin and T-cell receptor gene rearrangements in the international multicenter trial AIEOP-BFM ALL 2000 for childhood acute lymphoblastic leukemia. Leukemia

Flotho C, Coustan-Smith E, Pei D, Cheng C, Song G, Pui CH, Downing JR, Campana D (2007) A set of genes that regulate cell proliferation predicts treatment outcome in childhood acute lymphoblastic leukemia. Blood 110(4):1271–1277. doi:10.1182/blood-2007-01-068478

Ford AM, Fasching K, Panzer-Grumayer ER, Koenig M, Haas OA, Greaves MF (2001) Origins of "late" relapse in childhood acute lymphoblastic leukemia with TEL-AML1 fusion genes. Blood 98(3):558–564

Ford AM, Ridge SA, Cabrera ME, Mahmoud H, Steel CM, Chan LC, Greaves M (1993) In utero rearrangements in the trithorax-related oncogene in infant leukaemias. Nature 363(6427):358–360. doi:10.1038/363358a0

Gandemer V, Rio AG, de Tayrac M, Sibut V, Mottier S, Ly Sunnaram B, Henry C, Monnier A, Berthou C, Le Gall E, Le Treut A, Schmitt C, Le Gall JY, Mosser J, Galibert MD (2007) Five distinct biological processes and 14 differentially expressed genes characterize TEL/AML1-positive leukemia. BMC Genomics 8:385. doi:10.1186/1471-2164-8-385

Greaves M (1999) Molecular genetics, natural history and the demise of childhood leukaemia. Eur J Cancer 35(14):1941–1953 S0959-8049(99)00296-8 [pii]

Greaves M (2006) Infection, immune responses and the aetiology of childhood leukaemia. Nat Rev Cancer 6(3):193–203. doi:10.1038/nrc1816

Greaves MF, Wiemels J (2003) Origins of chromosome translocations in childhood leukaemia. Nat Rev Cancer 3(9):639–649. doi:10.1038/nrc1164

Houlston RS (2010) Low-penetrance susceptibility to hematological malignancy. Curr Opin Genet Dev 20(3):245–250. doi:10.1016/j.gde.2010.03.004

Hunger SP, Raetz EA, Loh ML, Mullighan CG (2011) Improving outcomes for high-risk ALL: translating new discoveries into clinical care. Pediatr Blood Cancer 56(6):984–993. doi:10.1002/pbc.22996

Iacobucci I, Lonetti A, Paoloni F, Papayannidis C, Ferrari A, Storlazzi CT, Vignetti M, Cilloni D, Messa F, Guadagnuolo V, Paolini S, Elia L, Messina M, Vitale A, Meloni G, Soverini S, Pane F, Baccarani M, Foa R, Martinelli G (2010) The PAX5 gene is frequently rearranged in BCR-ABL1-positive acute lymphoblastic leukemia but is not associated with outcome. A rep behalf GIMEMA Acute Leuk Work Party. Haematol 95(10):1683–1690. doi:10.3324/haematol.2009.020792

Jansen MW, Corral L, van der Velden VH, Panzer-Grumayer R, Schrappe M, Schrauder A, Marschalek R, Meyer C, den Boer ML, Hop WJ, Valsecchi MG, Basso G, Biondi A, Pieters R, van Dongen JJ (2007) Immunobiological diversity in infant acute lymphoblastic leukemia is related to the occurrence and type of MLL gene rearrangement. Leukemia 21(4):633–641

Kaatsch P (2010) Epidemiology of childhood cancer. Cancer Treat Rev 36(4):277–285. doi:10.1016/j.ctrv.2010.02.003

Kang H, Chen IM, Wilson CS, Bedrick EJ, Harvey RC, Atlas SR, Devidas M, Mullighan CG, Wang X, Murphy M, Ar K, Wharton W, Borowitz MJ, Bowman WP, Bhojwani D, Carroll WL, Camitta BM, Reaman GH, Smith MA, Downing JR, Hunger SP, Willman CL (2010) Gene expression classifiers for relapse-free survival and minimal residual disease improve risk classification and outcome prediction in pediatric B-precursor acute lymphoblastic leukemia. Blood 115(7):1394–1405. doi:10.1182/blood-2009-05-218560

Knudson AG Jr (1971) Mutation and cancer: statistical study of retinoblastoma. Proc Natl Acad Sci U S A 68(4):820–823

Konrad M, Metzler M, Panzer S, Ostreicher I, Peham M, Repp R, Haas OA, Gadner H, Panzer-Grumayer ER (2003) Late relapses evolve from slow-responding subclones in t(12;21)-positive acute lymphoblastic leukemia: evidence for the persistence of a preleukemic clone. Blood 101(9):3635–3640. doi:10.1182/blood-2002-10-3252

Kraszewska MD, Dawidowska M, Kosmalska M, Sedek L, Grzeszczak W, Szczepanski T, Witt M (2012a) Immunoglobulin/T-cell receptor gene rearrangements in the diagnostic paradigm of pediatric T-cell acute lymphoblastic leukemia patients. Leuk Lymphoma. doi:10.3109/10428194.2011.654338

Kraszewska MD, Dawidowska M, Larmonie NS, Kosmalska M, Sedek L, Szczepaniak M, Grzeszczak W, Langerak AW, Szczepanski T, Witt M (2011) DNA methylation pattern is altered in childhood T-cell acute lymphoblastic leukemia patients as compared with normal thymic subsets: insights into CpG island methylator phenotype in T-ALL. Leukemia. doi:10.1038/leu.2011.208

Kraszewska MD, Dawidowska M, Szczepanski T, Witt M (2012b) T-cell acute lymphoblastic leukaemia: recent molecular biology findings. Br J Haematol 156(3):303–315. doi:10.1111/j.1365-2141.2011.08957.x

Langerak AW, Wolvers-Tettero IL, van den Beemd MW, van Wering ER, Ludwig WD, Hahlen K, Necker A, van Dongen JJ (1999) Immunophenotypic and immunogenotypic characteristics of TCRgammadelta + T cell acute lymphoblastic leukemia. Leukemia 13(2):206–214

Liedtke M (2010) MLL. Homo sapiens myeloid/lymphoid or mixed-lineage leukemia (trithorax homolog, Drosophila)

Malyukova A, Dohda T, von der Lehr N, Akhoondi S, Corcoran M, Heyman M, Spruck C, Grander D, Lendahl U, Sangfelt O (2007) The tumor suppressor gene hCDC4 is frequently mutated in human T-cell acute lymphoblastic leukemia with functional consequences for Notch signaling. Cancer Res 67(12):5611–5616. doi:10.1158/0008-5472.CAN-06-4381

Martinelli G, Iacobucci I, Storlazzi CT, Vignetti M, Paoloni F, Cilloni D, Soverini S, Vitale A, Chiaretti S, Cimino G, Papayannidis C, Paolini S, Elia L, Fazi P, Meloni G, Amadori S, Saglio G, Pane F, Baccarani M, Foa R (2009) IKZF1 (Ikaros) deletions in BCR-ABL1-positive acute lymphoblastic leukemia are associated with short disease-free survival and high rate of cumulative incidence of relapse: a GIMEMA AL WP report. J Clin Oncol 27(31):5202–5207. doi:10.1200/JCO.2008.21.6408

Matsuoka S, Oike Y, Onoyama I, Iwama A, Arai F, Takubo K, Mashimo Y, Oguro H, Nitta E, Ito K, Miyamoto K, Yoshiwara H, Hosokawa K, Nakamura Y, Gomei Y, Iwasaki H, Hayashi Y, Matsuzaki Y, Nakayama K, Ikeda Y, Hata A, Chiba S, Nakayama KI, Suda T (2008) Fbxw7 acts as a critical fail-safe against premature loss of hematopoietic stem cells and development of T-ALL. Genes Dev 22(8):986–991. doi:10.1101/gad.1621808

Meyer C, Kowarz E, Hofmann J, Renneville A, Zuna J, Trka J, Ben Abdelali R, Macintyre E, De Braekeleer E, De Braekeleer M, Delabesse E, de Oliveira MP, Cave H, Clappier E, van Dongen JJ, Balgobind BV, van den Heuvel-Eibrink MM, Beverloo HB, Panzer-Grumayer R, Teigler-Schlegel A, Harbott J, Kjeldsen E, Schnittger S, Koehl U, Gruhn B, Heidenreich O, Chan LC, Yip SF, Krzywinski M, Eckert C, Moricke A, Schrappe M, Alonso CN, Schafer BW, Krauter J, Lee DA, Zur Stadt U, Te Kronnie G, Sutton R, Izraeli S, Trakhtenbrot L, Lo Nigro L, Tsaur G, Fechina L, Szczepanski T, Strehl S, Ilencikova D, Molkentin M, Burmeister T, Dingermann T, Klingebiel T, Marschalek R (2009) New insights to the MLL recombinome of acute leukemias. Leukemia 23(8):1490–1499. doi:10.1038/leu.2009.33

Milano J, McKay J, Dagenais C, Foster-Brown L, Pognan F, Gadient R, Jacobs RT, Zacco A, Greenberg B, Ciaccio PJ (2004) Modulation of notch processing by gamma-secretase inhibitors causes intestinal goblet cell metaplasia and induction of genes known to specify gut secretory lineage differentiation. Toxicol Sci 82(1):341–358. doi:10.1093/toxsci/kfh254

Mullighan CG (2009) Genomic analysis of acute leukemia. Int J Lab Hematol 31(4):384–397. doi:10.1111/j.1751-553X.2009.01167.x

Mullighan CG (2010) Genetic variation and the risk of acute lymphoblastic leukemia. Leuk Res 34(10):1269–1270. doi:10.1016/j.leukres.2010.05.013

Mullighan CG, Downing JR (2009a) Genome-wide profiling of genetic alterations in acute lymphoblastic leukemia: recent insights and future directions. Leukemia 23(7):1209–1218. doi:10.1038/leu.2009.18

Mullighan CG, Downing JR (2009b) Global genomic characterization of acute lymphoblastic leukemia. Semin Hematol 46(1):3–15. doi:10.1053/j.seminhematol.2008.09.005

Mullighan CG, Su X, Zhang J, Radtke I, Phillips LA, Miller CB, Ma J, Liu W, Cheng C, Schulman BA, Harvey RC, Chen IM, Clifford RJ, Carroll WL, Reaman G, Bowman WP, Devidas M, Gerhard DS, Yang W, Relling MV, Shurtleff SA, Campana D, Borowitz MJ, Pui CH, Smith M, Hunger SP, Willman CL, Downing JR (2009a) Deletion of IKZF1 and prognosis in acute lymphoblastic leukemia. N Engl J Med 360(5):470–480. doi:10.1056/NEJMoa0808253

Mullighan CG, Zhang J, Harvey RC, Collins-Underwood JR, Schulman BA, Phillips LA, Tasian SK, Loh ML, Su X, Liu W, Devidas M, Atlas SR, Chen IM, Clifford RJ, Gerhard DS, Carroll WL, Reaman GH, Smith M, Downing JR, Hunger SP, Willman CL (2009b) JAK mutations in high-risk childhood acute lymphoblastic leukemia. Proc Natl Acad Sci U S A 106(23):9414–9418. doi:10.1073/pnas.0811761106

Nachman JB, Heerema NA, Sather H, Camitta B, Forestier E, Harrison CJ, Dastugue N, Schrappe M, Pui CH, Basso G, Silverman LB, Janka-Schaub GE (2007) Outcome of treatment in children with hypodiploid acute lymphoblastic leukemia. Blood 110(4):1112–1115. doi:10.1182/blood-2006-07-038299

O'Neil J, Grim J, Strack P, Rao S, Tibbitts D, Winter C, Hardwick J, Welcker M, Meijerink JP, Pieters R, Draetta G, Sears R, Clurman BE, Look AT (2007) FBW7 mutations in leukemic cells mediate NOTCH pathway activation and resistance to gamma-secretase inhibitors. J Exp Med 204(8):1813–1824. doi:10.1084/jem.20070876

Pastorczak A, Gorniak P, Sherborne A, Hosking F, Trelinska J, Lejman M, Szczepanski T, Borowiec M, Fendler W, Kowalczyk J, Houlston RS, Mlynarski W (2011) Role of 657del5 NBN mutation and 7p12.2 (IKZF1), 9p21 (CDKN2A), 10q21.2 (ARID5B) and 14q11.2 (CEBPE) variation and risk of childhood ALL in the Polish population. Le. Leuk Res 35(11):1534–1536. doi:10.1016/j.leukres.2011.07.034

Piccaluga PP, Paolini S, Martinelli G (2007) Tyrosine kinase inhibitors for the treatment of Philadelphia chromosome-positive adult acute lymphoblastic leukemia. Cancer 110(6): 1178–1186. doi:10.1002/cncr.22881

Pieters R, Schrappe M, De Lorenzo P, Hann I, De Rossi G, Felice M, Hovi L, LeBlanc T, Szczepanski T, Ferster A, Janka G, Rubnitz J, Silverman L, Stary J, Campbell M, Li CK, Mann G, Suppiah R, Biondi A, Vora A, Valsecchi MG (2007) A treatment protocol for infants younger than 1 year with acute lymphoblastic leukaemia (Interfant-99): an observational study and a multicentre randomised trial. Lancet 370(9583):240–250. doi:10.1016/S0140-6736(07)61126-X

Pongers-Willemse MJ, Seriu T, Stolz F, d'Aniello E, Gameiro P, Pisa P, Gonzalez M, Bartram CR, Panzer-Grumayer ER, Biondi A, San Miguel JF, van Dongen JJ (1999) Primers and protocols for standardized detection of minimal residual disease in acute lymphoblastic leukemia using immunoglobulin and T cell receptor gene rearrangements and TAL1 deletions as PCR targets: report of the BIOMED-1 CONCERTED ACTION: investigation of minimal residual disease in acute leukemia. Leukemia 13(1):110–118

Prasad RB, Hosking FJ, Vijayakrishnan J, Papaemmanuil E, Koehler R, Greaves M, Sheridan E, Gast A, Kinsey SE, Lightfoot T, Roman E, Taylor M, Pritchard-Jones K, Stanulla M, Schrappe M, Bartram CR, Houlston RS, Kumar R, Hemminki K (2010) Verification of the susceptibility loci on 7p12.2, 10q21.2, and 14q11.2 in precursor B-cell acute lymphoblastic leukemia of childhood. Blood 115(9):1765–1767. doi:10.1182/blood-2009-09-241513

Pui CH (2010) Recent research advances in childhood acute lymphoblastic leukemia. J Formos Med Assoc 109(11):777–787. doi:10.1016/S0929-6646(10)60123-4

Pui CH, Carroll WL, Meshinchi S, Arceci RJ (2011) Biology, risk stratification, and therapy of pediatric acute leukemias: an update. J Clin Oncol 29(5):551–565. doi:10.1200/JCO.2010.30.7405

Pui CH, Gaynon PS, Boyett JM, Chessells JM, Baruchel A, Kamps W, Silverman LB, Biondi A, Harms DO, Vilmer E, Schrappe M, Camitta B (2002) Outcome of treatment in childhood acute lymphoblastic leukaemia with rearrangements of the 11q23 chromosomal region. Lancet 359(9321):1909–1915. doi:10.1016/S0140-6736(02)08782-2

Pui CH, Jeha S (2007) New therapeutic strategies for the treatment of acute lymphoblastic leukaemia. Nat Rev Drug Discov 6(2):149–165. doi:10.1038/nrd2240

Real PJ, Tosello V, Palomero T, Castillo M, Hernando E, de Stanchina E, Sulis ML, Barnes K, Sawai C, Homminga I, Meijerink J, Aifantis I, Basso G, Cordon-Cardo C, Ai W, Ferrando A (2009) Gamma-secretase inhibitors reverse glucocorticoid resistance in T cell acute lymphoblastic leukemia. Nat Med 15(1):50–58. doi:10.1038/nm.1900

Roman-Gomez J, Jimenez-Velasco A, Agirre X, Prosper F, Heiniger A, Torres A (2005) Lack of CpG island methylator phenotype defines a clinical subtype of T-cell acute lymphoblastic leukemia associated with good prognosis. J Clin Oncol 23(28):7043–7049. doi:10.1200/JCO.2005.01.4944

Roman-Gomez J, Jimenez-Velasco A, Castillejo JA, Agirre X, Barrios M, Navarro G, Molina FJ, Calasanz MJ, Prosper F, Heiniger A, Torres A (2004) Promoter hypermethylation of cancer-related genes: a strong independent prognostic factor in acute lymphoblastic leukemia. Blood 104(8):2492–2498. doi:10.1182/blood-2004-03-0954

Ross ME, Zhou X, Song G, Shurtleff SA, Girtman K, Williams WK, Liu HC, Mahfouz R, Raimondi SC, Lenny N, Patel A, Downing JR (2003) Classification of pediatric acute lymphoblastic leukemia by gene expression profiling. Blood 102(8):2951–2959. doi:10.1182/blood-2003-01-0338

Schafer E, Irizarry R, Negi S, McIntyre E, Small D, Figueroa ME, Melnick A, Brown P (2010) Promoter hypermethylation in MLL-r infant acute lymphoblastic leukemia: biology and therapeutic targeting. Blood 115(23):4798–4809. doi:10.1182/blood-2009-09-243634

Schlissel MS (2003) Regulating antigen-receptor gene assembly. Nat Rev Immunol 3(11):890–899. doi:10.1038/nri1225nri1225

Schrappe M (2003) Prognostic factors in childhood acute lymphoblastic leukemia. Indian J Pediatr 70(10):817–824

Schultz KR, Bowman WP, Aledo A, Slayton WB, Sather H, Devidas M, Wang C, Davies SM, Gaynon PS, Trigg M, Rutledge R, Burden L, Jorstad D, Carroll A, Heerema NA, Winick N, Borowitz MJ, Hunger SP, Carroll WL, Camitta B (2009) Improved early event-free survival with imatinib in Philadelphia chromosome-positive acute lymphoblastic leukemia: a children's oncology group study. J Clin Oncol: Off J Am Soc Clin Oncol 27(31): 5175–5181. doi:10.1200/JCO.2008.21.2514

Stam RW, Schneider P, Hagelstein JA, van der Linden MH, Stumpel DJ, de Menezes RX, de Lorenzo P, Valsecchi MG, Pieters R (2010) Gene expression profiling-based dissection of MLL translocated and MLL germline acute lymphoblastic leukemia in infants. Blood 115(14):2835–2844. doi:10.1182/blood-2009-07-233049

Stumpel DJ, Schneider P, van Roon EH, Boer JM, de Lorenzo P, Valsecchi MG, de Menezes RX, Pieters R, Stam RW (2009) Specific promoter methylation identifies different subgroups of MLL-rearranged infant acute lymphoblastic leukemia, influences clinical outcome, and provides therapeutic options. Blood 114(27):5490–5498. doi:10.1182/blood-2009-06-227660

Stumpel DJ, Schotte D, Lange-Turenhout EA, Schneider P, Seslija L, de Menezes RX, Marquez VE, Pieters R, den Boer ML, Stam RW (2011) Hypermethylation of specific microRNA genes in MLL-rearranged infant acute lymphoblastic leukemia: major matters at a micro scale. Leukemia 25(3):429–439. doi:10.1038/leu.2010.282

Sutcliffe MJ, Shuster JJ, Sather HN, Camitta BM, Pullen J, Schultz KR, Borowitz MJ, Gaynon PS, Carroll AJ, Heerema NA (2005) High concordance from independent studies by the Children's Cancer Group (CCG) and Pediatric Oncology Group (POG) associating favorable prognosis with combined trisomies 4, 10, and 17 in children with NCI Standard-Risk B-precursor Acute Lymphoblastic Leukemia: a Children's Oncology Group (COG) initiative. Leukemia 19(5):734–740. doi:10.1038/sj.leu.2403673

Szczepanski T, Harrison CJ, van Dongen JJ (2010) Genetic aberrations in paediatric acute leukaemias and implications for management of patients. Lancet Oncol 11(9):880–889. doi:10.1016/S1470-2045(09)70369-9

Szczepanski T, Langerak AW, Wolvers-Tettero IL, Ossenkoppele GJ, Verhoef G, Stul M, Petersen EJ, de Bruijn MA, van't Veer MB, van Dongen JJ (1998) Immunoglobulin and T cell receptor gene rearrangement patterns in acute lymphoblastic leukemia are less mature in adults than in children: implications for selection of PCR targets for detection of minimal residual disease. Leuk: Off J Leuk Soc Am Leuk Res Fund, UK 12(7):1081–1088

Szczepański T, Pongers-Willemse MJ, Langerak AW, Harts WA, Wijkhuijs AJ, van Wering ER, van Dongen JJ (1999a) Ig heavy chain gene rearrangements in T-cell acute lymphoblastic leukemia exhibit predominant DH6-19 and DH7-27 gene usage, can result in complete V-D-J rearrangements, and are rare in T-cell receptor alpha beta lineage. Blood 93(12):4079–4085

Szczepański T, Pongers-Willemse MJ, Langerak AW, van Dongen JJ (1999b) Unusual immunoglobulin and T-cell receptor gene rearrangement patterns in acute lymphoblastic leukemias. Curr Top Microbiol Immunol 246:205–213 (discussion 214–205)

Szczepański T, van der Velden VH, Raff T, Jacobs DC, van Wering ER, Bruggemann M, Kneba M, van Dongen JJ (2003) Comparative analysis of T-cell receptor gene rearrangements at diagnosis and relapse of T-cell acute lymphoblastic leukemia (T-ALL) shows high stability of clonal markers for monitoring of minimal residual disease and reveals the occurrence of second T-ALL. Leukemia 17(11):2149–2156

Szczepański T, Willemse MJ, Brinkhof B, van Wering ER, van der Burg M, van Dongen JJ (2002) Comparative analysis of Ig and TCR gene rearrangements at diagnosis and at relapse of childhood precursor-B-ALL provides improved strategies for selection of stable PCR targets for monitoring of minimal residual disease. Blood 99(7):2315–2323

Szczepański T, Willemse MJ, van Wering ER, van Weerden JF, Kamps WA, van Dongen JJ (2001) Precursor-B-ALL with D(H)-J(H) gene rearrangements have an immature immunogenotype with a high frequency of oligoclonality and hyperdiploidy of chromosome 14. Leukemia 15(9):1415–1423

Tamai H, Inokuchi K (2010) 11q23/MLL acute leukemia : update of clinical aspects. J Clin Exp Hematop 50(2):91–98 JST.JSTAGE/jslrt/50.91 [pii]

van der Velden VH, Bruggemann M, Hoogeveen PG, de Bie M, Hart PG, Raff T, Pfeifer H, Luschen S, Szczepanski T, van Wering ER, Kneba M, van Dongen JJ (2004) TCRB gene rearrangements in childhood and adult precursor-B-ALL: frequency, applicability as MRD-PCR target, and stability between diagnosis and relapse. Leukemia 18(12):1971–1980

van der Velden VH, Szczepanski T, Wijkhuijs JM, Hart PG, Hoogeveen PG, Hop WC, van Wering ER, van Dongen JJ (2003) Age-related patterns of immunoglobulin and T-cell receptor gene rearrangements in precursor-B-ALL: implications for detection of minimal residual disease. Leukemia 17(9):1834–1844

van der Velden VH, van Dongen JJ (2009) MRD detection in acute lymphoblastic leukemia patients using Ig/TCR gene rearrangements as targets for real-time quantitative PCR. Methods Mol Biol 538:115–150. doi:10.1007/978-1-59745-418-6_7

van Dongen JJ, Comans-Bitter WM, Wolvers-Tettero IL, Borst J (1990) Development of human T lymphocytes and their thymus-dependency. Thymus 16(3–4):207–234

van Dongen JJ, Langerak AW, Bruggemann M, Evans PA, Hummel M, Lavender FL, Delabesse E, Davi F, Schuuring E, Garcia-Sanz R, van Krieken JH, Droese J, Gonzalez D, Bastard C, White HE, Spaargaren M, Gonzalez M, Parreira A, Smith JL, Morgan GJ, Kneba M, Macintyre EA (2003) Design and standardization of PCR primers and protocols for detection of clonal immunoglobulin and T-cell receptor gene recombinations in suspect lymphoproliferations: report of the BIOMED-2 concerted action BMH4-CT98-3936. Leukemia 17(12): 2257–2317

van Dongen JJ, Wolvers-Tettero IL (1991) Analysis of immunoglobulin and T cell receptor genes. Part I: Basic and technical aspects. Clin Chim Acta 198(1–2):1–91

Vardiman JW, Thiele J, Arber DA, Brunning RD, Borowitz MJ, Porwit A, Harris NL, Le Beau MM, Hellstrom-Lindberg E, Tefferi A, Bloomfield CD (2009) The 2008 revision of the World Health Organization (WHO) classification of myeloid neoplasms and acute leukemia: rationale and important changes. Blood 114(5):937–951. doi:10.1182/blood-2009-03-209262

Varnum-Finney B, Xu L, Brashem-Stein C, Nourigat C, Flowers D, Bakkour S, Pear WS, Bernstein ID (2000) Pluripotent, cytokine-dependent, hematopoietic stem cells are immortalized by constitutive Notch1 signaling. Nat Med 6(11):1278–1281. doi:10.1038/81390

Waanders E, van der Velden VH, van der Schoot CE, van Leeuwen FN, van Reijmersdal SV, de Haas V, Veerman AJ, van Kessel AG, Hoogerbrugge PM, Kuiper RP, van Dongen JJ (2011) Integrated use of minimal residual disease classification and IKZF1 alteration status accurately predicts 79 % of relapses in pediatric acute lymphoblastic leukemia. Leukemia 25(2):254–258. doi:10.1038/leu.2010.275

Weng AP, Ferrando AA, Lee W, Morris JP, Silverman LB, Sanchez-Irizarry C, Blacklow SC, Look AT, Aster JC (2004) Activating mutations of NOTCH1 in human T cell acute lymphoblastic leukemia. Science (New York, NY) 306(5694):269–271

Wilson A, MacDonald HR, Radtke F (2001) Notch 1-deficient common lymphoid precursors adopt a B cell fate in the thymus. J Exp Med 194(7):1003–1012

Yang JJ, Cheng C, Yang W, Pei D, Cao X, Fan Y, Pounds SB, Neale G, Trevino LR, French D, Campana D, Downing JR, Evans WE, Pui CH, Devidas M, Bowman WP, Camitta BM, Willman CL, Davies SM, Borowitz MJ, Carroll WL, Hunger SP, Relling MV (2009) Genome-wide interrogation of germline genetic variation associated with treatment response in childhood acute lymphoblastic leukemia. JAMA 301(4):393–403. doi:10.1001/jama.2009.7

Yeoh EJ, Ross ME, Shurtleff SA, Williams WK, Patel D, Mahfouz R, Behm FG, Raimondi SC, Relling MV, Patel A, Cheng C, Campana D, Wilkins D, Zhou X, Li J, Liu H, Pui CH, Evans WE, Naeve C, Wong L, Downing JR (2002) Classification, subtype discovery, and prediction of outcome in pediatric acute lymphoblastic leukemia by gene expression profiling. Cancer Cell 1(2):133–143 S1535610802000326 [pii]

Zuurbier L, Homminga I, Calvert V, Winkel MT, Buijs-Gladdines JG, Kooi C, Smits WK, Sonneveld E, Veerman AJ, Kamps WA, Horstmann M, Petricoin EF, 3rd, Pieters R, Meijerink JP (2010) NOTCH1 and/or FBXW7 mutations predict for initial good prednisone response but not for improved outcome in pediatric T-cell acute lymphoblastic leukemia patients treated on DCOG or COALL protocols. Leukemia. doi:10.1038/leu.2010.204

Chapter 2
Genetic Mechanisms and Molecular Markers of Neoplastic Transformation in Acute Myeloid Leukemia

Agata A. Filip, Marta Libura, Sebastian Giebel and Olga Haus

Abstract Acute myeloid leukemia (AML) constitutes a group of diseases heterogeneous with regard to clinical course, response to therapy as well as genetic features that contribute to disease pathogenesis, progression, and outcome. Numerous molecular lesions found in AML patients serve as prognostic and predictive factors; some of these markers have been included in the latest WHO classification. The analysis of cryptic genomic changes and alterations of gene expression is particularly important in cytogenetically normal AML patients. *NPM1* and biallelic *CEBPA* mutations are favorable prognostic factors, while *MLL* and *FLT3* duplications, *WT1*, *IDH1/IDH2*, *KIT*, *TET2*, and *DNMT3A* mutations, as well

A. A. Filip (✉)
Department of Cancer Genetics, Medical University of Lublin,
Radziwiłłowska 11, 20-950 Lublin, Poland
e-mail: a.filip@umlub.pl

M. Libura
Department of Hematology, Oncology and Internal Medicine,
Medical University of Warsaw,
Banacha 1a, 02-097 Warsaw, Poland
e-mail: marta.libura@gmail.com

S. Giebel
Department of Bone Marrow Transplantation,
Maria Skłodowska-Curie Memorial Cancer Center and Institute of Oncology,
Wybrzeze Armii Krajowej 15, 44-101 Gliwice, Poland
e-mail: sgiebel@poczta.onet.pl

O. Haus
Department of Clinical Genetics, Ludwik Rydygier Collegium Medicum in Bydgoszcz
Nicolaus Copernicus University in Toruń, Skłodowska-Curie 9, 85-094 Bydgoszcz, Poland
e-mail: haus@cm.umk.pl

O. Haus
Department of Hematology, Wrocław Medical University,
Pasteura 4, 50-367 Wrocław, Poland

M. Witt et al. (eds.), *Molecular Aspects of Hematologic Malignancies*,
Principles and Practice, DOI: 10.1007/978-3-642-29467-9_2,

as overexpression of *BAALC*, *ERG*, or *MN1* have an adverse prognostic impact. Aside from aberrations involving structural genes, mutations of microRNAs, copy number alterations, and altered methylation of gene promoter regions also influence the development and progression of AML.

2.1 Introduction

Acute myeloid leukemia (AML) constitutes a broad range of disorders with marked clinical and biological heterogeneity. It is defined as a clonal proliferation of immature hematopoietic progenitors (myeloblasts) with varying degree of myeloid differentiation in the bone marrow, peripheral blood, or extramedullary tissues (Vardiman et al. 2008). AML accounts for 25 % of all cases of leukemia and shows a bimodal distribution across age groups, with a small peak of incidence very early in life, and then a much more prominent peak in older patients (Zuo et al. 2009). The characterization of the individual subtype of AML, crucial for therapeutic decisions, is nowadays based mainly on cytogenetic and molecular alterations of blast cells, or on morphology and immunophenotype in the absence of a specific genetic marker. The identification of genetic lesions, including gene expression changes, provides the basis for risk stratification and allows for effective treatment design.

2.2 Genetic Pathomechanisms of Acute Myeloid Leukemia

Genetic changes, recognized as primary alterations in AML, fall into two categories: chromosome aberrations, revealed by GTG-banding (*G* bands by *T*rypsin using *G*iemsa) in about 60 % of AML and submicroscopic changes, which occur both in cytogenetically normal AML (CN-AML) and in cytogenetically abnormal AML (CA-AML) patients (Grimwade and Hills 2009).

2.2.1 Classical "Two Hits" Model of AML Transformation

It is now commonly recognized that a cell which becomes an AML blast acquires two distinct kinds of mutations (Gilliland 2001).

Class I mutations confer proliferation and survival advantage. They involve genes coding for receptor and nonreceptor protein tyrosine kinases like *FLT3*, *JAK2*, *C-KIT*, *ABL1* (*C-ABL* oncogene 1, nonreceptor tyrosine kinase), as well as for proteins of GTPase activity such as *N-RAS* and *K-RAS* (see Sect. 2.5), which alterations affect proliferative signaling pathways, causing abnormal growth of leukemic cells.[1]

Class II mutations lead to impaired differentiation of myeloid progenitor cells by affecting genes of transcription factors (TFs). They block the differentiation with minimal effect on proliferation. These mutations occur earlier in leukemogenesis (primary lesions) than class I mutations. Genes encoding TFs become disrupted either by their fusion, as a result of chromosome aberration (*CBF*, *MLL*, *EVI1*, *TEL* also named *ETV6*—ets variant 6, *RARA*—retinoic acid receptor, alfa), or by point mutation (*CEBPA* and *NPM1*) (Deguchi and Gilliland 2002; Kelly and Gilliland 2002).

While occurring separately, the aforementioned mutations cause excessive myeloproliferation (class I) or differentiation arrest (class II) of hematopoietic progenitors, resulting in the development of myeloproliferative syndrome or myelodysplasia, respectively. However, when occurring sequentially in a single cell, these "two hits" lead to a fully penetrating AML (Kelly and Gilliland 2002).

2.2.2 Extension of "Two Hits" Model by Other Mechanisms Leading to Leukemogenesis

The classical model of leukemogenesis proposed by Gilliland implies only lesions in the genes directly involved in the activation of proliferation and block of differentiation (Gilliland 2001). However, it has been recently shown that other gene classes might also be mutated in AML (Metzeler et al. 2011). These include genes which encode regulators of:

- Genomic stability and DNA repair, e.g.: tumor protein p53 (*TP53*),
- Transcription, e.g.: *TET2*, *IDH1/IDH2*, *DNMT3A*—DNA(cytosine-5)-methyltransferase 3 alpha
- Translation (microRNAs),
- Protein turnover, e.g.: *C-CBL*—Cas-Br-M(murine) ectopic retroviral transforming sequence.

Mutations of these genes indirectly contribute to AML transformation by the alteration of either structure or expression of final effector genes, which results in proliferation advantage and differentiation arrest. Thus, the updated version of "two hits" model should comprise any structural or quantitative gene aberration, which deregulates growth and differentiation of hematopoietic cells (Ko et al. 2010; Makishima et al. 2009; Marcucci et al. 2010; Yan et al. 2011).

[1] Unless included in the text, the names of the genes are presented in the descriptions in Tables 2.1 and 2.2. This refers to the whole chapter.

Table 2.1 Cryptic genetic alterations in AML and their prognostic impact

Gene/mutation	Chromosome localization	AML type/comment	Prognosis	Reference
FLT3-ITD	13q12	CN-AML	Poor	Whitman et al. (2010), Smith et al. (2011)
FLT3-TKD	13q12	CN-AML	Unclear	Whitman et al. (2010), Smith et al. (2011)
NPM1	5q35	CN-AML, distinct WHO entity (provisional)	*NPM1*(+)/*FLT3*-ITD(−)—favorable, *NPM1*(+)/*FLT3*-ITD(+)—intermediate, *NPM1*(−)/*FLT3*-ITD(−)—intermediate, *NPM1*(−)/*FLT3*-ITD(+)—poor	Bacher et al. (2010a), Becker et al. (2010), Thiede et al. (2006)
CEBPA	19q13.1	CN-AML, occurs as mono (sm) or biallelic (dm) mutation, distinct WHO entity (provisional)	dm—favorable, sm—intermediate	Dufour et al. (2010), Taskesen et al. (2011)
MLL-PTD	11q23.3	Mostly CN-AML, may associate with trisomy 11	Poor	Bacher et al. (2010a), Foran (2010), Mrózek et al. (2007)
IDH1	2q33.3	CN-AML	Poor in patients with *NPM1*(−)	Walker and Marcucci (2011)
IDH2	15q26.1	CN-AML	Poor in older patients	Walker and Marcucci (2011)
TET2	4q24	CN-AML	Poor, worsens prognosis in $CEBPA^{dm}$(+) AML, worsens prognosis in *NPM1*(+) AML	Metzeler et al. (2011)
WT1	11p13	CN-AML	Poor, especially poor in *FLT3*-ITD(+) patients	Betz and Hess (2010), Foran (2010), Gulley et al. (2010), Walker and Marcucci (2011)
N-RAS	1p13	CA-AML, associates with CBF leukemias	Neutral, may sensitize to cytarabine	Gulley et al. (2010), Smith et al. (2011)
C-KIT	4q12	CBF-AML	Poor	Betz and Hess (2010), Paschka et al. (2010)
BAALC	8q22.3	CN-AML	Overexpression—poor, especially poor in *FLT3*-ITD(+) patients, especially poor in *CEBPA*(−) patients	Bienz et al. (2005)

(continued)

Table 2.1 (continued)

Gene/ mutation	Chromosome localization	AML type/comment	Prognosis	Reference
ERG	21q22.3	May correlate with Down syndrome-associated leukemia	Overexpression—poor	Marcucci et al. (2005), (2007), (2009)
MN1	22q12.1	CN-AML	Overexpression—poor	Langer et al. (2009)
EVI1	3q26.2	–	Overexpression—poor	Walker and Marcucci (2011)
MIR-181a	9q33.3	Overexpression correlates with *CEBPA* mutation	Overexpression—favorable	Schwind et al. (2010a), Marcucci et al. (2011) Walker and Marcucci (2011)
MIR-191	3p21.31	–	Overexpression—poor	Garzon et al. (2008)
MIR-199a	19p13.2	–	Overexpression—poor	Garzon et al. (2008)

CN-AML cytogenetically normal AML; CA-AML cytogenetically abnormal AML; *FLT3* fms-related tyrosine kinase 3; *NPM1* nucleophosmin; *CEBPA* CCAAT/enhancer binding protein (C/EBP), alpha; *MLL* myeloid/lymphoid or mixed-lineage leukemia factor (trithorax homolog, Drosophila); *IDH1* isocitrate dehydrogenase 1 (NADP +), soluble; *IDH2* isocitrate dehydrogenase 2 (NADP +), mitochondrial; *TET2* tet methylcytosine dioxygenase 2; *WT1* Wilms tumor 1; *NRAS* neuroblastoma RAS viral (v-ras) oncogene homolog; *KIT* v-kit Hardy-Zuckerman 4 feline sarcoma viral oncogene homolog; *BAALC* brain and acute leukemia, cytoplasmic; *ERG* v-ets erythroblastosis virus E26 oncogene homolog (avian); *MN1* meningioma (disrupted in balanced translocation) 1; *EVI1* (*MECOM*) MDS1 and EVI1 complex locus

Table 2.2 Guidelines for cytogenetic and molecular risk group stratification in AML according to the European LeukemiaNet (after Döhner et al. 2010, modified)

Genetic risk group	Subsets	AML patients (%)
Favorable	t(8;21)(q22;q22); *RUNX1–RUNX1T1*(*AML1-ETO*)	27
	inv(16)(p13.1q22) or t(16;16)(p13.1;q22); *CBFB-MYH11*	
	Mutated *NPM1* without *FLT3*-ITD (normal karyotype)	
	Mutated *CEBPA* (normal karyotype)[a]	
Intermediate-I[b]	Mutated *NPM1* and *FLT3*-ITD (normal karyotype)	31
	Wild-type *NPM1* and *FLT3*-ITD (normal karyotype)[c]	
	Wild-type *NPM1* and *FLT3* (normal karyotype)	
Intermediate-II	t(9;11)(p22;q23); *MLLT3-MLL*	19
	Cytogenetic abnormalities not classified as favorable or adverse	
Adverse	inv(3)(q21q26.2) or t(3;3)(q21;q26.2); *RPN1-EVI1*	23
	t(6;9)(p23;q34); *DEK-NUP214*(*CAN*)	
	t(v;11)(v;q23)[d]; *MLL* rearranged	
	–5 or del(5q); –7; 17p abnormalities[e]; complex karyotype[f]	

[a] double (biallelic) mutated *CEBPA*

[b] includes all CN-AMLs, except for those included in the favorable subgroup. The aberrations are associated with intermediate or poor prognosis. However, they should be reported separately because of the potential different response to treatment

[c] NPM1(−)*FLT3*-ITD(+) AML is associated with poor prognosis, but it has been included in intermediate I group because of potential response to targeted treatment

[d] v, chromosome breakpoint other than 9p22

[e] with the rearrangement or deletion of *TP53* locus

[f] at least three chromosome aberrations, in the absence of one of the WHO designated recurrent balanced aberrations, i.e. t(15;17), t(8;21), inv/t(16)(q22), t(9;11), other 11q23 translocations, t(6;9), inv/t(3)(q26)

RUNX1(*AML1*) runt-related transcription factor 1; *RUNX1T1* (*ETO*) runt-related transcription factor 1, translocated to, 1 (cyclin D-related); *MYH11* myosin, heavy chain 11, smooth muscle; *NPM1* nucleophosmin; *FLT3* fms-related tyrosine kinase 3; *CEBPA* CCAAT/enhancer binding protein (C/EBP), alpha; *MLLT3* myeloid/lymphoid, or mixed-lineage leukemia (trithorax homolog, Drosophila) translocated to, 3; *MLL* myeloid/lymphoid or mixed-lineage leukemia factor (trithorax homolog, Drosophila); *RPN1* ribophorin I; *EVI1* (*MECOM*) MDS1 and EVI1 complex locus; *DEK*- DEK oncogene; *NUP214* (*CAN*) nucleoporin 214 kDa

2.3 Gross Genetic Alterations in AML

AML-associated chromosome aberrations often affect the components of the core binding factor (CBF) complex, i.e., RUNX1 (CBFA2, AML1) and core-binding factor, beta subunit (CBFB) proteins. This protein complex physiologically activates a number of genes critical for normal myeloid development. The resulting fusion genes include: *RUNX1–RUNX1T1* (*AML1-ETO*) due to t(8;21)(q22;q22), *CBFB-MYH11* due to inv(16)(p13.1q22) or t(16;16)(p13.1;q22), and *RUNX1–EVI1* due to t(3;21)(q26;q22). The first three aberrations are the cytogenetic markers of so-called CBF-AML, the last one is associated with therapy-related AML (Maki et al. 2008; Martens and Stunnenberg 2010). All these chimeric proteins act as dominant negative forms of the CBF complex, leading to differentiation blockade.

RUNX1–RUNX1T1 fusion protein, found in 10 % of AML cases, constitutively represses genes usually activated by RUNX1 transcription factor, including *C-FMS* (*CSF1R*—colony stimulating factor 1 receptor), *P14ARF* (*CDKN2A*—cyclin-dependent kinase inhibitor 2A) and *CEBPA*, thus inhibiting normal myeloid differentiation (Martens and Stunnenberg 2010).

CBFB-MYH11, the result of chromosome 16 inversion/translocation, occurs in 5 % of AML cases and encodes protein that fuses first 165 amino acids of CBFB to the *C*-terminal coiled-coil region of a smooth muscle myosin heavy chain (MYH11). In normal cells, CBFB interacts with the RUNX1, increasing its affinity to DNA, and thus stimulating its activity. CBFB-MYH11 protein interferes with normal RUNX1 activity, which results in the repression of transcription of target genes by the recruitment of corepressors, such as histone deacetylases (HDACs) (Martens and Stunnenberg 2010).

Despite the lesions caused by t(8;21) or inv/t(16), CBF-AMLs are associated with relatively good prognosis in comparison to CN-AML.

Another aberration contributing to differentiation arrest is t(15;17)(q22;q21), which results in *PML–RARA* fusion. It is specific for acute promyelocytic leukemia (APL), which covers approximately 10 % of all AML cases. In normal cells, promyelocytic leukemia (PML) localizes in nuclear bodies where it functions as a transcription factor and tumor suppressor. *RARA* encodes retinoic acid (RA) receptor alpha. Chimeric PML–RARA protein fails to respond to RA concentration changes, acquiring constitutive transcriptional repressor activity. Additionally, *PML–RARA* rearrangement results in the disruption of nuclear bodies, thus inducing a maturation block. As a result, the cells are blocked at the promyelocytic stage of differentiation and self-renewal. Interestingly, the spectrum of PML–RARA targeted genes is wider as compared to wild-type RARA targets, thus potential implications of this fusion may be much more complex.

Both all-*trans*-retinoic acid (ATRA) and arsenic trioxide (ATO), used in APL treatment, directly target PML–RARA-mediated transcriptional repression, and protein stability, inducing rapid differentiation of the promyelocytes and complete clinical remission in most APL patients (Licht and Sternberg 2005). Some variant translocations of chromosome 17, involving *RARA locus*, preserve ATRA sensitivity:

- t(15;17)(q35;q21)/*NPM1–RARA*,
- t(11;17)(q13;q21)/*NUMA1–RARA NUMA1*—nuclear mitotic apparatus protein 1,
- t(4;17)(q12;q21)/*FIP1L1–RARA FIP1L1*—FIP1 like 1 (*S. cerevisiae*).

Other aberrations yield an ATRA—resistant form of disease (Gulley et al. 2010; Licht and Sternberg 2005):

- interstitial duplication of chromosome 17 resulting in *STAT5B–RARA* fusion *STAT5B*—signal transducer and activator of transcription 5B
- t(11;17)(q23;q21)/*PLZF–RARA*
  PLZF also named *ZBTB16*—zinc finger and BTB domain containing 16

Various abnormalities of chromosome 11, involving mixed-lineage leukemia (MLL) gene *locus* at 11q23.3, i.e.

- t(11;19)(q23;p13)/*MLL-MLLT1*
  MLLT1—myeloid/lymphoid or mixed-lineage leukemia (trithorax homolog, Drosophila), translocated to, 1
- t(9;11)(p22;q23)/*MLL-MLLT3*
  are found in about 4 % of adult AML cases and in 15–20 % of pediatric AMLs (Balgobind et al. 2011).

MLL may fuse to one of over 50 partner genes, which results in chimeric proteins of oncogenic potential. The *N*-terminal MLL region of such a chimera is responsible for DNA-binding, and the fusion protein partner serves as strong transactivator of target genes (Martens and Stunnenberg 2010). The direct genomic targets of MLL fusion proteins remain largely unknown; however, gene expression profiling showed that AMLs with 11q23/*MLL* rearrangements are characterized by the deregulation of homeobox (HOX) genes (Bacher et al. 2010a). *MLL* aberrations are particularly common in patients with a history of treatment with topoisomerase II inhibitors (e.g. etoposide), and are generally related to adverse outcome, with the exception of t(9;11)/*MLL-MLLT3*, which is associated with intermediate prognosis (Bacher et al. 2010b; Betz and Hess 2010).

Another *MLL* alteration found in AML is its amplification (reviewed by Haus et al. 2009). It may present in variable forms, including hsr (homogenously stained region), dmin (double minute chromosomes), derivative 11q, and others. *MLL* is the second most frequently amplified gene in AML and myelodysplastic syndrome (MDS), with the incidence of less than 1 % of CA-AML, after *C-MYC* [*C-MYC*–v-myc myelocytomatosis viral oncogene homolog (avian)]. The number of *MLL* copies ranges from 5 to 50 per cell (Mohamed 2010). Both *MLL* amplification and its rearrangements result in the inhibition of myeloid differentiation. Additionally, over 90 % of AML/MDS cases with *MLL* amplification show an inactivation of *TP53* by deletion or mutation (Mohamed 2010). Some abnormalities involving *MLL* gene are cryptic, not detectable by classical cytogenetics.

C-MYC (8q24) amplification, presenting in the form of hsr or dmin, is observed in about 1 % of AML, but is rare as compared with solid tumors (Haus et al. 2009; Mohamed 2010). C-MYC is one of the pivotal TFs regulating hematopoiesis, which expression decreases during differentiation. However, *C-MYC* amplification does not necessarily lead to its higher expression. In pediatric AML, high expression of *C-MYC* associates with 11q23 rearrangements, while in adults it is related to *RUNX1–RUNX1T1*, *PML–RARA*, and *PLZF–RARA* fusions (Delgado and Leon 2010; Schotte et al. 2011).

Main gross genetic alterations in AML and their clinical relevance are presented in Table 10.1.

2.4 Cryptic Molecular Alterations Associated with Cytogenetically Normal AML

Aside from gross chromosomal rearrangements resulting in gene fusions, an increasing number of submicroscopic alterations have been identified which are essential for AML pathogenesis and serve as independent prognostic factors (Bacher et al. 2010b; Smith et al. 2011). Among 40 % of AML patients without cytogenetic abnormalities, more than 85 % have submicroscopic genetic alterations (Bacher et al. 2010b). Cryptic rearrangements may also be found in other cytogenetically defined subgroups of AML and may influence the outcome (Table 2.2).

2.4.1 Intragenic Aberrations

2.4.1.1 *FLT3*

The *FLT3* gene (fms-like tyrosine kinase receptor 3), located on chromosome 13q12, encodes the class III transmembrane tyrosine kinase receptor (Zuo et al. 2009). *FLT3* is normally expressed by hematopoietic stem cells, early myeloid and lymphoid precursors and both immature and mature monocytic cells. After activation by its ligand (FL), FLT3 supports the proliferation and survival of hematopoietic progenitors (Betz and Hess 2010).

Mutations in the *FLT3* gene are documented in approximately 30 % of all AML cases, across all French-American-British (FAB) subtypes, with an increased incidence in CN-AML, *MLL* partial tandem duplication (*MLL*-PTD)-positive AML, APL, and *DEK-CAN*(+) AML (Libura et al. 2003). They fall into two categories: internal tandem duplications of the 3–400 bp gene fragment (*FLT3*-ITD), that involve mainly the juxtamembrane (JM) domain (35–45 % of CN-AML; incidence in total AML population: 25 % for adults and 15 % for children) and less frequent point mutations (15 % of all *FLT3* mutations; 5 % of adult and 3 %

of pediatric AML), involving the kinase domain (*FLT3*-TKD) (Meshinchi et al. 2008). Both *FLT3*-ITD and *FLT3*-TKD result in ligand independent, constitutive activation of FLT3 (Gulley et al. 2010; Betz and Hess 2010).

FLT3-ITD has an adverse effect on relapse risk (RR) and overall survival (OS) of AML patients, even in prognostically favorable cytogenetic subtypes (e.g., APL with *PML–RARA* fusion gene), while little effect on remission induction is described. Prognostic significance of *FLT3*-TKD mutation remains unclear (Whitman et al. 2010; Smith et al. 2011).

2.4.1.2 *NPM1*

The nucleophosmin 1 gene (*NPM1*) is located on chromosome 5q35. Its mutations occur in 55 % of adult CN-AML cases and 30 % of the whole adult AML group. Their incidence is lower in pediatric AML (7.5 %) (Bacher et al. 2010b). NPM1 is a multifunctional protein shuttling between nuclear compartments and cytoplasm. It is localized predominantly within nucleolus, taking part in ribosome assembly and the regulation of ARF (CDKN2A—cyclin-dependent kinase inhibitor 2A) and p53 tumor suppressor function (Betz and Hess 2010). *NPM1* frameshift mutations retain the protein in the cytoplasm, which inhibits the ARF-p53 pathway (Mardis et al. 2009; Zuo et al. 2009). *NPM1* mutations are associated with an increased white blood cells count and leukemia of a monocytic M4/M5 lineage. Mutations of *NPM1* commonly coexist with *FLT3*-ITD. Only *NPM1*(+)/*FLT3*-ITD(−) configuration is recognized as a favorable prognostic factor, especially in patients aged ≥70 years. AML with *NPM1*(−)/*FLT3*-ITD(+) is associated with the worst outcome, while *NPM1*(+)/*FLT3*-ITD(+) and *NPM1*(−)/*FLT3*-ITD(−) AML—with the intermediate outcome (Bacher et al. 2010b; Becker et al. 2010; Thiede et al. 2006). *NPM1*-mutated AML presents distinct gene and microRNA expression profiles, and is provisionally recognized by the revised WHO classification (4th edition, 2008) as a separate entity (Becker et al. 2010; Vardiman et al. 2009).

2.4.1.3 *CEBPA*

The *CEBPA* gene maps to chromosome band 19q13.1 and encodes a CCAAT/enhancer binding protein (C/EBP) alpha, a transcription factor important in the regulation of myelopoiesis (Zuo et al. 2009). CEBPA regulates the transcription of genes encoding for interleukin 6 (IL-6), granulocyte colony-stimulating factor (G-CSF) receptor, myeloperoxidase, and others (Dufour et al. 2010). *CEBPA* mutations occur in approximately 5–15 % of CN-AML (Foran 2010). A frameshift and nonsense mutations in the *N*-terminal region result in a truncated, dominant negative protein. In-frame mutations involve a leucine zipper motif at the

C-terminus of CEBPA, which impairs dimerization and DNA-binding ability (Zuo et al. 2009).

Two-thirds of *CEBPA*(+) AML cases harbor mutations affecting both *C*- and *N*-terminal region simultaneously, each occurring at a different allele (dm, double allele mutation). The remaining *CEBPA*(+) AML cases exhibit mutation of only one allele (sm, single allele mutation). *CEBPA* double mutant cases present a unique gene expression signature, are rarely associated with *FLT3*-ITD and confer a favorable prognosis, as compared with *CEBPA*^{sm}(+), and *CEBPA*(−) AML. This suggests that *CEBPA*^{dm}(+) AML constitutes a distinct disease entity and it has been provisionally recognized as such in the latest WHO classification (Dufour et al. 2010; Taskesen et al. 2011).

2.4.1.4 MLL

Partial tandem duplications of *MLL* were the first molecular change recognized to be of prognostic value in CN-AML. They are found in 5–10 % of cases and have a negative impact on disease outcome, especially in older patients (Whitman et al. 2007). In CA-AML, *MLL*-PTD is frequently associated with chromosome 11 trisomy (Bacher et al. 2010b; Foran 2010; Mrózek et al. 2007).

2.4.1.5 *IDH1/2*

IDH1 and *IDH2* genes, located at 2q33.3 and 15q26.1, encode two isoforms of isocitrate dehydrogenase (NADP+), the enzyme associated with the tricarboxylic acid (TCA) cycle. Genome sequencing of de novo CN-AML showed the prevalence of *IDH1* and *IDH2* mutations of 16 and 14–15 %, respectively (Marcucci et al. 2010; Mardis et al. 2009). In pediatric AML mutations of *IDH* genes are rare (3 %) (Paschka et al. 2010; Smith et al. 2011; Walker and Marcucci 2011).

The precise role of *IDH* point mutations in AML pathogenesis is not clear, but they have been shown to alter DNA and the histone methylation profile, as well as to have an adverse prognostic impact in some groups of patients (see Table 2.1) (Dang et al. 2010; Figueroa et al. 2010a; Walker and Marcucci 2011).

2.4.1.6 *TET2*

Mutations in tet oncogene family member 2 (*TET2*) were recently described in several myeloproliferative neoplasms. *TET2 locus* at 4q24 is involved in some AML-associated aberrations, such as t(3;4)(q26;q24). Additionally, many different *TET2* point mutations that spread over the whole gene were discovered in 10–26 % of MDS or secondary AML and 12 % of de novo AML (Nibourel et al. 2010). Recent studies revealed that *TET2* encodes methylcytosine dioxygenase, an enzyme involved in the epigenetic regulation of myelopoiesis. TET2 influences the promoter methylation profile, changing the expression of target genes. *TET2* missense or nonsense mutations, resulting in a truncated or sequence-altered protein, lead to a promoter hypermethylation of target genes, and their silencing (Mohr et al. 2011). Similarly, *IDH1/IDH2* point mutations result in hypermethylation phenotype which suggests that both *IDH1/2* and *TET2* mutations represent a third type of genetic alteration important for AML leukemogenesis, different from class I and class II mutations (Figueroa et al. 2010a; Walker and Marcucci 2011).

TET2 mutations were found to have an adverse impact on the prognosis of CN-AML patients who have $CEBPA^{dm}$ and/or mutated *NPM1* without *FLT3*-ITD, classified by European LeukemiaNet (ELN) to the favorable-risk group (Metzeler et al. 2011).

2.4.1.7 Other Intragenic Aberrations Associated with CN-AML

Many other genes were found to be mutated in AML, i.e. *WT1*, *DNMT3A*, *ASXL1* [additional sex combs like 1 (Drosophila)], *CBL*, *HOXA9* (homeobox A9), *PTPN11* (protein tyrosine phosphatase, nonreceptor type 11), and *RUNX1* (*AML1*). Mutations of *WT1* are observed in 10 % of CN-AML and associate with the worse OS and primary chemotherapy resistance. Recently, mutations in *DNMT3A* gene encoding DNA methyltransferase were found in about 30 % of patients with intermediate-prognosis AML. They confer a poor prognosis that may be partially attributed to simultaneous *FLT3* and *IDH* mutations (Ley et al. 2010). Point mutations in *RUNX1* gene, found in 7–15 % of de novo AML, mainly of intermediate prognosis, are inversely correlated with NPM1 mutations and worsens the prognosis, especially in relation to event-free survival (EFS) (Gaidzik et al. 2011). The precise role of other aforementioned gene mutations in AML pathogenesis and their prognostic significance has to be further clarified.

2.4.2 Gene Overexpression

Overexpression of several genes involved in the regulation of normal hematopoiesis was shown to be an important prognostic factor in CN-AML. These include Brain and acute leukemia, cytoplasmic (*BAALC*), ETS-related gene (*ERG*), and *MN1*.

2.4.2.1 *BAALC*

Brain and acute leukemia, cytoplasmic gene (8q22.3) expression in normal hematopoietic precursors is downregulated during differentiation, which may point at its role in leukemogenesis (Gregory et al. 2009). Its overexpression is associated with the *HOX* gene family and *HOX* gene embedded microRNAs downregulation

(Schwind et al. 2010b). Many studies revealed poor prognostic significance of this marker in CN-AML. The strongest prognostic impact of *BAALC* overexpression seems to be restricted to patients lacking both *CEBPA* mutations, and *FLT3*-ITD (Bienz et al. 2005). It was suggested that dichotomization of CN-AML cases with regard to *BAALC* expression and *FLT3* mutation status presents the best risk stratification approach (Baldus et al. 2006).

2.4.2.2 *ERG*

ETS-related gene (21q22.3) is a member of the ETS family of TFs. High *ERG* expression correlates with the upregulation of many genes involved in cell proliferation, differentiation, apoptosis, and DNA methylation (Gregory et al. 2009; Schwind et al. 2010b). It was shown that *ERG* overexpression determines lower complete remission (CR) rate, as well as shorter disease-free survival (DFS), and OS (Marcucci et al. 2005). *ERG* expression provides additional prognostic information for patients who were already stratified according to *NPM1* and *FLT3*-ITD status, excluding the high risk *FLT3*-ITD(+)/*NPM1*(−) group (Marcucci et al. 2007; Metzeler et al. 2009).

Overexpression of both, *BAALC* and *ERG* predicts an adverse clinical outcome in de novo CN-AML. It is also associated with distinct gene and miRNA expression signatures (Schwind et al. 2010b).

2.4.2.3 *MN1*

Transcriptional coactivator MN1 is encoded by the meningioma-1 gene (*MN1*), mapped to 22q12.1. Like *BAALC*, *MN1* expression in normal hematopoietic cells depends on the stage of differentiation (Gregory et al. 2009). Constitutive overexpression of *MN1* in murine bone marrow rapidly induces myeloid leukemia, which is accompanied by an early-onset severe anemia, suggesting that *MN1* alone efficiently blocks megakaryocyte-erythroid differentiation (Gregory et al. 2009). Additionally, *MN1* gene is involved in translocation t(12;22)(p13;q12), resulting in *MN1-TEL*(*ETV6*) fusion.

In multivariate analysis, the overexpression of *MN1* in adult CN-AML was an independent marker of poor prognosis (Langer et al. 2009). It has strong prognostic value for CN-AML patients, especially in cases other than *NPM1*(+)/*FLT3*-ITD(−) (Heuser et al. 2006). *MN1* overexpression is commonly found together with overexpression of *BAALC* and with expression of wild-type *NPM1*. It was found that patients with overexpression of *BAALC* or *MN1* show similar gene expression signatures, which may suggest potential functional interplay between these genes in myeloid leukemogenesis (Langer et al. 2009).

2.5 Intragenic Aberrations Associated with Cytogenetically Abnormal AML

C-KIT (*SCFR*—stem cell factor receptor, *C-KIT* proto-oncogene; 4q12), *N-RAS* (neuroblastoma RAS viral oncogene homolog; 1p13), and *K-RAS* (Kirsten rat sarcoma viral oncogene homolog; 12p12) mutations in AML belong to class I mutations (Betz and Hess 2010). They were found to be associated with CBF leukemias, where they present the "second hit" in the course of transformation.

2.5.1 C-KIT

C-KIT protooncogene encodes type III receptor tyrosine kinase, important for signal transduction in normal hematopoiesis. Gain-of-function *C-KIT* mutations, involving mainly exons 8 and 17 (mut*KIT*8 and mut*KIT*17), were found in 2 % of overall AML, and in over 30 % of CBF-AML (Foran 2010). Both mutations confer higher RR for otherwise favorable CBF-leukemias; however, mut*KIT*17 has stronger adverse impact, which is more evident in inv(16)/*CBFB-MYH11*(+)AML (Betz and Hess 2010; Paschka et al. 2010).

2.5.2 N-RAS **and** *K-RAS*

RAS proteins have been shown to influence proliferation, differentiation, transformation, and apoptosis by transmitting mitogenic and growth signals into the cytoplasm and the nucleus. Usually inactive in normal cells, RAS molecules become activated by substitutions. Overall *N-* and *K-RAS* mutations (most commonly seen at codons 12, 13, and 61) are observed in about 15 % of AML and associate with inv(3) or inv(16) (Gulley et al. 2010). They may enhance the response to high dose cytarabine, but their general prognostic impact seems to be neutral (Gulley et al. 2010; Smith et al. 2011).

Beside *RAS* and *C-KIT* mutations, the aforementioned *FLT3* alterations also represent an additional type of activating mutations in CBF-AML and are indicators of poor prognosis. In practical terms, as *RAS*(+) CBF-leukemias retain their profile of prognostically favorable AML, identification of *C-KIT* and *FLT3* mutations enables prognostic restratification of CBF-AML patients.

2.6 MicroRNAs in AML

MicroRNAs (miRNAs) are small (18–25 nucleotides), noncoding RNAs that negatively regulate gene expression on a posttranscriptional level. miRNAs hybridize to the 3′-untranslated (3′-UTR) regions of protein-coding, messenger RNAs (mRNAs), and lead to their degradation or inhibition of translation (Seca et al. 2010). It is estimated that over 30 % of structural genes are regulated by miRNAs. They are involved in all crucial physiological processes, like proliferation, differentiation, apoptosis, signal transduction, etc.

As regulators of expression of structural genes miRNA may function indirectly, both as oncogenes (*oncomirs*) or tumor suppressors. Some miRNAs are localized in genomic regions associated with cancer, e.g. breakpoint regions in specific chromosome aberrations, hot-spots, minimal regions of loss of heterozygosity (LOH), and minimal regions of amplification (Marcucci et al. 2011).

Alterations of miRNA expression were described in many types of solid tumors and leukemias. It has been shown that miRNA expression profiles better characterize particular cancer subtypes than gene expression profiles (Seca et al. 2010). miRNA signatures were found to distinguish normal cells from AML blasts and AML from ALL cases. In AML they have also been shown to be associated with several chromosome aberrations, e. g. t(15;17), t(8;21), inv(16), t(11q23)/*MLL*, with *FLT3*-ITD, mutations in *NPM1* and *CEBPA*, as well as *BAALC* and *MN1* overexpression (Marcucci et al. 2011). Many miRNAs target genes inhibiting differentiation and apoptosis, or promoting cell proliferation. While downregulated they contribute to leukemogenesis (Schotte et al. 2011). These include:

- *miR-34b* targeting cyclin-dependent kinase 4 (*CDK4*) and cyclin E2 (*CCNE2*),
- *miR-15a* targeting *BCL2* (B-cell CLL/lymphoma 2; apoptosis regulator),
- *let-7* family targeting oncogenes *RAS* and *MYC*.

Microarray studies have shown that miRNA profiles are also associated with the outcome of AML patients. Overexpression of any of the following: *miR-20a*, *miR-25*, *miR-191*, *miR-199a*, or *miR-199b* was an independent adverse prognostic factor in intermediate and poor-risk cytogenetic groups (Garzon et al. 2008). On the contrary, high *miR-182* expression was found to improve prognosis in cytogenetically normal, poor molecular risk patients with *FLT3*-ITD, and/or wild-type *NPM1* (Schwind et al. 2010a). Sequential miRNA profiling may also be helpful in monitoring the response to therapy (Marcucci et al. 2011).

Although miRNA studies in AML are still at the initial stage, novel technologies enable quick transfer of the results from the bench to the clinic. Importantly, miRNA expression should not only be considered as putative prognostic factor, but also as potential target for novel therapeutic strategies.

2.7 Acquired Copy Number Alterations Identified by SNP Arrays

An important limitation of conventional cytogenetics is the inability to detect genomic alterations below 5 Mb. High resolution genomic single nucleotide arrays (aSNP) enable the measurement of gene copy number and the distinction of individual genotypes to detect a LOH. Although, like other array-based methods, SNP arrays are not useful for the detection of balanced aberrations, or changes present in <25 % cells, they facilitate refining karyotype-based risk stratification by identification of subtle acquired Copy Number Alterations (CNAs) and acquired copy neutral LOH (ACN-LOH) (Parkin et al. 2010). ACN-LOH, which may be caused by acquired somatic uniparental disomy (AS-UPD), arises during the development of the neoplastic clone, when a segment (partial UPD), or a whole chromosome is lost and replaced by its homolog. In any case it may result in LOH, thus influencing the outcome.

In AML, acquired CNAs of regions important for cell survival and differentiation, including both subchromosomal, or entire chromosome gains/losses, may associate with other molecular markers: most UPD(+) patients harbor also *NPM1* or *CEBPA* mutations (Bullinger et al. 2010; Heinrichs et al. 2010; Parkin et al. 2010). The presence of CNAs was shown to worsen the prognosis of AML patients with regard to OS, EFS, and progression-free survival (PFS) (Tiu et al. 2011).

2.8 Epigenetic Mechanisms in AML

The epigenetic control of gene expression, mainly DNA methylation, plays an important role in determining the biology of the cell. The addition of methyl groups to cytosines at the palindromic CpG sites clustered in promoter regions may alter gene expression by creating new binding sites for methylation-dependent repressor molecules, or by impairing the affinity of TFs to their target sequences (Figueroa et al. 2010b). The alterations in gene methylation, i.e. hypermethylation resulting in the silencing of particular tumor suppressor genes, as well as hypomethylation reactivating stem cell phenotype, may contribute to carcinogenesis (Alvarez et al. 2010; Ko et al. 2010). In most cases, AML blasts show a very strong hypermethylation signature compared to normal bone marrow CD34+ cells; however, some genes are hypomethylated. As different cytogenetic and molecular AML subtypes were found to display a unique methylation profile, the epigenetic changes seem to represent an important step in leukemic transformation. Mutations of genes involved in DNA methylation, like *TET2*, *IDH1*, *IDH2* and *DNMT3A*, were recently identified in AML patients (Alvarez et al. 2010; Figueroa et al. 2010a). By microarray genome-wide screening, the number of aberrantly methylated genes in AML patients was found to increase at relapse (Kroeger et al. 2008).

Since the methylation status of some genes, such as:

- *E2F1* E2F transcription factor 1,
- *SMG6* smg-6 homolog, nonsense mediated mRNA decay factor (*C. elegans*),
- *CXCR5* chemokine (C-X-C motif) receptor 5; CD185,
- *LCK* lymphocyte-specific protein tyrosine kinase; p56lck, and
- *DBC1* deleted in bladder cancer 1

associates with OS of AML patients, the analysis of a methylation profile may be helpful in the design of clinical trials with demethylating agents (Alvarez et al. 2010; Figueroa et al. 2010a).

2.9 Clinical Implications of Molecular Genetics in AML

The detection of cytogenetic and molecular alterations may be used for personalized therapeutic approach, adjusting the mode and intensity of treatment for individual patients. This strategy includes three different aspects: (1) the stratification of patients according to the estimated risk of relapse based on initial findings, (2) the implementation of novel agents targeting particular molecular pathways, (3) making therapeutic decisions based on the monitoring of minimal residual disease (MRD).

2.9.1 Risk Stratification Based on Cytogenetic and Molecular Features of AML

The initial treatment of AML patients consists of remission induction followed by intensive consolidation. The postconsolidation approach may include either allogeneic or autologous hematopoietic stem cell transplantation (HSCT). Standard induction regimens based on the combination of anthracyclines and cytarabine result in up to 70 % CR rate. However, the majority of patients who achieved CR experience relapse, which potentially could be prevented by strongly invasive allogeneic HSCT.

Blast cell karyotype is considered the most important, clinically relevant prognostic parameter in AML. The Medical Research Council (MRC) and the Southwest Oncology Group (SWOG) proposed stratification systems distinguishing patients with favorable, intermediate, and adverse karyotype (Grimwade et al. 1998; Slovak et al. 2000). Both systems were validated in subsequent studies, leading to the implementation of classical cytogenetics in standard procedures in AML (Döhner et al. 2010). Unlike patients with favorable karyotype, those with adverse cytogenetic features become candidates for allogeneic HSCT in the first

CR. Unfortunately, two-thirds of AML patients belong to the intermediate group, mostly CN-AML, without clear treatment recommendations.

The identification of molecular alterations influencing AML outcome allowed for the modification of the stratification system. As proposed in 2010 by the ELN, CN-AML patients that are *NPM1*(+) and *FLT3*-ITD(−) as well as those *CEBPA*^{dm}(+) are now classified as the favorable group (Döhner et al. 2010). The intermediate group has been further divided into subgroups I and II. The intermediate-I group displays better, *NPM1*(+)*FLT3*(+) or worse, *NPM1* (−)*FLT3*(+), prognosis, but in both cases a good response to targeted treatment is anticipated. The intermediate-II group has generally worse outcome. The adverse risk group remains unchanged (Table 2.2). The classification does not include APL.

The new system allows for precise discrimination of patients ≤60 years with regard to the probability of relapse, relapse free survival, and OS. It must be emphasized that, according to current recommendations, examination of *NPM1*, *CEBPA*, and *FLT3*-ITD is obligatory within clinical trials and recommended in the routine treatment of CN-AML patients (Röllig et al. 2011).

2.9.2 Targeted Therapy of AML

Although knowledge concerning the molecular background of AML is rapidly increasing; until now, the only subtype with established indications for targeted treatment has been APL. Before the introduction of ATRA, this subtype was associated with high risk of therapy-related mortality. The use of standard cytostatics causes a rapid destruction of leukemic cells that release procoagulation factors, leading to the development of disseminated intravascular coagulation (DIC) syndrome. Administration of ATRA results in rapid differentiation of leukemic promyelocytes, allowing achievement of CR while avoiding the risk of DIC. However, ATRA does not destroy leukemic stem cells, which makes it insufficient as a single agent in APL treatment. Current strategies are based on the combinations of ATRA with chemotherapy during remission induction, followed by consolidation, and maintenance (Sanz et al. 2009). Results are excellent, with the cure rate approaching 90 %; patients who relapse may be offered second-line protocols incorporating ATO.

The use of targeted therapies in other AML subtypes is under intense investigation. Of particular interest are patients with *FLT3*-ITD, associated with decreased DFS, and OS rates. Several *FLT3*-selective tyrosine kinase inhibitors have been developed, including midostaurin, lestaurtinib, and sunitinib (Weisberg et al. 2002; Levis et al. 2002; O'Farrell et al. 2003). All these agents have been shown to reduce the tumor burden in relapsed or refractory AML. However, responses were short term, suggesting that targeting *FLT3* as a sole therapy is not sufficient (Zarrinkar et al. 2009).

AML with leukemic cells harboring *MLL* gene rearrangement is associated with shorter remission duration and shorter survival. It has been recently suggested that reversing complex epigenetic processes with demethylating agents such as azacitidine and decitabine or with histone deacetylase inhibitors may play a role in *MLL*(+) AML treatment (Altucci and Minucci 2009). This hypothesis requires verification in clinical trials.

Since AML is a heterogeneous disease with a complex molecular background, it is unlikely that targeting a single molecular pathway can be sufficiently effective. Thus, targeted treatment, adjusted for individual patient genetic profile would be a preferred part of broader therapeutic strategy.

2.9.3 Monitoring of Minimal Residual Disease

Conventional cytogenetic methods allow for the evaluation of remission status at the level of 5 % of blasts in bone marrow. The application of more sensitive methods, including multiparametric flow cytometry, or RT-RQ-PCR enables the detection of MRD with the sensitivity of $<10^{-4}$.

Molecular monitoring of *PML–RARA* is widely used in APL. While the detection of this fusion gene after remission induction is not of clinical relevance, the achievement of molecular remission after consolidation is considered a major treatment objective (Sanz et al. 2009). It is well documented that patients with the disease persistent or recurrent at the molecular level, confirmed by two consecutive assays after completion of consolidation, will invariably relapse, unless additional therapy is given (Breccia et al. 2004). The suggested therapy for patients with documented molecular relapse may include ATO, which prevents hematological relapse in the majority of patients (Grimwade et al. 2009).

More recently, RQ-PCR has been utilized in the monitoring of *NPM1* mutations. It has been shown that $NPM1^{mut}$ transcript levels were significantly associated with prognosis after each treatment cycle and that its higher level after consolidation therapy was a significant factor for an increased risk of relapse and death. Serial posttreatment assessments of MRD allowed for early detection of relapse (Krönke et al. 2011).

2.10 Conclusions

Due to its cytogenetic and molecular complexity of prognostic significance, AML is nowadays the focus of intensive research. Apart from class I and II mutations resulting in increased proliferation/survival and impaired differentiation of AML blasts, respectively, alterations of genes regulating DNA repair, transcription, translation, and protein turnover were also shown to contribute to leukemogenesis. While chromosome aberrations are mainly large enough to be detected by conventional cytogenetics, the identification of cryptic changes requires sophisticated methods of molecular biology. Some of the aforementioned alterations are well-known prognostic or predictive factors in AML; others, such as *IDH1/2* mutations or *KIT* and *RAS* aberrations, have to be further examined to definitively establish their prognostic significance. miRNA and epigenetic changes were proven to be important for AML leukemogenesis, but their prognostic value similarly requires further investigation.

The knowledge about molecular pathogenesis of AML coupled with novel, genome-wide screening methods, has significant clinical implications for more precise risk stratification, response to therapy and MRD monitoring, as well as targeted therapies development.

Acknowledgments The authors would like to thank Dorothy Michalowski for proofreading and editing assistance.

References

Altucci L, Minucci S (2009) Epigenetic therapies in haematological malignancies: searching for true targets. Eur J Cancer 45:1137–1145

Alvarez S, Suela J, Valencia A, Fernández A, Wunderlich M, Agirre X, Prósper F, Martín-Subero JI, Maiques A, Acquadro F, Rodriguez Perales S, Calasanz MJ, Roman-Gómez J, Siebert R, Mulloy JC, Cervera J, Sanz MA, Esteller M, Cigudosa JC (2010) DNA methylation profiles and their relationship with cytogenetic status in adult acute myeloid leukemia. PLoS ONE 5(8):e12197. doi:10.1371/journal.pone.0012197

Bacher U, Kohlmann A, Haferlach T (2010a) Gene expression profiling for diagnosis and therapy in acute leukaemia and other hematologic malignancies. Cancer Treat Rev 36:637–646

Bacher U, Schnitter S, Haferlach T (2010b) Molecular genetics in acute myeloid leukemia. Curr Opin Oncol 22:646–655

Baldus CD, Thiede C, Soucek S, Bloomfield CD, Thiel E, Ehninger G (2006) BAALC expression and FLT3 internal tandem duplication mutations in acute myeloid leukemia patients with normal cytogenetics: prognostic implications. J Clin Oncol 24:790–797

Balgobind BV, Zwaan CM, Pieters R, Van den Heuvel-Eibrink MM (2011) The heterogeneity of pediatric MLL-rearranged acute myeloid leukemia. Leukemia 25:1239–1248

Becker H, Marcucci G, Maharry K, Radmacher MD, Mrózek K, Margeson D, Whitman SP, Wu YZ, Schwind S, Paschka P, Powell BL, Carter TH, Kolitz JE, Wetzler M, Carroll AJ, Baer MR, Caligiuri MA, Larson RA, Bloomfield CD (2010) Favorable prognostic impact of NPM1 mutations in older patients with cytogenetically normal de novo acute myeloid leukemia and associated gene- and microRNA-expression signatures: a Cancer and Leukemia Group B study. J Clin Oncol 28:596–604

Betz BL, Hess JL (2010) Acute myeloid leukemia diagnosis in the 21st century. Arch Pathol Lab Med 134:1427–1433

Bienz M, Ludwig M, Leibundgut EO, Mueller BU, Ratschiller D, Solenthaler M, Fey MF, Pabst T (2005) Risk assessment in patients with acute myeloid leukemia and a normal karyotype. Clin Cancer Res 11:1416–1424

Breccia M, Diverio D, Noguera NI, Visani G, Santoro A, Locatelli F, Damiani D, Marmont F, Vignetti M, Petti MC, Lo Coco F (2004) Clinico-biological features and outcome of acute promyelocytic leukemia patients with persistent polymerase chain reaction detectable disease after the AIDA front-line induction and consolidation therapy. Haematologica 89:29–33

Bullinger L, Krönke J, Schön C, Radtke I, Urlbauer K, Botzenhardt U, Gaidzik V, Carió A, Senger C, Schlenk RF, Downing JR, Holzmann K, Döhner K, Döhner H (2010) Identification of acquired copy number alterations and uniparental disomies in cytogenetically normal acute myeloid leukemia using high-resolution single-nucleotide polymorphism analysis. Leukemia 24:438–449

Dang L, Jin S, Su SM (2010) IDH mutations in glioma and acute myeloid leukemia. Trends Mol Med 16:287–397

Deguchi K, Gilliland DG (2002) Cooperativity between mutations in tyrosine kinases and in hematopoietic transcription factors in AML. Leukemia 16:740–744

Delgado MD, Leon J (2010) Myc roles in hematopoiesis and leukemia. Genes Cancer 1:605–616

Döhner H, Estey EH, Amadori S, Appelbaum FR, Büchner T, Burnett AK, Dombret H, Fenaux P, Grimwade D, Larson RA, Lo-Coco F, Naoe T, Niederwieser D, Ossenkoppele GJ, Sanz MA, Sierra J, Tallman MS, Löwenberg B, Bloomfield CD (2010) Diagnosis and management of acute myeloid leukemia in adults: recommendations from an international expert panel, on behalf of the European LeukemiaNet. Blood 115:453–474

Dufour A, Schneider F, Metzeler KH, Hoster E, Schneider S, Zellmeier E, Benthaus T, Sauerland MC, Berdel WE, Buchner T, Wormann B, Braess J, Hiddemann W, Bohlander SK, Spiekemann K (2010) Acute myeloid leukemia with biallelic CEBPA gene mutations and normal karyotype represents a distinct genetic entity associated with a favorable clinical outcome. J Clin Oncol 28:570–577

Figueroa ME, Abdel-Wahab O, Lu C, Ward PS, Patel J, Shih A, Li Y, Bhagwat N, Vasanthakumar A, Fernandez HF, Tallman MS, Sun Z, Wolniak K, Peeters JK, Liu W, Choe SE, Fantin VR, Paietta E, Löwenberg B, Licht JD, Godley LA, Delwel R, Valk PJ, Thompson CB, Levine RL, Melnick A (2010a) Leukemic IDH1 and IDH2 mutations result in a hypermethylation phenotype, disrupt TET2 function, and impair hematopoietic differentiation. Cancer Cell 18:553–567

Figueroa ME, Lugthart S, Li Y, Erpelinck-Verschueren C, Deng X, Christos PJ, Schifano E, Booth J, van Putten W, Skrabanek L, Campagne F, Mazumdar M, Greally JM, Valk PJ, Löwenberg B, Delwel R, Melnick A (2010b) DNA methylation signatures identify biologically distinct subtypes in acute myeloid leukemia. Cancer Cell 17:13–27

Foran JM (2010) New prognostic markers in acute myeloid leukemia: perspective from the clinic. Hematol Am Soc Hematol Educ Program 2010:47–55

Gaidzik VI, Bullinger L, Schlenk RF, Zimmermann AS, Röck J, Paschka P, Corbacioglu A, Krauter J, Schlegelberger B, Ganser A, Späth D, Kündgen A, Schmidt-Wolf IG, Götze K, Nachbaur D, Pfreundschuh M, Horst HA, Döhner H, Döhner K (2011) RUNX1 mutations in acute myeloid leukemia: results from a comprehensive genetic and clinical analysis from the AML Study Group. J Clin Oncol 29:1364–1372

Garzon R, Volinia S, Liu CG, Fernandez-Cymering C, Palumbo T, Pichiorri F, Fabbri M, Coombes K, Alder H, Nakamura T, Flomenberg N, Marcucci G, Calin GA, Kornblau SM, Kantarjian H, Bloomfield CD, Andreeff M, Croce CM (2008) MicroRNA signatures associated with cytogenetics and prognosis in acute myeloid leukemia. Blood 111:3183–3189

Gilliland DG (2001) Hematologic malignancies. Curr Opin Hematol 8:189–191

Gregory TK, Wald D, Chen Y, Vermaat JM, Xiong Y, Tse W (2009) Molecular prognostic markers for adult acute myeloid leukemia with normal cytogenetics. J Hematol Oncol 2:23. doi:10.1186/1756-8722-2-23

Grimwade D, Hills RK (2009) Independent prognostic factors for AML outcome. Hematol Am Soc Hematol Educ Program 2009(1):385–395

Grimwade D, Jovanovic JV, Hills RK, Nugent EA, Patel Y, Flora R, Diverio D, Jones K, Aslett H, Batson E, Rennie K, Angell R, Clark RE, Solomon E, Lo-Coco F, Wheatley K, Burnett AK (2009) Prospective minimal residual disease monitoring to predict relapse of acute promyelocytic leukemia and to direct pre-emptive arsenic trioxide therapy. J Clin Oncol 27:3650–3658

Grimwade D, Walker H, Oliver F, Wheatley K, Harrison C, Harrison G, Rees J, Hann I, Stevens R, Burnett A, Goldstone A (1998) The importance of diagnostic cytogenetics on outcome in AML: analysis of 1,612 patients entered into the MRC AML 10 trial. The Medical Research Council Adult and Children's Leukaemia Working Parties. Blood 92:2322–2333

Gulley ML, Shea TC, Fedoriw Y (2010) Genetic tests to evaluate prognosis and predict therapeutic response in acute myeloid leukemia. J Mol Diagn 12:3–16

Haus O, Duszeńko E, Jaśkowiec A, Skonieczka K (2009) Gene amplification in hematologic malignancies [Polish]. Acta Haem Pol 40:313–319

Heinrichs S, Li C, Look AT (2010) SNP array analysis in hematologic malignancies: avoiding false discoveries. Blood 115:4157–4161

Heuser M, Beutel G, Krauter J, Döhner K, von Neuhoff N, Schlegelberger B, Ganser A (2006) High meningioma 1 (MN1) expression as a predictor for poor outcome in acute myeloid leukemia with normal cytogenetics. Blood 108:3898–3905

Kelly LM, Gilliland DG (2002) Genetics of myeloid leukemias. Annu Rev Genomics Hum Genet 3:179–198

Ko M, Huang Y, Jankowska AM, Pape UJ, Tahiliani M, Bandukwala HS, An J, Lamperti ED, Koh KP, Ganetzky R, Liu XS, Aravind L, Agarwal S, Maciejewski JP, Rao A (2010) Impaired hydroxylation of 5-methylcytosine in myeloid cancers with mutant TET2. Nature 468:839–843

Kroeger H, Jelinek J, Estécio MR, He R, Kondo K, Chung W, Zhang L, Shen L, Kantarjian HM, Bueso-Ramos CE, Issa JP (2008) Aberrant CpG island methylation in acute myeloid leukemia is accentuated at relapse. Blood 112:1366–1373

Krönke J, Schlenk RF, Jensen KO, Tschürtz F, Corbacioglu A, Gaidzik VI, Paschka P, Onken S, Eiwen K, Habdank M, Späth D, Lübbert M, Wattad M, Kindler T, Salih HR, Held G, Nachbaur D, von Lilienfeld-Toal M, Germing U, Haase D, Mergenthaler HG, Krauter J, Ganser A, Göhring G, Schlegelberger B, Döhner H, Döhner K (2011) Monitoring of minimal residual disease in NPM1-mutated acute myeloid leukemia: a study from the German-Austrian Acute Myeloid Leukemia Study Group. J Clin Oncol 29:2709–2716

Langer C, Marcucci G, Holland KB, Radmacher MD, Maharry K, Paschka P, Whitman SP, Mrózek K, Baldus CD, Vij R, Powell BL, Carroll AJ, Kolitz JE, Caligiuri MA, Larson RA, Bloomfield CD (2009) Prognostic importance of MN1 transcript levels, and biologic insights from MN1-associated gene and microRNA expression signatures in cytogenetically normal acute myeloid leukemia: a Cancer and Leukemia Group B study. J Clin Oncol 27:3198–3204

Levis M, Allebach J, Tse KF, Zheng R, Baldwin BR, Smith BD, Jones-Bolin S, Ruggeri B, Dionne C, Small D (2002) A FLT3-targeted tyrosine kinase inhibitor is cytotoxic to leukemia cells in vitro and in vivo. Blood 99:3885–3891

Ley TJ, Ding L, Walter MJ, McLellan MD, Lamprecht T, Larson DE, Kandoth C, Payton JE, Baty J, Welch J, Harris CC, Lichti CF, Townsend RR, Fulton RS, Dooling DJ, Koboldt DC, Schmidt H, Zhang Q, Osborne JR, Lin L, O'Laughlin M, McMichael JF, Delehaunty KD, McGrath SD, Fulton LA, Magrini VJ, Vickery TL, Hundal J, Cook LL, Conyers JJ, Swift GW, Reed JP, Alldredge PA, Wylie T, Walker J, Kalicki J, Watson MA, Heath S, Shannon WD, Varghese N, Nagarajan R, Westervelt P, Tomasson MH, Link DC, Graubert TA, DiPersio JF, Mardis ER, Wilson RK (2010) DNMT3A mutations in acute myeloid leukemia. N Engl J Med 363:2424–2433

Libura M, Asnafi V, Tu A, Delabesse E, Tigaud I, Cymbalista F, Bennaceur-Griscelli A, Villarese P, Solbu G, Hagemeijer A, Beldjord K, Hermine O, Macintyre E (2003) FLT3 and MLL intragenic abnormalities in AML reflect a common category of genotoxic stress. Blood 102:2198–2204

Licht JD, Sternberg DW (2005) The molecular pathology of acute myeloid leukemia. Hematol Am Soc Hematol Educ Program 2005(1):137–142

Maki K, Yamagata T, Mitani K (2008) Role of the RUNX1-EVI1 fusion gene in leukemogenesis. Cancer Sci 99:1878–1883

Makishima H, Cazzolli H, Szpurka H, Dunbar A, Tiu R, Huh J, Muramatsu H, O'Keefe C, Hsi E, Paquette RL, Kojima S, List AF, Sekeres MA, McDevitt MA, Maciejewski JP (2009) Mutations of e3 ubiquitin ligase cbl family members constitute a novel common pathogenic lesion in myeloid malignancies. J Clin Oncol 27:6109–6116

Marcucci G, Baldus CD, Ruppert AS, Radmacher MD, Mrózek K, Whitman SP, Kolitz JE, Edwards CG, Vardiman JW, Powell BL, Baer MR, Moore JO, Perrotti D, Caligiuri MA,

Carroll AJ, Larson RA, de la Chapelle A, Bloomfield CD (2005) Overexpression of the ETS-related gene, ERG, predicts a worse outcome in acute myeloid leukemia with normal karyotype: a Cancer and Leukemia Group B study. J Clin Oncol 23:9234–9242

Marcucci G, Maharry K, Whitman SP, Vukosavljevic T, Paschka P, Langer C, Mrózek K, Baldus CD, Carroll AJ, Powell BL, Kolitz JE, Larson RA, Bloomfield CD (2007) High expression levels of the ETS-related gene, ERG, predict adverse outcome and improve molecular risk-based classification of cytogenetically normal acute myeloid leukemia: a Cancer and Leukemia Group B study. J Clin Oncol 25:3337–3343

Marcucci G, Maharry K, Wu YZ, Radmacher MD, Mrózek K, Margeson D, Holland KB, Whitman SP, Becker H, Schwind S, Metzeler KH, Powell BL, Carter TH, Kolitz JE, Wetzler M, Carroll AJ, Baer MR, Caligiuri MA, Larson RA, Bloomfield CD (2010) IDH1 and IDH2 gene mutations identify novel molecular subsets within de novo cytogenetically normal acute myeloid leukemia: a Cancer and Leukemia Group B study. J Clin Oncol 28:2348–2355

Marcucci G, Mrózek K, Radmacher MD, Garzon R, Bloomfield CD (2011) The prognostic and functional role of microRNAs in acute myeloid leukemia. Blood 117:1121–1129

Mardis ER, Ding L, Dooling DJ, Larson DE, McLellan MD, Chen K, Koboldt DC, Fulton RS, Delehaunty KD, McGrath SD, Fulton LA, Locke DP, Magrini VJ, Abbott RM, Vickery TL, Reed JS, Robinson JS, Wylie T, Smith SM, Carmichael L, Eldred JM, Harris CC, Walker J, Peck JB, Du F, Dukes AF, Sanderson GE, Brummett AM, Clark E, McMichael JF, Meyer RJ, Schindler JK, Pohl CS, Wallis JW, Shi X, Lin L, Schmidt H, Tang Y, Haipek C, Wiechert ME, Ivy JV, Kalicki J, Elliott G, Ries RE, Payton JE, Westervelt P, Tomasson MH, Watson MA, Baty J, Heath S, Shannon WD, Nagarajan R, Link DC, Walter MJ, Graubert TA, DiPersio JF, Wilson RK, Ley TJ (2009) Recurring mutations found by sequencing an acute myeloid leukemia genome. N Engl J Med 361:1058–1066

Martens JH, Stunnenberg HG (2010) The molecular signature of oncofusion proteins in acute myeloid leukemia. FEBS Lett 584:2662–2669

Meshinchi S, Stirewalt DL, Alonzo TA, Boggon TJ, Gerbing RB, Rocnik JL, Lange BJ, Gilliland DG, Radich JP (2008) Structural and numerical variation of FLT3/ITD in pediatric AML. Blood 111:4930–4933

Metzeler KH, Dufour A, Benthaus T, Hummel M, Sauerland MC, Heinecke A, Berdel WE, Büchner T, Wörmann B, Mansmann U, Braess J, Spiekermann K, Hiddemann W, Buske C, Bohlander SK (2009) ERG expression is an independent prognostic factor and allows refined risk stratification in cytogenetically normal acute myeloid leukemia: a comprehensive analysis of ERG, MN1, and BAALC transcript levels using oligonucleotide microarrays. J Clin Oncol 27:5031–5038

Metzeler KH, Maharry K, Radmacher MD, Mrózek K, Margeson D, Becker H, Curfman J, Holland KB, Schwind S, Whitman SP, Wu YZ, Blum W, Powell BL, Carter TH, Wetzler M, Moore JO, Kolitz JE, Baer MR, Carroll AJ, Larson RA, Caligiuri MA, Marcucci G, Bloomfield CD (2011) TET2 mutations improve the new European LeukemiaNet risk classification of acute myeloid leukemia: a Cancer and Leukemia Group B study. J Clin Oncol 29:1373–1381

Mohamed A (2010) MLL amplification in leukemia. Atlas Genet Cytogenet Oncol Haematol. http://AtlasGeneticsOncology.org/Anomalies/MLLampliID1547.html. Cited 22 Dec 2011

Mohr F, Döhner K, Buske C, Rawat VP (2011) TET genes: new players in DNA demethylation and important determinants for stemness. Exp Hematol 39:272–281

Mrózek K, Marcucci G, Paschka P, Whitman SP, Bloomfield CD (2007) Clinical relevance of mutations and gene expression changes in adult acute myeloid leukemia with normal cytogenetics: are we ready for a prognostically prioritized molecular classification? Blood 109:431–448

Nibourel O, Kosmider O, Cheok M, Boissel N, Renneville A, Philippe N, Dombret H, Dreyfus F, Quesnel B, Geffroy S, Quentin S, Roche-Lestienne C, Cayuela JM, Roumier C, Fenaux P, Vainchenker W, Bernard OA, Soulier J, Fontenay M, Preudhomme C (2010) Incidence and prognostic value of TET2 alterations in de novo acute myeloid leukemia achieving complete remission. Blood 116:1132–1135

O'Farrell A-M, Abrams TJ, Yuen HA, Ngai TJ, Louie SG, Yee KW, Wong LM, Hong W, Lee LB, Town A, Smolich BD, Manning WC, Murray LJ, Heinrich MC, Cherrington JM (2003) SU11248 is a novel FLT3 tyrosine kinase inhibitor with potent activity in vitro and in vivo. Blood 101:3597–3605

Parkin B, Erba H, Ouillette P, Roulston D, Purkayastha A, Karp J, Talpaz M, Kujawski L, Shakhan S, Li C, Shedden K, Malek SN (2010) Acquired genomic copy number aberrations and survival in adult acute myelogenous leukemia. Blood 116:4958–4967

Paschka P, Schlenk RF, Gaidzik VI, Habdank M, Krönke J, Bullinger L, Späth D, Kayser S, Zucknick M, Götze K, Horst HA, Germing U, Döhner H, Döhner K (2010) IDH1 and IDH2 mutations are frequent genetic alterations in acute myeloid leukemia and confer adverse prognosis in cytogenetically normal acute myeloid leukemia with NPM1 mutation without FLT3 internal tandem duplication. J Clin Oncol 28:3636–3643

Röllig C, Bornhäuser M, Thiede C, Taube F, Kramer M, Mohr B, Aulitzky W, Bodenstein H, Tischler HJ, Stuhlmann R, Schuler U, Stölzel F, von Bonin M, Wandt H, Schäfer-Eckart K, Schaich M, Ehninger G (2011) Long-term prognosis of acute myeloid leukemia according to the new genetic risk classification of the European LeukemiaNet recommendations: evaluation of the proposed reporting system. J Clin Oncol 29:2758–2765

Sanz MA, Grimwade D, Tallman MS, Lowenberg B, Fenaux P, Estey EH, Naoe T, Lengfelder E, Büchner T, Döhner H, Burnett AK, Lo-Coco F (2009) Management of acute promyelocytic leukemia: recommendations from an expert panel on behalf of the European LeukemiaNet. Blood 113:1875–1891

Schotte D, De Menezes RX, Akbari Moqadam F, Mohammadi Khankahdani L, Lange-Turenhout E, Chen C, Pieters R, Den Boer ML (2011) MicroRNAs characterize genetic diversity and drug resistance in pediatric acute lymphoblastic leukemia. Haematologica 96:703–711

Schwind S, Maharry K, Radmacher MD, Mrózek K, Holland KB, Margeson D, Whitman SP, Hickey C, Becker H, Metzeler KH, Paschka P, Baldus CD, Liu S, Garzon R, Powell BL, Kolitz JE, Carroll AJ, Caligiuri MA, Larson RA, Marcucci G, Bloomfield CD (2010a) Prognostic significance of expression of a single microRNA, miR-181a, in cytogenetically normal acute myeloid leukemia: a Cancer and Leukemia Group B study. J Clin Oncol 28:5257–5264

Schwind S, Marcucci G, Maharry K, Radmacher MD, Mrózek K, Holland KB, Margeson D, Becker H, Whitman SP, Wu YZ, Metzeler KH, Powell BL, Kolitz JE, Carter TH, Moore JO, Baer MR, Carroll AJ, Caligiuri MA, Larson RA, Bloomfield CD (2010b) BAALC and ERG expression levels are associated with outcome and distinct gene and microRNA expression profiles in older patients with de novo cytogenetically normal acute myeloid leukemia: a Cancer and Leukemia Group B study. Blood 116:5660–5669

Seca H, Almeida GM, Guimarães JE, Vasconcelos MH (2010) miR signatures and the role of miRs in acute myeloid leukaemia. Eur J Cancer 46:1520–1527

Slovak ML, Kopecky KJ, Cassileth PA, Harrington DH, Theil KS, Mohamed A, Paietta E, Willman CL, Head DR, Rowe JM, Forman SJ, Appelbaum FR (2000) Karyotypic analysis predicts outcome of preremission and postremission therapy in adult acute myeloid leukemia: a Southwest Oncology Group/Eastern Cooperative Oncology Group Study. Blood 96:4075–4083

Smith ML, Hills RK, Grimwade D (2011) Independent prognostic variables in acute myeloid leukaemia. Blood Rev 25:39–51

Taskesen E, Bullinger L, Corbacioglu A, Sanders M, Erpelinck CA, Wouters BJ, van der Poel-van de Luytgaarde SC, Damm F, Krauter J, Ganser A, Schlenk RF, Löwenberg B, Delwel R, Dohner H, Valk PJ, Dohner K (2011) Prognostic impact, concurrent genetic mutations and gene expression features of AML with CEBPA mutations in a cohort of 1182 cytogenetically normal AML: further evidence for CEBPA double mutant AML as a distinctive disease entity. Blood 117:2469–2475

Thiede C, Koch S, Creutzig E, Steudel C, Illmer T, Schaich M, Ehninger G (2006) Prevalence and prognostic impact of NPM1 mutations in 1485 adult patients with acute myeloid leukemia (AML). Blood 107:4011–4020

Tiu RV, Gondek LP, O'Keefe CL, Elson P, Huh J, Mohamedali A, Kulasekararaj A, Advani AS, Paquette R, List AF, Sekeres MA, McDevitt MA, Mufti GJ, Maciejewski JP (2011) Prognostic impact of SNP array karyotyping in myelodysplastic syndromes and related myeloid malignancies. Blood 117:4552–4560

Vardiman JW, Brunning RD, Arber DA (2008) Introduction and overview of the classification of the myeloid neoplasms. In: Swerdlow SH, Campo E, Harris NL et al (eds) WHO classification of tumours of haematopoietic and lymphoid tissues. IARC Press, Lyon, pp 18–30

Vardiman JW, Thiele J, Arber DA, Brunning RD, Borowitz MJ, Porwit A, Harris NL, Le Beau MM, Hellström-Lindberg E, Tefferi A, Bloomfield CD (2009) The 2008 revision of the World Health Organization (WHO) classification of myeloid neoplasms and acute leukemia: rationale and important changes. Blood 114:937–951

Walker A, Marcucci G (2011) Impact of molecular prognostic factors in cytogenetically normal acute myeloid leukemia at diagnosis and relapse. Haematologica 96:640–643

Weisberg E, Boulton C, Kelly LM, Manley P, Fabbro D, Meyer T, Gilliland DG, Griffin JD (2002) Inhibition of mutant FLT3 receptors in leukemia cells by the small molecule tyrosine kinase inhibitor PKC412. Cancer Cell 1:433–443

Whitman SP, Maharry K, Radmacher MD, Becker H, Mrózek K, Margeson D, Holland KB, Wu YZ, Schwind S, Metzeler KH, Wen J, Baer MR, Powell BL, Carter TH, Kolitz JE, Wetzler M, Moore JO, Stone RM, Carroll AJ, Larson RA, Caligiuri MA, Marcucci G, Bloomfield CD (2010) FLT3 internal tandem duplication associates with adverse outcome and gene- and microRNA-expression signatures in patients 60 years of age or older with primary cytogenetically normal acute myeloid leukemia: a Cancer and Leukemia Group B study. Blood 116:3622–3626

Whitman SP, Ruppert AS, Marcucci G, Mrózek K, Paschka P, Langer C, Baldus CD, Wen J, Vukosavljevic T, Powell BL, Carroll AJ, Kolitz JE, Larson RA, Caligiuri MA, Bloomfield CD (2007) Long-term disease-free survivors with cytogenetically normal acute myeloid leukemia and MLL partial tandem duplication: a Cancer and Leukemia Group B study. Blood 109:5164–5167

Yan XJ, Xu J, Gu ZH, Pan CM, Lu G, Shen Y, Shi JY, Zhu YM, Tang L, Zhang XW, Liang WX, Mi JQ, Song HD, Li KQ, Chen Z, Chen SJ (2011) Exome sequencing identifies somatic mutations of DNA methyltransferase gene DNMT3A in acute monocytic leukemia. Nat Genet 43:309–315

Zarrinkar PP, Gunawardane RN, Cramer MD, Gardner MF, Brigham D, Belli B, Karaman MW, Pratz KW, Pallares G, Chao Q, Sprankle KG, Patel HK, Levis M, Armstrong RC, James J, Bhagwat SS (2009) AC220 is a uniquely potent and selective inhibitor of FLT3 for the treatment of acute myeloid leukemia (AML). Blood 114:2984–2992

Zuo Z, Chandra P, Wen YH, Koeppen H (2009) Molecular diagnostics of acute myeloid leukaemia. Diagn Histopathol 15:531–539

Chapter 3
Molecular Pathogenesis of Aggressive B-cell Lymphomas

Przemysław Juszczyński and Krzysztof Warzocha

Abstract B-cell lymphomas are tumors arising from B-lymphoid cells at different stages of their development. In this chapter, we discuss the molecular pathogenesis of these tumors, specifically highlighting processes generating functional immunoglobulin genes that are associated with increased risk of genetic errors leading to lymphomagenesis. We review and summarize the enormous progress in understanding the pathologic, molecular, and clinical heterogeneity of these tumors that has been made during the past decades with the aid of high-throughput, platform-based gene expression, and associated functional studies. Finally, we discuss the translational consequences of these studies and review the emerging therapeutic strategies in aggressive lymphomas.

3.1 Introduction

Lymphomas are tumors arising from lymphoid B or T cells; approximately 90 % of lymphomas are of B cell origin. There are 20 new lymphoma cases diagnosed per 100,000 people every year in the Western World, but the frequency of this disease has been increasing over the last 20 years. Lymphomas are a highly heterogeneous group of disorders, comprising multiple pathologic subtypes distinguished in the current World Health Organization (WHO) classification of tumors

P. Juszczyński (✉) · K. Warzocha
Institute of Hematology and Transfusion Medicine,
Indiry Gandhi 14, 02-776 Warsaw, Poland
e-mail: pjuszczynski@ihit.waw.pl

K. Warzocha
e-mail: warzocha@ihit.waw.pl

M. Witt et al. (eds.), *Molecular Aspects of Hematologic Malignancies*,
Principles and Practice, DOI: 10.1007/978-3-642-29467-9_3,

of hematopoietic and lymphoid tissues (Swerdlow et al. 2008). Classification of B-cell malignancies reflects the enormous progress in understanding the pathologic, molecular, and clinical heterogeneity of these tumors that has been made during the past decades. For most B-cell lymphomas, they appear to recapitulate normal stages of B cell differentiation and arise as a consequence of errors in unique biological processes generating functional immunoglobulin genes. Numerous genetic lesions and signaling pathways have been identified as drivers or at least propellers of oncogenic transformation. In addition, it is becoming increasingly clear that B-cell tumors are not solely dependent on these abnormalities, but also rely on other factors supporting malignant growth of most B-cell lymphomas, including microenvironmental cues, infectious agents, and antigenic stimulation—key factors that are crucial also for normal B cell differentiation and survival. For these reasons, identification and characterization of lesions and processes leading to malignant phenotype might provide a platform in the development of modern targeted therapies, hitting the "Achilles' heel" of the tumor. In this chapter, we review the cellular origin and molecular pathogenesis of lymphoid malignancies, focusing specifically on diffuse large B-cell lymphoma (DLBCL). Finally, we discuss key translational consequences of these studies.

3.2 Cellular Origin of B-cell Lymphomas

Understanding normal B-lineage lymphocyte development and specific DNA editing processes leading to generation of functional immunoglobulin (Ig) genes is critical for understanding the molecular pathogenesis and structure of chromosomal translocations involving Ig genes in specific lymphoma categories. Development of B cell begins in the bone marrow and occurs in distinct differentiation steps leading to maturation and specific structure of the B-cell receptor (BCR) (Fig. 3.1a). The process of Ig genes rearrangements is initiated at the stage of early lymphoid progenitors with the assembly of variable regions of Ig heavy (IgH) and light (IgL) chains genes in a process called variable-diversity-joining (*VDJ*) gene recombination (Fig. 3.1b) (Busslinger 2004; Schatz and Ji 2011). This process is mediated by products of recombination activating gene 1 (RAG1) and RAG2. DNA breaks introduced by these enzymes are ligated by an error-prone non-homologous end joining (NHEJ) mechanism, facilitating translocations (Fugmann et al. 2000; Schatz and Ji 2011). During *VDJ* recombination, terminal deoxynucleotidyl transferase (TdT) mediates templateless insertions of nucleotides at junction sites between the rearranged genes (Schatz and Ji 2011). Cells with productive rearrangements of IgH and IgL chains, presenting IgM/IgD (immunoglobulin class M/D) on the surface, leave the bone marrow microenvironment, and populate the peripheral lymphoid organs. Upon na B cell contact with an antigen, the lymphocyte undergoes rapid proliferation and forms germinal center (GC). GCs are specialized structures where editing of Ig genes continues and is mediated by two distinct mechanisms: class-switch recombination (CSR) and

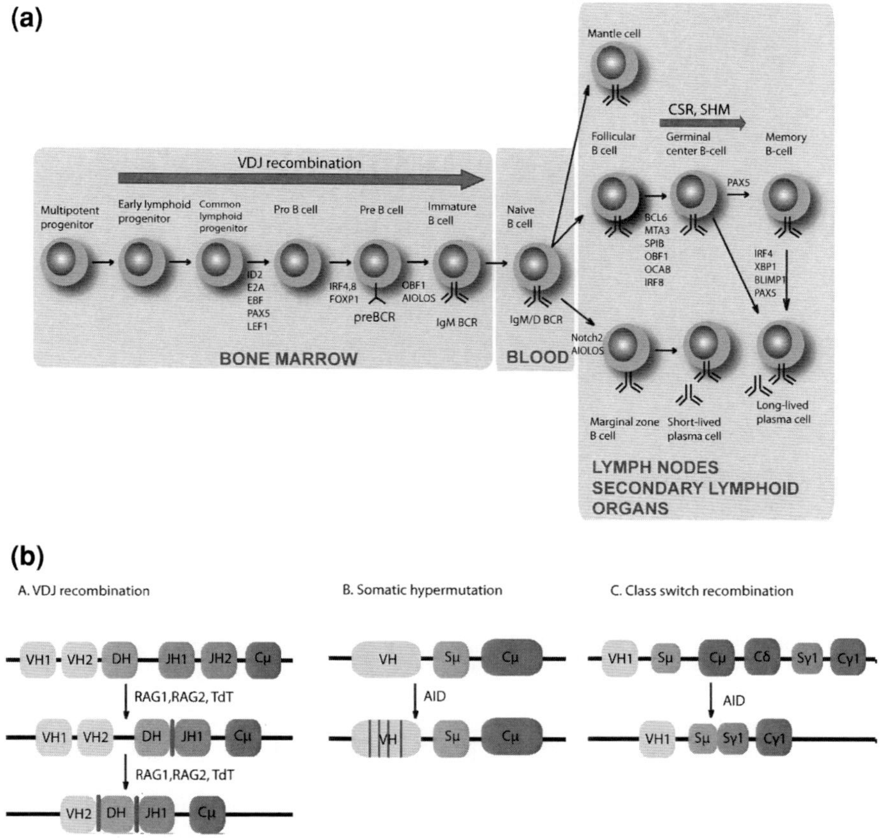

Fig. 3.1 Development of normal B cells. Development of B cells is initiated in the bone marrow, where editing of immunoglobulin heavy (*IGH*) and light (*IGL*) genes begins (*VDJ* recombination, **a** and **b**). This stage of B cell development is antigen-independent and requires RAG1 and RAG2 recombinases. During *VDJ* recombination, TdT incorporates nucleotides that are not encoded in the germline DNA (**b**, *left panel*, *vertical bars*). Immature B cells leave the bone marrow and upon contact with antigen, form germinal centers of secondary lymphoid organs, where editing of Ig genes continues in the process of Ig class-switch recombination (CSR), and somatic hypermutation (SHM) (**a** and **b**, medium, and *right panels*). These mechanisms require the activation-induced cytidine deaminase (AID). Cells expressing favorable antibody variants are positively selected, expanded and released into the periphery as plasma cells, or memory B cells. Critical transcription factors regulating B cell ontogenesis are indicated in **a** (Martinez-Climent et al. 2010)

somatic hypermutation (SHM) (Klein and Dalla-Favera 2008). During CSR, B-cells change the isotype of the expressed BCR, while SHM introduces nucleotide changes resulting in the generation of antibody variants. Both CSR and SHM require activity of the activation-induced cytidine deaminase (AID) (Muramatsu et al. 2000). During the GC reaction, cells with non-productive Ig edits, leading to loss of BCR expression or reduced affinity of the receptor are eliminated by

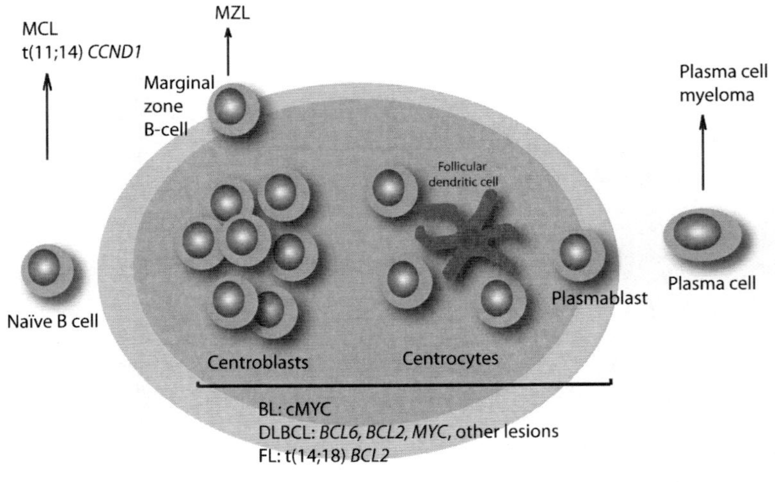

Fig. 3.2 Germinal center and lymphomagenesis. Majority of B-cell lymphomas derive from germinal- or postgerminal B cells and harbor chromosomal translocations or mutations that deregulate expression of certain oncogenes. Due to different stages of B cell differentiation, they acquire distinct oncogenic abnormalities and are reliant on different survival pathways (see text for details). *MZL* marginal zone lymphoma, *MCL* mantle cell lymphoma, *BL* Burkitt lymphoma, *CCND1* cyclin D1, *DLBCL* diffuse large B-cell lymphoma, *FL* follicular lymphoma, *BCL2* B-cell CLL/lymphoma 2, *BCL6* B-cell CLL/lymphoma 6, *MYC* myelocytomatosis viral oncogene homolog

apoptosis. In contrast, cells with increased antigen affinity are positively selected, expanded, and released into the periphery as antibody secreting plasma cells or long-lived memory B-cells (Klein and Dalla-Favera 2008; Rajewsky 1996).

Physiology of the GC reaction, combining rapid proliferation of antigen-exposed cells with extensive DNA editing processes results in development of a cell with highly specialized biology, but is inevitably associated with increased risk of editing errors. In fact, majority of B-cell lymphomas derive from germinal- or postgerminal B cells and harbor chromosomal translocations or mutations that deregulate expression of certain oncogenes (Fig. 3.2) (Abramson and Shipp 2005; Klein et al. 1998; Kramer et al. 1998; Pasqualucci et al. 2008). The absence of analogous stage in the development of T cells might explain much lower frequency of T-cell lymphomas. A subset of tumors also exhibits aberrant SHM of genes that are not targeted by this editing process in normal GC B cells (Pasqualucci et al. 2001).

3.3 Transforming Events in B-cell Lymphomas

Chromosomal translocations are the most common structural abnormalities in B-cell lymphomas. Many of the resulting aberrations are sufficient to drive lymphomagenesis in murine models, highlighting their dominant role, whereas others require additional lesions. In line with their pathogenetic role, specific recurrent translocations are an integral part of the lymphoma entity definitions, such as follicular lymphoma (FL), marginal zone B-cell lymphoma (MZL), mucosa-associated lymphoid tissue (MALT)-type, and mantle cell lymphoma (MCL).

Consistent with the active editing of Ig genes, reciprocal chromosomal translocations in lymphomas in most cases involve one of the Ig loci and a proto-oncogene. As a consequence of such translocations, the oncogene is brought under the control of the Ig enhancer and is constitutively expressed. This mechanism is clearly different in lymphomas than in leukemias, where reciprocal translocations usually lead to a formation of a fusion gene and a resulting fusion protein, combining fragments of two proteins, which exhibit constitutive kinase, or transcriptional modulator activity.

Detailed analysis of the structure of Ig-oncogene breakpoints can indicate the stage of B-cell development, at which the lesion has occurred. Some translocations, such as the *BCL2-IGH* translocation (*BCL2*; B-cell CLL/lymphoma 2), associated with FL or DLBCL, have breakpoints in the proximity of *IGHJ* genes (immunoglobulin heavy joining group) or adjacent to *IGHD/IGHJ* junctions. These breakpoints are often characterized by nucleotide deletions and insertions at the junction sites, a typical feature of *VDJ* recombination. In case of other translocations, breakpoints are located in the IgH switch regions, in which DNA breaks are introduced during class switching. The third group of translocations involves breakpoints within or close to rearranged *VDJ* genes. *IGHV* in such cases are always somatically mutated, suggesting that such translocations occur as a consequence of double-strand breaks introduced by SHM process (Kuppers and Dalla-Favera 2001; Goossens et al. 1998; Bross et al. 2000; Papavasiliou and Schatz 2000). Consistent with the role of AID in mediating CSR and SHM, this enzyme is required for GC-derived lymphomagenesis and *AID* deficiency in mice prevents *BCL6* (B-cell CLL/lymphoma 6)-dependent, GC-derived lymphomas (Pasqualucci et al. 2008). AID is also required for spontaneous *MYC* (myelocytomatosis viral oncogene homolog)-*IGH* translocations into switch regions during CSR (Ramiro et al. 2004). Furthermore, a subset of DLBCLs characterized by the activated B cell-like DLBCL transcriptional profile (see below) is characterized by high AID expression and high frequency of switch translocations (Lenz et al. 2007).

The process of SHM can be also involved in pathogenesis of lymphomas by mutating non-Ig genes. Such a process, called aberrant SHM, targets multiple loci, including *PIM1* (proviral integration site-1), *MYC, RhoH/TTF* (Ras homolog gene family, member H), *FAS* (TNF superfamily member 6), and *PAX5* (paired box gene 5) in more than 50 % of DLBCL (Pasqualucci et al. 2001; Muschen et al. 2002). Aberrant SHMs are also present in other GC or postGC derived lymphomas, including acquired immunodeficiency syndrome (AIDS)-related lymphomas, FL, primary mediastinal large B-cell lymphomas, and MZL (Gaidano et al. 2003; Mottok et al. 2009; Deutsch et al. 2009; Gagyi et al. 2008). Finally, in addition to translocations and SHM of oncogenes, lymphomas exhibit frequent somatic mutations and copy number alterations in transcriptional modulator genes, genes coding for proteins involved in critical signal transduction pathways, and tumor suppressors (Lenz et al. 2008c; Pasqualucci et al. 2006; Morin et al. 2010; Yap et al. 2011; Pasqualucci et al. 2011; Green et al. 2010; Lenz and Staudt 2010; Nogai et al. 2011). These structural abnormalities are usually associated with specific lymphoma subtypes.

3.4 Molecular Heterogeneity of DLBCL

DLBCLs, the most common type of lymphoma in adults, constitute clinically, pathologically, and genetically heterogeneous group of tumors. The pathogenetic heterogeneity of this disease is reflected by the clinical variability in the disease course. Although approximately 50–55 % of DLBCL patients can be cured with modern therapy, the remaining patients succumb to their disease (Abramson and Shipp 2005). Clinical prognostic models, such as the International Prognostic Index (IPI), can be used to robustly identify patients who are less likely to be cured with standard chemotherapy (Shipp 1993). Although such models were proven extremely useful clinically, they provide solely descriptive risk assessment and do not provide specific insights into tumor cell biology, which could facilitate the use of alternative, more effective treatment strategies, or guide the identification of novel therapeutic targets. Enormous progress in understanding of molecular heterogeneity of these tumors has been achieved with the platform based gene expression technologies. Following sections will highlight the results of these studies and present their translational consequences.

3.4.1 Similarities of DLBCL Cells to Putative Cell of Origin (COO Classification)

In the early studies utilizing cDNA microarrays to analyze heterogeneity of DLBCL, these tumors were classified according to their similarities to either GC B cells (GCB-type DLBCL) or in vitro activated B cells (ABC-type DLBCL) (Alizadeh et al. 2000; Rosenwald et al. 2002; Wright et al. 2003). The gene expression profiles of these subtypes suggest that they arise from B cells at various stages of differentiation. GCB-type DLBCLs express many genes specific for GC B lymphocytes and are thought to derive from GC B cells. In contrast, ABC DLBCLs seem to be derived from B cells that are in the process of differentiating into plasma cells (Rosenwald et al. 2002), but due to certain genetic lesions, are unable to fully differentiate (Pasqualucci et al. 2006; Tam et al. 2006). Consistent with distinct ontogenetic level of transformed lymphocyte, GCB, and ABC DLBCLs are associated with different pathogenetic and oncogenic mechanisms. GCB-type tumors are characterized by higher expression of *BCL6* and exhibit ongoing SHM of Ig gene rearrangements. A frequent genetic abnormality, present in about 45 % of GCB DLBCLs is the t(14;18) translocation juxtaposing the *BCL2* gene and the *IGH* locus and deregulating the antiapoptotic BCL2 protein (Rosenwald et al. 2002). GCB DLBCL exhibit more frequent genetic aberrations that might deregulate PTEN/PI3K/AKT (phosphatase and tensin homolog/phosphoinositide-3-kinase/v-akt murine thymoma viral oncogene homolog) pathway and more frequent amplifications of 12q, including *MDM2* (mdm2 p53 binding homolog) locus (Lenz et al. 2008c). Amplification of MDM2, a p53 E3 ubiquitin ligase, functionally inactivates p53 (Lenz et al. 2008c). GCB tumors also exhibit recurrent somatic mutations affecting the polycomb-group oncogene *EZH2* (enhancer of zeste homolog 2 [Drosophila]), which encodes a histone methyltransferase responsible for trimethylating lysine 27 of histone H3 (H3K27), occuring in over 20 % of these DLBCLs and are absent in DLBCLs of ABC type (Morin et al. 2010). Mutations in *CREBBP* (CREB binding protein) and *EP300* (E1A binding protein p300) acetyltransferases are also more frequent in GCB-DLBCLs than in ABC-type tumors (Pasqualucci et al. 2011). These two highly related histone and nonhistone acetyltransferases act as transcriptional co-activators in multiple signaling pathways. Mutations in these genes are usually hemizygotic and mutually exclusive with deletions, suggesting haploinsufficient mechanism of action. These lesions are thought to induce specific defects in acetylation-mediated inactivation of BCL6 and activation of the p53 tumor suppressor (Pasqualucci et al. 2011). However, given the physiological role of *CREBBP* and *EP300* in modulating activity of multiple transcription factors, these lesions are likely to play much broader role in lymphomagenesis.

The most characteristic feature of DLBCLs exhibiting ABC phenotype is constitutive activity of NFκB (nuclear factor of κ light polypeptide gene enhancer in B cells) (Davis et al. 2001; Compagno et al. 2009). Nuclear localization and constitutive activity of NFκB is present in over 60 % of ABC-DLBCLs (Compagno et al. 2009). In normal B cells, activation of this transcription factor is regulated by engagement of surface receptors such as BCR and CD40 (Jost and Ruland 2007). CD40 engagement and activation of NFκB induces expression of IRF4 (interferon regulatory factor 4) and downregulates BCL6, which terminate GC reaction, and promote plasma cell differentiation. ABC-type DLBCLs exhibit constitutive activity of NFκB and expression of IRF4 and also have lower expression of BCL6, indicating that they derive from a postgerminal lymphocyte. However, full plasma cell differentiation seems to be blocked due to structural or functional inactivation of BLIMP-1, which is encoded by *PRDM1* (PR domain containing-1), a transcriptional repressor that is required for plasmacytic differentiation (Pasqualucci et al. 2006; Klein and Dalla-Favera 2008). Inactivating mutations and deletions of *PRDM1* have been detected in approximately one quarter of ABC DLBCLs and additional quarter of DLBCLs have amplifications of *SPIB* (Spi-B transcription factor, Spi-1/PU.1 related), a transcriptional modulator that represses BLIMP-1 expression and blocks differentiation (Pasqualucci et al. 2006; Lenz et al. 2008c; Schmidlin et al. 2008). Activity of NFκB in ABC-DLBCLs can be induced by multiple mechanisms. A major reason of uncontrolled activation of the pathway are somatic mutations in multiple genes regulating activity of NFκB, including *A20* (*TNFAIP3,* tumor necrosis factor alpha induced protein 3*), RANK* (*TNFRSF11A*, tumor necrosis factor receptor superfamily, member 11a)*, TRAF2* (TNF receptor-associated factor 2)*, TRAF5* (TNF receptor-associated factor 5)*, MAP3K7* (mitogen-activated protein kinase 7), and *CARD11* (caspase recruitment domain family, member 11) (Compagno et al. 2009). These mutations are present in over 50 % of ABC-type tumors. CARD11 is a component of CBM complex (CARD11-BCL10-MALT1), indispensable for NFκB activation by BCR (Bidere et al. 2009; Lenz et al. 2008a; Ngo et al. 2006). Activating mutations in *CARD11* coiled-coil domain are present in approximately 10 % of ABC DLBCL samples (Lenz et al. 2008a; Ngo et al. 2006) and RNA-interference mediated silencing of either CARD11, MALT1, or BCL10 was toxic to ABC, but not to GCB DLBCL cell lines. Alternative mechanism inducing NFκB activity in ABC-DLBCLs is BCR signaling that activates the CBM complex. As a consequence, ABC-DLBCLs with constitutive activity of NFκB exhibit higher expression of NFκB-regulated genes (Feuerhake et al. 2005).

Different cell of origin and distinct biological characteristics of GCB- and ABC-type DLBCLs largely determine their clinical behavior. Tumors with GCB-like gene expression profile have better prognosis than ABC-type tumors. These differences are present both in patients treated with standard combination chemotherapy (CHOP—cyclophosphamide, doxorubicin, vincristine, prednisone) and CHOP-like regimens combined with anti-CD20 antibody (rituximab) (Alizadeh et al. 2000; Fu et al. 2008; Choi et al. 2009; Rosenwald et al. 2002).

It should be noted, however, that the COO classification of DLBCLs assigns tumors to two categories, GCB- and ABC- types, leaving a fraction of tumors unassigned. This is of particular importance because this unspecified group includes 17–40 % of tumors (Rosenwald et al. 2002; Wright et al. 2003; Monti et al. 2005). These observations suggest additional complexity of DLBCLs beyond the GCB and ABC distinction. Additional substructure can be also inferred from the gene expression studies highlighting the prognostic signatures of DLBCLs that are largely independent of cell of origin category and stratify patients also within GCB and ABC classes (Lenz et al. 2008b; Rosenwald et al. 2002). These prognostic signatures reflect cellular proliferation, GC reaction process, and interactions with microenvironment (MHC II, lymph node, and stromal signatures). Except for proliferation and GC signatures, associated with ABC- and GCB-DLBCLs; respectively, the microenvironment-related signatures are independent of COO subclasses, but remain associated with prognosis (Lenz et al. 2008b; Rosenwald et al. 2002). As the COO classification is based on the similarities of tumor cells to isolated B lymphocytes, the role of microenvironment is by definition excluded. Taken together, these observations suggest additional complexity of DLBCLs.

3.4.2 Classification of DLBCLs Without a Priori Assumptions (Comprehensive Clusters Classification, CCC)

To unveil this molecular substructure in an unbiased way, a genome-wide genetic profiling, and multiple clustering methods (hierarchical clustering, probabilistic clustering, and self-organizing maps) have been applied to 176 newly identified DLBCL patients (Monti et al. 2005). Using an approach that assessed an agreement among these three clustering algorithms and selected the most stable numbers of clusters with each algorithm, three biologically robust clusters were defined that were independent of prior COO distinction (Monti et al. 2005; Rosenwald et al. 2002; Wright et al. 2003). Within each cluster, overexpressed genes and pathways were identified and analyzed to indicate the most likely biological background of the subset and provide clues to lymphomagenesis. The first cluster, termed "Host Response" (HR) was largely determined by the host inflammatory response and microenvironment, rather than tumor cells themselves. In HR tumors, overexpressed genes included those involved in T-cell receptor signaling, T-cell, natural killer (NK) cell and monocyte/macrophage activation, complement pathway proteins, inflammatory cytokines, and cytokine receptors such as interferon gamma (IFN-γ), tumor necrosis factor (TNF)-related proteins, and adhesion molecules (Monti et al. 2005). Consistent with this signature, primary HR DLBCLs contain significantly higher numbers of morphologically distinct tumor-infiltrating CD2+/CD3+ lymphocytes and S100+/GILT+ (gamma-interferon-inducible lysosomal thiol reductase) CD1a-CD123- interdigitating dendritic cells (Monti et al. 2005). In addition to the prominent, brisk inflammatory infiltrate, these tumors exhibit less frequent recurrent genetic abnormalities, which may suggest alternative, possibly antigen-driven, pathogenetic mechanisms in this group (Monti et al. 2005; Takahashi et al. 2006). Consistent with an inflammatory environment, lymphoma cells in HR tumors frequently exhibit constitutive activity and nuclear localization of NFκB transcription factor (Monti et al. 2005; Feuerhake et al. 2005). The T-cell and dendritic-cell infiltrates in HR tumors resemble those of a histologically defined WHO subtype of DLBCL, namely T-cell/histiocyte-rich B-cell lymphoma (T/HRBCL). In spite of the brisk inflammatory infiltrates in HR (and T/HRBCL) tumors, patients with these DLBCLs do not have a more favorable outcome (Monti et al. 2005).

The second cluster, termed "Oxidative Phosphorylation" (OxPhos), showed increased expression of genes involved in mitochondrial function and electron transport, suggesting important role of these mitochondrial processes in their pathogenesis (Monti et al. 2005). OxPhos lymphomas had more frequent abnormalities in expression or structure of genes involved in execution of exogenous and endogenous apoptotic pathways, such as more frequent t(14;18), and higher expression of mitochondrial antiapoptotic members of *BCL2* family, including *BCL2A1* (BCL2-related protein A1, *BFL-1/A1),* and more frequent deletions of *FAS* death domain (Monti et al. 2005; Takahashi et al. 2006).

The third cluster, accounting for more than 50 % of DLBCLs, was characterized primarily by increased expression of components of the BCR signaling cascade, including SYK (spleen tyrosine kinase) and BLNK (B-cell linker) and certain B-cell-specific transcription factors, such as BCL6. Of note, these tumors had also more frequent standalone *BCL6* translocations, suggesting that these tumors likely rely on the BCR signaling cascade and BCL6 transcriptional program (Monti et al. 2005). Cell lines exhibiting transcriptional signature of BCR tumors and primary isolated viable tumor cells obtained from a subset of DLBCL patients exhibit constitutive, antigen-independent ("tonic") activity of the SYK kinase and phosphorylation of its direct target, adapter protein BLNK. Ablation of SYK activity, either by small-molecule, ATP-competitive inhibitor of SYK or by overexpression of a SYK phosphatase PTPROt (protein tyrosine phosphatase, receptor type, O, truncated) was toxic to BCR-type lymphoma cells, suggesting that these tumors are reliant on tonic, antigen-independent BCR signaling for their survival. Consistent with more frequent standalone translocations of *BCL6*, genes regulated by this oncogene were clearly differentially regulated in BCR tumors (Polo et al. 2007). Since BCL6 modulates the strength and duration of BCR signaling by repressing the SYK phosphatase, these observations suggest that BCL6 transcriptional program is at least in part responsible for the biological characteristic of this group (Polo et al. 2007).

3.5 Translating Basic Science to New Molecularly Targeted Therapies

Recognition of the molecular structure and pathogenetic mechanisms of aggressive B-cell lymphomas and discovery of critical survival pathways associated with tumor growth provided new insights refining molecular taxonomy of these malignancies and identified new rational therapeutic targets. Ideally, a good "candidate" mechanism for therapeutic targeting should be specific and exhibit an important role in the pathogenesis of the tumor. Inhibition/modulation of such mechanism should have well characterized, clear-cut consequences that explain therapeutic effect. Finally, it should be targetable with selective compounds.

Emerging therapeutic targets in lymphomas, at least partially meeting these requirements, include BCR signaling and BCR signaling-associated signal transduction pathways, certain transcription factors such as NFκB and BCL6, and deregulated apoptotic mechanisms.

BCR signaling can be exploited therapeutically by targeting critical downstream pathway components, including SYK, BTK (Bruton tyrosine kinase), PKCβ1 (protein kinase C beta 1)-dependent activation of NFκB, PI3K/AKT/mTOR pathway, and MAPK (mitogen activated protein kinase) cascade. As SYK represents proximal component of the BCR complex involved in transmission and amplification of the signal, it is also an attractive therapeutic target (Dal Porto et al. 2004; Monroe 2006). In vitro inhibition of this kinase with a specific, ATP-competitive small molecule inhibitor (R406, fostamatinib), eliminated tonic and antigen-induced receptor activity and led to apoptosis of BCR-dependent lymphoma cell lines (Chen et al. 2008). Fostamatinib exhibited also a promising clinical activity in a phase I/II trial of relapsed/refractory DLBCL patients (Friedberg et al. 2010). BTK is another candidate for therapeutic intervention blocking BCR activity (Honigberg et al. 2010). Inhibition of this kinase kills ABC cells with chronic active B cell-receptor signaling, but not the cells with *CARD11* coiled-coil mutations and constitutive NFκB signaling (Davis et al. 2010).

As BCR signal is transmitted downstream to NFκB via PKCβ1, inhibition of this kinase represents complementary therapeutic strategy. Overexpression of PKCβ1 in tumor cells is clinically associated with higher aggressiveness of the tumor, further highlighting its pathogenetic role (Shipp et al. 2002). Selective PKCβ1 inhibitor, enzastaurin has been tested initially in a phase I/II trial in relapsed/refractory DLBCL patients and used in monotherapy exhibited modest clinical activity (Robertson et al. 2007). Enzastaurin maintenance therapy is currently tested in DLBCL patients that completed standard CHOP-rituximab immunochemotherapy.

Activation of NFκB is an important mechanism mediating growth and apoptosis resistance in DLBCLs. Clinically available, indirect strategy inhibiting NFκB is proteasome inhibition with small-molecule inhibitors of this protease complex, such as bortezomib. Proteasome inhibition leads to unspecific accumulation of IκBα/ε (inhibitor of NFκB alpha/epsilon) and cytosolic sequestration of NFκB (Adams 2004). In pilot phase II trial, bortezomib combined with chemotherapy was tested in patients with relapsed/refractory DLBCLs and induced higher response rate in patients with the ABC subtype than in those with the GCB tumors (85 vs. 13 %) (Dunleavy et al. 2009). Given the antiapoptotic role of NFκB, such combination might have additive or synergistic effect in therapy of this highly selected and defined group of patients (Dunleavy et al. 2009). More recently, MALT1 (mucosa associated lymphoid tissue lymphoma translocation gene 1), a paracaspase required for NFκB signaling and survival of ABC lymphoma cells has emerged as a therapeutic target in this pathway (Bidere et al. 2009; Ferch et al. 2009; Ruefli-Brasse et al. 2003).

Deregulation of BCL2 family components and associated resistance to apoptotic signals is another attractive therapeutic target. Preclinical data from lymphoma cell lines and primary tumors indicate that inhibition of BCL2 with small molecule inhibitor ABT-737 exhibits high efficacy against these tumors (Deng et al. 2007).

BCL6, the most frequently deregulated gene in DLBCL is another attractive therapeutic target (Polo et al. 2007; Ci et al. 2009). BCL6 for its transcriptional repressor function requires certain corepressors recruited by BCL6 BTB domain (bric-a-brac, tramtrack, broad complex domain). Disruption of this interaction with specific peptide inhibitors (BPI, BCL6 peptide inhibitor) eliminates BCL6 transcriptional repressor activity and oncogenic potential (Cerchietti et al. 2009; Polo et al. 2004). More recently, a small molecule inhibitor of BCL6 BTB domain has been developed and demonstrated promising antitumor activity in in vitro and mouse models (Cerchietti et al. 2010).

3.6 Conclusions

Significant progress in the understanding of the molecular pathogenesis and cellular origin of B-cell lymphomas has been made in the past several years, largely owing to the advent of high-throughput gene expression profiling methods and coupled functional studies. Results of these investigations begin to enter clinical diagnostics and clinical trials in the setting of molecularly targeted therapies guided by biomarkers that identify patients potentially sensitive to tested drugs.

As technological progress in biosciences continues, we begin to appreciate the far more complex nature of mature B-cell malignancies than emerged originally from gene expression studies. The true complexity of these malignancies involves multiple levels of cellular structure and function, such as DNA structural changes, epigenome, expression of noncoding RNAs, cellular proteome and kinome (entire set of protein kinases), metabolic pathways, and other processes with their mutual interactions. As the understanding of this complexity increases, we can expect further refinements in pathologic classification of lymphomas and new personalized treatment options used in the context of mechanisms active in individual patients.

References

Abramson JS, Shipp MA (2005) Advances in the biology and therapy of diffuse large B-cell lymphoma: moving toward a molecularly targeted approach. Blood 106(4):1164–1174

Adams J (2004) The proteasome: a suitable antineoplastic target. Nat Rev Cancer 4(5):349–360

Alizadeh AA, Eisen MB, Davis RE, Ma C, Lossos IS, Rosenwald A, Boldrick JC, Sabet H, Tran T, Yu X, Powell JI, Yang L, Marti GE, Moore T, Hudson J Jr, Lu L, Lewis DB, Tibshirani R, Sherlock G, Chan WC, Greiner TC, Weisenburger DD, Armitage JO, Warnke R, Levy R, Wilson W, Grever MR, Byrd JC, Botstein D, Brown PO, Staudt LM (2000) Distinct types of diffuse large B-cell lymphoma identified by gene expression profiling. Nature 403(6769): 503–511

Bidere N, Ngo VN, Lee J, Collins C, Zheng L, Wan F, Davis RE, Lenz G, Anderson DE, Arnoult D, Vazquez A, Sakai K, Zhang J, Meng Z, Veenstra TD, Staudt LM, Lenardo MJ (2009) Casein kinase 1alpha governs antigen-receptor-induced NF-kappaB activation and human lymphoma cell survival. Nature 458(7234):92–96

Bross L, Fukita Y, McBlane F, Demolliere C, Rajewsky K, Jacobs H (2000) DNA double-strand breaks in immunoglobulin genes undergoing somatic hypermutation. Immunity 13(5): 589–597

Busslinger M (2004) Transcriptional control of early B cell development. Annu Rev Immunol 22:55–79

Cerchietti LC, Ghetu AF, Zhu X, Da Silva GF, Zhong S, Matthews M, Bunting KL, Polo JM, Fares C, Arrowsmith CH, Yang SN, Garcia M, Coop A, Mackerell AD Jr, Prive GG, Melnick

A (2010) A small-molecule inhibitor of BCL6 kills DLBCL cells in vitro and in vivo. Cancer Cell 17(4):400–411

Cerchietti LC, Yang SN, Shaknovich R, Hatzi K, Polo JM, Chadburn A, Dowdy SF, Melnick A (2009) A peptomimetic inhibitor of BCL6 with potent antilymphoma effects in vitro and in vivo. Blood 113(15):3397–3405

Chen L, Monti S, Juszczynski P, Daley J, Chen W, Witzig TE, Habermann TM, Kutok JL, Shipp MA (2008) SYK-dependent tonic B-cell receptor signaling is a rational treatment target in diffuse large B-cell lymphoma. Blood 111(4):2230–2237

Choi WW, Weisenburger DD, Greiner TC, Piris MA, Banham AH, Delabie J, Braziel RM, Geng H, Iqbal J, Lenz G, Vose JM, Hans CP, Fu K, Smith LM, Li M, Liu Z, Gascoyne RD, Rosenwald A, Ott G, Rimsza LM, Campo E, Jaffe ES, Jaye DL, Staudt LM, Chan WC (2009) A new immunostain algorithm classifies diffuse large B-cell lymphoma into molecular subtypes with high accuracy. Clin Cancer Res 15(17):5494–5502

Ci W, Polo JM, Cerchietti L, Shaknovich R, Wang L, Yang SN, Ye K, Farinha P, Horsman DE, Gascoyne RD, Elemento O, Melnick A (2009) The BCL6 transcriptional program features repression of multiple oncogenes in primary B cells and is deregulated in DLBCL. Blood 113(22):5536–5548

Compagno M, Lim WK, Grunn A, Nandula SV, Brahmachary M, Shen Q, Bertoni F, Ponzoni M, Scandurra M, Califano A, Bhagat G, Chadburn A, Dalla-Favera R, Pasqualucci L (2009) Mutations of multiple genes cause deregulation of NF-kappaB in diffuse large B-cell lymphoma. Nature 459(7247):717–721

Dal Porto JM, Gauld SB, Merrell KT, Mills D, Pugh-Bernard AE, Cambier J (2004) B cell antigen receptor signaling 101. Mol Immunol 41(6–7):599–613

Davis RE, Brown KD, Siebenlist U, Staudt LM (2001) Constitutive nuclear factor kappaB activity is required for survival of activated B cell-like diffuse large B cell lymphoma cells. J Exp Med 194(12):1861–1874

Davis RE, Ngo VN, Lenz G, Tolar P, Young RM, Romesser PB, Kohlhammer H, Lamy L, Zhao H, Yang Y, Xu W, Shaffer AL, Wright G, Xiao W, Powell J, Jiang JK, Thomas CJ, Rosenwald A, Ott G, Muller-Hermelink HK, Gascoyne RD, Connors JM, Johnson NA, Rimsza LM, Campo E, Jaffe ES, Wilson WH, Delabie J, Smeland EB, Fisher RI, Braziel RM, Tubbs RR, Cook JR, Weisenburger DD, Chan WC, Pierce SK, Staudt LM (2010) Chronic active B-cell-receptor signalling in diffuse large B-cell lymphoma. Nature 463(7277):88–92

Deng J, Carlson N, Takeyama K, Dal Cin P, Shipp M, Letai A (2007) BH3 profiling identifies three distinct classes of apoptotic blocks to predict response to ABT-737 and conventional chemotherapeutic agents. Cancer Cell 12(2):171–185

Deutsch AJ, Fruhwirth M, Aigelsreiter A, Cerroni L, Neumeister P (2009) Primary cutaneous marginal zone B-cell lymphomas are targeted by aberrant somatic hypermutation. J Invest Dermatol 129(2):476–479

Dunleavy K, Pittaluga S, Czuczman MS, Dave SS, Wright G, Grant N, Shovlin M, Jaffe ES, Janik JE, Staudt LM, Wilson WH (2009) Differential efficacy of bortezomib plus chemotherapy within molecular subtypes of diffuse large B-cell lymphoma. Blood 113(24):6069–6076

Ferch U, Kloo B, Gewies A, Pfander V, Duwel M, Peschel C, Krappmann D, Ruland J (2009) Inhibition of MALT1 protease activity is selectively toxic for activated B cell-like diffuse large B cell lymphoma cells. J Exp Med 206(11):2313–2320

Feuerhake F, Kutok JL, Monti S, Chen W, LaCasce AS, Cattoretti G, Kurtin P, Pinkus GS, de Leval L, Harris NL, Savage KJ, Neuberg D, Habermann TM, Dalla-Favera R, Golub TR, Aster JC, Shipp MA (2005) NFkappaB activity, function, and target-gene signatures in primary mediastinal large B-cell lymphoma and diffuse large B-cell lymphoma subtypes. Blood 106(4):1392–1399

Friedberg JW, Sharman J, Sweetenham J, Johnston PB, Vose JM, Lacasce A, Schaefer-Cutillo J, De Vos S, Sinha R, Leonard JP, Cripe LD, Gregory SA, Sterba MP, Lowe AM, Levy R, Shipp MA (2010) Inhibition of Syk with fostamatinib disodium has significant clinical activity in non-Hodgkin lymphoma and chronic lymphocytic leukemia. Blood 115(13):2578–2585

Fu K, Weisenburger DD, Choi WW, Perry KD, Smith LM, Shi X, Hans CP, Greiner TC, Bierman PJ, Bociek RG, Armitage JO, Chan WC, Vose JM (2008) Addition of rituximab to standard chemotherapy improves the survival of both the germinal center B-cell-like and non-germinal center B-cell-like subtypes of diffuse large B-cell lymphoma. J Clin Oncol 26(28):4587–4594

Fugmann SD, Lee AI, Shockett PE, Villey IJ, Schatz DG (2000) The RAG proteins and V(D)J recombination: complexes, ends, and transposition. Annu Rev Immunol 18:495–527

Gagyi E, Balogh Z, Bodor C, Timar B, Reiniger L, Deak L, Csomor J, Csernus B, Szepesi A, Matolcsy A (2008) Somatic hypermutation of IGVH genes and aberrant somatic hypermutation in follicular lymphoma without BCL-2 gene rearrangement and expression. Haematologica 93(12):1822–1828

Gaidano G, Pasqualucci L, Capello D, Berra E, Deambrogi C, Rossi D, Maria Larocca L, Gloghini A, Carbone A, Dalla-Favera R (2003) Aberrant somatic hypermutation in multiple subtypes of AIDS-associated non-Hodgkin lymphoma. Blood 102(5):1833–1841

Goossens T, Klein U, Kuppers R (1998) Frequent occurrence of deletions and duplications during somatic hypermutation: implications for oncogene translocations and heavy chain disease. Proc Natl Acad Sci U S A 95(5):2463–2468

Green MR, Monti S, Rodig SJ, Juszczynski P, Currie T, O'Donnell E, Chapuy B, Takeyama K, Neuberg D, Golub TR, Kutok JL, Shipp MA (2010) Integrative analysis reveals selective 9p24.1 amplification, increased PD-1 ligand expression, and further induction via JAK2 in nodular sclerosing Hodgkin lymphoma and primary mediastinal large B-cell lymphoma. Blood 116(17):3268–3277

Honigberg LA, Smith AM, Sirisawad M, Verner E, Loury D, Chang B, Li S, Pan Z, Thamm DH, Miller RA, Buggy JJ (2010) The Bruton tyrosine kinase inhibitor PCI-32765 blocks B-cell activation and is efficacious in models of autoimmune disease and B-cell malignancy. Proc Natl Acad Sci U S A 107(29):13075–13080

Jost PJ, Ruland J (2007) Aberrant NF-kappaB signaling in lymphoma: mechanisms, consequences, and therapeutic implications. Blood 109(7):2700–2707

Klein U, Dalla-Favera R (2008) Germinal centres: role in B-cell physiology and malignancy. Nat Rev Immunol 8(1):22–33

Klein U, Goossens T, Fischer M, Kanzler H, Braeuninger A, Rajewsky K, Kuppers R (1998) Somatic hypermutation in normal and transformed human B cells. Immunol Rev 162:261–280

Kramer MH, Hermans J, Wijburg E, Philippo K, Geelen E, van Krieken JH, de Jong D, Maartense E, Schuuring E, Kluin PM (1998) Clinical relevance of BCL2, BCL6, and MYC rearrangements in diffuse large B-cell lymphoma. Blood 92(9):3152–3162

Kuppers R, Dalla-Favera R (2001) Mechanisms of chromosomal translocations in B cell lymphomas. Oncogene 20(40):5580–5594

Lenz G, Davis RE, Ngo VN, Lam L, George TC, Wright GW, Dave SS, Zhao H, Xu W, Rosenwald A, Ott G, Muller-Hermelink HK, Gascoyne RD, Connors JM, Rimsza LM, Campo E, Jaffe ES, Delabie J, Smeland EB, Fisher RI, Chan WC, Staudt LM (2008a) Oncogenic CARD11 mutations in human diffuse large B cell lymphoma. Science 319(5870):1676–1679

Lenz G, Nagel I, Siebert R, Roschke AV, Sanger W, Wright GW, Dave SS, Tan B, Zhao H, Rosenwald A, Muller-Hermelink HK, Gascoyne RD, Campo E, Jaffe ES, Smeland EB, Fisher RI, Kuehl WM, Chan WC, Staudt LM (2007) Aberrant immunoglobulin class switch recombination and switch translocations in activated B cell-like diffuse large B cell lymphoma. J Exp Med 204(3):633–643

Lenz G, Staudt LM (2010) Aggressive lymphomas. N Engl J Med 362(15):1417–1429

Lenz G, Wright G, Dave SS, Xiao W, Powell J, Zhao H, Xu W, Tan B, Goldschmidt N, Iqbal J, Vose J, Bast M, Fu K, Weisenburger DD, Greiner TC, Armitage JO, Kyle A, May L, Gascoyne RD, Connors JM, Troen G, Holte H, Kvaloy S, Dierickx D, Verhoef G, Delabie J, Smeland EB, Jares P, Martinez A, Lopez-Guillermo A, Montserrat E, Campo E, Braziel RM, Miller TP, Rimsza LM, Cook JR, Pohlman B, Sweetenham J, Tubbs RR, Fisher RI, Hartmann E, Rosenwald A, Ott G, Muller-Hermelink HK, Wrench D, Lister TA, Jaffe ES, Wilson WH, Chan WC, Staudt LM (2008b) Stromal gene signatures in large-B-cell lymphomas. N Engl J Med 359(22):2313–2323

Lenz G, Wright GW, Emre NC, Kohlhammer H, Dave SS, Davis RE, Carty S, Lam LT, Shaffer AL, Xiao W, Powell J, Rosenwald A, Ott G, Muller-Hermelink HK, Gascoyne RD, Connors JM, Campo E, Jaffe ES, Delabie J, Smeland EB, Rimsza LM, Fisher RI, Weisenburger DD, Chan WC, Staudt LM (2008c) Molecular subtypes of diffuse large B-cell lymphoma arise by distinct genetic pathways. Proc Natl Acad Sci U S A 105(36):13520–13525

Martinez-Climent JA, Fontan L, Gascoyne RD, Siebert R, Prosper F (2010) Lymphoma stem cells: enough evidence to support their existence? Haematologica 95(2):293–302

Monroe JG (2006) ITAM-mediated tonic signalling through pre-BCR and BCR complexes. Nat Rev Immunol 6(4):283–294

Monti S, Savage KJ, Kutok JL, Feuerhake F, Kurtin P, Mihm M, Wu B, Pasqualucci L, Neuberg D, Aguiar RC, Dal Cin P, Ladd C, Pinkus GS, Salles G, Harris NL, Dalla-Favera R, Habermann TM, Aster JC, Golub TR, Shipp MA (2005) Molecular profiling of diffuse large B-cell lymphoma identifies robust subtypes including one characterized by host inflammatory response. Blood 105(5):1851–1861

Morin RD, Johnson NA, Severson TM, Mungall AJ, An J, Goya R, Paul JE, Boyle M, Woolcock BW, Kuchenbauer F, Yap D, Humphries RK, Griffith OL, Shah S, Zhu H, Kimbara M, Shashkin P, Charlot JF, Tcherpakov M, Corbett R, Tam A, Varhol R, Smailus D, Moksa M, Zhao Y, Delaney A, Qian H, Birol I, Schein J, Moore R, Holt R, Horsman DE, Connors JM, Jones S, Aparicio S, Hirst M, Gascoyne RD, Marra MA (2010) Somatic mutations altering EZH2 (Tyr641) in follicular and diffuse large B-cell lymphomas of germinal-center origin. Nat Genet 42(2):181–185

Mottok A, Renne C, Seifert M, Oppermann E, Bechstein W, Hansmann ML, Kuppers R, Brauninger A (2009) Inactivating SOCS1 mutations are caused by aberrant somatic hypermutation and restricted to a subset of B-cell lymphoma entities. Blood 114(20): 4503–4506

Muramatsu M, Kinoshita K, Fagarasan S, Yamada S, Shinkai Y, Honjo T (2000) Class switch recombination and hypermutation require activation-induced cytidine deaminase (AID), a potential RNA editing enzyme. Cell 102(5):553–563

Muschen M, Rajewsky K, Kronke M, Kuppers R (2002) The origin of CD95-gene mutations in B-cell lymphoma. Trends Immunol 23(2):75–80

Ngo VN, Davis RE, Lamy L, Yu X, Zhao H, Lenz G, Lam LT, Dave S, Yang L, Powell J, Staudt LM (2006) A loss-of-function RNA interference screen for molecular targets in cancer. Nature 441(7089):106–110

Nogai H, Dorken B, Lenz G (2011) Pathogenesis of non-Hodgkin's lymphoma. J Clin Oncol 29(14):1803–1811

Papavasiliou FN, Schatz DG (2000) Cell-cycle-regulated DNA double-stranded breaks in somatic hypermutation of immunoglobulin genes. Nature 408(6809):216–221

Pasqualucci L, Bhagat G, Jankovic M, Compagno M, Smith P, Muramatsu M, Honjo T, Morse HC, Nussenzweig MC, Dalla-Favera R (2008) AID is required for germinal center-derived lymphomagenesis. Nat Genet 40(1):108–112

Pasqualucci L, Compagno M, Houldsworth J, Monti S, Grunn A, Nandula SV, Aster JC, Murty VV, Shipp MA, Dalla-Favera R (2006) Inactivation of the PRDM1/BLIMP1 gene in diffuse large B cell lymphoma. J Exp Med 203(2):311–317

Pasqualucci L, Dominguez-Sola D, Chiarenza A, Fabbri G, Grunn A, Trifonov V, Kasper LH, Lerach S, Tang H, Ma J, Rossi D, Chadburn A, Murty VV, Mullighan CG, Gaidano G, Rabadan R, Brindle PK, Dalla-Favera R (2011) Inactivating mutations of acetyltransferase genes in B-cell lymphoma. Nature 471(7337):189–195

Pasqualucci L, Neumeister P, Goossens T, Nanjangud G, Chaganti RS, Kuppers R, Dalla-Favera R (2001) Hypermutation of multiple proto-oncogenes in B-cell diffuse large-cell lymphomas. Nature 412(6844):341–346

Polo JM, Dell'Oso T, Ranuncolo SM, Cerchietti L, Beck D, Da Silva GF, Prive GG, Licht JD, Melnick A (2004) Specific peptide interference reveals BCL6 transcriptional and oncogenic mechanisms in B-cell lymphoma cells. Nat Med 10(12):1329–1335

Polo JM, Juszczynski P, Monti S, Cerchietti L, Ye K, Greally JM, Shipp M, Melnick A (2007) Transcriptional signature with differential expression of BCL6 target genes accurately identifies BCL6-dependent diffuse large B cell lymphomas. Proc Natl Acad Sci U S A 104(9):3207–3212

Rajewsky K (1996) Clonal selection and learning in the antibody system. Nature 381(6585): 751–758

Ramiro AR, Jankovic M, Eisenreich T, Difilippantonio S, Chen-Kiang S, Muramatsu M, Honjo T, Nussenzweig A, Nussenzweig MC (2004) AID is required for c-myc/IgH chromosome translocations in vivo. Cell 118(4):431–438

Robertson MJ, Kahl BS, Vose JM, de Vos S, Laughlin M, Flynn PJ, Rowland K, Cruz JC, Goldberg SL, Musib L, Darstein C, Enas N, Kutok JL, Aster JC, Neuberg D, Savage KJ, LaCasce A, Thornton D, Slapak CA, Shipp MA (2007) Phase II study of enzastaurin, a protein kinase C beta inhibitor, in patients with relapsed or refractory diffuse large B-cell lymphoma. J Clin Oncol 25(13):1741–1746

Rosenwald A, Wright G, Chan WC, Connors JM, Campo E, Fisher RI, Gascoyne RD, Muller-Hermelink HK, Smeland EB, Giltnane JM, Hurt EM, Zhao H, Averett L, Yang L, Wilson WH, Jaffe ES, Simon R, Klausner RD, Powell J, Duffey PL, Longo DL, Greiner TC, Weisenburger DD, Sanger WG, Dave BJ, Lynch JC, Vose J, Armitage JO, Montserrat E, Lopez-Guillermo A, Grogan TM, Miller TP, LeBlanc M, Ott G, Kvaloy S, Delabie J, Holte H, Krajci P, Stokke T, Staudt LM (2002) The use of molecular profiling to predict survival after chemotherapy for diffuse large-B-cell lymphoma. N Engl J Med 346(25):1937–1947

Ruefli-Brasse AA, French DM, Dixit VM (2003) Regulation of NF-kappaB-dependent lymphocyte activation and development by paracaspase. Science 302(5650):1581–1584

Schatz DG, Ji Y (2011) Recombination centres and the orchestration of V(D)J recombination. Nat Rev Immunol 11(4):251–263

Schmidlin H, Diehl SA, Nagasawa M, Scheeren FA, Schotte R, Uittenbogaart CH, Spits H, Blom B (2008) Spi-B inhibits human plasma cell differentiation by repressing BLIMP1 and XBP-1 expression. Blood 112(5):1804–1812

Shipp MA (1993) A predictive model for aggressive non-Hodgkin's lymphoma. The International Non-Hodgkin's Lymphoma Prognostic Factors Project. N Engl J Med 329(14):987–994

Shipp MA, Ross KN, Tamayo P, Weng AP, Kutok JL, Aguiar RC, Gaasenbeek M, Angelo M, Reich M, Pinkus GS, Ray TS, Koval MA, Last KW, Norton A, Lister TA, Mesirov J, Neuberg DS, Lander ES, Aster JC, Golub TR (2002) Diffuse large B-cell lymphoma outcome prediction by gene-expression profiling and supervised machine learning. Nat Med 8(1):68–74

Swerdlow SH, International Agency for Research on Cancer, World Health Organization (2008) WHO classification of tumours of haematopoietic and lymphoid tissues. World health organization classification of tumours, 4th edn. International Agency for Research on Cancer, Lyon, France

Takahashi H, Feuerhake F, Kutok JL, Monti S, Dal Cin P, Neuberg D, Aster JC, Shipp MA (2006) FAS death domain deletions and cellular FADD-like interleukin 1beta converting enzyme inhibitory protein (long) overexpression: alternative mechanisms for deregulating the extrinsic apoptotic pathway in diffuse large B-cell lymphoma subtypes. Clin Cancer Res 12(11 Pt 1):3265–3271

Tam W, Gomez M, Chadburn A, Lee JW, Chan WC, Knowles DM (2006) Mutational analysis of PRDM1 indicates a tumor-suppressor role in diffuse large B-cell lymphomas. Blood 107(10):4090–4100

Wright G, Tan B, Rosenwald A, Hurt EH, Wiestner A, Staudt LM (2003) A gene expression-based method to diagnose clinically distinct subgroups of diffuse large B cell lymphoma. Proc Natl Acad Sci U S A 100(17):9991–9996

Yap DB, Chu J, Berg T, Schapira M, Cheng SW, Moradian A, Morin RD, Mungall AJ, Meissner B, Boyle M, Marquez VE, Marra MA, Gascoyne RD, Humphries RK, Arrowsmith CH, Morin GB, Aparicio SA (2011) Somatic mutations at EZH2 Y641 act dominantly through a mechanism of selectively altered PRC2 catalytic activity, to increase H3K27 trimethylation. Blood 117(8):2451–2459

Chapter 4
Molecular Biology and Classification of Multiple Myeloma

Anna Dmoszyńska and Norbert Grząśko

Abstract In recent years, significant progress has been made in understanding the molecular pathogenesis of multiple myeloma (MM). MM is characterized by the sequential multistage progressive accumulation of genetic abnormalities which lead to deregulation of key regulatory pathways. Numeric chromosomal abnormalities are present in almost all MM patients. Primary translocations occur early in MM pathogenesis, whereas secondary translocations are involved in progression. Chromosomal abnormalities include full or partial deletion of chromosome 13 and 17, amplification of chromosome 1, and recurrent 14q32 translocations. Hyperdiploidy is present in 45 % of patients. From the clinical point of view, the knowledge of MM molecular biology is important in making decisions about therapeutic choices and in designing novel molecule targeted drugs.

4.1 Introduction

Multiple myeloma (MM) is a clonal B-cell disorder characterized by: (1) production of monoclonal protein containing one type of immunoglobulin heavy chain (IgG or IgA) and one type of immunoglobulin light chain (kappa or lambda), (2) plasma cell proliferation and accumulation in bone marrow leading to cytopenias and bone resorption. Almost all cases of MM are preceded by monoclonal gammopathy of

A. Dmoszyńska (✉) · N. Grząśko
Department of Haematooncology and Bone Marrow Transplantation, Medical University of Lublin, Staszica 11, 20-081 Lublin, Poland
e-mail: annadmosz@wp.pl

N. Grząśko
e-mail: norbertgrzasko@gmail.com

M. Witt et al. (eds.), *Molecular Aspects of Hematologic Malignancies*, Principles and Practice, DOI: 10.1007/978-3-642-29467-9_4,

undetermined significance (MGUS). At the stage of MGUS, one or more of the genes encoding for cyclin D, are mutated, and it is suggested to be an early oncogenic event in MGUS and MM. MM is a very heterogeneous disease with survival time varying from a few months to 10 years or longer. Numerous studies indicate that this heterogeneity is associated with different and specific molecular cytogenetic changes detected in MM patients.

In 2009, the International Myeloma Working Group (IMWG) proposed new working genetic classification of MM based on detected molecular cytogenetic changes (Fonseca et al. 2009). Detailed classification with characteristic clinical and laboratory features is presented in Table 4.1.

4.2 Hyperdiploid and Non-hyperdiploid Multiple Myeloma

Chromosomal aberrations are present in about 80–85 % of MM patients. The chromosome content reflects at least two pathways of pathogenesis. Generally, MM can be divided into two major subtypes: hyperdiploid (H-MM) and non-hyperdiploid (NH-MM), comprising about 55 and 45 % of cases, respectively (Wuilleme et al. 2005; Carrasco et al. 2006). The ploidy category is stable over the course of the disease. Moreover, identical subtypes were documented also in MGUS, indicating two different pathogenetic pathways of plasma cell dyscrasias (Chng et al. 2005; Chng et al. 2006a).

Hyperdiploid genotype in MM is the result of harboring chromosomal trisomies, usually of chromosomes 3, 5, 7, 9, 11, 15, 19, and 21. The number of chromosomes in patients with H-MM varies from 48 to 74 with the median of 53. NH-MM can be divided into: hypoploid with a chromosome number less than 46, pseudodiploid with a chromosome number of 46, and additional structural aberrations. The most common aberrations present in NH-MM are: monosomy of chromosome 13, chromosome 8p deletion, additional copies of chromosome 1q, and translocations of *IGH* (immunoglobulin heavy chain) genes (Fonseca et al. 2003a; Carrasco et al. 2006). Generally, patients with NH-MM have poorer prognosis than H-MM cases (Fassas et al. 2002; Debes-Marun et al. 2003). The overall survival (OS) in NH-MM was reported to be 18.2 versus 36.8 months in H-MM ($p < 0.04$) (Smadja et al. 2001).

4.3 Mutations of Immunoglobulin Heavy Chain Gene

IGH genes are located in chromosome 14q32. Aberrations of this region are detected in about 13 % of MM patients with the use of classical cytogenetic methods and in about 60–70 % with the use of fluorescence in situ hybridization (FISH). Usually, *IGH* translocations are associated with NH-MM and a less favorable outcome. The most common aberrations of the *IGH* locus include:

Table 4.1 Molecular cytogenetic classification of multiple myeloma according to International Myeloma Working Group (Fonseca et al. 2009)

Multiple myeloma subtype	Proportion of patients (%)	Characteristic features
Hyperdiploid	45	More favorable prognosis, monoclonal protein IgG-kappa, older patients
Non-hyperdiploid	40	Unfavorable prognosis, monoclonal protein IgA-lambda, younger patients
1. Cyclin D translocation	18	
• t(11;14)(q13;q32)	16	Upregulation of *CCND1*, favorable prognosis, bone lesions, two subtypes by GEP
• t(6;14)(p21;q32)	2	Probably same features as t(11;14)(q13;q32)
• t(12;14)(p13;q32)	<1	Rare
2. *MMSET* translocation	15	
• t(4;14)(p16;q32)	15	Upregulation of *MMSET*, upregulation of *FGFR3* in 75 % of cases, unfavorable prognosis with conventional therapy, bone lesions less frequent
3. *MAF* translocation	8	Unfavorable prognosis
• t(14;16)(q32;q23)	5	Reported as aggressive by at least two series
• t(14;20)(q32;q11)	2	One series shows more aggressive disease
• t(8;14)(q24;q32)	1	Unknown effect on outcome but presumed aggressive
Unclassified (other)	15	

CCND1–cyclin D1, GEP—gene expression profiling, *MMSET*—multiple myeloma SET domain, *FGFR3*—fibroblast growth factor receptor 3, *MAF*—musculoaponeurotic fibrosarcoma oncogene family

t(11;14)(q13;q32), t(4;14)(p16;q32), t(14;16)(q32;q23), t(6;14)(p21;q32), t(14;20)(q32;q11), and t(8;14)(q24;q32) (Avet-Loiseau et al. 2007; Fonseca et al. 2003b; Moreau et al. 2002).

4.3.1 Translocation t(11;14)(q13;q32)

Translocation t(11;14)(q13;q32) is one of the most common aberrations in MM detected in about 15–18 % of patients (Fonseca et al. 2003b). It is also observed in MGUS cases with a similar incidence (Fonseca et al. 2002a). The translocation results in upregulation of *CCND1* (cyclin D1) and *MYEOV* (myeloma overexpressed gene in a subset of t(11;14)-positive multiple myelomas) genes. Characteristic features of MM with t(11;14)(q13;q32) are: lymphoplasmacytic morphology of plasma cells, CD20 expression, hyposecretory disease with low monoclonal protein production, light chain disease, and light chain lambda involvement (Hoyer et al. 2000; Garand et al. 2003).

In the majority of reports, the presence of t(11;14)(q13;q32) was associated with a better prognosis, although this effect was not statistically significant. Additionally, in some cases, MM with the presence of this translocation manifested as an aggressive disease, such as plasma cell leukemia (Moreau et al. 2002). More recently, reports did not support positive influence of t(11;14)(q13;q32) on survival (Gertz et al. 2005; Avet-Loiseau et al. 2007).

4.3.2 Translocation t(4;14)(p16;q32)

Translocation t(4;14)(p16;q32) is only detectable with the use of FISH or reverse transcriptase polymerase chain reaction (PCR) and cannot be shown in classical cytogenetic studies (Sawyer et al. 2001). It is specific for MM and can be found in about 15 % of MM patients, especially in cases with heavy chain IgA and light chain lambda. There is a very high incidence of chromosome 13 abnormalities coexisting with t(4;14)(p16;q32) (Avet-Loiseau et al. 2002). The translocation can be present in premalignant stages of MM, although it is less common in MGUS than in smoldering (asymptomatic) MM (SMM) (Avet-Loiseau et al. 1999a; Fonseca et al. 2002a). This can explain more aggressive course of the disease progressing from SMM. The consequence of the translocation is the overexpression of two genes: *FGFR3* (fibroblast growth factor receptor 3) and *MMSET* (multiple myeloma SET domain) (Chesi et al. 1998a). In about 25 % of cases, t(4;14)(p16;q32) is imbalanced, which results in the loss of derivative chromosome 14 and, consequently, the loss of *FGFR3* expression (Keats et al. 2003).

The presence of t(4;14)(p16;q32) was shown in several series to be associated with a poor prognosis and shorter survival (Moreau et al. 2002; Gertz et al. 2005). Patients with t(4;14)(p16;q32) had a short duration of response after high-dose therapy with autologous stem cell transplantation (HDT/ASCT) and usually relapsed during the first year after HDT-ASCT (Chang et al. 2004a; Chang et al. 2005).

4.3.3 Translocation t(14;16)(q32;q23) and Other MAF Translocations

MAF genes (musculoaponeurotic fibrosarcoma oncogene family) are located at a fragile site of chromosome 16 and encode for small protein molecules acting as transcription factors (Chesi et al. 1998b). Translocations involving *MAF* genes are detectable in about 5–7 % of MM patients and arise from *IGH* rearrangements with chromosome 16. The most common *MAF* translocation is t(14;16)(q32;q23) involving *C-MAF*. Similar to t(4;14)(p16;q32), it is specific for MM and can be detected with the use of FISH or reverse transcriptase-PCR but not with classical cytogenetic methods. The presence of *C-MAF* translocation is associated with a more aggressive course of the disease, heavy chain IgA, light chain lambda, and chromosome 13 deletion (Fonseca et al. 2003b; Shaughnessy et al. 2007).

4.3.4 Other Chromosome 14q32 Translocations

Translocation t(6;14)(p21;q32) results in activation of *CCND3* gene (cyclin D3) and can be detected in about 5 % of MM patients (Shaughnessy et al. 2001). This translocation results in the upregulation of cyclin D3. The clinical significance of t(6;14)(p21;q32) is similar to that of t(11;14)(q13;q32), which is in line with almost identical gene expression profiles in these two MM subsets (Bergsagel et al. 2005). It is also detected in MGUS cases with a similar incidence (Fonseca et al. 2002a). Other chromosome 14q32 translocations, such as t(14;20)(q32;q11) or t(8;14)(q24;q32) are rare, and their clinical significance is not clear.

4.4 Chromosome 13 Abnormalities

About two-thirds of cases with chromosome 13 abnormalities are present between patients with NH-MM and one-third in patients with H-MM. Patients with chromosome 13 abnormalities and NH-MM have shortened OS and time to progression (TTP) (Fonseca et al. 2003b), but direct influence of these aberrations is unclear. It may reflect the coincidence of chromosome 13 monosomy or deletion with other genetic changes related to poor prognosis, like t(4;14)(p16;q32) or del17p13 (Chiecchio et al. 2006; Avet-Loiseau et al. 2007). In patients with H-MM, chromosome 13 abnormalities have no prognostic value (Chang et al. 2006b). It is noteworthy that chromosome 13 abnormalities have an important role in the clonal expansion of plasma cells, and almost 90 % of cases with t(4;14)(p16;q32) gain chromosome 13 deletions during the course of the disease (Avet-Loiseau et al. 1999b; Fonseca et al. 2002b).

4.5 Chromosome 1 Abnormalities

The majority of chromosome 1 abnormalities involve pericentromeric regions (Sawyer et al. 1998; Sawyer et al. 2005). In many cases, 1q gain and 1p loss are closely related and difficult to differentiate (Carrasco et al. 2006). Chromosome 1q amplification is frequently associated with other abnormalities, such as t(4;14)(p16;q32) or t(14;16)(q32;q23), and with a high proliferation index. In cases with chromosome 1q21 amplification, there is enhanced expression of *CKS1B* gene (cyclin kinase subunit 1B), which is responsible for a high proliferation rate, although it has been suggested that *CKS1B* overexpression is simply the consequence of an advanced and genetically instable disease.

Chromosome 1 abnormalities are regarded as a major prognostic factor in MM, and their presence was shown to be associated with an unfavorable disease course, shorter progression-free survival (PFS), and shorter OS (Chang et al. 2006; Shaughnessy et al. 2007).

4.6 Chromosome 17p13 Deletion

The deletion of chromosome 17p13, involving the locus of tumor-suppressor gene *p53*, is not specific for MM and can be found in other malignances. It is the most significant adverse molecular cytogenetic prognostic factor in MM, detected in 10 % of patients at diagnosis, in 18 % at first relapse, and in 33 % at further relapses (Molnar et al. 2008). It is worth noting that the deletion of 17p13 is rare in MGUS. The presence of 17p13 deletion is associated with shorter OS, more aggressive disease, hypercalcemia, involvement of central nervous system, higher incidence of plasma cell leukemia, and extramedullary plasmacytomas (Fonseca et al. 2003b; Chang et al. 2004b; Avet-Loiseau et al. 2007; Chng et al. 2007; Tiedemann et al. 2008). The deletion of 17p13 with defective function of *p53* is detectable in most cases of plasma cell leukemia, suggesting that extramedullary disease and plasma cell survival in extramedullary sites are the result of *p53* abnormalities.

In all tested series, 17p13 deletion was confirmed to have a significantly adverse effect on survival (Drach et al. 1998; Fonseca et al. 2003b; Avet-Loiseau et al. 2007). It was also associated with short remission duration after HDT/ASCT (Chang et al. 2005). The negative influence of 17p13 deletion on disease course was not overcome even by allogeneic stem cell transplantation. In one study, the overall complete response (CR) rate was 50 %, and none of the genetic abnormalities resulted in worse response rate, except for the deletion of 17p13 (7 % CR in patients carrying del(17p13) versus 56 % CR in patients with other genetic abnormalities). Similarly, event-free survival (EFS) was significantly shorter for patients carrying del(17p13) (Schilling et al. 2008).

4.7 Chromosome 12p Deletions

Recently, deletions of chromosome 12 were detected in about 12 % of MM patients using a single nucleotide polymorphism array-based approach for detection of copy number alterations (Avet-Loiseau et al. 2009). The deletions were localized in the short arm of the chromosome, and their size was variable. However, they always involved the gene encoding CD27 molecule (member of the tumor necrosis factor receptor family. The presence of 12p deletions was associated with shortened EFS and OS. Other studies showed that the low expression of CD27 on myeloma cells was an adverse prognostic factor in MM patients (Moreau et al. 2006).

4.8 Chromosome 16q Abnormalities

Abnormalities of chromosome 16q are important and recurrent aberrations in MM, detected in 20 % of cases by single nucleotide polymorphism microarrays (Walker et al. 2006). The *WWOX* gene (WW domain-containing oxidoreductase), localized in 16q, acts as a tumor-suppressor gene. In addition, biallelic 16q deletion of is probably associated with poor prognosis (Jenner et al. 2007). However, these findings need confirmation in further studies.

4.9 Activation of NF-κB

NF-κB (nuclear factor kappa-light-chain-gene-enhancer in B cells)–a transcription factor regulating immune response, proliferation, cell cycle, and apoptosis—plays a crucial role in MM pathogenesis. Activation of NF-κB can be detected by gene expression profiling. It has been proven recently that there is a constitutive activation of the NF-κB pathway with NF-κB nuclear hyperactivity in about 50 % of MM patients (Annunziata et al. 2007; Keats et al. 2007). The activation is caused by multiple genetic mechanisms, such as inactivation of NF-κB suppressors (consequence of biallelic deletion or deletion/mutation combination) and NF-κB hyperactivity (consequence of amplification or chromosome translocations). It is present in all major genetic subtypes of MM, which suggests its secondary character.

4.10 *RAS* Mutations

It was shown that *RAS* (rat sarcoma) mutation status was associated with progression of MGUS to MM (Rasmussen et al. 2005). *K-RAS*, but not *N-RAS*, mutations predicted adverse outcomes in MM patients (Liu et al. 1996). *RAS* mutations can be detected more frequently in patients with t(11;14)(q13;q32) and they are probably predictive factors of disease progression in this subtype of MM (Bezieau et al. 2001; Chng et al. 2008).

4.11 Methylation of p16 and Inactivation of p18

The importance of p16 protein in MM pathogenesis is associated with the regulation of cell cycle. The inactivation of *p16* gene, mainly by promoter region methylation and rarely by deletion, was detected in almost 50 % of MM patients (Mateos et al. 2002; Gonzalez-Paz et al. 2007). It is involved in MM pathogenesis but has limited prognostic value (Sarasquete et al. 2006).

The product of *p18* gene is crucial for the development of normal plasma cells, and its inactivation likely plays an important role in increased monoclonal plasma cell proliferation. The increased expression of p18 can almost completely inhibit proliferation and induce apoptosis in myeloma cell lines by inhibition of the *CCND1* pathway (Kulkarni et al. 2002). Biallelic *p18* gene deletions were found in 10 % of MM patients (Tasaka et al. 1997).

4.12 MicroRNAs

MicroRNAs (miRNAs) are short, noncoding, single-strand RNA molecules of 19–25 nucleotides in length. They are involved in cell differentiation, proliferation, and apoptosis. They regulate other genes expression by pairing to their target mRNA complementary sites, which induce translation inhibition and degradation of target mRNA. Recently, published studies indicate that miRNAs may contribute to the pathogenesis of MM. The expression of miRNAs was profiled using miRNA microarrays and reverse transcriptase-PCR in human myeloma cell lines and plasma cells derived from MM patients, MGUS patients and normal donors. Results showed that miR-21, miR-106b ~25, miR-181a, and miR-181b are expressed in MM and MGUS but not in normal plasma cells. Moreover, miR-32 and miR-17 ~92 were upregulated in MM when compared with MGUS and normal plasma cells (Pichiorri et al. 2008). Changes in miRNAs expression are associated with other molecular abnormalities. For instance, the expression of miR-1 and miR-133a was selectively upregulated in MM patients with t(14;16), while the expression of miR-125a ~5p, miR-99b, and let-7e was upregulated in patients with t(4;14) (Lionetti et al. 2009; Gutiérrez et al. 2010).

The role of miRNAs in the pathogenesis of MM is complex. It was shown that the expression of miR-21 made myeloma cell lines growth independent of the presence of interleukin-6, a potent growth factor of myeloma cells (Löffler et al. 2007). MiRNAs can also act through the reduction of expression of *PCAF* (p300/CBP-associated factor), which is a positive p53 regulator (Pichiorri et al. 2008). These data suggest an important role of miRNAs in the pathogenesis of MM but need further confirmation.

4.13 *MYC* Abnormalities

The family of genes encoding for MYC transcription factors consists of three genes: *C-MYC*, *N-MYC*, and *L-MYC*. Translocations of *C-MYC* gene, localized in chromosome 8q24, seem to be important in MM progression. They are rare in MGUS and reflect advanced disease stage. Translocations involving *C-MYC* were detected in 15 % of MM patients, in 44 % of patients with advanced MM, and in 90 % of NH-MM cases. There are also rare MM cases presented with upregulated expression of *N-MYC* and *L-MYC*. The prognostic value of *C-MYC* translocations is not clear, and there are reports showing both negative and neutral impact on survival (Avet-Loiseau et al. 2007; Chesi et al. 2008).

4.14 Conclusions

Cytogenetic and molecular changes play an important role in myeloma pathogenesis. The heterogeneous disease course reflects different genetic aberrations found in MM patients. There are two major subtypes of MM: H-MM associated with a better prognosis, longer survival, and a more indolent course; and NH-MM associated with less favorable outcomes. Patients with NH-MM carry additional aberrations more frequently. Aberrations of immunoglobulin heavy chain genes, localized in locus 14q32, are characteristic for MM, the most common being: t(4;14)(p16;q32), t(6;14)(p21;q32), t(8;14)(q24;q32), t(11;14)(q13;q32), t(14;16)(q32;q23), and t(14;20)(q32;q11). Among them, t(4;14)(p16;q32) and t(14;16)(q32;q23) are regarded as the most adverse prognostic factors. Other genetic aberrations associated with an unfavorable disease course, lower response rate, and shorter survival are: chromosome 17p13 deletion, chromosome 13 monosomy or deletion, and chromosome 1q21 changes. Chromosome 17p13 deletion, resulting in the loss of function of tumor-suppressor gene *p53,* is not specific for MM, but it remains the most significant of cytogenetic prognostic factors associated with aggressive disease course and poor prognosis. MM patients may also display such genetic abnormalities as chromosome 12 deletion, chromosome 16q aberrations, activation of NF-κB, *K-RAS* mutations, methylation of p16, inactivation of p18, changes of miRNAs, and *MYC* abnormalities. The impact of these abnormalities on MM course needs further investigation.

References

Annunziata CM, Davis RE, Demchenko Y, Bellamy W, Gabrea A, Zhan F, Lenz G, Hanamura I, Wright G, Xiao W, Dave S, Hurt EM, Tan B, Zhao H, Stephens O, Santra M, Williams DR, Dang L, Barlogie B, Shaughnessy JD Jr, Kuehl WM, Staudt LM (2007) Frequent engagement of the classical and alternative NF-kappaB pathways by diverse genetic abnormalities in multiple myeloma. Cancer Cell 12:115–130

Avet-Loiseau H, Facon T, Daviet A, Godon C, Rapp MJ, Harousseau JL, Grosbois B, Bataille R (1999a) 14q32 translocations and monosomy 13 observed in monoclonal gammopathy of undetermined significance delineate a multistep process for the oncogenesis of multiple myeloma, Intergroupe Francophone du Myelome. Cancer Res 59:4546–4550

Avet-Loiseau H, Li JY, Morineau N, Facon T, Brigaudeau C, Harousseau JL, Grosbois B, Bataille R (1999b) Monosomy 13 is associated with the transition of monoclonal gammopathy of undetermined significance to multiple myeloma. Intergroupe Francophone du Myelome. Blood 94:2583–2589

Avet-Loiseau H, Facon T, Grosbois B, Magrangeas F, Rapp MJ, Harousseau JL, Minvielle S, Bataille R (2002) Oncogenesis of multiple myeloma: 14q32 and 13q chromosomal abnormalities are not randomly distributed, but correlate with natural history, immunological features, and clinical presentation. Blood 99:2185–2191

Avet-Loiseau H, Attal M, Moreau P, Charbonnel C, Garban F, Hulin C, Leyvraz S, Michallet M, Yakoub-Agha I, Garderet L, Marit G, Michaux L, Voillat L, Renaud M, Grosbois B, Guillerm G, Benboubker L, Monconduit M, Thieblemont C, Casassus P, Caillot D, Stoppa AM, Sotto JJ, Wetterwald M, Dumontet C et al (2007) Genetic abnormalities and survival in multiple myeloma: the experience of the Intergroupe Francophone du Myelome. Blood 109:3489–3495

Avet-Loiseau H, Li C, Magrangeas F, Gouraud W, Charbonnel C, Harousseau JL, Attal M, Marit G, Mathiot C, Facon T, Moreau P, Anderson KC, Campion L, Munshi NC, Minvielle S (2009) Prognostic significance of copy-number alterations in multiple myeloma. J Clin Oncol 27:4585–4590

Bergsagel PL, Kuehl WM, Zhan F, Sawyer J, Barlogie B, Shaughnessy J Jr (2005) Cyclin D dysregulation: an early and unifying pathogenic event in multiple myeloma. Blood 106:296–303

Bezieau S, Devilder MC, Avet-Loiseau H, Mellerin MP, Puthier D, Pennarun E, Rapp MJ, Harousseau JL, Moisan JP, Bataille R (2001) High incidence of N and K-Ras activating mutations in multiple myeloma and primary plasma cell leukemia at diagnosis. Human Mutat 18:212–224

Carrasco DR, Tonon G, Huang Y, Zhang Y, Sinha R, Feng B, Stewart JP, Zhan F, Khatry D, Protopopova M, Protopopov A, Sukhdeo K, Hanamura I, Stephens O, Barlogie B, Anderson KC, Chin L, Shaughnessy JD Jr, Brennan C, Depinho RA (2006) High-resolution genomic profiles define distinct clinico-pathogenetic subgroups of multiple myeloma patients. Cancer Cell 9:313–325

Chang H, Sloan S, Li D, Zhuang L, Yi QL, Chen CI, Reece D, Chun K, Keith Stewart A (2004a) The t(4;14) is associated with poor prognosis in myeloma patients undergoing autologous stem cell transplant. Br J Haematol 125:64–68

Chang H, Sloan S, Li D, Keith Stewart A (2004b) Multiple myeloma involving central nervous system: high frequency of chromosome 17p13.1 (p53) deletions. Br J Haematol 127:280–284

Chang H, Qi XY, Samiee S, Yi QL, Chen C, Trudel S, Mikhael J, Reece D, Stewart AK (2005) Genetic risk identifies multiple myeloma patients who do not benefit from autologous stem cell transplantation. Bone Marrow Transplant 36:793–796

Chang H, Qi X, Trieu Y, Xu W, Reader JC, Ning Y, Reece D (2006) Multiple myeloma patients with CKS1B gene amplification have a shorter progression-free survival post-autologous stem cell transplantation. Br J Haematol 135:486–491

Chesi M, Nardini E, Lim RS, Smith KD, Kuehl WM, Bergsagel PL (1998a) The t(4;14) translocation in myeloma dysregulates both FGFR3 and a novel gene, MMSET, resulting in IgH/MMSET hybrid transcripts. Blood 92:3025–3034

Chesi M, Bergsagel PL, Shonukan OO, Martelli ML, Brents LA, Chen T, Schröck E, Ried T, Kuehl WM (1998b) Frequent dysregulation of the c-maf proto-oncogene at 16q23 by translocation to an Ig locus in multiple myeloma. Blood 91:4457–4463

Chesi M, Robbiani DF, Sebag M, Chng WJ, Affer M, Tiedemann R, Valdez R, Palmer SE, Haas SS, Stewart AK, Fonseca R, Kremer R, Cattoretti G, Bergsagel PL (2008) AID-dependent activation of a MYC transgene induces multiple myeloma in a conditional mouse model of post-germinal center malignancies. Cancer Cell 13:167–180

Chiecchio L, Protheroe RK, Ibrahim AH, Cheung KL, Rudduck C, Dagrada GP, Cabanas ED, Parker T, Nightingale M, Wechalekar A, Orchard KH, Harrison CJ, Cross NC, Morgan GJ, Ross FM (2006) Deletion of chromosome 13 detected by conventional cytogenetics is a critical prognostic factor in myeloma. Leukemia 20:1610–1617

Chng WJ, Van Wier SA, Ahmann GJ, Winkler JM, Jalal SM, Bergsagel PL, Chesi M, Trendle MC, Oken MM, Blood E, Henderson K, Santana-Dávila R, Kyle RA, Gertz MA, Lacy MQ, Dispenzieri A, Greipp PR, Fonseca R (2005) A validated FISH trisomy index demonstrates the hyperdiploid and nonhyperdiploid dichotomy in MGUS. Blood 106:2156–2161

Chng WJ, Winkler JM, Greipp PR, Jalal SM, Bergsagel PL, Chesi M, Trendle MC, Ahmann GJ, Henderson K, Blood E, Oken MM, Hulbert A, Van Wier SA, Santana-Dávila R, Kyle RA, Gertz MA, Lacy MQ, Dispenzieri A, Fonseca R (2006a) Ploidy status rarely changes in myeloma patients at disease progression. Leuk Res 30:266–271

Chng WJ, Santana-Dávila R, Van Wier SA, Ahmann GJ, Jalal SM, Bergsagel PL, Chesi M, Trendle MC, Jacobus S, Blood E, Oken MM, Henderson K, Kyle RA, Gertz MA, Lacy MQ, Dispenzieri A, Greipp PR, Fonseca R (2006b) Prognostic factors for hyperdiploid-myeloma: effects of chromosome 13 deletions and IgH translocations. Leukemia 20:807–813

Chng WJ, Price-Troska T, Gonzalez-Paz N, Van Wier S, Jacobus S, Blood E, Henderson K, Oken M, Van Ness B, Greipp P, Rajkumar SV, Fonseca R (2007) Clinical significance of TP53 mutation in myeloma. Leukemia 21:582–584

Chng WJ, Gonzalez-Paz N, Price-Troska T, Jacobus S, Rajkumar SV, Oken MM, Kyle RA, Henderson KJ, Van Wier S, Greipp P, Van Ness B, Fonseca R (2008) Clinical and biological significance of RAS mutations in multiple myeloma. Leukemia 22:2280–2284

Debes-Marun CS, Dewald GW, Bryant S, Picken E, Santana-Dávila R, González-Paz N, Winkler JM, Kyle RA, Gertz MA, Witzig TE, Dispenzieri A, Lacy MQ, Rajkumar SV, Lust JA, Greipp PR, Fonseca R (2003) Chromosome abnormalities clustering and its implications for pathogenesis and prognosis in myeloma. Leukemia 17:427–436

Drach J, Ackermann J, Fritz E, Krömer E, Schuster R, Gisslinger H, DeSantis M, Zojer N, Fiegl M, Roka S, Schuster J, Heinz R, Ludwig H, Huber H (1998) Presence of a p53 gene deletion in patients with multiple myeloma predicts for short survival after conventional-dose chemotherapy. Blood 92:802–809

Fassas AB, Spencer T, Sawyer J, Zangari M, Lee CK, Anaissie E, Muwalla F, Morris C, Barlogie B, Tricot G (2002) Both hypodiploidy and deletion of chromosome 13 independently confer poor prognosis in multiple myeloma. Br J Haematol 118:1041–1047

Fonseca R, Bailey RJ, Ahmann GJ, Rajkumar SV, Hoyer JD, Lust JA, Kyle RA, Gertz MA, Greipp PR, Dewald GW (2002a) Genomic abnormalities in monoclonal gammopathy of undetermined significance. Blood 100:1417–1424

Fonseca R, Harrington D, Oken MM, Dewald GW, Bailey RJ, Van Wier SA, Henderson KJ, Blood EA, Rajkumar SV, Kay NE, Van Ness B, Greipp PR (2002b) Biologic and prognostic significance of interphase FISH detection of chromosome 13 abnormalities (D13) in multiple myeloma: an Eastern Cooperative Oncology Group (ECOG) Study. Cancer Res 62:715–720

Fonseca R, Debes-Marun CS, Picken EB, Dewald GW, Bryant SC, Winkler JM, Blood E, Oken MM, Santana-Dávila R, González-Paz N, Kyle RA, Gertz MA, Dispenzieri A, Lacy MQ, Greipp PR (2003a) The recurrent IgH translocations are highly associated with nonhyperdiploid variant multiple myeloma. Blood 102:2562–2567

Fonseca R, Blood E, Rue M, Harrington D, Oken MM, Kyle RA, Dewald GW, Van Ness B, Van Wier SA, Henderson KJ, Bailey RJ, Greipp PR (2003b) Clinical and biologic implications of recurrent genomic aberrations in myeloma. Blood 101:4569–4575

Fonseca R, Bergsagel PL, Drach J, Shaughnessy J, Gutierrez N, Stewart AK, Morgan G, Van Ness B, Chesi M, Minvielle S, Neri A, Barlogie B, Kuehl WM, Liebisch P, Davies F, Chen-Kiang S, Durie BG, Carrasco R, Sezer O, Reiman T, Pilarski L, Avet-Loiseau H (2009)

International Myeloma working group molecular classification of multiple myeloma: spotlight review. Leukemia 23:2210–2221
Garand R, Avet-Loiseau H, Accard F, Moreau P, Harousseau JL, Bataille R (2003) t(11;14) and t(4;14) translocations correlated with mature lymphoplasmocytoid and immature morphology, respectively, in multiple myeloma. Leukemia 17:2032–2035
Gertz MA, Lacy MQ, Dispenzieri A, Greipp PR, Litzow MR, Henderson KJ, Van Wier SA, Ahmann GJ, Fonseca R (2005) Clinical implications of t(11;14)(q13;q32), t(4;14)(p16.3;q32) and -17p13 in myeloma patients treated with high-dose therapy. Blood 106:2837–2840
Gonzalez-Paz N, Chng WJ, McClure RF, Blood E, Oken MM, Van Ness B, James CD, Kurtin PJ, Henderson K, Ahmann GJ, Gertz M, Lacy M, Dispenzieri A, Greipp PR, Fonseca R (2007) Tumor suppressor p16 methylation in multiple myeloma: biological and clinical implications. Blood 109:1228–1232
Gutiérrez NC, Sarasquete ME, Misiewicz-Krzeminska I, Delgado M, De Las Rivas J, Ticona FV, Fermiñán E, Martín-Jiménez P, Chillón C, Risueño A, Hernández JM, García-Sanz R, González M, San Miguel JF (2010) Deregulation of microRNA expression in the different genetic subtypes of multiple myeloma and correlation with gene expression profiling. Leukemia 24:629–637
Hoyer JD, Hanson CA, Fonseca R, Greipp PR, Dewald GW, Kurtin PJ (2000) The (11;14) (q13;q32) translocation in multiple myeloma. A morphologic and immunohistochemical study. Am J Clin Pathol 113:831–837
Jenner MW, Leone PE, Walker BA, Ross FM, Johnson DC, Gonzalez D, Chiecchio L, Dachs Cabanas E, Dagrada GP, Nightingale M, Protheroe RK, Stockley D, Else M, Dickens NJ, Cross NC, Davies FE, Morgan GJ (2007) Gene mapping and expression analysis of 16q loss of heterozygosity identifies WWOX and CYLD as being important in determining clinical outcome in multiple myeloma. Blood 110:3291–3300
Keats JJ, Reiman T, Maxwell CA, Taylor BJ, Larratt LM, Mant MJ, Belch AR, Pilarski LM (2003) In multiple myeloma, t(4;14)(p16;q32) is an adverse prognostic factor irrespective of FGFR3 expression. Blood 101:1520–1529
Keats JJ, Fonseca R, Chesi M, Schop R, Baker A, Chng WJ, Van Wier S, Tiedemann R, Shi CX, Sebag M, Braggio E, Henry T, Zhu YX, Fogle H, Price-Troska T, Ahmann G, Mancini C, Brents LA, Kumar S, Greipp P, Dispenzieri A, Bryant B, Mulligan G, Bruhn L, Barrett M et al (2007) Promiscuous mutations activate the noncanonical NF-kappaB pathway in multiple myeloma. Cancer Cell 12:131–144
Kulkarni MS, Daggett JL, Bender TP, Kuehl WM, Bergsagel PL, Williams ME (2002) Frequent inactivation of the cyclin-dependent kinase inhibitor p18 by homozygous deletion in multiple myeloma cell lines: ectopic p18 expression inhibits growth and induces apoptosis. Leukemia 16:127–134
Lionetti M, Biasiolo M, Agnelli L, Todoerti K, Mosca L, Fabris S, Sales G, Deliliers GL, Bicciato S, Lombardi L, Bortoluzzi S, Neri A (2009) Identification of microRNA expression patterns and definition of a microRNA/mRNA regulatory network in distinct molecular groups of multiple myeloma. Blood 114:e20–e26
Liu P, Leong T, Quam L, Billadeau D, Kay NE, Greipp P, Kyle RA, Oken MM, Van Ness B (1996) Activating mutations of N- and K-ras in multiple myeloma show different clinical associations: analysis of the Eastern Cooperative Oncology Group Phase III Trial. Blood 88:2699–2706
Löffler D, Brocke-Heidrich K, Pfeifer G, Stocsits C, Hackermüller J, Kretzschmar AK, Burger R, Gramatzki M, Blumert C, Bauer K, Cvijic H, Ullmann AK, Stadler PF, Horn F (2007) Interleukin-6 dependent survival of multiple myeloma cells involves the Stat3-mediated induction of micro-RNA-21 through a highly conserved enhancer. Blood 110:1330–1333
Mateos MV, García-Sanz R, López-Pérez R, Moro MJ, Ocio E, Hernández J, Megido M, Caballero MD, Fernández-Calvo J, Bárez A, Almeida J, Orfão A, González M, San Miguel JF (2002) Methylation is an inactivating mechanism of the p16 gene in multiple myeloma associated with high plasma cell proliferation and short survival. Br J Haematol 118:1034–1040
Molnar S, Zepeda VJJ, Van Wier S, Braggio E, Keats J, Kuehl M, Price-Troska T, Ahmann G, Rempel R, Henderson K, Rajkumar SV, Greipp PR, Auclair D, Carpten J, Baker A, Stewart K, Bergsagel L,

Chng WJ, Fonseca R (2008) Loss of p53 is a marker of progression in plasma cell neoplasias and is a negative prognostic factor in relapsed disease. Blood (ASH Annu Meet Abstr) 112:1663

Moreau P, Facon T, Leleu X, Morineau N, Huyghe P, Harousseau JL, Bataille R, Avet-Loiseau H (2002) Recurrent 14q32 translocations determine the prognosis of multiple myeloma, especially in patients receiving intensive chemotherapy. Blood 100:1579–1583

Moreau P, Robillard N, Jégo G, Pellat C, Le Gouill S, Thoumi S, Avet-Loiseau H, Harousseau JL, Bataille R (2006) Lack of CD27 in myeloma delineates different presentation and outcome. Br J Haematol 132:168–170

Pichiorri F, Suh SS, Ladetto M, Kuehl M, Palumbo T, Drandi D, Taccioli C, Zanesi N, Alder H, Hagan JP, Munker R, Volinia S, Boccadoro M, Garzon R, Palumbo A, Aqeilan RI, Croce CM (2008) MicroRNAs regulate critical genes associated with multiple myeloma pathogenesis. Proc Natl Acad Sci USA 105:12885–12890

Rasmussen T, Kuehl M, Lodahl M, Johnsen HE, Dahl IM (2005) Possible roles for activating RAS mutations in the MGUS to MM transition and in the intramedullary to extramedullary transition some plasma cell tumors. Blood 105:317–323

Sarasquete ME, García-Sanz R, Armellini A, Fuertes M, Martín-Jiménez P, Sierra M, Del Chillón Carmen M, Alcoceba M, Balanzategui A, Ortega F, Hernández JM, Sureda A, Palomera L, González M, San Miguel JF (2006) The association of increased p14ARF/p16INK4a and p15INK4a gene expression with proliferative activity and the clinical course of multiple myeloma. Haematologica 91:1551–1554

Sawyer JR, Tricot G, Mattox S, Jagannath S, Barlogie B (1998) Jumping translocations of chromosome 1q in multiple myeloma: evidence for a mechanism involving decondensation of pericentromeric heterochromatin. Blood 91:1732–1741

Sawyer JR, Lukacs JL, Thomas EL, Swanson CM, Goosen LS, Sammartino G, Gilliland JC, Munshi NC, Tricot G, Shaughnessy JD Jr, Barlogie B (2001) Multicolour spectral karyotyping identifies new translocations and a recurring pathway for chromosome loss in multiple myeloma. Br J Haematol 112:167–174

Sawyer JR, Tricot G, Lukacs JL, Binz RL, Tian E, Barlogie B, Shaughnessy J Jr (2005) Genomic instability in multiple myeloma: evidence for jumping segmental duplications of chromosome arm 1q. Genes Chromosomes Cancer 42:95–106

Schilling G, Hansen T, Shimoni A, Zabelina T, Perez-Simon JA, Gutierrez NC, Bethge W, Liebisch P, Schwerdtfeger R, Bornhauser M, Otterstetter S, Penas EM, Dierlamm J, Ayuk F, Atanackovic D, Bacher U, Bokemeyer C, Zander A, San Miguel J, Nagler A, Kröger N (2008) Impact of genetic abnormalities on survival after allogeneic hematopoietic stem cell transplantation in multiple myeloma. Leukemia 22:1250–1255

Shaughnessy J Jr, Gabrea A, Qi Y, Brents L, Zhan F, Tian E, Sawyer J, Barlogie B, Bergsagel PL, Kuehl M (2001) Cyclin D3 at 6p21 is dysregulated by recurrent chromosomal translocations to immunoglobulin loci in multiple myeloma. Blood 98:217–223

Shaughnessy JD Jr, Zhan F, Burington BE, Huang Y, Colla S, Hanamura I, Stewart JP, Kordsmeier B, Randolph C, Williams DR, Xiao Y, Xu H, Epstein J, Anaissie E, Krishna SG, Cottler-Fox M, Hollmig K, Mohiuddin A, Pineda-Roman M, Tricot G, van Rhee F, Sawyer J, Alsayed Y, Walker R, Zangari M et al (2007) A validated gene expression model of high-risk multiple myeloma is defined by deregulated expression of genes mapping to chromosome 1. Blood 109:2276–2284

Smadja NV, Bastard C, Brigaudeau C, Leroux D, Fruchart C (2001) Hypodiploidy is a major prognostic factor in multiple myeloma. Blood 98:2229–2238

Tasaka T, Berenson J, Vescio R, Hirama T, Miller CW, Nagai M, Takahara J, Koeffler HP (1997) Analysis of the p16INK4A, p15INK4B and p18INK4C genes in multiple myeloma. Br J Haematol 96:98–102

Tiedemann RE, Gonzalez-Paz N, Kyle RA, Santana-Davila R, Price-Troska T, Van Wier SA, Chng WJ, Ketterling RP, Gertz MA, Henderson K, Greipp PR, Dispenzieri A, Lacy MQ, Rajkumar SV, Bergsagel PL, Stewart AK, Fonseca R (2008) Genetic aberrations and survival in plasma cell leukemia. Leukemia 22:1044–1052

Walker BA, Leone PE, Jenner MW, Li C, Gonzalez D, Johnson DC, Ross FM, Davies FE, Morgan GJ (2006) Integration of global SNP-based mapping and expression arrays reveals key regions, mechanisms, and genes important in the pathogenesis of multiple myeloma. Blood 108:1733–1743
Wuilleme S, Robillard N, Lodé L, Magrangeas F, Beris H, Harousseau JL, Proffitt J, Minvielle S, Avet-Loiseau H (2005) Ploidy, as detected by fluorescence in situ hybridization, defines different subgroups in multiple myeloma. Leukemia 19:275–278

Chapter 5
Chronic Lymphocytic Leukemia

Anton W. Langerak and Yorick Sandberg

Abstract Human chronic lymphocytic leukemia (CLL) is the most common form of leukemia in the Western world. CLL has long been believed to be a single disease, but recent insights underline the biological and clinical heterogeneity of CLL. Recognition of CLL subgroups with a completely different pathophysiology and clinical course, has paved the way to better define high-risk CLL patients based on prognostic factors, to predict response to therapy, and to estimate progression-free and overall survival. Moreover, knowledge of different aspects of the (immuno) pathogenesis of CLL (genomic and epigenetic aberrations, antigenic stimulation, microenvironmental stimuli) has greatly increased. These insights are key to further develop preventive strategies and to design innovative therapeutic strategies.

5.1 Introduction

Chronic lymphocytic leukemia (CLL) is the most common form of leukemia in the Western world. The incidence of CLL is estimated to be almost 4/100,000 individuals, whereas every year 15,000 (US)—20,000 (Europe) new CLL patients are diagnosed (Zenz et al. 2010). Incidence rates differ significantly between men and

A. W. Langerak (✉) · Y. Sandberg
Department of Immunology, Erasmus MC, University Medical Center Rotterdam, Dr. Molewaterplein 50, 3015, GE, Rotterdam, The Netherlands
e-mail: a.langerak@erasmusmc.nl

Y. Sandberg
Department of Internal Medicine, Erasmus MC, University Medical Center Rotterdam, Rotterdam, The Netherlands

M. Witt et al. (eds.), *Molecular Aspects of Hematologic Malignancies*, Principles and Practice, DOI: 10.1007/978-3-642-29467-9_5,

women, with CLL occurring twice as often in males. With a median age at diagnosis of >70 years, CLL typically is a disease of the elderly.

For a very long time no new insights into CLL pathogenesis were obtained, whereas progress in therapy was hardly reached. Two major developments have changed this. First, the clinical recognition that CLL is not a single disease but is rather heterogeneous in its presentation and disease course, was substantiated by new insights into prognostically relevant biological factors. This has resulted in much more attention for molecular pathogenesis and prognostication in CLL, with many new markers being evaluated and implemented. Second, the application of therapeutic antibodies, either as monotherapy, but mostly in combination with other drugs (chemo-immunotherapy), has caused enormous improvement in progression-free and overall survival.

Hence, there is a growing interest in studying CLL in both basic and translational research, as well as clinical trials. In this chapter the current concepts of CLL molecular (immuno) pathogenesis are discussed in view of their translational and clinical implications.

5.2 Clinical Heterogeneity and CLL Pathogenesis

CLL is characterized by the accumulation in the blood of small, rounded lymphocytes with scanty cytoplasm, and a typical immunophenotype ($CD5^{+}$, $CD23^{+}$, $CD20^{dim}$, $CD79^{dim}$, surface immunoglobulin $[sIg]^{dim}$) (Dighiero and Hamblin 2008). Circulating CLL cells are arrested in the G0/G1 phase of the cell cycle and show a low proliferation rate. Proliferation of CLL typically occurs in proliferation centers (pseudo-follicles) in bone marrow or lymph nodes. Upon exit from bone marrow or nodes, the circulating CLL cells accumulate due to disturbances in apoptosis.

Despite the seemingly homogeneous nature of CLL cells, CLL is not a single disease entity. Rather, CLL is characterized by a remarkable heterogeneity, with some patients being asymptomatic at diagnosis, and others presenting with lymph node enlargement, bone marrow failure, or other features (e.g. fatigue, autoimmune hemolytic anemia). A considerable fraction of CLL patients shows a relatively indolent clinical course over a period of 10–20 years, often without requiring any type of therapy ("watch and wait"). This group of patients will eventually die with CLL, but not from CLL. Other CLL patients have a clinically more aggressive disease for which therapy is needed. The two major complications that CLL patients suffer from are cytopenia (anemia, thrombocytopenia) and (secondary) immunodeficiency (related to low serum Ig levels).

CLL patients are generally classified according to clinical staging systems, named after Binet and Rai. Both the Binet (A–C) and Rai (0–IV) classifications take into account the extent of the disease in predicting tumor aggressiveness and survival. Age, co-morbidity, and performance status are also clear predictors of survival (Table 5.1). Although these clinical classifications have their prognostic

Table 5.1 Prognostic factors in CLL

Classical prognostic factors	Recent (biological) prognostic factors
Age	Soluble CD23 levels
Rai (0–IV) or Binet (A-C) stage	Membrane markers (CD38, ZAP70)
Performance status	Chromosomal aberrations
Co-morbidity	IGHV mutational status
Serum markers (lactate dehydrogenase, β2-microglobulin, thymidine kinase)	Molecular markers (LPL, ADAM29, SNPs)
Bone marrow infiltration pattern	Minimal residual disease (MRD)
Lymphocyte doubling time	

ADAM29, a disintegrin and metalloprotease domain family 29; *CD*, cluster of differentiation; *LPL*, lipoprotien lipase; *SNP*, single nucleotide polymorphism; *ZAP70*, zeta–associated protien 70

value, a further search has been conducted for biological parameters with a predictive value at diagnosis (Table 5.1).

Collectively, these markers point to a complex pathophysiology. Although the biological features and mechanisms are beginning to be disclosed, the exact underlying pathogenic mechanisms in CLL are still incompletely understood. In spite of that, it is now generally accepted that both *intrinsic* (genomic aberrations and mutations, epigenetic modifications) and *external* (B-cell receptor (BCR)-mediated antigenic stimulation, microenvironmental stimuli) events contribute to CLL pathogenesis (Zenz et al. 2010).

5.3 Genetics and Epigenetics

5.3.1 Genetic Susceptibility

CLL shows a strong familial predisposition (elevated risk of 7 % in first-degree relatives), but studies identifying involved loci are scarce. In one of the few large studies on familial CLL, several associated chromosome regions were identified, but definition of involved loci was lacking (Sellick et al. 2005). Large-scale genome-wide association studies of CLL patients and controls using single nucleotide polymorphisms (SNPs) have revealed 10 CLL risk loci at several different chromosomal regions (Di Bernardo et al. 2008, Crowther-Swanepoel et al. 2010). So far no high-penetrance (causative) genes have been identified, thus supporting a polygenic model of several low-penetrance susceptibility loci. In another susceptibility study, the main focus was on mapping SNPs in genes involved in the DNA damage response and in cell cycle pathways (Rudd et al. 2006). Based on the idea of a possible etiological role of (in-) directly mutagenic chemical agents in CLL (Blair et al. 2007), SNPs in genes implicated in the three main DNA repair pathways were recently studied. Clear differences were found for SNPs in *ERCC2* (excision-repair complementing defective in Chinese hamster 2;

Table 5.2 Most relevant characteristics of recurrent genomic aberrations in CLL

Chromosomal aberration	Gene(s) involved	Overall incidence (%)[a]	Incidence in refractory CLL (%)[b]	Overall survival (months)[a]
11q23 deletion	*ATM*, other (?)	18	25	79
Trisomy 12	Unknown	16	12	114
13q14 deletion	*miR-15a*, *miR-16-1*	55	25	133
17p13 deletion	*TP53*	7	31	32
No clear aberration	?	~18	Unknown	111

[a] According to Döhner et al. (2000)
[b] According to Zenz et al. (2010)

a component of nucleotide-excision repair) and *XRCC1* (X-ray repair complementing defective in Chinese hamster 1; a component of base-excision repair system) loci between CLL patients with unfavorable cytogenetic aberrations and controls, which suggests that DNA repair SNPs could be related to outcome in CLL (Ganster et al. 2009).

5.3.2 Genomic Aberrations and Epigenetics

Based on limited karyotypic data (only for 40–50 % of CLL cases enough metaphases are obtained) mostly complemented by fluorescence in situ hybridization data, it has become evident that there are no recurrent CLL translocations. Rather, CLL is characterized by multiple chromosomal aberrations that together occur in approximately 80 % of cases. These especially concern deletions of chromosomal regions 17p, 11q or 13q, and trisomy of chromosome 12 (Table 5.2). The presence of these aberrations correlates with the clinical heterogeneity of CLL (Döhner et al. 2000; Zenz et al. 2010), corroborating the idea that CLL is not a single disease.

Deletions of chromosome band 13q14 are the most frequent genetic events in CLL (roughly 50 %), correlating with a more favorable prognosis (Table 5.2). The 13q14 region encompasses the *miR15a* and *miR16-1* microRNA genes, which target the survival factor BCL2 (B-cell CLL/Lymphoma 2) (Calin et al. 2002). Loss of these miRs would give rise to high BCL2 levels, and thus to enhanced survival. Interestingly, mice with deletion/mutation in the *miR15a/16-1* cluster region develop a human CLL-like disease (Raveche et al. 2007; Klein et al. 2010). Trisomy 12 occurs in ~15 % of CLL, but the genes relevant for CLL pathogenesis are unknown. Initially, trisomy 12 was suggested to be associated with a shorter time to progression, but this has not been convincingly confirmed in later studies. The median overall survival is very similar to CLL with 13q14 deletions (Table 5.2).

Another frequent deletion concerns (part of) the long arm of chromosome 11 (in 10–20 % of early stage CLL to >20 % of refractory CLL), which identifies a CLL subgroup with a clearly inferior outcome (Table 5.2). The *ATM* (ataxia-telangiectasia mutated) gene has been identified as the most important candidate gene in this region (Austen et al. 2007). *ATM* mutations are known to occur in approximately 12 % of CLL; in about one-third of CLL with a 11q23 deletion they are present on the second allele (Austen et al. 2007). ATM dysfunction leads to loss of cell cycle control and p53 dysfunction, resulting in disturbed apoptosis. Interestingly, the *TP53* (tumor protein) gene itself is the primary gene implicated in deletions involving band 17p13. Strikingly, in >80 % of cases the second allele harbors *TP53* mutations, thus leading to a functional loss of p53 activity (Zenz et al. 2010). CLL with 17p aberrations form a minor subgroup in early CLL (around 5 %), but its proportion increases in refractory CLL (>30 %) (Table 5.2). Defects in either ATM or p53, which collectively may occur in up to 30 % of CLL patients, lead to impaired DNA damage response and are correlated to therapy resistance and poor survival. In this CLL subgroup impairment in the activation of p53 is the common event underlying resistance to drugs such as fludarabine through disrupted apoptosis induction.

Finally, epigenetic analysis of sporadic CLL has revealed global DNA hypomethylation possibly resulting in genomic instability, in combination with CpG island hypermethylation of particular genes (Zenz et al. 2010). Moreover, genome-wide methylation analysis suggests differential methylation patterns between different CLL subgroups (Kanduri et al. 2010).

5.4 Antigenic Stimulation and B-Cell Receptor (BCR) Sinaling

5.4.1 IGHV SHM Status

At the end of the 1990s it was shown in two independent seminal studies that the somatic hypermutation (SHM) status of the rearranged immunoglobulin heavy variable (IGHV) genes is a very informative prognostic parameter in CLL (Damle et al. 1999; Hamblin et al. 1999). SHM formation is a physiological process in germinal centers (GC) of lymph node follicles, characterized by random introduction of mutations within rearranged genes at rates of $\sim 10^{-5}$–10^{-3} mutations per base pair per generation ($\sim 10^{6}$-fold higher than spontaneous mutation rate). It is now well-established that CLL cases can be categorized into two clinically meaningful subsets using the IGHV SHM status; one subset with mutated IGHV genes (<98 % identity to closest germline IGHV gene) showing a more favorable outcome; and a second subset with unmutated IGHV genes (≥98 % identity) generally showing a poor response to therapy and an inferior overall survival. CLL with a 17p deletion often shows therapy resistance, which is in keeping with their poor survival. Not surprisingly, 11q and 17p deletions were almost exclusively found in unmutated CLL (see below), whilst 13q14 deletions are clearly overrepresented in mutated CLL; trisomy 12 cases are divided over both groups (Kröber et al. 2002). IGHV SHM status even seems to have prognostic value independent of the Binet and Rai clinical stage (Dighiero and Hamblin 2008). This has led to its utilization for inclusion or stratification of CLL patients in many clinical protocols.

Several surrogate markers for IGHV SHM status have been evaluated, such as CD38 (cyclic ADP ribose hydrolase), ZAP70 (zeta-chain-associated protein kinase 70), and LPL (lipoprotein lipase) (Oppezzo et al. 2005; Heintel et al. 2005). None of them has so far replaced IGHV SHM status as reliable and robust marker for multicentre studies. IGHV SHM status, though cumbersome, still is the most informative marker (Chap. 26 on IGHV gene analysis). Another argument for IGHV SHM status analysis is that important prognostic information resides in BCR molecules. For example, CLL cases with IGHV3-21 usage are mostly mutated but show poorer overall survival than mutated CLL as a whole (Tobin et al. 2002; Lin et al. 2003; Thorsélius et al. 2006). This has revitalized in-depth studies on the role of the BCR in CLL.

5.4.2 Stereotyped BCRs

Already more than a decade ago, it was hypothesized that CLL cells are selected by antigenic pressure (pathogenic bacteria, apoptotic cells, or even auto-antigens) (Johnson et al. 1997). This hypothesis emerged from early studies showing that the IGHV gene repertoire of CLL is highly restricted and biased as compared to the normal adult B-cell repertoire (Kipps et al. 1989; Schroeder and Dighiero 1994). In unmutated CLL, increased usage of IGHV1-69 was observed, whereas IGHV4-34, IGHV3-23, and IGHV3-7 were more frequently seen in mutated CLL (Fais et al. 1998). Since CLL typically occurs in elderly patients, it was evaluated whether similar shifts in IGHV usage appear in normal B cells upon aging. IGHV1-69 is not found to be increased in normal elderly, whereas IGHV4-34 can be, probably related to herpes virus reactivation. Also, clear associations between IGHV and IGHJ genes have been found in CLL, e.g., IGHV3-7 and IGHJ4 (~90 %), IGHV4-34 and IGHJ6 (~50 %), IGHV1-69 and IGHJ6 (Fais et al. 1998; Widhopf and Kipps 2001; Potter et al. 2003). In addition, an almost exclusive association with the same light chain (IGKV3-20) was noted for the IGHV1-69/IGHJ6 subgroup. Another striking example is IGHV3-21 usage in combination IGLV3-21 usage in a subset of CLL patients (Tobin et al. 2003).

Another important observation on the role of the BCR in CLL biology was the finding that up to 30 % of CLL cases show very similar gene usage and homologous IGH antigen-recognition complementarity determining region 3 (HCDR3) motifs. This phenomenon is referred to as *stereotyped BCR* (Fig. 5.1),

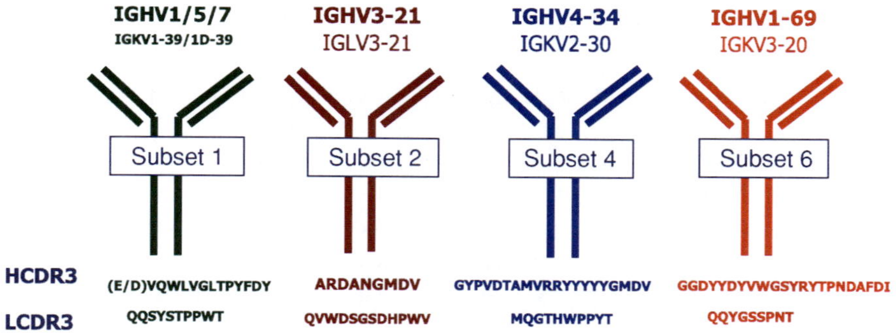

Fig. 5.1 Clinico-biologically relevant stereotyped CLL subsets. Indicated are the characteristic IGHV and IGKV / IGLV genes per stereotyped subset, as well as the amino acid residues in the respective CDR3 motifs, HCDR3 and LCDR3. Stereotyped subsets are based on data obtained by (Stamatopoulos 2007) and (Murray et al. 2008). Figure obtained from Dr. R. Rosenquist, Uppsala, Sweden and reproduced with permission

(Stamatopoulos et al. 2007; Murray et al. 2008; Darzentas et al. 2010). Interestingly, the frequency of stereotypy varies between different CLL groups, ranging from 11 % in mutated CLL to >40 % in unmutated CLL, and being high in, e.g., IGHV3-21, and IGHV1-69 CLL cases. Moreover, even CLL-biased deletions and particular SHM patterns were found to be associated with stereotyped CLL subsets (Belessi et al. 2006; Murray et al. 2008). Thus, CLL can now largely be divided into two categories: one (consisting of approximately 30 % of primarily unmutated CLL cases) with a very restricted repertoire and BCR stereotypy (clustered cases); a second with a heterogeneous BCR (nonclustered cases).

Importantly, stereotyped BCRs not only have biological impact but also seem to confer prognostic information in addition to, but also independently of, IGHV SHM status (Ghia et al. 2005; Stamatopoulos et al. 2007). This is particularly true for IGHV3-21/IGLV3-21 expressing CLL, which showed more progressive disease than other IGHV3-21 cases (heterogeneous HCDR3 and variable light chain gene usage) (Ghia et al. 2005). Interestingly, stereotyped IGHV4-34 CLL seem to have a better prognosis than heterogeneous IGHV4-34 cases.

Collectively, the current data strongly point toward a model that CLL development is not so much a random event in the elderly B-cell population, but rather represents a stepwise process in which BCR-mediated antigen stimulation is clearly implicated (Stamatopoulos 2009). BCR stimulation could act as a factor triggering initial transformation and further promoting acquisition of additional genetic lesions (Chiorazzi and Ferrarini 2011). The importance of BCR signaling is even further underscored by the recent observation of intraclonal diversity in an IGHV4-34 expressing stereotypic subset, which is suggestive of ongoing antigenic stimulation via the BCR (Sutton et al. 2009).

5.4.3 Nature of Antigens Recognized by BCRs

The idea that antigen-specificity of the BCR seems a critical factor in CLL biology and clinical course, has prompted the quest for the antigen(s) implicated in BCR stimulation. This might disclose the etiology and immunopathogenesis of CLL, and potentially provide clues to prevention and/or treatment of the disease.

It may not be surprising that unmutated and mutated CLL would recognize different types of antigens, given the differences in SHM levels of their BCR. Mutated CLL generally express oligo-/monoreactive antibodies that most likely develop in a T-cell-dependent manner. In contrast, unmutated CLL tend to express BCR with long HCDR3 motifs and amino acid residues that favor polyreactivity, thus resembling natural antibodies. Natural antibodies are associated with autoreactivity and are often stereotyped, a feature most frequently seen in unmutated CLL. However, polyreactivity is certainly not restricted to stereotyped antigen-binding sites. It has actually been suggested that both unmutated and mutated CLL originate from auto-reactive B-cell precursors, but that SHM plays an important role in mutated CLL to alter this original BCR auto-reactivity (Hervé et al. 2005).

Certain stereotyped BCR are known to recognize antigenic structures on apoptotic cells (Chu et al. 2008), which might reflect an intrinsic property of such B cells to clear cellular debris and/or dead microorganisms. In other cases, the BCR encoded by the CLL cells shares features with auto-antibodies; one example is the similarity between rheumatoid factor and the BCR in unmutated CLL of the IGHV1-69/IGKV3-20 subset. Another example is the mutated IGHV4-34 CLL subset, which shows a stereotyped BCR that is characterized by a long, positively charged HCDR3 (Murray et al. 2008). As IGHV4-34 antibodies constitute a considerable fraction of the characteristic anti-DNA antibodies in systemic lupus erythematodes patients, the IGHV4-34 CLL subset may thus have originated from a progenitor cell with anti-DNA specificity, although this reactivity could have been abrogated in the CLL cells through SHM-based editing.

It has been shown that $\sim$60 % of CLL BCR molecules were polyreactive and bound to apoptotic cell surfaces (Catera et al. 2008). Structures recognized typically comprised two types of antigens: (1) native molecules, relocated to the external cell surface during apoptosis; (2) neoantigens, generated by oxidation during apoptosis. Some of the oxidized epitopes appeared to be similar to microbial epitopes.

Although the exact antigens are not yet known for all CLL cases, a picture is now beginning to emerge that often CLL may derive from normal B cells that function to remove cellular debris, and/or provide a first defense line against pathogens. Sustained antigenic stimulation via their BCR and an activated cell state are key steps in CLL leukemogenesis, a process in which additional genetic lesions are subsequently acquired.

5.4.4 Cell of Origin

Initially, it was hypothesized that unmutated CLL are derived from antigen-inexperienced naïve B cells, and mutated CLL would stem from memory B cells that have undergone a germinal center reaction. However, gene expression profiling experiments have shown that the transcriptome of both CLL subgroups is not that different and mostly resembles that of memory cells (Klein et al. 2001; Rosenwald et al. 2001). Both CLL subgroups are thus believed to be derived from antigen-experienced B cells, which differ in their SHM level and especially in the way they are selected for their antigen-specificity (Chiorazzi and Ferrarini 2011). In this model, mutated CLL could be considered as the counterparts of memory B cells that mostly have developed from a GC-dependent developmental pathway, or alternatively from a marginal zone (MZ) pathway. Unmutated CLL would also originate from antigen-experienced memory-like B cells, the difference being that such cells had not been able to alter their BCR by mutation during differentiation.

Based on detailed bioinformatic analysis, it has also been hypothesized that different CLL categories might have a distinct ontogeny. CLL cases with a heterogeneous BCR likely derive from precursor cells of the conventional B-cell pool, whereas cases with a stereotyped BCR could originate from progenitor cells that are intermediate between the true innate and the conventional adaptive B-cell immune system (Darzentas et al. 2010).

5.4.5 BCR Signaling

An important effect of antigen binding to the BCR is the activation of downstream signaling pathways resulting in further proliferation and survival of the cells. However, upon interaction with antigen the surface IgM molecule is downregulated, thus suggesting that CLL that just entered circulation could show lower BCR responsiveness than CLL cells in the tissue sites. Following reexpression in the circulation, CLL cells may enter the tissues again with increased responsiveness. Despite this reversible pattern of surface IgM expression, circulating mutated and unmutated CLL cells persistently differ intrinsically in their BCR responsiveness. Unmutated CLL have retained signaling capacity via the BCR, whereas mutated CLL are anergized by downregulation of the surface IgM molecules (Mockridge et al. 2007). The state of anergy in mutated CLL most probably reflects a real difference in the type and length of antigen stimulation in tissues between unmutated and mutated CLL.

5.5 Signals from the Microenvironment

It is well documented that CLL cells undergo spontaneous apoptosis in vitro, despite their accumulation in vivo. This underlines the importance of external signals that allow CLL cells to survive and expand in vivo (Burger 2011). Such external signals are transmitted by various cell types that are collectively referred to as the microenvironment: T cells, antigen presenting cells (APC), and stromal cells (monocyte-derived nurse-like cells, NLC; mesenchymal stromal cells, MSC; follicular dendritic cells). CLL cells are involved in a spectrum of cellular and molecular interactions with cells in the leukemia microenvironment, which results in their survival, expansion, and protection.

Similar to their normal counterparts, CLL cells have the capacity to enter tissue microenvironments via adhesion molecules and chemokine receptors (Burger 2011). VLA-4 (integrin alpha 4) is an important integrin molecule on CLL cells that binds the VCAM-1 (vascular cell adhesion molecule 1) on endothelial cells. Interactions between CD38 on CLL cells and CD31 (platelet endothelial cell adhesion molecule; PECAM-1) on NLC provide an important survival signal. CLL cells show high expression of the chemokine receptor CXCR4 (chemokine cxc motif receptor 4), which binds CXCL12 (chemokine cxc motif ligand 12) that is secreted by NLC and MSC in the microenvironment. Expression levels of another chemokine receptor (CXCR3) might be variable on CLL cells, with low expression being associated with advanced stage CLL and poor survival (Ocana et al. 2007). Chemokine receptors are G-protein coupled receptors with downstream signaling molecules, similar to the kinases downstream of the BCR. Studies with small molecule inhibitors for these signaling kinases are underscoring the importance of these molecules for CLL tissue homing and retention. Administration of the inhibitors causes a transient increase in CLL cells in the circulation through mobilization effects. Collectively, adhesion molecules and chemokine receptors thus mediate migration of CLL cells into the tissue microenvironment and adhesion to stromal cells.

Importantly, CLL cells themselves also secrete chemokines (CCL3, CCL4; chemokine CC motif ligand 3 and 4, respectively) which attract monocytes and particularly T-lymphocytes. CCL3/CCL4 secretion is increased upon BCR stimulation of CLL cells or in vitro through co-culture with NLC (Burger et al. 2009). Of note, high CCL3 plasma levels seem to be correlated to poor prognostic markers (Sivina et al. 2011); whether this is directly related to the attraction of T-cells remains to be established. Another important molecular communication between CLL cells and T-cells concerns the CD40 ligand (on T)—CD40 (costimulatory protein on CLL cells) interaction, which provides a survival signal in vitro and perhaps mediates tissue events in vivo (Wierda et al. 2000). In CLL patients normal T-cell function seems to be compromised by the tumor or by reactivated viruses (Mackus et al. 2003). Still, the exact role of T-cells as accessory cells in CLL is not completely understood.

5.6 Prognostic and Therapeutic Implications

As discussed, many different molecular features and cellular processes underlie CLL biology and clinical behavior. Although all these factors impact, to some extent, the survival of CLL patients, the most relevant biological prognostic markers in CLL clinical management seem to be cytogenetic features (i.e., genomic aberrations), and IGHV SHM status. According to the international workshop on CLL (iwCLL) guidelines (Hallek et al. 2008), only cytogenetic analysis is recommended for CLL patients in routine practice, but in clinical trials cytogenetic analysis as well as IGHV SHM analysis (along with CD38 and ZAP70) are considered mandatory pretreatment tests. Importantly, in some trials IGHV3-21 usage is considered an independent predictor of poor prognosis. It remains to be shown whether other stereotyped BCR should also be considered as independent prognostic markers. Currently, much effort is put in defining the prognostic value of subgroups with such stereotyped BCR in large international CLL cohorts. Multivariate analyses will eventually disclose the most relevant independent prognostic factors to be used in future CLL classification.

Prognostic information is currently being exploited in two different ways in CLL. First, to define high-risk CLL patients for inclusion in clinical trials. This is mostly done based on 17p deletions, *TP53* mutations, 11q deletions, and/or an unmutated IGH SHM status. Second, to identify patients that might benefit from other treatment strategies. A good example is the ultra high-risk CLL patients (with 17p deletions and/or *TP53* mutations), who show a high risk of early relapse or progression upon FCR (fludarabine, cyclophosphamide, and rituximab = monoclonal antibody against B-lymphocyte CD20 antigen) therapy. Due to their disrupted p53 activity, these patients are refractory to fludarabine and possibly also to other forms of chemotherapy that depend on a good functioning of response to DNA damage. Hence, such patients could benefit from novel treatment modalities that are not dependent on proper p53 action.

Results from the German CLL8 trial have shown that for CLL patients in first-line treatment chemo-immunotherapy (FCR) is superior over chemotherapy alone (Hallek et al. 2010). FCR has now become the gold standard for comparing new treatment modalities. As CLL patients with 17p deletions or *TP53* mutations do not seem to benefit from FCR therapy, other therapeutic options might be chosen upfront for those patients, such as CamPath (alemtuzumab, monoclonal antibody for CD52 antigen) or CamPath plus prednisolone. Also in refractory patients alemtuzumab could be an alternative, as might be allogeneic stem cell transplantation (Dreger et al. 2010), or novel agents (see below). Another approach in CLL patients refractory to fludarabine and alemtuzumab is the use of ofatumumab (Wierda et al. 2010). Ofatumumab is a new generation type I CD20 monoclonal antibody that shows a higher complement-dependent cytotoxicity (CDC) and a slower CD20 off-rate than rituximab. The new glycoengineered (type II) CD20 monoclonal antibody GA101 shows a much better antibody-dependent cell death

Table 5.3 Novel therapeutic targets in CLL

Target	Agent	Type of agent
CD20 antigen	Rituximab	(type I) antibody
	Ofatumumab	(type I) antibody
	GA101	(type II) antibody
CD52 antigen	Alemtuzumab (CamPath)	Antibody
CXCR4	Plerixafor (AMD3100)	Small molecule inhibitor
VLA-4	Natalizumab	Antibody
Syk	Fostamatinib disodium	Small molecule inhibitor
Btk	PCI-32765	Small molecule inhibitor
PI3 K-δ	CAL-101	Small molecule inhibitor

Btk, Bruton's tyrosine kinase, *PI3 K-*δ, phosphatidyl inositol 3 kinase–delta; *Syk*, spleen tyrosine kinase

(ADCC) and apoptosis than type I CD20 monoclonal antibodies. Phase III trials are ongoing to establish its effect on survival in CLL patients.

Apart from optimization of CD20 antibody therapies, novel agents against biological targets are being evaluated (Table 5.3). These include CXCR4 antagonists, but also small molecules inhibiting kinases downstream of the BCR (Andritsos et al. 2010; Friedberg et al. 2010; Honigberg et al. 2010; Lannuti et al. 2011). Interestingly, these kinase inhibitors often result in a transient lymphocytosis in the first weeks after treatment. This possibly reflects CLL cell mobilization from the protective tissue environment into the blood, making the cells more vulnerable to the effects of therapeutic agents, next to direct inhibitory effects on BCR signaling. Although the true value of these novel therapeutic targets remains to be determined, many options exist thanks to the increased knowledge of CLL biology.

5.7 Conclusions

Human CLL has evolved over the last 10–15 years from a poorly studied, incurable disease into a disease that is extensively studied by many researchers worldwide. At the basis of this interest is the pivotal finding that CLL is biologically and clinically much more heterogeneous than was initially assumed. Recognition of CLL subgroups with a completely different pathophysiology and clinical course, has paved the way to better define high-risk CLL patients based on prognostic factors, to predict response to therapy, and to estimate progression-free and overall survival. Moreover, knowledge of various intrinsic and external features of the (immuno) pathogenesis of CLL (genomic and epigenetic aberrations, BCR stimulation and antigen type, microenvironmental stimuli) has greatly increased. These insights are key to further develop preventive strategies (avoidance of external stimuli) and to design innovative therapeutic strategies. In that respect many potential targets have been identified, for which small molecule inhibitors or antibodies are being tested in models or being evaluated in phase I/II trials. Agents modifying methylation and acetylation patterns might also become interesting options.

The main challenge will now be to develop treatment modalities that include multiple agents, preferably in a tailored strategy in which eligibility of patients is defined by prognostic markers. With the expected improvements in CLL survival through such strategies, cure can become a realistic goal in at least a proportion of CLL patients. Minimal residual disease analysis via PCR or preferably multicolor flow cytometry will be essential to monitor leukemia kinetics (in view of risk group stratification) and to predict relapse (in view of adaptation of treatment strategy).

References

Andritsos LA, Byrd JC, Hewes B, Kipps TJ, Johns D, Burger JA (2010) Preliminary results from a phase I/II dose escalation study to determine the maximum tolerated dose of plerixafor in combination with rituximab in patients with relapsed chronic lymphocytic leukemia. Haematologica 95:A772

Austen B, Skowronska A, Baker C, Powel JE, Gardiner A, Oscier D, Majid A, Dyer M, Siebert R, Taylor AM, Moss PA, Stankovic T (2007) Mutation status of the residual ATM allele is an important determinant of the cellular response to chemotherapy and survival in patients with chronic lymphocytic leukemia containing an 11q deletion. J Clin Oncol 25:5448–5457

Belessi CJ, Davi FB, Stamatopoulos KE, Degano M, Andreou TM, Moreno C, Merle-Béral H, Crespo M, Laoutaris NP, Montserrat E, Caligaris-Cappio F, Anagnostopoulos AZ, Ghia P (2006) IGHV gene insertions and deletions in chronic lymphocytic leukemia: "CLL-biased" deletions in a subset of cases with stereotyped receptors. Eur J Immunol 36:1963–1974

Blair A, Purue MP, Weisenburger DD, Baris D (2007) Chemical exposures and risk of chronic lymphocytic leukemia. Br J Haematol 139:753–761

Burger JA, Quiroga MP, Hartmann E, Burkle A, Wierda WG, Keating MJ, Rosenwald A (2009) High-level expression of T-cell chemokines CCL3 and CCL4 by chronic lymphocytic leukemia B cells in nurse like cell cocultures and after BCR stimulation. Blood 113: 3050–3058

Burger JA (2011) Mechanisms of leukemia cell trafficking, homing, and tissue retention in CLL. Hematol Education 5:91–99

Chiorazzi N, Ferrarini M (2011) Cellular origin(s) of chronic lymphocytic leukemia: cautionary notes and additional considerations and possibilities. Blood 117:1781–1791

Calin GA, Dumitru CD, Shimizu M, Bichi R, Zupo S, Noch E, Aldler H, Rattan S, Keating M, Rai K, Rassenti L, Kipps T, Negrini M, Bullrich F, Croce CM (2002) Frequent deletions and down-regulation of miR15 and miR16 at 13q14 in chronic lymphocytic leukemia. Proc Natl Acad Sci USA 99:15524–15529

Catera R, Silverman GJ, Hatzi K, Seiler T, Didier S, Zhang L, Hervé M, Meffre E, Oscier DG, Vlassara H, Scofield RH, Chen Y, Allen SL, Kolitz J, Rai KR, Chu CC, Chiorazzi N (2008) Chronic lymphocytic leukemia cells recognize conserved epitopes associated with apoptosis and oxidation. Mol Med 14:665–674

Chu CC, Catera R, Hatzi K, Yan XJ, Zhang L, Wang XB, Fales HM, Allen SL, Kolitz JE, Rai KR, Chiorazzi N (2008) Chronic lymphocytic leukemia antibodies with a common stereotypic rearrangement recognize nonmuscle myosin heavy chain IIA. Blood 112:5122–5129

Crowther-Swanepoel D, Broderick P, Di Bernardo MC, Dobbins SE, Torres M, Mansouri M, Ruiz-Ponte C, Enjuanes A, Rosenquist R, Carracedo A, Jurlander J, Campo E, Juliusson G, Montserrat E, Smedby KE, Dyer MJS, Matutues E, Dearden C, Sunter NJ, Hall AG, Mainou-

Fowler T, Jackson GH, Summerfield G, Harris RJ, Pettitt AR, Allsup DJ, Bailey JR, Pratt G, Pepper C, Fegan C, Parker A, Oscier D, Allan JM, Catovsky D, Houlston RS (2010) Common variants at 2q37.3, 8q24.21, 15q21.3 and 16q24.1 influence chronic lymphocytic leukemia risk. Nat Genet 42:132–136

Damle RN, Wasil T, Fais F, Ghiotto F, Valetto A, Allen SL, Buchbinder A, Budman D, Dittmar K, Kolitz J, Lichtman SM, Schulman P, Vinciguerra VP, Rai KR, Ferrarini M, Chiorazzi N (1999) Ig V gene mutation status and CD38 expression as novel prognostic indicators in chronic lymphocytic leukemia. Blood 94:1840–1847

Darzentas N, Hadzidimitriou A, Murray F, Hatzi K, Josefsson P, Laoutaris N, Moreno C, Anagnostopoulos A, Jurlander J, Tsaftaris A, Chiorazzi N, Belessi C, Ghia P, Rosenquist R, Davi F, Stamatopoulos K (2010) A different ontogenesis for chronic lymphocytic leukemia cases carrying stereotyped antigen receptors: molecular and computational evidence. Leukemia 24:125–132

Di Bernardo MC, Crowther-Swanepoel D, Broderick P, Webb E, Sellick G, Wild R, Sullivan K, Vijayakrishnan J, Wang Y, Pittman AM, Sunter NJ, Hall AG, Dyer MJS, Matutues E, Dearden C, Mainou-Fowler T, Jackson GH, Summerfield G, Harris RJ, Pettitt AR, Hillmen P, Allsup DJ, Bailey JR, Pratt G, Pepper C, Fegan C, Allan JM, Catovsky D, Houlston RS (2008) A genome-wide association study identifies six susceptibility loci for chronic lymphocytic leukemia. Nat Genet 40:1204–1210

Dighiero G, Hamblin TJ (2008) Chronic lymphocytic leukaemia. Lancet 371:1017–1029

Döhner H, Stilgenbauer S, Benner A, Leupot E, Krober A, Bullinger L, Döhner K, Bentz M, Lichter P (2000) Genomic aberrations and survival in chronic lymphocytic leukemia. N Engl J Med 343:1910–1916

Dreger P, Döhner H, Ritgen M, Böttcher S, Busch R, Dietrich S, Bunjes D, Cohen S, Schubert J, Hegenbart U, Beelen D, Zeis M, Stadler M, Hasenkamp J, Uharek L, Scheid C, Humpe A, Zenz T, Winkler D, Hallek M, Kneba M, Schmitz N, Stilgenbauer S (2010) Allogeneic stem cell transplantation provides durable disease control in poor-risk chronic lymphocytic leukemia: long-term clinical and MRD results of the German CLL study group CLL3X trial. Blood 116:2438–2447

Fais F, Ghiotto F, Hashimoto S, Sellars B, Valetto A, Allen SL, Schulman P, Vinciguerra VP, Rai K, Rassenti LZ, Kipps TJ, Dighiero G, Schroeder HW Jr, Ferrarini M, Chiorazzi N (1998) Chronic lymphocytic leukemia B cells express restricted sets of mutated and unmutated antigen receptors. J Clin Invest 102:1515–1525

Friedberg JW, Sharman J, Sweetenham J, Johnston PB, Vose JM, Lacasce A, Schaefer-Cutillo J, De Vos S, Sinha R, Leonard JP, Cripe LD, Gregory SA, Sterba MP, Lowe AM, Levy R, Shipp MA (2010) Inhibition of Syk with fostamatinib disodium has significant clinical activity in non-Hodgkin lymphoma and chronic lymphocytic leukemia. Blood 115:2578–2585

Ganster C, Neesen J, Zehetmeyer S, Jager U, Esterbauer H, Mannhalter C, Kluge B, Fonatsch C (2009) DNA repair polymorphisms associated with cytogenetic subgroups in B-cell chronic lymphocytic leukemia. Genes Chromosom Cancer 48:760–767

Ghia P, Stamatopoulos K, Belessi C, Moreno C, Stella S, Guida G, Michel A, Crespo M, Laoutaris N, Montserrat E, Anagnostopoulos A, Dighiero G, Fassas A, Caligaris-Cappio F, Davi F (2005) Geographic patterns and pathogenetic implications of IGHV gene usage in chronic lymphocytic leukemia: the lesson of the IGHV3-21 gene. Blood 105:1678–1685

Hallek M, Fischer K, Fingerle-Rowson G, Fink AM, Busch R, Mayer J, Hensel M, Hopfinger G, Hess G, von Grünhagen U, Bergmann M, Catalano J, Zinzani PL, Caligaris-Cappio F, Seymour JF, Berrebi A, Jäger U, Cazin B, Trneny M, Westermann A, Wendtner CM, Eichhorst BF, Staib P, Bühler A, Winkler D, Zenz T, Böttcher S, Ritgen M, Mendila M, Kneba M, Döhner H, Stilgenbauer S (2010) Addition of rituximab to fludarabine and cyclophosphamide in patients with chronic lymphocytic leukaemia: a randomised, open-label, phase 3 trial. Lancet 376:1164–1174

Hallek M, Cheson BD, Catovsky D, Caligaris-Cappio F, Dighiero G, Döhner H, Hillmen P, Keating MJ, Montserrat E, Rai KR, Kipps TJ (2008) Guidelines for the diagnosis and treatment of chronic lymphocytic leukemia: a report from the International Workshop on

Chronic Lymphocytic Leukemia updating the National Cancer Institute-Working Group 1996 guidelines. Blood 111:5446–5456

Hamblin TJ, Davis Z, Gardiner A, Oscier DG, Stevenson FK (1999) Unmutated Ig V(H) genes are associated with a more aggressive form of chronic lymphocytic leukemia. Blood 94:1848–1854

Heintel D, Kienle D, Shehata M, Kröber A, Kroemer E, Schwarzinger I, Mitteregger D, Le T, Gleiss A, Mannhalter C, Chott A, Schwarzmeier J, Fonatsch C, Gaiger A, Döhner H, Stilgenbauer S, Jäger U (2005) High expression of lipoprotein lipase in poor risk B-cell chronic lymphocytic leukemia. Leukemia 19:1216–1223

Hervé M, Xu K, Ng YS, Wardemann H, Albesiano E, Messmer BT, Chiorazzi N, Meffre E (2005) Unmutated and mutated chronic lymphocytic leukemias derive from self-reactive B cell precursors despite expressing different antibody reactivity. J Clin Invest 115:1636–1643

Honigberg LA, Smith AM, Sirisawad M, Verner E, Loury D, Chang B, Li S, Pan Z, Thamm DH, Miller RA, Buggy JJ (2010) The Bruton tyrosine kinase inhibitor PCI-32765 blocks B-cell activation and is efficacious in models of autoimmune disease and B-cell malignancy. Proc Natl Acad Sci USA 107:13075–13080

Johnson TA, Rassenti LZ, Kipps TJ (1997) Ig VH1 genes expressed in B cell chronic lymphocytic leukemia exhibit distinctive molecular features. J Immunol 158:235–246

Kanduri M, Cahill N, Goransson H, Enström C, Ryan F, Isaksson A, Rosenquist R (2010) Differential genome-wide array-based methylation profiles in prognostic subsets of chronic lymphocytic leukemia. Blood 115:296–305

Kipps TJ, Tomhave E, Pratt LF, Duffy S, Chen PP, Carson DA (1989) Developmentally restricted immunoglobulin heavy chain variable region gene expressed at high frequency in chronic lymphocytic leukemia. Proc Natl Acad Sci USA 86:5913–5917

Klein U, Tu Y, Stolovitzky GA, Mattioli M, Cattoretti G, Husson H, Freedman A, Inghirami G, Cro L, Baldini L, Neri A, Califano A, Dalla-Favera R (2001) Gene expression profiling of B cell chronic lymphocytic leukemia reveals a homogenous phenotype related to memory B cells. J Exp Med 194:1625–1638

Klein U, Lia M, Crespo M, Siegel R, Shen Q, Mo T, Ambesi-Impiombato A, Califano A, Migliazza A, Bhagat G, Dalla-Favera R (2010) The DLEU2/miR-15a/16-1 cluster controls B cell proliferation and its deletion leads to chronic lymphocytic leukemia. Cancer Cell 17:28–40

Kröber A, Seiler T, Benner A, Bullinger L, Brückle E, Lichter P, Döhner H, Stilgenbauer S (2002) V(H) mutation status, CD38 expression level, genomic aberrations, and survival in chronic lymphocytic leukemia. Blood 100:1410–1416

Lannuti BJ, Meadows SA, Herman SE, Kashishian A, Steiner B, Johnson AJ, Byrd JC, Tyner JW, Loriaux MM, Deininger M, Druker BJ, Puri KD, Ulrich RG, Giese NA (2011) CAL-101, a p110delta selective phosphatidylinositol-3-kinase inhibitor for the treatment of B-cell malignancies, inhibits PI3 K signalling and cellular viability. Blood 117:591–594

Lin K, Manocha S, Harris RJ, Matrai Z, Sherrington PD, Pettitt AR (2003) High frequency of p53 dysfunction and low level of VH mutation in chronic lymphocytic leukemia patients using the VH3-21 gene segment. Blood 102:1145–1146

Mackus WJ, Frakking FN, Grummels A, Gamadia LE, De Bree GJ, Hamann D, Van Lier RA, Van Oers MH (2003) Expansion of CMV-specific CD8 + CD45RA + CD27- T-cells in B-cell chronic lymphocytic leukemia. Blood 102:1057–1063

Mockridge CI, Potter KN, Wheatley I, Neville LA, Packham G, Stevenson FK (2007) Reversible anergy of sIgM-mediated signaling in two subsets of CLL defined by VH-gene mutational status. Blood 109:4424–4431

Murray F, Darzentas N, Hadzidimitriou A, Tobin G, Boudjogra M, Scielzo C, Laoutaris N, Karlsson K, Baran-Marzsak F, Tsaftaris A, Moreno C, Anagnostopoulos A, Caligaris-Cappio F, Vaur D, Ouzounis C, Belessi C, Ghia P, Davi F, Rosenquist R, Stamatopoulos K (2008) Stereotyped patterns of somatic hypermutation in subsets of patients with chronic lymphocytic leukemia: implications for the role of antigen selection in leukemogenesis. Blood 111:1524–1533

Ocana E, Delgado-Perez L, Campos-Caro A, Munoz J, Paz A, Franco R, Brieva JA (2007) The prognostic role of CXCR3 expression by chronic lymphocytic leukemia B cells. Haematologica 92:349–356

Oppezzo P, Vasconcelos Y, Settegrana C, Jeannel D, Vuillier F, Legarff-Tavernier M, Kimura EY, Bechet S, Dumas G, Brissard M, Merle-Béral H, Yamamoto M, Dighiero G, Davi F (2005) The LPL/ADAM29 expression ratio is a novel prognosis indicator in chronic lymphocytic leukemia. Blood 106:650–657

Potter KN, Orchard J, Critchley E, Mockridge CI, Jose A, Stevenson FK (2003) Features of the overexpressed V1-69 genes in the unmutated subset of chronic lymphocytic leukemia are distinct from those in the healthy elderly repertoire. Blood 101:3082–3084

Raveche ES, Salerno E, Scaglione BJ, Manohar V, Abbasi F, Lin YC, Fredrickson T, Landgraf P, Ramachandra S, Huppi K, Toro JR, Zenger VE, Metcalf RA, Marti GE (2007) Abnormal microRNA-16 locus with synteny to human 13q14 linked to CLL in NZB mice. Blood 109:5079–5086

Rosenwald A, Alizadeh AA, Widhopf G, Simon R, Davis RE, Yu X, Yang L, Pickeral OK, Rassenti LZ, Powell J, Botstein D, Byrd JC, Grever MR, Cheson BD, Chiorazzi N, Wilson WH, Kipps TJ, Brown PO, Staudt LM (2001) Relation of gene expression phenotype to immunoglobulin mutation genotype in B cell chronic lymphocytic leukemia. J Exp Med 194:1639–1647

Rudd MF, Sellick GS, Webb EL, Catovsky D, Houlston RS (2006) Variants in the ATM-BRCA2-CHEK2 axis predispose to chronic lymphocytic leukemia. Blood 108:638–644

Schroeder HW Jr, Dighiero G (1994) The pathogenesis of chronic lymphocytic leukemia: analysis of the antibody repertoire. Immunol Today 15:288–294

Sellick GS, Webb EL, Allinson R, Matutes E, Dyer MJS, Jønsson V, Langerak AW, Mauro FR, Fuller S, Wiley J, Lyttelton M, Callea V, Yuille M, Catovsky D, Houlston RS (2005) A high-density SNP genomewide linkage scan for chronic lymphocytic leukemia susceptibility loci. Am J Hum Genet 77:420–429

Sivina M, Hartmann E, Kipps TJ, Rassenti L, Krupnik D, Lerner S, LaPushin R, Xiao L, Huang X, Werner L, Neuberg D, Kantarjian H, O'Brien S, Wierda WG, Keating MJ, Rosenwald A, Burger JA (2011) CCL3 (MIP-1α) plasma levels and the risk for disease progression in chronic lymphocytic leukemia. Blood 117:1662–1669

Stamatopoulos K, Belessi C, Moreno C, Boudjograh M, Guida G, Smilevska T, Belhoul L, Stella S, Stavroyianni N, Crespo M, Hadzidimitriou A, Sutton L, Bosch F, Laoutaris N, Anagnostopoulos A, Montserrat E, Fassas A, Dighiero G, Caligaris-Cappio F, Merle-Béral H, Ghia P, Davi F (2007) Over 20 % of patients with chronic lymphocytic leukemia carry stereotyped receptors: pathogenetic implications and clinical correlations. Blood 109:259–270

Stamatopoulos K (2009) Stereotyped B cell receptors in CLL. In: Ghia P, Rosenquist R, Davi F (eds) Immunoglobulin gene analysis in chronic lymphocytic leukemia. Wolters Kluwer Health Italy Ltd, Milan, pp 95–111

Sutton LA, Kostareli E, Hadzidimitriou A, Darzentas N, Tsaftaris A, Anagnostopoulos A, Rosenquist R, Stamatopoulos K (2009) Extensive intraclonal diversification in a subgroup of chronic lymphocytic leukemia patients with stereotyped IGHV4-34 receptors: implications for ongoing interactions with antigen. Blood 114:4460–4468

Thorsélius M, Kröber A, Murray F, Thunberg U, Tobin G, Bühler A, Kienle D, Albesiano E, Maffei R, Dao-Ung LP, Wiley J, Vilpo J, Laurell A, Merup M, Roos G, Karlsson K, Chiorazzi N, Marasca R, Döhner H, Stilgenbauer S, Rosenquist R (2006) Strikingly homologous immunoglobulin gene rearrangements and poor outcome in VH3-21-utilizing chronic lymphocytic leukemia independent of geographical origin and mutational status. Blood 107:2889–2894

Tobin G, Thunberg U, Johnson A, Thörn I, Söderberg O, Hultdin M, Botling J, Enblad G, Sällström J, Sundström C, Roos G, Rosenquist R (2002) Somatically mutated Ig V(H)3-21 genes characterize a new subset of chronic lymphocytic leukemia. Blood 99:2262–2264

Tobin G, Thunberg U, Johnson A, Eriksson I, Söderberg O, Karlsson K, Merup M, Juliusson G, Vilpo J, Enblad G, Sundström C, Roos G, Rosenquist R (2003) Chronic lymphocytic leukemias utilizing the VH3-21 gene display highly restricted Vlambda2-14 gene use and homologous CDR3 s: implicating recognition of a common antigen epitope. Blood 101:4952–4957

Widhopf GF 2nd, Kipps TJ (2001) Normal B cells express 51p1-encoded Ig heavy chains that are distinct from those expressed by chronic lymphocytic leukemia B cells. J Immunol 166:95–102

Wierda WG, Cantwell MJ, Woods SJ, Rassenti LZ, Prussak CE, Kipps TJ (2000) CD40 ligand (CD154) gene therapy for chronic lymphocytic leukemia. Blood 96:2917–2924

Wierda WG, Kipps TJ, Mayer J, Stilgenbauer S, Williams CD, Hellmann A, Robak T, Furman RR, Hillmen P, Trneny M, Dyer MJ, Padmanabhan S, Piotrowska M, Kozak T, Chan G, Davis R, Losic N, Wilms J, Russell CA, Osterborg A (2010) Ofatumumab as single-agent CD20 immunotherapy in fludarabine-refractory chronic lymphocytic leukemia. J Clin Oncol 28:1749–1755

Zenz T, Mertens D, Küppers R, Döhner H, Stilgenbauer S (2010) From pathogenesis to treatment of chronic lymphocytic leukemia. Nat Rev Cancer 10:37–50

Chapter 6
Molecular Biology of Chronic Myeloid Leukemia

Tomasz Sacha, Kajetana Foryciarz and Aleksander B. Skotnicki

Abstract Chronic myeloid leukemia (CML) is a clonal myeloproliferative disorder resulting from an acquired genetic aberration t(9;22)(q34;q11) (Philadelphia chromosome) in stem cells. As a result the *BCR/ABL* fusion gene is formed which encodes a specific mRNA, translated into BCR/ABL proteins with an abnormally high tyrosine kinase activity, playing a crucial role in leukemic transformation and neoplastic proliferation of hematopoietic stem cells. BCR/ABL protein activates a number of transcription factors and gene promoters; however, its expression does not explain all the biological mechanisms of the origin of CML and its progression. Trisomy of chromosome 8, 19, isochromosome 17, and an additional Ph chromosome are the most frequent additional chromosomal abnormalities detected in course of CML progression. Suppressor genes dysfunction may play a role in the progression of CML. There is a considerable heterogeneity of the molecular mechanism and the genes involved in the development and progression of CML.

T. Sacha (✉) · A. B. Skotnicki
Department of Hematology, Jagiellonian University Hospital in Kraków, Kopernika 17, 31-501 Kraków, Poland
e-mail: sachatom@gmail.com

A. B. Skotnicki
e-mail: alekskot@cm-uj.krakow.pl

K. Foryciarz
Pharmaceutical Research Associates Sp. z o.o., Al. Wyścigowa 6, 02-681 Warsaw, Poland
e-mail: kajetana@foryciarz.com

M. Witt et al. (eds.), *Molecular Aspects of Hematologic Malignancies*, Principles and Practice, DOI: 10.1007/978-3-642-29467-9_6,

6.1 Introduction

Chronic myeloid leukemia (CML) is a clonal myeloproliferative disorder resulting from an acquired genetic aberration in pluripotential stem cells, described for the first time in 1960 (Nowell and Hungerford 1960) as the Philadelphia chromosome (Ph)—a recurrent chromosomal abnormality detectable in more than 90 % of patients suffering from this type of leukemia. CML accounts for approximately 15 % of diagnosed leukemias, with an annual incidence of 1–2:100 000 in the general population and most common presentation in the fifth and sixth decades of life (Altekruse et al. 2010).

6.2 Clinical Features

CML usually presents with anemia, a high number of blood granulocytes and their precursors, a large proportion of mature neutrophils, absolute basophilia, normal or elevated platelet counts, and frequently, splenomegaly. Typical symptoms are those characteristic of anemia (fatigue, weakness, headache, dizziness), loss of appetite, and weight loss, and—in consequence of splenomegaly—pain, bloating, and satiety. Occasionally, the patient presents with bone pains or hyperviscosity associated with a very high white cell count. CML is usually diagnosed in the chronic phase (CP). After a period of stability in CP, the patient progresses to the accelerated phase (AP), which is associated with deterioration of the patient's health and the need for more intense therapy to control the increased white cell count and progressive splenomegaly. According to the WHO definition, the most advanced phase of CML is blast crisis (BC) characterized by $\geq$20 % of blasts in bone marrow or peripheral blood and/or extramedullary infiltrates of leukemic cells and symptoms typical of acute leukemia. BC still represents an important clinical problem and is often characterized by a short median survival time (O'Brien et al. 2007).

6.3 Chromosomal and Genetic Aberrations in CML

The Ph is the result of a reciprocal translocation between the long arm fragment (9q34) of chromosome 9 containing the *ABL* proto-oncogene—a human homologue of v-abl oncogene carried by the Abelson murine leukemia virus (A-MuLV) (Abelson and Rabstein 1970) and a part of the long arm of chromosome 22, which breaks in a specific breakpoint cluster region (BCR). As a result the shortened chromosome 22q− (Ph) is formed with the *BCR/ABL* fusion gene in the region of a junction on chromosome 22, and the *ABL/BCR* gene on the elongated chromosome 9q+ (see Fig. 6.1).

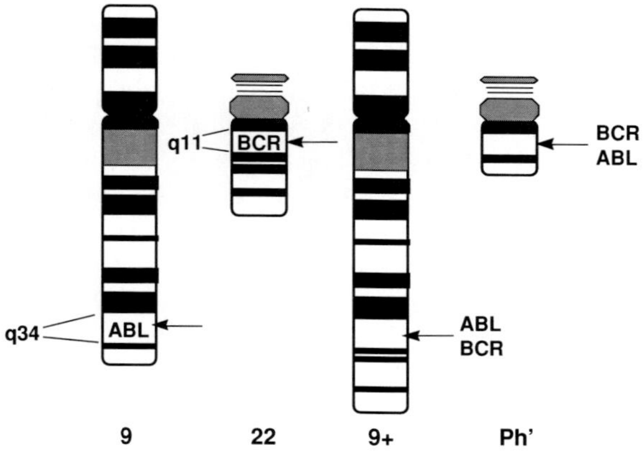

Fig. 6.1 Formation of the Philadelphia chromosome

The classic t(9;22)(q34;q11) translocation is detected by conventional cytogenetic methods in approximately 85 % of patients suffering from CML. In 5 % of patients, the Ph chromosome is the result of a complex exchange of genetic material, usually between three or more chromosomes, but in most cases chromosomes 9 and 22 are involved (Kessel et al. 1981). Conventional cytogenetics fails to detect the Ph chromosome in the remaining 10 % of CML patients. In more than 50 % of those patients, the *BCR/ABL* gene could be detected by molecular methods—fluorescence in situ hybridization (FISH), Southern blotting, or reverse transcriptase-polymerase chain reaction (RT-PCR) (Groffen et al. 1984). In less than 5 % of patients presenting with symptoms typical for CML, the commonly used cytogenetic and molecular techniques are unable to detect the Ph chromosome and the *BCR/ABL* gene (Shepherd et al. 1987; Wiedemann et al. 1988). In those patients, a CML-like disease, which in some cases may be classified as a myeloproliferative–myelodysplastic disorder, could be diagnosed (Kurzrock et al. 1990; Costello et al. 1995). The pathogenesis of this disease is still unclear (Cogswell et al. 1989; Melo 1996a, b; Selleri et al. 1990). The consequence of the t(9;22) is also a chromosome 9q+ with the *ABL–BCR* fusion gene detected in approximately 60–70 % of patients with CML. It results from the junction of one of the first ABL exons (usually exon Ib) with an exon b3 or b4 of the *BCR* gene (Konopka and Witte 1985; Melo 1996a, b) and its product is detectable by RT-PCR with an incidence similar to the occurrence of the 9q+ chromosome (Melo 1996a, b). The *ABL/BCR* gene formation does not play any important role in the development and progression of CML. It is expressed both in the chronic and blastic phase (Konopka and Witte 1985; Melo 1996a, b).

The expression of the p210 protein (the product of the *BCR/ABL* gene) by itself does not explain all the biological mechanisms of the origin of CML and its progression. It is hypothesized that the *BCR/ABL* translocation is one of the molecular events in the complex process of CML oncogenesis (Cannistra 1990), although other cooperating genetic lesions responsible for the emergence of the disease have not been discovered until now. Additional acquired genetic aberrations are relatively rare at the time of diagnosis and usually accompanied by the evolution of the disease to the accelerated or blastic phase (Apperley 2007). An intriguing question is why the Ph chromosome appears first in the course of the disease. A genetic predisposition could be one of the possible answers. Detection of the *BCR/ABL* gene using a very sensitive modified nested RT-PCR method in approximately 25 % of healthy volunteers aged over 55 years could confirm this hypothesis (Biernaux et al. 1995; Bose et al. 1998). The occurrence of the Ph chromosome may be the result of an increased genetic instability, or the progressive accumulation of genotoxic agents, both correlated with age. The epidemiological data indicate, however, that the incidence of CML is significantly lower than the frequency of *BCR/ABL* gene detection in healthy volunteers. Based on the current state of knowledge it is, therefore, assumed that the detection of a small number of *BCR/ABL* gene copies using very sensitive methodology in an individual without symptoms of the disease has no clinical significance. The second crucial observation concerns the presence of chromosomal abnormalities in Ph-negative cells in approximately 5 % of patients with CML in complete cytogenetic remission (CCgR) defined as the absence of Ph-positive metaphases in conventional cytogenetic analysis (Bumm et al. 2003; O'Dwyer et al. 2003). It should be noted, however, that the incidence of cytogenetic abnormalities in healthy populations is unknown.

6.4 Cytogenetic Aberrations in Progression of CML

The most frequent additional chromosomal abnormalities in Ph-positive cells detected by conventional cytogenetic analysis in progression of CML are: trisomy of chromosome 8 (+8) and 19 (+19), isochromosome 17 [i(17q)], and an additional Ph chromosome. Trisomy 8 is quite common in patients with CML in the blastic phase (approximately 40 %). It results in the increased expression of the *c-MYC* oncogene (Avian myelocytomatosis virus oncogene cellular homolog) located within the band 8q24 which is associated with many human cancers, often with a poor prognosis. The proto-oncogene *c-MYC* is implicated in cell growth, proliferation, loss of differentiation, and apoptosis. Deregulated expression of *c-MYC* in CML may be associated with the disease progression. The blocking of *c-MYC* by antisense oligonucleotides in vitro results in inhibition of leukemic transformation dependent on the *BCR/ABL* gene. Moreover, a very high expression of *c-MYC* was detected in cells of patients with CML in BC. Interestingly, trisomy 8 occurs as a marker of a cytogenetic clonal evolution (defined as the presence of karyotypic abnormalities in addition to the Ph) in patients with CML in CCgR treated with imatinib. It is, however, detected in Ph (−) cells and since the course of the disease in these patients is usually benign, trisomy 8 is supposed not to be necessary for the progression of leukemia, especially if it occurs in Ph(−) cells. Isochromosome 17, i(17q), is detected in Ph(+) cell clones in approximately 20 % of patients with CML in BC. As a consequence of the i(17q) formation, one copy of *TP53* (tumor suppressor p53 gene) is lost. A decreased activity of this gene may lead to reduced apoptosis and impaired DNA repair mechanisms, which results in disease progression. Occurrence of i(17q) could unmask the effect of an existing mutation of *TP53* in the other allele. In CML BC, the reported incidence of *TP53* mutations is variable and somewhat contradictory with the average frequency being 11 % (8–25 %) (Nakai and Misawa 1995; Feinstein et al. 1991). The *TP53* mutation in CML patients in BC with i(17q) was detected (22 %); however, direct link of diminished activity or *TP53* mutation with i(17q) and progression to BC is not as clear (Radich 2007). An additional Ph chromosome and trisomy 19 occurs in 30 and 12 % of patients with CML in the blastic phase, respectively. Other aberrations, which play a role in the progression of CML to BC are: the loss of the *Y* chromosome, trisomy 21, and monosomy 7 (each found in a small percentage of patients) (Radich 2007). Additional cytogenetic aberrations in Ph(+) cells may occur at different frequencies in myeloid and lymphoid type of BC. At least one of the above-mentioned genetic aberrations is reported in about 75 % of patients with CML in the AP or BC (Melo 1996a, b). Translocations of known oncogenes in BC occur rarely (<5 %). Translocations t(3;21) and t(7;11) involve *AML-1/EVI-1* (acute myeloid leukemia-1/ecotropic virus integration site 1 protein homolog) genes and *NUP98/HOXA9* (nucleoporin 98 kD/homeobox9) genes, coding for transcription factors. Disturbances in the expression of these genes lead to maturation arrest (*AML-1/EVI-1*) or increased cell proliferation (*NUP98/HOXA9*). However, the frequency of aberrant expression of these genes in BC, with no relation to the above-mentioned translocations, is not known (Radich 2007). Such a multiplicity of possible disturbances suggests that the underlying cause of maturation arrest in the BC of CML, playing a crucial role in the progression of CML, is the genetic instability of cell clones.

6.5 Molecular Aberrations in the Course of CML

6.5.1 Formation of the BCR/ABL Gene

The chimeric *BCR/ABL* gene is formed as the result of the fusion of the *BCR* and *ABL* gene parts. The rupture of the *ABL* gene may occur anywhere in the region of more than 300 kb, located within its 5′ end. The gene breakpoint may be located upstream from the first exon Ib, between the exons Ib and Ia, as well as downstream of the exon Ia (Melo 1996a). Several possible breakpoints within the *BCR* gene were found. In the vast majority of patients with CML and in approximately one-third of patients with acute lymphoblastic leukemia (ALL), the breakpoint is located within a fragment of 5.8 kb (*major breakpoint cluster region*, M-bcr). This leads to separation of five exons, b1–b5, according to the latest nomenclature called 12–16. In this case, regardless of where the *ABL* gene breaks, the result of the *BCR/ABL* chimeric gene formation is the synthesis of a hybrid *BCR/ABL*

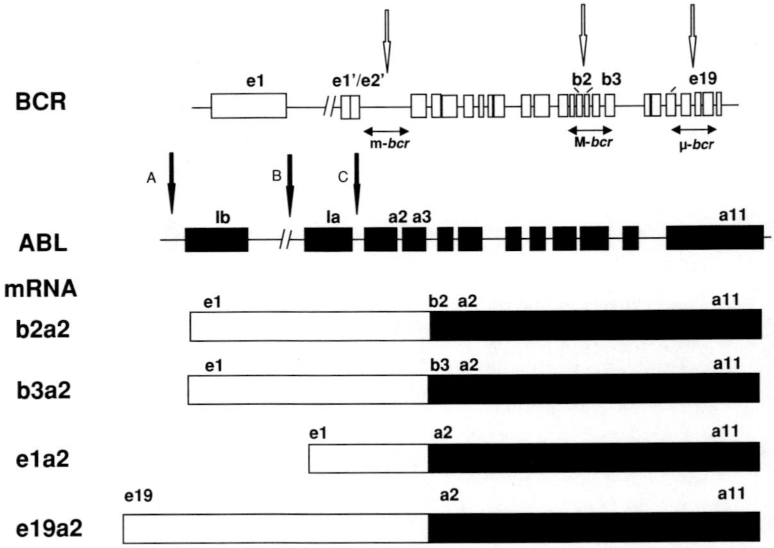

b2a2, b3a2, e1a2, e19a2: possible types of mRNA BCR/ABL transcripts

possible *ABL* gene break points location: A - upstream from exon Ib, B - between exons Ib and Ia, C - downstream of exon Ia

possible *BCR* gene break points location: *m-bcr, M-bcr* or *μ-bcr* region

Ib – first exon b, Ia – first exon a of *ABL* gene
e1, e1', e2', b2, b3, e19 - exons of *BCR* gene

Fig. 6.2 Formation of the *BCR–ABL* fusion gene

mRNA, with a junction at b2a2 or b3a2, which codes for the protein p210 (see Fig. 6.2).

In most patients with ALL (approximately two-thirds) and in rare cases of CML and acute myeloid leukemia (2 %), the breakpoint of the *BCR* gene is located within a long intron (54.4 kb), between the exons e2′ and e2 (*minor breakpoint cluster region, m-bcr*) (Chissoe et al. 1995). In these cases, the transcript of the *BCR/ABL* gene containing the e1a2 junction is translated into a smaller (185–190 kDa) protein (p190) (see Fig. 6.2). The occurrence of the p190 protein is associated with increased monocytosis, which may suggest a similarity to chronic myelomonocytic leukemia (CMML), classified among myeloproliferative–myelodysplastic syndromes. In these cases the *BCR/ABL* gene is not detected (Melo et al. 1994). In very rare cases the *BCR* gene breakpoint may be close to the 3′ end (*micro breakpoint cluster region, μ-bcr*), which results in the formation of a longer *BCR/ABL* gene and an mRNA transcript with a junction at e19a2. The resulting p230 protein of the *BCR/ABL* gene contains additional 180 amino acids, as compared to the p210 protein and, similar to the p210 and p190 proteins, possesses excessive tyrosine kinase activity. Patients suffering from CML with this type of translocation present with significant thrombocythemia. The clinical course of this rare type of CML may resemble chronic neutrophilic leukemia (CNL) (Pane et al. 1996). Detection of breaks in the *BCR* gene, located outside the three locations listed above, as well as an unusual breakage of the *ABL* gene is rare. The effect of this type of translocation is the formation of an atypical *BCR/ABL* transcript with b2a3 or b3a3 junctions or with different junctions, containing intron sequences of differing lengths (see Fig. 6.2) (Melo 1996a, b). The resulting transcripts also exhibit oncogenic potential and increased tyrosine kinase activity. There is a potential risk that these unusual products of the *BCR/ABL* translocation remain undetected with the use of primers commonly applied in RT-PCR tests, which do not cover the entire region of the translocation. Extremely rare genetic test results may occur in this situation, where the Ph chromosome is detected in the karyotype, while the absence of the *BCR/ABL* translocation is revealed by RT-PCR test. Application of multiplex RT-PCR with the use of multiple primer pairs may prevent such disparities and therefore should be used in a routine molecular diagnostics of CML.

6.5.2 The Role of the BCR–ABL Gene in CML Pathogenesis

The chimeric *BCR/ABL* gene, formed on chromosome 22, encodes a specific mRNA, which is translated into $p210^{BCR\text{–}ABL}$, $p190^{BCR\text{–}ABL}$, $p230^{BCR\text{–}ABL}$ proteins with an abnormally high tyrosine kinase activity. This activity has a crucial role in leukemic transformation and the mechanisms controlling autonomous neoplastic proliferation of hematopoietic stem cells (Melo 1996a, b). In contrast to normal cells, those with *BCR/ABL* gene expression, show an enhanced proliferation in response to minimal concentrations of growth factors, delayed apoptosis in the event of growth factors, absence in in vitro cultures, and a decreasing ability of maturation in subsequent divisions (Carella et al. 1997). Numerous interactions of the chimeric gene product with other cellular proteins have been reported (Cohen et al. 1995).

The BCR/ABL protein kinase substrates can be grouped according to their physiological role into:

- adapter molecules, such as Crkl and p62DOK,
- proteins with catalytic function, such as Fes (tyrosine-protein kinase Fes/Fps, involved in the regulation of the actin cytoskeleton, microtubule assembly, cell attachment, and cell spreading) or Syp (synapthophysin, a nonreceptor protein tyrosine phosphatase, possibly involved in organizing membrane components),
- proteins responsible for the cytoskeleton and cell membrane formation, such as paxillin (see also Fig. 6.3).

The BCR/ABL protein kinase activity in leukemic progenitor cells results in decreased adhesion to stroma cells and extracellular matrix (Gordon et al. 1987; Kothari et al. 1986), activation of mitogenic signals (Puil et al. 1994), decreased apoptosis (Bedi et al. 1994), and proteasome-mediated degradation of Abl

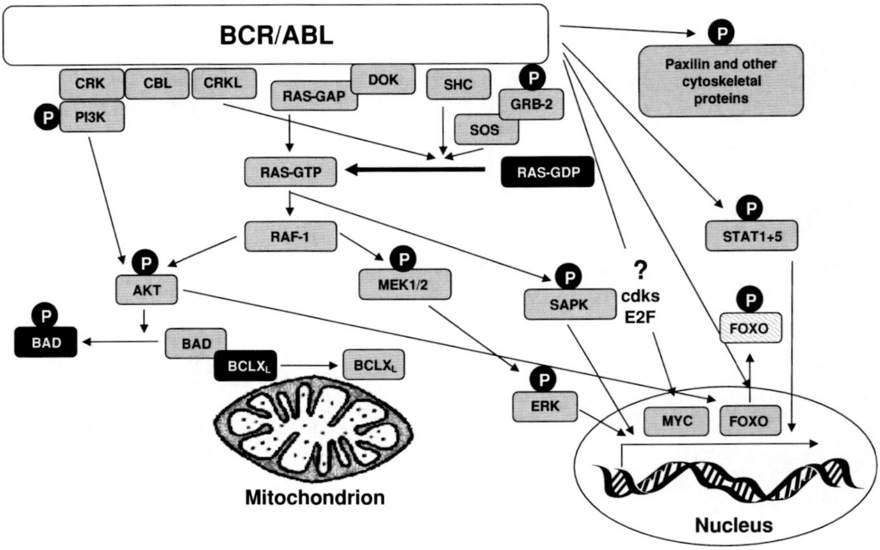

Fig. 6.3 BCR/ABL protein kinase activity in leukemic progenitor cells. CRKL—Crk-like protein, may mediate the transduction of intracellular signals, shown to activate the JUN and RAS kinase signaling pathways and to transform fibroblasts; p62DOK—enzymatically inert adaptor or scaffolding protein, provides a docking platform for the assembly of multimolecular signaling complexes, modulates integrin activation; SHC—Src homology-2 containing proteins, signaling adapter that couples activated receptor tyrosine kinases to Ras via the recruitment of the GRB2/SOS complex and implicated in the cytoplasmic propagation of mitogenic signals; SOS—Son of sevenless homolog, promotes the exchange of Ras-bound GDP by GTP; CBL—Casitas B-lineage lymphoma proto-oncogene, adapter oncoprotein that functions as a negative regulator of many signaling pathways that are triggered by activation of cell surface receptors; GRB2—Growth factor receptor-bound protein 2, adapter protein that provides a critical link between cell surface growth factor receptors and the Ras signaling pathway; PI3 K—Phosphatidylinositol-4-phosphate 3-kinase, has a role in several intracellular trafficking events, its activation by BCR/ABL results in reduced apoptosis; AKT—RAC-alpha serine/threonine-protein kinase, which regulate many processes, including metabolism, proliferation, cell survival, growth, and angiogenesis; BAD—Bcl2 antagonist of cell Heath, promotes cell death acts as a link between growth factor receptor signaling and the apoptotic pathways; BCLX—Bcl-2-like protein 1, potent inhibitor of cell death, inhibits activation of caspases; RAS—Alternate between an inactive form bound to GDP and an active form bound to GTP, plays a role in GTPase-mediated signal transduction; SAPK—Stress-activated map kinase, serine/threonine-protein kinase involved in various processes, such as cell proliferation, differentiation, migration, transformation, and programmed cell death; RAF—1-RAF proto-oncogene serine/threonine-protein kinase, involved in the transduction of mitogenic signals from the cell membrane to the nucleus. Part of the Ras-dependent signaling pathway from receptors to the nucleus; MEK1/2—Dual specificity mitogen-activated protein kinase 2, catalyzes the concomitant phosphorylation of a threonine and a tyrosine residue in a Thr-Glu-Tyr sequence located in MAP kinases; activates the ERK1 and ERK2 MAP kinases; ERK 1—Mitogen-activated protein kinase 3, involved in both the initiation and regulation of meiosis, mitosis, and postmitotic functions in differentiated cells by phosphorylating a number of transcription factors; MYC—Myc proto-oncogene protein, participates in the regulation of gene transcription; binds DNA in a non-specific manner, seems to activate the transcription of growth-related genes; FOXO—Forkhead box protein O, transcriptional activator which triggers apoptosis in the absence of survival factors; STAT1 + 5—Signal transducer and activator of transcription, carries out a dual function: signal transduction and activation of transcription; Paxillin—Cytoskeletal protein involved in actin-membrane attachment at sites of cell adhesion to the extracellular matrix (focal adhesion)

inhibitory proteins (Dai and Pendergast 1995) in those cells. CRK-like protein (Crkl) is one of the regulators of integrin-mediated cell adhesion and cell motility. Phosphorylated by BCR/ABL kinase may initiate contact between the BCR/ABL and paxilline, as well as the entire complex of adhesion molecules, which results in decreased adhesion. Phosphorylated Crkl also activates the Ras-dependent and JNK pathways, which initiates a signaling transduction leading ultimately to the activation of gene transcription (activation of Ras and subsequently Sapk and Raf kinases) (see Fig. 6.3. For explanation of protein names—see Fig. 6.3 legend) (Sawyers et al. 1995; Cortez et al. 1996) and is required for malignant transformation (activation of the Jnk/Sapk pathway). The proliferative signal from the BCR/ABL kinase is transduced into the nucleus and activates the *MYC* promoter. It is suggested that cyclin-dependent kinases (cdks) and E2F transcription factors are involved in this process.

Reduced apoptosis is the result of activation of several mechanisms. Constitutive phosphorylation of Stat transcription factors (Stat1 and Stat5) by *BCR/ABL* results in transcriptional activation of BCLX-potent inhibitor of cell death, which also contributes to malignant transformation. Activation of PI3 kinase in the complex formed by BCR/ABL with Cbl, Crk, and Crkl leads to the activation of the serine–threonine kinase Akt. Akt phosphorylates the pro-apoptotic protein Bad, which becomes inactive because it is no longer able to bind anti-apoptotic proteins such as BCLX. PI3 K/Akt may phosphorylate, in the nucleus, the fork-head O transcription factors (FOXO) (involved in the transcription of genes encoding pro-apoptotic molecules and inhibitors of the cell cycle) which induces their migration from the nucleus to the cytoplasm and subsequent degradation (Cilloni et al. Cilloni et al. 2008; Naka et al. 2010).

It was found that *BCR/ABL* can induce the proteasome-mediated degradation of Abl interactor 1 (Abi-1) and Abl interactor 2 (Abi-2)—two proteins with inhibitory function. Abi-1 plays a critical function in actin cytoskeleton dynamics, Abi-2 is a substrate of c-Abl, plays a dual role as the regulator and the potential effector of the c-Abl protein, and may function as a tumor suppressor in mammalian cells. The degradation of Abi-1 and Abi-2 is specific for Ph-positive acute leukemias and is not seen in Ph-negative cells. Since the experimental data refer to acute leukemias and not to CP CML the significance of this finding remains to be confirmed.

6.5.3 Molecular Aberrations in the Progression of CML

The mechanisms underlying the evolution of CML to the accelerated and blastic phase are not fully understood. The progression of CML is closely related to genetic instability. Proliferation stimulation by the activated *Ras* oncogene (Sawyers et al. 1995), increased transcriptional activity of STAT, decreased apoptosis resulting from activation of PI3 K/Akt, and cellular adhesion defect to actin, are certainly involved in CML development (Carella et al. 1997). However, the question of their role in the progression to more advanced phases remains unanswered. Cell lines with activated tyrosine kinase BCR/ABL accumulate damaged DNA to a greater extent than other cells due to enhanced "spontaneous" DNA damage and defects in the repair mechanisms leading to misrepair (Nowicki et al. 2004). Additionally, BCR/ABL caused increased anti-apoptotic *BCL2* and *BCL-XI* (B-cell lymphoma 2 and B-cell lymphoma XI) genes expression causes the delay of the G2/M cell cycle phase. As a result, the process of eliminating cells with damaged DNA can be arrested (Slupianek et al. 2002). An additional mechanism of DNA damage is related to BCR/ABL-mediated generation of reactive oxygen species (ROS) by the mitochondrial respiratory chain (MRC) (Sattler et al. 2000). These mechanisms are likely to cause genetic instability and stimulate mutagenesis (Koptyra et al. 2006). A characteristic feature of AP and BC is an increased level of *BCR/ABL* mRNA and BCR/ABL protein (approximately three-fold), which is accompanied by a strong activation of the signal transduction (reflected for example in increased CRKL phosphorylation) (Barnes et al. 2005). It appears that progression to AP or BC should involve inhibition of the tumor suppressor genes and activation of new oncogenes. However, the participation of TP53 is assessed in only 20–30 % of cases, although it is not certain whether or not there are functional changes of the genes involved in p53-mediated function. The homozygous deletion of exon 2 of *INK4A/ARF* gene (also referred to as *CDKN2A/ARF*, cyclin-dependent kinase inhibitor 2a/alternate reading frame product of the *CDKN2A* locus gene) is detected in about 50 % of the cases of CML lymphoblastic crisis. This deletion eliminates two proteins that normally control the *G1/S* phase and up-regulate *p*53.Another suppressor gene whose dysfunction may play a role in the progression of CML is *PP2A* (protein phosphatase 2A), a gene which is involved in the regulation of proliferation, apoptosis, and cell maturation and contributes to the degradation of the BCR/ABL protein in the proteasome. It was found in in vitro studies that *BCR/ABL* is able to stimulate expression of the nuclear oncogene SET (a cyclin B-interacting protein involved in the regulation of G2/M transition, apoptosis, transcription, nucleosome assembly, and histone binding, which possesses a protein phosphatase inhibitor activity and is a negative regulator of *PP2A*). A lowered activity of *PP2A* results in reduced degradation and persistence of BCR/ABL (Radich 2007).

6.6 Conclusions

CML is probably one of the best studied malignant disorders. A considerable heterogeneity of the molecular mechanisms and the involvement of numerous genes in the development and progression of CML are probably due to the appearance of the *BCR/ABL* chimeric gene, causing genetic instability, abnormal proliferation, differentiation, and apoptosis, resulting in an uncontrolled proliferation of hematopoietic cells. Precise understanding of the molecular pathogenesis was required to develop a rationally designed therapy. The discovery of the Ph, and subsequent identification of the BCR/ABL tyrosine kinase as the causative molecular event of CML allowed to design and synthesize specific inhibitors of this kinase. The clinical trials demonstrated remarkable results achieved with tyrosine kinase inhibitors. In this way the results of basic studies on molecular pathogenesis of CML have been translated into extremely successful anticancer therapies.

References

Abelson HT, Rabstein LS (1970) Lymphosarcoma: virus- induced thymic-independent disease in mice. Cancer Res 30:2213–2222

Altekruse SF, Kosary CL, Krapcho M, Neyman N, Aminou R, Waldron W, Ruhl J, Howlader N, Tatalovich Z, Cho H, Mariotto A, Eisner MP, Lewis DR, Cronin K, Chen HS, Feuer EJ, Stinchcomb DG, Edwards BK (eds) (2010) SEER cancer statistics review, 1975–2007, National Cancer Institute. Bethesda. http://seer.cancer.gov/csr/1975_2007/, based on November 2009 SEER data submission, posted to the SEER web site

Apperley J (2007) Part I: mechanisms of resistance to imatinib in chronic myeloid leukaemia. Lancet Oncol 8:1018–1029

Barnes DJ, Palaiologou D, Panousopoulou E, Schultheis B, Yong AS, Wong A, Pattacini L, Goldman JM, Melo JV (2005) BCR-ABL expression levels determine the rate of development of resistance to imatinib mesylate in chronic myeloid leukemia. Cancer Res 65:8912–8919

Bedi A, Zehnbauer BA, Barber JP, Sharkis SJ, Jones RJ (1994) Inhibition of apoptosis by BCR-ABL in chronic myeloid leukemia. Blood 83:2038–2044

Biernaux C, Loos M, Sels A, Huez G, Stryckmans P (1995) Detection of major BCR-ABL gene expression at a very low level in blood cells of some healthy individuals. Blood 86:3118–3122

Bose S, Deininger M, Gora-Tybor J, Goldman JM, Melo JV (1998) The presence of typical and atypical BCR-ABL fusion genes in leukocytes of normal individuals: biologic significance and implications for the assessment of minimal residual disease. Blood 92:3362–3367

Bumm T, Müller C, Al-Ali HK, Kron K, Shepherd P, Schmidt E, Leiblein S, Franke C, Hennig E, Friedrich T, Krahl R, Niederwieser D, Deininger MWN (2003) Emergence of clonal cytogenetic abnormalities in Ph– cells in some CML patients in cytogenetic remission to imatinib but restoration of polyclonal hematopoiesis in the majority. Blood 101:1941–1949

Cannistra SA (1990) Chronic myelogenous leukaemia as a model for a genetic basis of cancer. Hematol Oncol Clin North Am 48:337–353

Carella AM, Frassoni F, Melo J, Sawyers C, Eaves C, Eaves A, Apperley J, Tura S, Hehlmann R, Reiffers J, Lerma E, Goldman J (1997) New insights in biology and current therapeutic options for patients with chronic myelogenous leukemia. Hematologica 82:478–495

Chissoe SL, Bodenteich A, Wang YF, Wang YP, Burian SW, Dennis C, Crabtree J, Freeman A, Iyer K, Jian L, Ma Y, McLaury HJ, Pan HQ, Sharan O, Toth S, Wong Z, Zhang G, Heisterkamp N, Groffen J, Roe BA (1995) Sequence and analysis of the human ABL gene, the BCR gene, and regions involved in the Philadelphia chromosomal translocation. Genomics 27:67–82

Cilloni D, Panuzzo C, Messa F, Arruga F, Bracco E, Bernardoni R, Carturan S, Pautasso M, Messa E, Morotti A, Pradotto M, Iacobucci I, Kalenic T, Martinelli G, Saglio G (2008) Imatinib induced re-activation of FoxO3 transcription factor in CML is responsible for the induction of a quiescent status of CD34 leukaemic progenitor cells. Blood 112:1090

Cogswell PC, Morgan R, Dunn M, Neubauer A, Nelson P, Poland-Johnston NK, Sandberg AA, Liu E (1989) Mutations of the Ras ptotooncogenes in chronic myelogenous leukemia: a high frequency of Ras mutations in bcr/abl rearrangement-negative chronic myelogenous leukemia. Blood 74:2629–2633

Cohen GB, Ren R, Baltimore D (1995) Modular binding domains in signal transduction proteins. Cell 80:237–248

Cortez D, Stoica G, Pierce JH, Pendergast AM (1996) The BCR-ABL tyrosine kinase inhibits apoptosis by activating a Ras-dependent signaling pathway. Oncogene 13:2589–2594

Costello R, Lafage M, Toiron Y, Brunel V, Sainty D, Arnoulet C, Mozziconacci MJ, Bouabdallah R, Gastaut J, Maraninchi D, Gabert J (1995) Philadelphia chromosome-negative chronic myeloid leukaemia: a report of 14 new cases. Br J Haematol 90:346–352

Dai Z, Pendergast AM (1995) Abi-2, a novel SH3-containing protein interacts with the c-Abl tyrosine kinase and modulates c-Abl transforming activity. Genes Dev 9:2569–2582

Feinstein E, Cimino G, Gale RP, Alimena G, Berthier R, Kishi K, Goldman J, Zaccaria A, Berrebi A, Canaani E (1991) p53 in chronic myelogenous leukemia in acute phase. Proc Natl Acad Sci U S A 88:6293–6297

Gordon MY, Dowding CR, Riley GP, Goldman JM, Greaves MF (1987) Altered adhesive interactions with marrow stroma of haematopoietic progenitor cells in chronic myeloid leukaemia. Nature 328:342–344

Groffen J, Stephenson JR, Heisterkamp N, de Klein A, Bartram CR, Grosveld G (1984) Philadelphia chromosomal breakpoints are clustered within a limited region, bcr, on chromosome 22. Cell 36:93–99

Kessel GAHM, van Agthoven AJ, de Groot PG, Hagemeijer A (1981) Characterization of a complex philadelphia translocation (1p−; 9q+; 22q−) by gene mapping. Human Genet 58:162–165

Konopka JB, Witte ON (1985) Detection of c-abl tyrosine kinase activity in vitro permits direct comparison of normal and altered abl gene products. Mol Cell Biol 5:3116–3123

Koptyra M, Falinski R, Nowicki MO, Stoklosa T, Majsterek I, Nieborowska-Skorska M, Blasiak J, Skorski T (2006) BCR/ABL kinase induces self-mutagenesis via reactive oxygen species to encode imatinib resistance. Blood 108:319–327

Kothari VC, Advani S, Rao SGA (1986) Growth factors in chronic myelogenous leukemias. Cancer Lett 32:285–292

Kurzrock R, Kantarjian HM, Shtalrid M, Gutterman JU, Talpaz M (1990) Philadelphia chromosome-negative chronic myelogenous leukemia without breakpoint cluster region rearrangement: a chronic myeloid leukemia with distinct clinical course. Blood 75:445–452

Melo JV (1996a) The molecular biology of chronic myeloid leukemia. Leukemia 10:751–756

Melo JV (1996b) The diversity of BCR-ABL fusion proteins and their relationship to leukemia phenotype. Blood 88:2375–2384

Melo JV, Myint H, Galton DA, Goldman JM (1994) P190BCR-ABL chronic myeloid leukemia: the missing link with chronic myelomonocytic leukemia? Leukemia 8:208–211

Naka K, Hoshii T, Muraguchi T, Tadokoro Y, Ooshio T, Kondo Y, Nakao S, Motoyama N, Hirao A (2010) TGF-beta-FOXO signalling maintains leukaemia-initiating cells in chronic myeloid leukaemia. Nature 463:676–680

Nakai H, Misawa S (1995) Chromosome 17 abnormalities and inactivation of the p53 gene in chronic myeloid leukemia and their prognostic significance. Leuk Lymphoma 19:213–221

Nowell PC, Hungerford DA (1960) A minute chromosome in human chronic granulocytic leukemia. Science 132:1497–1500

Nowicki MO, Falinski R, Koptyra M, Slupianek A, Stoklosa T, Gloc E, Nieborowska-Skorska M, Blasiak J, Skorski T (2004) BCR/ABL oncogenic kinase promotes unfaithful repair of the reactive oxygen species-dependent DNA double-strand breaks. Blood 104:3746–3753

O'Brien S, Berman E, Bhalla K, Copelan EA, Devetten MP, Emanuel PD, Erba HP, Greenberg PL, Moore JO, Przepiorka D, Radich JP, Schilder RJ, Shami P, Smith BD, Snyder DS, Soiffer RJ, Tallman MS, Talpaz M, Wetzler M (2007) Chronic myelogenous leukemia. J Natl Compr Canc Netw 5:474–496

O'Dwyer ME, Gatter KM, Loriaux M, Druker BJ, Olson SB, Magenis RE, Lawce H, Mauro MJ, Maziarz RT, Braziel RM (2003) Demonstration of Philadelphia chromosome negative abnormal clones in patients with chronic myelogenous leukemia during major cytogenetic responses induced by imatinib mesylate. Leukemia 17:481–487

Pane F, Frigeri F, Sindona M, Luciano L, Ferrara F, Cimino R, Meloni G, Saglio G, Salvatore F, Rotoli B (1996) Neutrophilic-chronic myeloid leukemia: a distinct disease with a specific molecular marker (BCR-ABL with C3/A2 junction). Blood 88:2410–2414

Puil L, Liu J, Gish G, Mbamalu G, Bowtell D, Pelicci PG, Arlinghaus R, Pawson T (1994) Bcr-Abl oncoproteins bind directly to activators of the Ras signaling pathway. EMBO J 13:764–773

Radich JP (2007) The biology of CML blast crisis. Hematol Am Soc Hematol Educ Program 1:384–391

Sattler M, Verma S, Shrikhande G, Byrne CH, Pride YB, Winkler T, Greenfield EA, Salgia R, Griffin JD (2000) The BCR/ABL tyrosine kinase induces production of reactive oxygen species in hematopoietic cells. J Biol Chem 275:24273–24278

Sawyers CL, McLaughlin J, Witte ON (1995) Genetic requirement for Ras in the transformation of fibroblasts and hematopoietic cells by the Bcr-Abl oncogene. J Exp Med 181:307–313

Selleri L, Emilia G, Luppi M, Temperani P, Zucchini P, Tagliafico E, Artusi T, Sarti M, Donelli A, Castoldi GL (1990) Chronic myelogenous leukemia with typical clinical and morphological features can be Philadelphia chromosome negative and 'bcr negative'. Hematol Pathol 4:67–77

Shepherd PCA, Ganesan TS, Galton DAG (1987) Haematological classification of the chronic myeloid leukemias. Baillieres Clin Haematol 1:887–906

Slupianek A, Hoser G, Majsterek I, Bronisz A, Malecki M, Blasiak J, Fishel R, Skorski T (2002) Fusion tyrosine kinases induce drug resistance by stimulation of homology-dependent recombination repair, prolongation of G(2)/M phase, and protection from apoptosis. Mol Cell Biol 22:4189–4201

Wiedemann LM, Karhi KK, Shivji MK, Rayter SI, Pegram SM, Dowden G, Bevan D, Will A, Galton DA, Chan LC (1988) The correlation of breakpoint cluster region rearrangement and p210 phl/abl expression with morphological analysis of Ph-negative chronic myeloid leukemia and other myeloproliferative diseases. Blood 71:349–355

Chapter 7
Molecular Biology of Myelodysplastic Syndromes

Francesc Solé

Abstract Cytogenetic aberrations, involving chromosomes 5 (5q-), 7 (−7 and 7q-), and 8 (trisomy), are detected with the use of classical cytogenetics in at least 50 % of patients with myelodysplastic syndromes (MDS). They are currently the most powerful predicting factors of overall survival and transformation to acute leukemia in MDS. The use of complementary methods, i.e., fluorescence in situ hybridization, comparative genomic hybridization (array CGH), or single nucleotide polymorphism arrays could reveal chromosomal aberrations in 20–40 % of cases without cytogenetically detectable aberrations. Recently, genome sequencing demonstrated that more than 80 % of MDS patients present with single gene mutations, but the prognostic impact of these mutations is still provisional.

7.1 Introduction

The myelodysplastic syndromes (MDS) comprise a set of chronic medullary insufficiencies, relatively common in daily practice. They generally occur in individuals aged above 50, usually manifesting as mono-, bi-, or pancytopenia with morphological and dyshematopoietic alterations, which evolve into acute leukemia (AL) in 20–30 % of cases. MDS were previously classified into five morphologic subtypes proposed by the French–American–British (FAB) cooperative group (Bennett et al. 1982): simple refractory anemia (RA), refractory anemia with ringed sideroblasts (RARS), refractory anemia with excess of blasts

F. Solé (✉)
Laboratori de Citogenètica Molecular, Servei de Patologia, Escola de Citologia Hematològica Soledad Woessner-IMAS, Hospital del Mar, Passeig Marítim 25-29, 08003 Barcelona, Spain
e-mail: fsole@parcdesalutmar.cat

M. Witt et al. (eds.), *Molecular Aspects of Hematologic Malignancies*, Principles and Practice, DOI: 10.1007/978-3-642-29467-9_7,

Table 7.1 Cytogenetic alterations in patients with de novo MDS

Cytogenetic alterations in de novo MDS	
Most frequent alterations	Other alterations
5q-, del(5q)	t(1;3)(p36;q21)
7q- or −7	t(1;7)(p11;p11)
+8	t(2;11)(p21;q23)
i(17)(q10)	inv(3)(q21q26), t(3;3)(q21;q26)
del(20)(q11q13)	del(9)(q13q22)
−Y	del(11q)
	+11
	12p-, del(12p)
	+13
	13q-
	−18/18q-
	−20
	+21

(RAEB), refractory anemia with excess of blasts in transformation (RAEB-t), and chronic myelomonocytic leukemia (CMML). The criteria for this classification are based on the percentage of blasts in bone marrow and peripheral blood, the absolute number of circulating monocytes, the presence of Auer rods, and the proportion of ringed sideroblasts, all along with variable morphological and dyshematopoietic characteristics. Recently, the World Health Organization (WHO) has proposed a new classification, which establishes the following entities: (1) refractory anemia with or without ringed sideroblasts; (2) refractory cytopenia with multiline myelodysplasia; (3) refractory anemia with excess of blasts; (4) 5q- syndrome (Brunning et al. 2008).

Regarding cytogenetic findings, the detection rate of chromosomal abnormalities in MDS patients varies between 30 and 50 % (Solé et al. 2005; Haase et al. 2007; Pozdnyakova et al. 2008). Chromosomal abnormalities reported in MDS are presented in Table 7.1. Notably, the most frequent abnormalities occur in the form of monosomy or deletion in chromosomes 5 and 7, and as trisomy 8. Other alterations involve 1q, 3q21–26, 11q, 12p, and 17p (Solé et al. 2005; Haase et al. 2007; Pozdnyakova et al. 2008). The detection of balanced translocations is very rare (<1 %) and the finding of complex karyotypes (three or more cytogenetic abnormalities) is observed in 25 % of cases with an abnormal karyotype.

Set out below are the morphological and clinical characteristics related to the most common cytogenetic abnormalities in patients with primary MDS.

7.1.1 3q21–3q26 Involvement

This abnormality could be observed in both MDS and AML (acute myeloid leukemia) patients (Brunning et al. 2008). The involvement of 3q21 and 3q26 regions in MDS is observed in approximately 2 % of patients. The most frequent

alterations involve: inv(3)(q21q26)/*EVI1* (EVI1, ecotropic viral integration site 1, encoding a transcriptional regulator), t(3;5)(q26; q34)/*EVI1-MLF1* (*MLF1*, myeloid leukemia factor 1, encoding a putative transcription factor involved in hematopoiesis),
t(3; 3)(q21; q26)/*MDS1-EVI1* (*MDS1,* myelodysplasia syndrome-associated protein 1, encoding a putative transcription factor). The location of the *EVI1* gene in band 3q26 is a remarkable sign at molecular level. Most patients present with an excess of blasts and a significant percentage (30–50 %) are patients with a history of a prior treatment with chemotherapy. A marked dysmegakaryopoiesis is a particular feature in a group of patients with this cytogenetic anomaly. In 50 % of these cases there is a normal platelet count, while 30 % present with an elevated platelet count. Response to treatment is low with a short survival prognosis (Schanz et al. 2012).

7.1.2 5q- Deletion

The 5q deletion is specific for patients with RA, usually women within an average age of 65. This cytogenetic abnormality is related to megakaryocytic hypolobulation (three or fewer nuclear lobes) or megakaryocytes with just one nucleus, normal or elevated platelet count, macrocytic anemia, red cell hypoplasia in bone marrow, and long survival (Van den Berghe et al. 1985; Solé et al. 2005; Haase et al. 2007; Brunning et al. 2008). In these patients, progression to acute leukemia is rare.

Patients with 5q deletion, as the only abnormality, present the typical characteristics of the so-called 5q-syndrome. This involves older women with macrocytic anemia, thrombocytosis, hypolobulated megakaryocytes, and favorable clinical progress. The experience of the Spanish cooperative group of hematological cytogenetics (Grupo Cooperativo Español de Citogenética Hematológica, GCECGH) confirms the good prognosis for individuals with this chromosomal abnormality, even in patients with RAEB, which is usually associated with an unfavorable clinical evolution. The study by Mallo et al. (2011) shows that the prognosis of patients with 5q- chromosome depends on the complexity of genetic alterations rather than on the percentage of involved blasts in bone marrow or other parameters. Thus, a higher number of accompanying alterations is related to worse prognosis. It should be noted, however, that patients with 5q-, as the only alteration, have the same prognosis as those with 5q- plus one additional alteration.

Recently, a new drug called Lenalidomide has shown a great efficacy in patients with MDS and 5q deletion, not only as a single abnormality, but also when associated with other cytogenetic abnormalities. Therefore, in patients with MDS in which no 5q deletion is observed by means of conventional cytogenetic methods, the implementation of the fluorescence in situ hybridization (FISH) with the 5q probe may be indicated in order to rule out 5q deletion (Mallo et al. 2008).

This molecular cytogenetic approach enables detection of 5q deletion in a greater number of patients.

7.1.3 Monosomy 7 and 7q Deletion

Monosomy 7 or 7q deletions are other very common abnormalities in MDS, reported in both children and adults. These aberrations are related to an initial phase of disease with hypoproliferative bone marrow and refractory cytopenia with defective neutrophils chemotaxis, recurrent infections, and gradual progression into a myeloproliferative syndrome, terminally progressing into AML (Solé et al. 2005; Haase et al. 2007). This alteration is very common in patients with MDS or AML secondary to the use of alkylating agents, such as cyclofosfamide. In the recent cytogenetic scoring system proposed by Schanz et al. (2012) patients with monosomy 7 have worse prognosis than those with deletion of chromosome 7q. These correlations were previously presented by Cordoba et al. (2012).

7.1.4 Trisomy 8

According to the recent literature data, trisomy 8 is the most common cytogenetic abnormality in MDS patients (Haase et al. 2007; Pozdnyakova et al. 2008). It is more common in women than in men (11 vs. 5 %), affecting mainly elderly patients, and it is more frequent in primary than in secondary MDS. This alteration can appear as a single abnormality or can be associated with other aberrations. Trisomy 8 was also reported as the most commonly observed numerical chromosomal abnormality in the Spanish population (Sole et al. 2005).

In some cases, the detection of trisomy 8 may be problematic due to inherent characteristics of chromosome 8 morphology or due to insufficient quality of the obtained metaphases. In these cases, the FISH technique is of use to confirm a suspected trisomy 8 when it is difficult to assess it by means of conventional cytogenetic methods.

MDS cases with trisomy of chromosome 8 are classified into intermediate cytogenetic prognosis group, both in the International Prognostic Scoring System (IPSS) (Greenberg et al. 1997), and in the most recent reports on results of cytogenetic study in MDS patients (Solé et al. 2005; Haase et al. 2007; Pozdnyakova et al. 2008).

7.1.5 12p Deletion

Another very common alteration observed in MDS is 12p deletion (5 %). It is particularly frequent in patients with RAEB, but it is also detected in secondary acute leukemia (5–10 %). This alteration is often associated with the presence of other cytogenetic abnormalities (Solé et al. 2005). In a group of 968 patients (Solé et al. 2005), deletion of chromosome 12, although observed in 13 patients with RAEB has been associated with a good prognosis. The good prognosis related to 12p-was recently confirmed in a larger series of patients (Pozdnyakova et al. 2008; Schanz et al. 2012)

7.1.6 Isochromosome 17q or i(17)(q10)

In the series of GCECGH, isochromosome i(17)(q10), as the sole cytogenetic abnormality, was detected in less than 5 % of patients (Solé et al. 2005). It is of note that i(17)(q10) is usually observed in complex karyotypes. A clinical and biological profile of patients with i(17)(q10) as a single anomaly, includes: older men with hepato or splenomegaly, hypercellular bone marrow, basophilia, eosinophilia, dysmorphic megakaryocytes, and a poor clinical response (most cases progressing into AL and having a very short survival) (Lai et al. 1995).

Regarding the prognostic value, the Spanish group (Solé et al. 2005) suggests a poor prognosis for patients with i(17)(q10) as a single anomaly while the German group (Haase et al. 2007) classifies it within intermediate prognosis. Finally, the new proposal of cytogenetic scoring system by Schanz et al. encompasses the i(17q) within intermediate prognosis.

7.2 Prognostic Value of the Cytogenetic Abnormalities

One of the main limitations of the IPSS (Greenberg et al. 1997) is the stratification of patients according to cytogenetic lesions into three groups only. This implies that in the intermediate prognosis category many cytogenetic abnormalities are included, some of which may entail good and others poor prognosis. To overcome this limitation, Solé et al. (2005) and Haase et al. (2007), in large cohorts of MDS patients, established a new stratification system, taking into account the less frequent cytogenetic alterations. This highlights the good prognosis related to the deletions del(11q), del(12p), and the poor prognosis related to the karyotypes with more than three cytogenetic abnormalities. Recently, Schanz et al. (2012) proposed a new cytogenetic scoring system of MDS, aimed at improvement of the IPSS (Greenberg et al. 1997) through classification of patients into five prognosis categories: very good, good, intermediate, poor, very poor (Table 7.2; Schanz

Table 7.2 Proposal of new cytogenetics *score* of MDS (Schanz et al. 2012)

Prognosis	Cytogenetic aberrations
Very good prognosis (>60.8 months)	del(11q), −Y
Good prognosis (48.5 months)	5q-, 5q-, +1, der(1;7), 12p-, 20q-, +21,
Intermediate prognosis (25 months)	2 alt., 7q-, +8, i(17)(q10), +19, −21, independent clones
Poor prognosis (15 months)	der(3)(q21/q26), −7 as a single alteration, karyotype with 3 cytogenetic alterations, double alterations with −7/7q-
Very poor prognosis (5.7 months)	Karyotype with >3 cytogenetic abnormalities (4 or more abnormalities)

et al. 2012). Moreover, Schanz et al. (2011) demonstrated in a recent study, that the significance of cytogenetics in relation to prognosis is greater than the significance of the proportion of blasts in bone marrow, assigned in the original IPSS. These results suggest a higher score for cytogenetics than for the percentage of bone marrow blasts. These preliminary results will be introduced in the revised IPSS (R-IPSS).

7.2.1 Implementation of FISH in the Study of MDS

Despite the absence of comprehensive regulations, most laboratories consider FISH indispensable in cases with less than 10 evaluable metaphases or with no divisions, as well as to assess minimal residual disease (Table 7.3). The recommended FISH probes are those specific for the most frequent cytogenetic aberrations in MDS, such as: 5q, 7q, *CEP8* (centromeric 8 chromosome), and 20q. Some laboratories suggest the use of additional probes specific for: 11q, 17p13 (*TP53*), and *CEPY* (centromeric FISH probe). These FISH probes could also be recommended in cases with normal cytogenetics in 20 analyzed metaphases, or in cases eligible for treatment according to cytogenetic results. For example, detection of 5q aberrations with the use of FISH in patients without 5q aberrations according to classical cytogenetics enables the use of Lenalidomide in a greater number of patients (Haferlach et al. 2008, Mallo et al. 2008).

On the other hand, in those cases where a complex karyotype is detected, the application of such techniques as multicolor FISH (M-FISH) or spectral karyotyping (SKY), enables the detection of a higher number of cytogenetic abnormalities (Table 7.3). The applications of these techniques could not be considered in the diagnosis and should be restricted to research interest (Table 7.3).

Table 7.3 Cytogenetic study protocol of MDS

Mandatory	Optional	Recommended
Conventional cytogenetic study ("gold standard") In cases with no divisions or less than 10 metaphases suitable for the analysis, apply FISH with 5q and 7q probes, centromeric of 8 and 20q or consider applying CGH/SNP array Apply FISH for monitoring of minimal residual disease Apply 5q- FISH probe in cases where 5q- is not detected, that meet the following requirements: Suspected 5q- syndrome Absence of metaphases suitable for the analysis Altered karyotype with chromosome 5 involvement but without evidence of 5q- (e.g., monosomy 5) Complex karyotype	In cases of complex karyotype, apply M-FISH or SKY	Conservation of biological samples in the Tumor/ Tissue Bank

7.2.2 CGH/SNP Arrays in MDS

Comparative genomic hybridization (CGH) or single nucleotide polymorphism (SNP) arrays are applied for detection of gains and losses of genetic material in cases with complex karyotype or marker chromosomes (Tiu et al. 2011). Recent studies with the use of SNP arrays have shown that 87 % of patients with MDS have cytogenetic abnormalities and that 60 % of patients with normal karyotype present gain or loss of genetic material (Gondek et al. 2008).

Both approaches, the array CGH and SNP arrays, will likely soon become a part of a routine diagnostics of hematological malignancies. The main advantages of these techniques include: independence of dividing cells, ability to detect gain and loss of genetic material (these are the most frequent alterations in patients with MDS), and higher resolution of the analysis, as compared to conventional cytogenetics (0.5 vs. 10 Mb, respectively). Additionally, a technique of SNP arrays enables the detection of UPD (uniparental disomy, which occurs when two copies of a chromosome, or a part of a chromosome, are received from one parent and no copies from the other, resulting in deletion of one allele and duplication of the other). However, array techniques also have certain limitations, among which the following should be noted: inability to detect genetic alterations of the pathological clone when a proportion of tumor cells is less than 30 %; inability to detect balanced translocations (rare in MDS, 1 % and very common in other diseases such as acute leukemia or lymphomas), and a higher cost, as compared to conventional cytogenetics, though similar to that of the use of four FISH probes.

Table 7.4 Major genes mutated in MDS and their prognostic significance (Bejar et al. 2011)

Gene	Incidence (%)	Prognosis
TET2	20	Good
ASXL1	14.4	Poor
RUNX1	8.7	Poor
TP53	7.5	Poor
EZH2	6.4	Poor
NRAS	3.6	Poor
JAK2	3	Intermediate
ETV6	2.7	Poor
CBL	2.3	Poor
IDH2	2.1	Poor
NPM1	1.8	Intermediate
IDH1	1.4	Good
KRAS	0.9	Intermediate
GNAS	0.7	Unknown
PTPN11	0.7	Unknown
BRAF	0.5	Unknown
PTEN	0.2	Unknown
CDKN2A	0.2	Unknown

TET2 ten eleven translocation-2; *ASXL1* additional sex-comb-like-1; *RUNX1* transcriptional core binding factor family name; *TP53* protein P53; *EZH2* enhancer of zeste homolog 2; *NRAS* neuroblastoma *RAS* viral (v-ras) oncogene homolog; *JAK2* janus kinase 2; *ETV6* ets variant; *CBL* casitas B-cell lymphoma; *IDH2* isocitrate dehydrogenase gene 2; *NPM1* nucleophosmin gene; *IDH1* isocitrate dehydrogenase gene 1; *KRAS* v-Ki-ras 2 Kirsten rat sarcoma viral oncogene homolog; *GNAS* GNAS complex locus; *PTPN11* protein tyrosine phosphatase, non-receptor type 11; *BRAF* v-raf murine sarcoma viral oncogene homolog B1; *PTEN* phosphatase and tensin homolog; *CDKN2A* cyclin-dependent kinase

Preliminary results of studies with the use of the above-mentioned methodology have already proven its usefulness. In 2008, Gondek et al. 2008 presented the outcomes of comparative analysis of cytogenetic alterations in MDS patients detected by means of conventional cytogenetics (karyotype) and SNP arrays. They found that SNP arrays enabled detection of cytogenetic abnormalities in 80 % of patients versus 50 % of patients as revealed through conventional cytogenetics. In addition, by means of SNP arrays cytogenetic abnormalities were detected in 68 % of patients with normal karyotypes according to classical cytogenetics, while 80 % of patients with no metaphases for conventional cytogenetics presented cytogenetic abnormalities detected by arrays. Additionally, 33 % of patients manifested loss of heterozygosity (LOH) or UPD.

In a recent study of genetic alterations in a group of 430 MDS patients analyzed with the use of SNP arrays, the authors conclude that the presence and the number of detected lesions are independent predictors of overall and event-free survival. The significant diagnostic and prognostic contribution of SNP-array-detected defects in MDS and related diseases underscore the utility of SNP arrays when combined with conventional cytogenetics in hematological malignancies (Tiu et al. 2011). The load of prognostic information obtained from the results of CGH and SNP arrays, relative to their economic input, do raise the need for the use of these techniques in MDS cases with no metaphases or with normal karyotype (Heinrichs et al. 2009; Thiel et al. 2011). At the moment, there are still too few studies to unequivocally establish the prognostic value of cytogenetic abnormalities detected by CGH/SNP arrays. Therefore, the new proposed revision of IPSS will be based solely on the aberrations detected by means of conventional cytogenetic methods.

7.3 Point Mutations

In the recent years the introduction of sequencing techniques into the study of MDS has demonstrated the implication of some genes in the etiology of this disease (Table 7.4). Recently, Bejar et al. (2011) presented a review of major genetic changes and their clinical implications in MDS patients. Of note are also further works, including those using full-genome sequencing, which reveal new genes involved in MDS, particularly highlighting mutations of *SF3B1* (splicing factor 3b, subunit 1, gene related with alternative splicing), with an incidence of nearly 75 % in the cases with ringed sideroblasts (Papaemmanuil et al. 2011; Yoshida et al. 2011).

7.4 Conclusions

The routine application of cytogenetic and molecular cytogenetic methods in the diagnostics of MDS provides complementary information to those of cytology, allowing to establish cytological-cytogenetic-based subgrouping of MDS patients. The results of numerous studies, including those performed in a large series of patients, with cytogenetic and clinical monitoring indicate that karyotype analysis has important clinical and therapeutic implications.

On the other hand, the continual learning on new cytogenetic alterations will allow establishing of new cytological entities with well-defined clinical characteristics. The implementation of array technology will reveal the molecular mechanisms involved in MDS, thus contributing to establishment of more specific therapeutic approaches. The application of whole genome sequencing already provides knowledge on additional genes involved in MDS pathomechanisms. However, for the moment, the study of these genes has been solely restricted to research activities and their potential implementation into diagnostic testing of the MDS requires further study.

Acknowledgments I want to thank the support received from Celgene (Spain) in the translation of the paper.

References

Bejar R, Stevenson K, Abdel-Wahab O, Galili N, Nilsson B, Garcia-Manero G, Kantarjian H, Raza A, Levine RL, Neuberg D, Ebert BL (2011) Clinical effect of point mutations in myelodysplastic syndromes. N Engl J Med 364:2496–2506

Bennett JM, Catovsky D, Daniel MT, Flandrin G, Galton DA, Gralnick HR, Sultan C (1982) The French–American–British co-operative group. Proposals for the classification of the myelodysplastic syndromes. Br J Haematol 51:189–199

Brunning RD, Orazi A, Germing U, Le Beau MM, Porwit A, Baumann I (2008) Myelodysplastic syndromes. In: Swerdlow SH, Campo E, Lee Harris N, Jaffe ES, Pileri SA, Stein H, Thiele J, Vardiman JW (eds) WHO classification of tumours of haematopoietic and lymphoid tissues. IARC, Lyon, pp 87–107

Cordoba I, Gonzalez Porras JR, Nomdedeu B, Luño E, De Paz R, Such E, Tormo M, Vallespi T, Collado R, Xicoy B, Andreu R, Muñoz JA, Solé F, Cervera J, Cañizo M (2012) Better prognosis for patients with del(7q) than those with monosomy 7 in myelodysyplastic syndromes. Cancer 118:127–133. doi:10.1002/cncr.26279

Gondek LP, Tiu R, O'Keefe CL, Sekeres MA, Theil KS, Maciejewski JP (2008) Chromosomal lesions and uniparental disomy detected by SNP arrays in MDS, MDS/MPD, and MDS-derived AML. Blood 111:1534–1542

Greenberg P, Cox C, Le Beau MM, Fenaux P, Morel P, Sanz G, Sanz M, Vallespí T, Hamblin T, Oscier D, Ohyashiki K, Toyama K, Aul C, Mufti G, Bennett J (1997) International scoring system for evaluating prognosis in myelodysplastic syndromes. Blood 89:2079–2088

Haase D, Germing U, Schanz J, Pfeilstöcker M, Nösslinger T, Hildebrandt B, Kundgen A, Lübbert M, Kunzmann R, Giagounidis AA, Aul C, Trümper L, Krieger O, Stauder R, Müller TH, Wimazal F, Valent P, Fonatsch C, Steidl C (2007) New insights into the prognostic impact of the karyotype in MDS and correlation with subtypes: evidence from a core dataset of 2124 patients. Blood 110:4385–4395

Haferlach C, Bacher U, Tiu R, Maciejewski JP, List A (2008) Myelodysplastic syndromes with del(5q) indications and strategies for cytogenetic testing. Cancer Genet Cytogenet 187(2):101–111

Heinrichs S, Kulkarni RV, Bueso-Ramos CE, Levine RL, Loh ML, Li C, Neuberg D, Kornblau SM, Issa JP, Gilliland DG, Garcia-Manero G, Kantarjian HM, Estey EH, Look AT (2009) Accurate detection of uniparental disomy and microdeletions by SNP array analysis in myelodysplastic syndromes with normal cytogenetics. Leukemia 23:1605–1613

Lai JL, Preudhomme C, Zandecki M, Flactif M, Vanrumbeke M, Lepelley P, Wattel E, Fenaux P (1995) Myelodysplastic syndromes and acute myeloid leukemia with 17p deletion. An entity characterized by specific dysgranulopoïesis and a high incidence of P53 mutations. Leukemia 9:370–381

Mallo M, Arenillas L, Espinet B, Salido M, Hernández JM, Lumbreras E, Del Rey M, Arranz E, Ramiro S, Font P, González O, Renedo M, Cervera J, Such E, Sanz GF, Luño E, Sanzo C, González M, Calasanz MJ, Mayans J, García-Ballesteros C, Amigo V, Collado R, Oliver I, Carbonell F, Bureo E, Insunza A, Yañez L, Muruzabal MJ, Gómez-Beltrán E, Andreu R, León P, Gómez V, Sanz A, Casasola N, Moreno E, Alegre A, Martín Ml, Pedro C, Serrano S, Florensa L, Solé F (2008) Fluorescence in situ hybridization improves the detection of 5q31 deletion in myelodysplastic syndromes without cytogenetic evidence of 5q-. Haematologica 93:1001–1008

Mallo M, Cervera J, Schanz J, Such E, García-Manero G, Luño E, Steidl C, Espinet B, Vallespí T, Germing U, Blum S, Ohyashiki K, Grau J, Pfeilstöcker P, Hernández JM, Noesslinger T, Giagounidis A, Aul C, Calasanz MJ, Martín Ml, Valent P, Collado R, Haferlach C, Fonatsch C, Lübbert M, Stauder R, Hildebrandt B, Krieger O, Pedro C, Arenillas L, Sanz MA, Valencia A, Florensa L, Sanz GF, Haase D, Solé F (2011) Impact of adjunct cytogenetic abnormalities for prognostic stratification in patients with myelodysplastic syndrome and deletion 5q. Leukemia 25:110–120

Morel P, Hebbar M, Lai JL, Duhamel A, Preudhomme C, Wattel E, Bauters F, Fenaux P (1993) Cytogenetic analysis has strong independent prognostic value in de novo myelodysplastic syndromes and can be incorporated in a new scoring system: a report on 408 cases. Leukemia 7:1315–1323

Papaemmanuil E, Cazzola M, Boultwood J, Malcovati L, Vyas P, Bowen D, Pellagatti A, Wainscoat JS, Hellstrom-Lindberg E, Gambacorti-Passerini C, Godfrey AL, Rapado I, Cvejic A, Rance R, McGee C, Ellis P, Mudie LJ, Stephens PJ, McLaren S, Massie CE, Tarpey PS, Varela I, Nik-Zainal S, Davies HR, Shlien A, Jones D, Raine K, Hinton J, Butler AP, Teague JW, Baxter EJ, Score J, Galli A, Della Porta MG, Travaglino E, Groves M, Tauro S, Munshi NC, Anderson KC, El-Naggar A, Fischer A, Mustonen V, Warren AJ, Cross NC, Green AR, Futreal PA, Stratton MR, Campbell PJ (2011) Chronic Myeloid Disorders Working Group of the International Cancer Genome Consortium. Somatic SF3B1 mutation in myelodysplasia with ring sideroblasts. N Engl J Med 365:1384–1395

Pozdnyakova O, Miron PM, Tang G, Walter O, Raza A, Woda B, Wang SA (2008) Cytogenetic abnormalities in a series of 1,029 patients with primary myelodysplastic syndromes: report from the US with a focus on some undefined single chromosomal abnormalities. Cancer 113:3331–3340

Schanz J, Tuechler H, Solé F, Mallo M, Luño E, Cervera J, Granada I, Hildebrandt B, Slovak Ml, Ohyashiki K, Steidl C, Fonatsch C, Pfeilstoecker M, Noesslinger T, Valent P, Giagounidis A, Aul A, Luebbert M, Stauder R, Krieger O, Garcia-Manero G, Faderl S, Pierce S, Le Beau MM, Bennett J, Greenberg P, Germing U, Haase D (2012) A new, comprehensive cytogenetic scoring system for primary myelodysplastic syndromes and oligoblastic AML leukemia following MDS derived from an international database merge. J Clin Oncol 30:820–829

Schanz J, Steidl C, Fonatsch C, Pfeilstöcker M, Nösslinger T, Tuechler H, Valent P, Hildebrandt B, Giagounidis A, Aul C, Lübbert M, Stauder R, Krieger O, Garcia-Manero G, Kantarjian H, Germing U, Haase D, Estey E (2011) Coalesced multicentric analysis of 2,351 patients with myelodysplastic syndromes indicates an underestimation of poor-risk cytogenetics of myelodysplastic syndromes in the international prognostic scoring system. J Clin Oncol 29:1963–1970

Solé F, Luño E, Sanzo C, Espinet B, Sanz GF, Cervera J, Calasanz MJ, Cigudosa JC, Millà F, Ribera JM, Bureo E, Marquez ML, Arranz E, Florensa L (2005) Identification of novel cytogenetic markers with prognostic significance in a series of 968 patients with primary myelodysplastic syndromes. Haematologica 90:1168–1178

Thiel A, Beier M, Ingenhag D, Servan K, Hein M, Moeller V, Betz B, Hildebrandt B, Evers C, Germing U, Royer-Pokora B (2011) Comprehensive array CGH of normal karyotype myelodysplastic syndromes reveals hidden recurrent and individual genomic copy number alterations with prognostic relevance. Leukemia 25:387–399

Tiu RV, Gondek LP, O'Keefe CL, Elson P, Huh J, Mohamedali A, Kulasekararaj A, Advani AS, Paquette R, List AF, Sekeres MA, McDevitt MA, Mufti GJ, Maciejewski JP (2011) Prognostic impact of SNP arrays karyotyping in myelodysplastic syndromes and related myeloid malignancies. Blood 117:4552–4560

Van Den Berghe H, Vermaelen K, Mecucci C, Barbieri D, Tricot G (1985) The 5q- anomaly. Cancer Genet Cytogenet 17:189–255

Toyama K, Ohyashiki K, Yoshida Y, Abe T, Asano S, Hirai H, Hirashima K, Hotta T, Kuramoto A, Kuriya SH, Miyazaki T, Kakishita E, Mizoguchi H, Okada M, Shirakawa SH, Takaku F, Tomonaga M, Uchino H, Yasunaga K, Nomura T (1993) Clinical implications of chromosomal abnormalities in 401 patients with myelodysplastic syndromes: a multicentric study in Japan. Leukemia 7:499–508

Yoshida K, Sanada M, Shiraishi Y, Nowak D, Nagata Y, Yamamoto R, Sato Y, Sato-Otsubo A, Kon A, Nagasaki M, Chalkidis G, Suzuki Y, Shiosaka M, Kawahata R, Yamaguchi T, Otsu M, Obara N, Sakata-Yanagimoto M, Ishiyama K, Mori H, Nolte F, Hofmann WK, Miyawaki S, Sugano S, Haferlach C, Koeffler HP, Shih LY, Haferlach T, Chiba S, Nakauchi H, Miyano S, Ogawa S (2011) Frequent pathway mutations of splicing machinery in myelodysplasia. Nature 478:64–69

Chapter 8
Myeloproliferative Neoplasms

Andrzej Hellmann, Maria Bieniaszewska, Witold Prejzner and Aleksandra Leszczyńska

Abstract This chapter presents the significance of achievements in molecular biology for the group of disorders called myeloproliferative neoplasms in the latest WHO classification. From a clinical point of view, the finding of specific point mutations or gene fusions has finally proven their neoplastic origin. Second, these findings have given clinicians a very useful tool that can simplify diagnostic procedures and make the final diagnosis more precise and reliable. Another advantage is the development of new drugs to target these mutations. While a separate chapter of this book is devoted to chronic myeloid leukemia, here we present the *JAK2* and *MPL* gene mutations in polycythemia vera, essential thrombocythemia, and primary myelofibrosis; the *PDGFRA* and *PDGFRB* fusion genes in chronic eosinophilic leukemia; and the *KIT* gene mutation in systemic mastocytosis. Some new discoveries in this still expanding field are also highlighted.

8.1 Introduction

The most recent, fourth edition of the World Health Organization (WHO) classification of tumors of hematopoietic and lymphoid tissues (2008) has updated the terminology and diagnostic criteria for the group of disorders known as myeloproliferative syndromes or disorders (Swerdlow et al. 2008). Initially, four of them, known now as the classic ones, were grouped together by Dameshek (1951).

A. Hellmann (✉) · M. Bieniaszewska · W. Prejzner · A. Leszczyńska
Department of Hematology and Transplantology, Medical University of Gdańsk, Dębinki 7, 80-952 Gdańsk, Poland
e-mail: klhem@gumed.edu.pl

M. Witt et al. (eds.), *Molecular Aspects of Hematologic Malignancies*, Principles and Practice, DOI: 10.1007/978-3-642-29467-9_8,

These include chronic myeloid leukemia (CML), polycythemia vera (PV), essential thrombocythemia (ET), and primary myelofibrosis (PMF). The WHO classification in 2001 added to this list some rare disorders, such as chronic eosinophilic leukemia (CEL) and chronic neutrophilic leukemia. In the latest WHO classification, mastocytosis is listed with all the above-mentioned disorders in the group of myeloproliferative neoplasms (MPNs). These changes in classification and terminology are the result of developments in molecular biology during the last 25 years. The concept of the neoplastic nature of these disorders (although not proven in 100 % of the cases) was confirmed by identification of specific molecular markers: either gene point mutations or gene fusions. In 1984, the *BCR-ABL* fusion gene, which results from a translocation between chromosomes 9 and 22, was described in CML (Groffen et al. 1984). In 1993, a mutation of the *KIT* gene, characteristic of systemic mastocytosis (SM), was found (Furitsu et al. 1993). In 2003, the *FIP1L1-PDGFRA* fusion gene characteristic of CEL was described (Cools et al. 2003). Two years later, a *JAK2* gene mutation was found in a majority of PV cases and in at least half of ET and PMF cases (James et al. 2005; Baxter et al. 2005; Levine et al. 2005; Kralovics et al. 2005). In 2006, an *MPL* gene mutation was found in ET and PMF patients (Pikman et al. 2006). A *TET2* mutation was first identified in 2009 in various myeloid neoplasms including MPNs (about 10 % of patients are positive for this mutation) (Delhommeau et al. 2009). This *TET2* mutation probably alters myeloid development via epigenetic modifications, and it usually precedes the *JAK2* mutation. Some recent studies, however, showed that the *TET2* mutation can also occur after the *JAK2* mutation (Schaub et al. 2010).

All of the above-mentioned genes, except for *TET2,* encode cytoplasmic or membrane-bound receptor protein tyrosine kinases. This results in the activation of signal transduction pathways, leading to an increase in cell proliferation. Thus, MPNs are clonal hematopoietic stem cell disorders characterized by the proliferation of one or more of the myeloid lineages: erythroid, megakaryocytic, neutrophil or eosinophil granulocytes, or mast cells. It is important to mention that fibrosis of the bone marrow, even in PMF, is not a clonal event, but the reaction to megakaryocyte or granulocyte proliferation. Initially, MPNs are characterized by increased cellularity of the bone marrow, where the percentage of blast cells is normal or slightly increased (by up to 10 %), and organopathy (splenomegaly) is often also present. Hematopoiesis is effective, with the normal maturation of cells, but blast transformation may form the final stage of these disorders. Before the era of molecular insights into MPN biology, the diagnosis of these disorders was sometimes difficult. In order to make a final diagnosis, it was necessary to meet many major or minor criteria based on clinical or laboratory findings. The starting point for the diagnosis of Ph-negative or *BCR/ABL*-negative classical myeloproliferative disorders (i.e. PV, ET, or PMF) was the exclusion of Ph chromosome positivity or *BCR/ABL* positivity. Nowadays, such procedures are only recommended in the case of *JAK2*, *MPL,* or another mutation negativity. The current numerical criteria in the case of platelet number or hemoglobin level in ET or PV could be lowered due to the molecular proof of neoplastic origin of these disorders.

With the use of molecular tools, it is quite easy to distinguish between almost all of the MPN entities from reactive causes of elevated blood counts (Hellmann and Bieniaszewska 2009).

However, it is sometimes difficult to make a differential diagnosis between classical MPNs that are positive for a *JAK2* mutation, i.e., PV, ET, and PMF. In such patients, a trephine biopsy of the bone marrow plays a crucial role in the final diagnosis. It is especially important for distinguishing between ET and the pre-fibrotic stage of PMF.

The evolving understanding of the molecular pathogenesis of MPNs has led to the development of so-called targeted therapies in these disorders. Tyrosine kinase inhibitors were successfully introduced in the treatment of CML (see Chap. 6) more than 10 years ago. These drugs are also successfully used in the therapy of CEL and aggressive forms of systemic mastocytosis (SM). Current clinical trials on targeted therapies for other MPNs are predominantly based on *JAK2* inhibitors, and began in 2007. The most important trials included such molecules as INCB 1824, TG 101348, SB 1518, and CEP 701 (Van Etten et al. 2011). These trials are mainly conducted on PMF patients, but also on PV and ET patients who are unresponsive to other therapies. These drugs reduce splenomegaly and constitutional symptoms common in PMF. However, some toxic effects (including anemia and thrombocytopenia) have been observed.

8.2 *JAK2* and *MPL* Gene Mutations

The Janus kinase 2 *(JAK2)* gene encodes cytoplasmic tyrosine kinase, which plays an important role in cytokine signaling pathways. A point mutation in exon 14 of this gene at nucleotide 1849 (G > T transversion) results in the substitution of phenylalanine for valine (V617F) in the JAK2 protein. This mutation induces its constitutive activation (Baxter et al. 2005; James et al. 2005; Kralovics et al. 2005; Levine et al. 2005).

Because the *JAK2* mutation causing V617F substitution (frequently shortened in the literature, however, improperly, to V617F *JAK2* gene mutation) has a gain-of-function character, the JAK/STAT signaling pathway is activated, even in the complete absence of receptor ligands, i.e., hematopoietic growth factors: thrombopoietin, or erythropoietin (EPO). This leads to erythropoietin-independent proliferation in vitro, to the maturation of erythropoietic progenitors in cell cultures, to uncontrolled proliferation of erythropoiesis in the bone marrow in vivo, and to an increase in the mature cell count in peripheral blood. The latter effect is also observed in irradiated mice transplanted with hematopoietic progenitors containing *JAK2* V617F cells, but not the wild-type *JAK2* (Wernig et al. 2006). This provides strong evidence that the *JAK2* mutation plays a causal or contributory role in the pathogenesis of PV, ET, and PMF.

The molecular findings concerning PV, ET, and PMF, lead to the most important question: how might the same mutation be responsible for three different phenotypes? This problem was investigated by many research teams. Three main explanations for this phenomenon have been postulated.

The first one is the so-called "dosage" hypothesis (Vannucchi et al. 2008). The key finding was the observation of differences in the level of allele burden in patients with PV, ET, and PMF. Duplication of the mutant allele at the single cell level, as a result of mitotic recombination, is more frequent in PV and PMF than in ET. Homozygosity might provide greater activation of the signaling pathway than that seen in cells with mutant and wild-type alleles (Scott et al. 2006). The lack of competition between normal and mutant alleles might also enhance the effect of mutant protein and contribute to the derangement of cellular function. Importantly, in many patients a differential diagnosis between PV, ET, and PMF can be made by assessing the burden of *JAK2*-positive alleles by quantitative measurements (RQ-PCR—real-time quantitative polymerase chain reaction).

The second hypothesis explaining the genotypic-phenotypic correlation suggests the possibility of another clonal event in preJAK mutated cells (Kralovics et al. 2006; Nussenzveig et al. 2007). This "first clonal hit" favors the acquisition of V617F *JAK2* or W515 *MPL* mutation. This possibility is mainly supported by the clinical observation that in patients with a transformation of MPN, leukemic cells are usually *JAK2* V617F negative (Theocharides et al. 2007). So far, this postulated primary mutation (clonal event) has remained unidentified. One of the candidates is the *TET2* gene mutation (Van Etten et al. 2011).

The last hypothesis explains the paradox of a single mutation with three clinical phenotypes by host-modifying influences (genetic background). There are some data suggesting that several single-nucleotide polymorphisms (SNPs) and haplotypes within *JAK2* show an association with only one disorder among the MPNs (Pardanani et al. 2008). A particular distribution of alleles determines the disease phenotype.

Another mutation that can be found in MPN patients negative for the *JAK2* V617F mutation (detected in about 15 % of these patients) is a point mutation in the juxtamembrane region of the thrombopoietin receptor (*MPL*) gene. The *MPL* gene mutations are mainly located in exon 10 (Siemiątkowska et al. 2009). The best method for detecting these mutations is high-resolution melt analysis (Pietra et al. 2011).

The *MPL* mutation affecting codon 505 was found for the first time in patients with familial hereditary thrombocytosis (Ding et al. 2004). In 1–3 % of patients with ET and 5–7 % with PMF, tryptophan (W) residue in 515 position is the most frequently mutated one. W515 is a key amino acid located in the unique domain of the MPL receptor that prevents its spontaneous activation. The substitution of tryptophan by leucine (W515L), lysine (W515 K), or alanine (W515A), changes the spatial conformation of MPL and activates the JAK2 signaling pathway. Expression of the *MPL* W515 allele, results in the cytokine-independent growth of cell lines, as in the case of the *JAK2* V617F mutation. However, in contrast to the *JAK2* V617F mutation, no growth of endogenous erythroid colonies in the *MPL*-mutated cell culture was observed. Coexistence of both the above-mentioned mutations is extremely rare. In one patient within our ET-cohort, coexistence of

JAK2 V617F and *MPL* W515 K was found (Hellmann et al., unpublished data). The same finding was recently described by another group (Pietra et al. 2011).

8.2.1 Polycythemia Vera

The *JAK2* V617F mutation located in exon 14 occurs in 96 % of PV patients (Vannucchi et al. 2007). In patients who meet the major clinical criterion for the diagnosis of PV (hemoglobin level), detection of mutations is sufficient to confirm the diagnosis. In a small percentage of patients, in whom no mutation of *JAK2* V617F is found, further diagnostic steps involve the search for other, less common mutations. The *JAK2* gene mutations of exon 12 are found in approximately 3 % of PV patients (Pardanani et al. 2007). Patients with these mutations are generally younger and have higher hemoglobin levels, lower serum erythropoietin, and predominantly erythroid myelopoiesis, in comparison to patients with typical mutations in exon 14.

About 5 years after identifying the *JAK2* V617F mutation in PV, this disease now appears to be, in some respects, similar to CML. Unfortunately, novel targeted therapy with JAK2 kinase inhibitors has not brought as promising results as the treatment with BCR/ABL kinase inhibitors in CML patients. One of the reasons is the fact that these tyrosine kinase inhibitors target not only the mutant but also the wild-type JAK2 (Chen and Prchal 2010).

8.2.2 Essential Thrombocythemia

ET is another disorder among MPNs, in which the *JAK2* mutation has been found. In this case, the mutation occurs only in about 50–60 % of patients. According to several studies, the genotype-phenotype correlation is evident in ET. Patients with *JAK2* V617F-positive ET are older, have a higher number of platelets, a higher leukocyte count, and a higher hemoglobin level upon diagnosis than those lacking the V617F mutation. These findings inspired the hypothesis that *JAK2* V617F-positive ET is the early stage (pre-PV stage) or a *forme fruste* of PV, rather than true ET (Campbell et al. 2005). The hypothesis is further supported by the fact that, so far, no case of conversion from the *JAK2* wild-type ET to the mutant-type of the disease has been described.

According to the data published from the large prospective Primary Thrombocythemia 1 (PT-1) study, the prevalence of typical *MPL* mutations in ET is 3.4 % (Beer et al. 2008). The clinical influence of the *MPL* mutation is unclear. In the PT-1 study, the ET patients who carried the *MPL* mutation were older than the *JAK2* V617F-negative patients and had lower hemoglobin and higher platelet levels than *JAK2* V617F-positive ET patients. Patients with *MPL*-mutant ET presented hypocellular bone marrow with reduced erythroid and granulocytic lineages, as compared to non-*MPL*-mutant patients (Beer et al. 2008).

8.2.3 *Primary Myelofibrosis*

Similar to ET, the *JAK2* V617F mutation is found in about 50 % of patients with PMF. However, unlike in ET, the genotypic-phenotypic correlations are controversial. In reviewing the studies on large cohorts of PMF patients, the presence of the *JAK2* V617F mutation was associated with lower survival rate, higher incidence of leukemic transformation, and higher leukocyte or hemoglobin levels in two independent studies (Barosi et al. 2007; Campbell et al. 2006). By contrast, in other studies no correlation between the *JAK2* V617F mutation and laboratory or clinical findings was noted (Tefferi et al. 2008a), but a low level of mutant allele burden, associated with a myelodepletive type of the disease, was regarded as an independent negative prognostic factor associated with shortened survival in PMF. In the future, this finding may have a critical influence on the choice of therapy, particularly for young patients with PMF. It could help to identify candidates with the early stage of the disease, who are eligible for bone marrow transplantation (Guglielmelli et al. 2009).

A mutation at codon 515 of the *MPL* gene is found in 7–10 % of *JAK2* V617F-negative patients with PMF. In some studies, the frequency of the *MPL* mutation is even higher. Because of limited clinical data, there is still controversy over the presence of genotype-phenotype correlations in PMF.

8.3 *PDGFRA* or *PDGFRB* Fusion Genes

The platelet-derived growth factor receptor alpha (*PDGFRA*) gene belongs to the tyrosine kinase family genes. Fusion of *FIP1L1* (FIP1-like 1 gene encoding a subunit of CPSF, the cleavage and polyadenylation specificity factor involved in pre-mRNA 3′-end processing) to the *PDGFRA* causes a constitutive tyrosine kinase activation of the resulting protein. This, in turn, activates downstream signaling regulating cell proliferation and survival (Stover et al. 2006). The most common clonal abnormality in eosinophilic proliferations is a cryptic deletion of chromosome 4q12, generating the *FIP1L1/PDGFRA* fusion gene. This is an 800-kb submicroscopic deletion, resulting in the fusion of the 5′ part of the *FIP1L1* gene to the 3′ part of *PDGFRA*. Since the deletion is only 800 kb in size, this genomic rearrangement remains undetectable by standard cytogenetic methods, but can be detected by fluorescence in situ hybridization (FISH). The breakpoints of the *FIP1L1* gene always appear within its introns. They are scattered over a 40-kb region encompassing introns 8–13. However, other breakpoints have also been described, e.g., in intron 16, outside the typical breakpoint cluster region (Lambert et al. 2007). The breakpoint in *PDGFRA* occurs exclusively in exon 12 (Cools et al. 2003).

The *FIP1L1/PDGFRA* fusion gene can be more sensitively identified by reverse transcriptase-polymerase chain reaction (RT-PCR) than by fluorescent in situ hybridization (FISH). In some patients, the fusion gene remains difficult to detect, which may be due to its low expression level and/or heterogeneity of *FIP1L1* breakpoints (Lambert et al. 2007). Therefore, a combination of RT-PCR and FISH provides the best chance of identifying *FIP1L1/PDGFRA*-positive patients (Apperley and Bain 2004). Due to the very good molecular response to treatment in most CEL patients, nested RT-PCR—when positive at the time of diagnosis—is the method of choice for assessments of treatment response (Halaburda et al. 2006).

Besides the *PDGFRA* gene rearrangement, eosinophilia with rearrangement of the platelet-derived growth factor receptor beta (*PDGFRB*) gene has also been observed. A distinctive type of myeloid neoplasm occurs in association with the rearrangement of *PDGFRB*, which is located on chromosome 5q31. Usually, the aberration t(5;12)(q31;p12) is detected. This translocation results in a fusion of *ETV6* (ets variant 6 gene, encoding an ETS family transcription factor) with *PDGFRB* gene. The hematological features are mostly those of chronic myelomonocytic leukemia (usually with eosinophilia). This disease, with rearrangements of *PDGFRB*, is similar to CEL in its sensitivity to the tyrosine kinase inhibitor imatinib. However, not all the cases of translocation of t(5;12)(q31;p12) lead to *ETV6-PDGFRB* gene fusion. Patients without the fusion gene do not respond to imatinib. Because of the therapeutic implications, FISH and RT-PCR should be used when *PDGFRB* rearrangements are suspected (Curtis et al. 2007).

8.3.1 Chronic Eosinophilic Leukemia

Chronic eosinophilic leukemia (CEL) is a myeloproliferative neoplasm in which an autonomous, clonal proliferation of eosinophil precursors results in a persistent increase in the number of eosinophils in peripheral blood, bone marrow, and tissues. Tissue infiltration by eosinophils and the release of cytokines from eosinophil granules leads to tissue damage in organs, such as the heart, lungs, liver, central nervous system, skin, and gastrointestinal tract. Diagnosis of CEL is based on an increased number of eosinophils ($\geq$1.5 G/L) and identification of the signs of eosinophil clonality, such as rearrangements of *PDGFRA* or an increased number of myeloblasts in the bone marrow (>2 %) or peripheral blood (>5 %). However, in many patients it is impossible to prove eosinophil clonality. In such patients, diagnosis of hypereosinophilic syndrome (HES) should be made. This syndrome is defined as eosinophilia ($\geq$1.5 G/L) persisting for at least 6 months, for which no underlying cause is found.

8.4 *KIT* Gene Mutations

Identification of the *KIT* (mast cell growth factor receptor gene) D816 V mutation has facilitated a better understanding of the molecular mechanisms of mastocytosis, contributed to improving its diagnosis, and promoted the search for new targeted therapies (Furitsu et al. 1993). In humans, the *KIT* gene is located on chromosome

4q12, adjacent to the *PDGFRA* gene. The human *KIT* gene spans approximately 88 kb and contains 21 exons coding for a type III tyrosine kinase receptor (Giebel et al. 1992). The *KIT* gene was first identified as a cellular homolog of the feline sarcoma viral oncogene *v-kit*. Human *KIT* is a proto-oncogene that encodes the transmembrane receptor with intrinsic tyrosine kinase activity. The *KIT* gene product is a tyrosine kinase receptor for stem cell factor (SCF) and is considered to serve as a key regulator of normal mast cell differentiation. At present it is known that activation of the SCF/KIT signaling pathway is associated with multiple biological effects, including cell proliferation, maturation, differentiation, and suppression of apoptosis. Furthermore, *KIT* activates several signal transduction pathways, such as the protein kinase C (PKC), mitogen-activated protein kinase (MAPK), PI-3 kinase, and Janus kinase (JAK) signaling. In most patients with SM, the *KIT* D816 V mutation in exon 17 is found, which results in substitution of valine for aspartic acid at 816 amino acid residue. The *KIT* D816 V mutation is associated with SCF-independent phosphorylation and activation of the protein product (KIT tyrosine kinase receptor), and it contributes to the autonomous differentiation and growth of neoplastic mast cells. Since the first description of the activating *KIT* gene mutation in human mast cell line in 1993, many different *KIT* mutations have been reported in patients with mastocytosis (Pignon et al. 1997). The D816 V mutation is found in more than 90 % of patients with this disease. The *KIT* mutations cluster in a relatively small region—most frequently in exon 17—and they lead to amino acid changes at the juxtamembrane and tyrosine kinase 2 domain of KIT. Less frequently, *KIT* mutations are detected in exons 2, 8, and 9 or in exons 11, 13, and 14 (Pignon et al. 1997; Mital et al. 2011).

The *KIT* mutations are also frequently observed in other neoplastic disorders. Interestingly, careful analysis of the *KIT* mutations shows a clear association between the type of *KIT* mutation and the specific disease. Except for mastocytosis, *KIT* mutations may be found in gastrointestinal tumors, acute myeloid leukemia, seminoma, and non-Hodgkin lymphoma. At present, the exact mechanisms leading to the association between specific *KIT* mutations and particular diseases remains unknown. It is supposed that such associations could be related to the up-regulation of different signal transduction pathways by different mutations. In contrast to adults, the *KIT* mutation occurring in exon 17, causing D816 V substitution in the resulting protein (again shortened to D816 V *KIT* mutation—see comment above) is infrequent in children with cutaneous mastocytosis. However, other types of somatic activating *KIT* mutations were identified, outside of exon 17, in 44 % of pediatric patients with cutaneous mastocytosis (CM) (Bodemer et al. 2010).

8.4.1 Systemic Mastocytosis

Mastocytosis is a group of rare diseases characterized by an excessive proliferation and accumulation of mast cells in one or more organs, such as the skin, alimentary tract, liver, spleen, bones, and bone marrow. Mastocytosis may occur at any age. In children, CM is the most prevalent form, whereas adults usually suffer from SM with mast cell infiltration of extracutaneous organs. In SM, bone marrow is infiltrated by mast cells. Thus, bone marrow cytology and trephine biopsy, combined with relevant immunohistochemical analyses, are the cornerstone of diagnosis. Additional tests used to confirm the presence of this disease (minor criteria) include immunophenotypic analyses of mast cells, determination of tryptase concentration, and molecular tests. According to the WHO, either one major criterion (the presence of dense infiltrates of >15 mast cells in bone marrow or in other extracutaneous organs, detected by immunohistochemical analysis) and one of the minor criteria (as mentioned above), or three minor criteria are required for the diagnosis of SM. Detection of the D816 V *KIT* gene mutation is a minor but very important criterion for the diagnosis of mastocytosis. In suspected SM, the diagnostic standard is to examine unfractionated bone marrow cells or mononuclear bone marrow cells for *KIT* mutations.

The most frequently used medications for the treatment of aggressive mast cell disorders are cladribine and interferon alpha 2b (Tefferi et al. 2008b). There have been several attempts to use tyrosine kinase inhibitors as targeted therapy. Unfortunately, imatinib did not give the expected response in SM patients with the D816 V *KIT* mutation. However, attempts with dasatinib (a second-generation tyrosine kinase inhibitor) have proved its beneficial effects. In patients without the typical D816 V *KIT* mutation, the search for other mutations by whole *KIT* gene sequencing should be prompted. Some of such rare mutations are targeted by imatinib, with a very good clinical response (Valent et al. 2007; Mital et al. 2011).

8.5 Conclusions

Although myeloproliferative neoplasms described in this chapter are well known to clinicians since the early twentieth century, most of the knowledge of their neoplastic origin, proved by gene expression studies, has been acquired in recent years. This knowledge should be used in everyday clinical hematological practice. In most patients, the only way to establish a certain diagnosis is to perform proper molecular studies. These investigations are also important because of the expanding possibilities of introducing novel targeted therapies in the treatment of these diseases. Molecular methods, like RT-PCR or RQ-PCR, are also important tools for monitoring the effects of such therapies.

References

Apperley J, Bain B (2004) The FIP1L1- PDGFRA syndrome: a case of mistaken identity? Blood 104:2999–3000

Barosi G, Bergamaschi G, Marchetti M, Vannucchi AM, Guglielmelli P, Antonioli E, Massa M, Rosti V, Campanell R, Villani L, Viarengo G, Gattoni E, Gerli G, Specchia G, Tinelli C, Rambaldi A, Barbui T (2007) *JAK2* V617F mutational status predicts progression to large splenomegaly and leukemic transformation in primary myelofibrosis. Blood 110:4030–4036

Baxter EJ, Scott LM, Campbell PJ, East C, Fourouclas N, Swanton S, Vassilliou GS, Bench AJ, Boyd EM, Curtim N, Scott MA, Erber WN, The Cancer Genome Project, Green AR (2005) Acquired mutation of the tyrosine kinase JAK2 in human myeloproliferative disorders. Lancet 365:1054–1061

Beer PA, Campbell PJ, Scott LM, Bench AJ, Erber WN, Bareford D, Wilkins BS, Reilly JT, Hasselbach HC, Bowman R, Wheatley K, Buck G, Harrison CN, Green AR (2008) MPL mutations in myeloproliferative disorders: analysis of the PT-1 cohort. Blood 112:141–149

Bodemer C, Hermine O, Palmérini F, Yang Y, Grandpeix-Guyodo C, Leventhal PS, Hadj-Rabia S, Nasca L, Georgin-Lavialle S, Cohen-Akenine A, Launay JM, Barete S, Feger F, Arock M, Catteau B, Sans B, Stalder JF, Skowron F, Thomas L, Lorette G, Plantin P, Bordigoni P, Lortholary O, de Prost Y, Moussy A, Sobol H, Dubreuil P (2010) Pediatric mastocytosis is a clonal disease associated with D816 V and other activating c-KIT mutations. J Invest Dermatol 130:804–815

Campbell PJ, Grisshammer M, Dohner K, Dohner H, Kusec R, Hasselbach HC, Larsen TS, Pallisgaard N, Giraudier S, Le Bousse-Kerdiles MC, Desterke C, Guerton B, Dupriez B, Bordessoule D, Fenaux P, Kiledijan JJ, Vialard JF, Briere J, Harrison CN, Green AR, Reilly JT (2006) V617F mutation in *JAK2* is associated with poorer survival in idiopathic myelofibrosis. Blood 107:2098–2100

Campbell PJ, Scott LM, Buck G, Wheatley K, East CL, Marsden JT, Duffy A, Boyd EM, Bench AJ, Scott MA, Vassiliou GS, Milligan DW, Smith SR, Erber WN, Bareford D, Wilkins BS, Reilly JT, Harrison CN, Green AR (2005) Definition of subtypes of essential thrombocythaemia and relation to polycythaemia vera based on *JAK2* V617F mutation status: a prospective study. Lancet 366:1945–1953

Chen AT, Prchal JT (2010) JAK 2 kinase inhibitors and myeloproliferative disorders. Curr Opin Hematol 17:110–116

Cools J, DeAngelo DJ, Gotlib J, Stover EH, Legare RD, Cortes J, Kutok J, Clark J, Galinsky I, Griffin JD, Cross NC, Tefferi A, Malone J, Alam R, Schrier SL, Schmid J, Rose M, Vandenberghe P, Verhoef G, Boogaerts M, Wlodarska I, Kantarjian H, Marynen P, Coutre SE, Stone R, Gilliland DG (2003) A tyrosine kinase created by fusion of the PDGFRA and FIP1L1 genes as a therapeutic target of imatinib in idiopathic hypereosinophilic syndrome. N Engl J Med 348:1201–1214

Curtis CE, Grand FH, Waghorn K, Sahoo TP, George J, Cross NC (2007) A novel ETV6-PDGFRB fusion transcript missed by standard screening in a patient with an imatinib responsive chronic myeloproliferative disease. Leukemia 21:1839–1841

Dameshek W (1951) Some speculations on the myeloproliferative syndromes. Blood 6:372–375

Delhommeau F, Dupont S, Della Valle V, James C, Trannoy S, Massé A, Kosmider O, Le Couedic JP, Robert F, Alberdi A, Lécluse Y, Plo I, Dreyfus FJ, Marzac C, Casadevall N, Lacombe C, Romana SP, Dessen P, Soulier J, Viguié F, Fontenay M, Vainchenker W, Bernard OA (2009) Mutation in TET2 in myeloid cancers. N Engl J Med 360:2289–2301

Ding A, Komatsu H, Wakita A, Kato-Uranishi M, Ito M, Satoh A, Tsuboi K, Nitta M, Miyazaki H, Iida S, Ueda R (2004) Familial essential thrombocythemia associated with dominant-positive activating mutation of c-MPL gene, which encodes for the receptor for thrombopoietin. Blood 103:4198–4200

Furitsu T, Tsujimura T, Tono T, Ikeda H, Kitayama H, Koshimizu U, Sugahara H, Butterfield JH, Ashman LK, Kanayama Y (1993) Identification of mutations in the coding sequence of the proto-oncogene c-kit in a human mast cell leukemia cell line causing ligand-independent activation of c-kit product. J Clin Invest 92:1736–1744

Giebel LB, Strunk KM, Holmes SA, Spritz RA (1992) Organization and nucleotide sequence of the human KIT (mast/stem cell growth factor receptor) proto-oncogene. Oncogene 7:2207–2217

Groffen J, Stephenson JR, Heisterkamp N, de Klein A, Bartrum CR, Grosveld G (1984) Philadelphia chromosomal breakpoints are clustered within limited region, bcr, on chromosome 22. Cell 36:93–99

Guglielmelli P, Barosi G, Speschia G, Rambaldi A, Lo Coco F, Antonoli E, Pieri L, Pancrazzi A, Delaini F, Longo G, Ammatuna E, Liso V, Bosi A, Barbui T, Vannucchi AM (2009) Identification of patients with poorer survival in primary myelofibrosis based on the burden of *JAK* V617F mutated allele. Blood 114:1477–1483

Halaburda K, Prejzner W, Szatkowski D, Limon J, Hellmann A (2006) Allogeneic bone marrow transplantation for hypereosinophilic syndrome: long-term follow-up with eradication of FIP1L1-PDGFRA fusion transcript. Bone Marrow Transpl 38:319–320

Hellmann A, Bieniaszewska M (2009) Myeloprolifarative neoplasms—classification, diagnostic and therapeutic options in the light of molecular findings. Eur Haematol (Touch Breifings) 3:57–60

James C, Ugo V, Le Couédic JP, Staerk J, Delhommeau F, Lacout C, Garçon L, Raslova H, Berger R, Bennaceur-Griscelli A, Villeval JL, Constantinescu SN, Casadevall N, Vainchenker W (2005) A unique clonal *JAK2* mutation leading to constitutive signalling causes polycythaemia vera. Nature 434:1144–1148

Kralovics R, Passamonti F, Buser AS, Teo SS, Tiedt R, Passweg JR, Tichelli A, Cazzola M, Skoda RC (2005) A gain-of-function mutation of *JAK2* in myeloproliferative disorders. N Engl J Med 352:1779–1790

Kralovics R, Teo SS, Li S, Theocharides A, Buser AS, Tichelli A, Skoda RC (2006) Acquisition of the V617F mutation of *JAK2* is a late genetic event in a subset of patients with myeloproliferative disorders. Blood 108:1377–1380

Lambert F, Heimann P, Herens C, Chariot A, Bours V (2007) A case of FIP1L1-PDGFRA—positive chronic eosinophilic leukemia with a rare FIP1L1 breakpoint. J Mol Diagn 9:414–419

Levine RL, Wadleigh M, Cools J, Ebert BL, Wernig G, Huntly BJ, Boggon TJ, Wlodarska I, Clark JJ, Moore S, Adelsperger J, Koo S, Lee JC, Gabriel S, Mercher T, D'Andrea A, Fröhling S, Döhner K, Marynen P, Vandenberghe P, Mesa RA, Tefferi A, Griffin JD, Eck MJ, Sellers WR, Meyerson M, Golub TR, Lee SJ, Gilliland DG (2005) Activating mutation of the tyrosine kinase JAK2 in polycythemia vera, essential thrombocythemia, and myeloid metaplasia with myelofibrosis. Cancer Cell 7:387–397

Mital A, Piskorz A, Lewandowski K, Wasąg B, Limon J, Hellmann A (2011) A case of mast cell leukaemia with exon 9 KIT mutation and good response to imatinib. Eur J Haematol 86: 531–535

Nussenzveig RH, Swierczek SI, Jelinek J, Gaikwad A, Liu E, Verstovsek S, Prchal JF, Prchal JT (2007) Polycythemia vera is not initiated by *JAK2*V617F mutation. Exp Hematol 35:32–38

Pardanani A, Fridley BL, Lashlo TL, Gilliland DF, Tefferi A (2008) Host genetic variation contributes to phenotypic diversity in myeloproliferative disorders. Blood 111:2785–2789

Pardanani A, Lashlo TL, Finke C, Hanson CA, Tefferi A (2007) Prevalence and clinicopathologic correlates of JAK2 exon 12 mutations in JAK2V617F-negative polycythemia vera. Leukemia 21:1960–1963

Pietra D, Brisci A, Rumi E, Boggi S, Elena C, Pietrelli A, Bordoni R, Ferrari M, Passamonti F, De Bellis G, Cremonesi L, Cazzola M (2011) Deep sequencing reveals double mutation in cis of MPL exon 10 in myeloproliferative neoplasms. Haematologica 96:607–611

Pignon J, Giraudier S, Duquesnoy P, Jouault H, Imbert M, Vainchenker W, Vernant J, Tulliez (1997) A new c-kit mutation in a case of aggressive mast cell disease. Br J Haematol 96: 374–376

Pikman Y, Lee BH, Mercher T (2006) MPLW515L is a novel somatic activating mutation in myelofibrosis with myeloid metaplasia. PloS Med 3:e270

Schaub FX, Looser R, LI S, HaoShen H, Lehmann T, Tichelli A, Skoda RC (2010) Clonal analysis of TET2 and JAK 2 mutations suggests that TET2 can be a late event in the progression of myeloproliferative neoplasms. Blood 115:2003–2007

Scott LM, Scott MA, Campbell PJ, Green AR (2006) Progenitors homozygous for the V617F mutation occur in most patients with polycythemia vera, but not essential thromocythemia. Blood 108:2435–2437

Siemiątkowska A, Bieniaszewska M, Hellmann A, Limon J (2009) *JAK2* and *MPL* mutations in V617F-negative myeloproliferative neoplasms. Leukemia Res 34:387–389

Stover EH, Chen J, Folens C, Lee BH, Mentens N, Marynen P, Williams IR, Gilliland DG, Cools J (2006) Activation of FIP1L1-PDGFRalpha requires disruption of the juxtamembrane domain of PDGFR alpha and is FIP1L1-independent. Proc Natl Acad Sci U S A 103:8078–8083

Swerdlow SH, Campo E, Harris NL, Jaffe ES, Pileri SA, Stein H, Thiele J, Vardiman JW (2008) WHO classification of tumours of haematopoietic and lymphoid tissues. IARC Press, Lyon

Tefferi A, Lasho TL, Huang J, Finke C, Hanson CA, Mesa RA, Li CY, Wu W, Hanson CA, Pardanani A (2008a) Low *JAK2*V617F allele burden in primary myelofibrosis, compared to either a higher allele burden or unmutated status, is associated with inferior overall and leukemia-free survival. Leukemia 22:756–761

Tefferi A, Verstovesk S, Pardanani A (2008b) How we diagnose and treat WHO-defined systemic mastocytosis in adults. Haematologica 3:6–9

Theocharides A, Boissinot M, Girodon F, Garand R, Teo SS, Lippert E, Talmant P, Tichelli A, Hermouet S, Skoda RC (2007) Leukemic blasts in transformed *JAK2*-V617F-positive myeloproliferative disorders are frequently negative for the *JAK2*-V617F mutation. Blood 110:375–379

Valent P, Akin C, Escribano L, Födinger M, Hartmann K, Brockow K, Castells M, Sperr WR, Kluin-Nelemans HC, Hamdy NA, Lortholary O, Robyn J, van Doormaal J, Sotlar K, Hauswirth AW, Arock M, Hermine O, Hellmann A, Triggiani M, Niedoszytko M, Schwartz LB, Orfao A, Horny HP, Metcalfe DD (2007) Standards and standardization in mastocytosis: consensus statements on diagnostics, treatment recommendations and response criteria. Eur J Clin Invest 37:435–453

Van Etten RA, Koschmieder S, Delhommeau F, Perrotti D, Holyoake T, Pardanani A, Mesa R, Green T, Ibrahim AR, Moghal T, Gale P, Goldman J (2011) The Ph-positive and Ph-negative myeloproliferative neoplasms: some topical pre-clinical and clinical issue. Haematologica 96:590–601

Vannucchi AM, Antonioli E, Guglielmelli P, Pardanani A, Tefferi A (2008) Clinical correlates of *JAK2*V617F presence or allele burden in myeloproliferative neoplasms: a critical reappraisal. Leukemia 22:1299–1307

Vannucchi AM, Antonioli E, Guglielmelli P, Rambaldi A, Barosi G, Marchioli R, Marfisi RA, Finazzi G, Guerini V, Fabris F, Randi ML, De Stefano V, Caberlon S, Tafuri A, Ruggeri M, Specchia G, Liso V, Rossi E, Pogliani E, Gugliotta L, Bosi A, Barbui T (2007) Clinical profile of homozygous *JAK2* 617 V > F mutation in patients with polycythemia vera and essential thrombocythemia. Blood 110:840–846

Wernig G, Mercher T, Okabe R, Levine RL, Lee BH, Gilliland DG (2006) Expression of Jak2V617F causes a polycythemia vera-like disease with associated myelofibrosis in a murine bone marrow transplant model. Blood 107:4274–4281

Part II
Diagnostics and Monitoring of Therapy of Hemato-oncologic Diseases

Chapter 9
Flow Cytometric Immunophenotyping as Diagnostic Tool of Hematopoietic Malignancies

Łukasz Sędek, Juan Flores-Montero, Joanna Bulsa, Susana Barrena, Julia Almeida, Alberto Orfao and Tomasz Szczepański

Abstract Flow cytometry is a diagnostic technique capable of distinguishing cells by their size, internal complexity, and antigen repertoire (phenotype) with the use of monoclonal antibodies conjugated with fluorescent dyes. Nowadays, flow cytometry has become a highly specific and fully reproducible method for the diagnosis of hematological malignancies. Flow cytometry allows for the analysis of any type of sample prepared as a single cell suspension, e.g., blood, bone marrow, cerebrospinal fluid, as well as homogenized solid tissues like lymph nodes. The detailed phenotypic features of the analyzed cells depend on the number of simultaneously used monoclonal antibodies, which is in turn dependent

Ł. Sędek (✉) · J. Bulsa · T. Szczepański
Department of Pediatric Hematology and Oncology, Medical University of Silesia, 3 Maja 13-15, 41-800 Zabrze, Poland
e-mail: lsedek@sum.edu.pl

J. Bulsa
e-mail: joannabulsa@gmail.com

T. Szczepański
e-mail: szczep57@poczta.onet.pl

J. Flores-Montero · S. Barrena · J. Almeida · A. Orfao
Department of Medicine, Cancer Research Center (IBMCC-CSIC-USAL) and Cytometry Service, University of Salamanca, Av. Universidad de Coimbra, Campus Miguel de Unamuno, 37007 Salamanca, Spain
e-mail: jflores@usal.es

S. Barrena
e-mail: subadelfa@usal.es

J. Almeida
e-mail: jalmeida@usal.es

A. Orfao
e-mail: orfao@usal.es

M. Witt et al. (eds.), *Molecular Aspects of Hematologic Malignancies*, Principles and Practice, DOI: 10.1007/978-3-642-29467-9_9,

on the flow cytometer specification. Flow cytometric assays, particularly immunophenotyping, have broad clinical applications, especially in the diagnostics of hematological malignancies (e.g., acute lymphoblastic leukemia—ALL, acute myeloid leukemia—AML and chronic lymphoproliferative disorders—CLPD), based on precise determination of the lineage, maturation stage and phenotypic aberrancies of tumor versus normal/reactive cells.

9.1 Introduction

Flow cytometry is a diagnostic technique enabling analysis of single cell suspensions. Distinguishing cell populations is possible through the usage of monoclonal antibodies conjugated with fluorescent dyes, which bind to specific epitopes revealing the cells' antigen repertoire (phenotype). Another parameter measured in flow cytometry is cell-driven light scatter providing information about the morphology of the cells, their size and internal complexity. After several decades, since the production of the earliest flow cytometry instruments, their applications have grown, along with the establishment and development of methods for the production of monoclonal antibodies and computerization. Nowadays, flow cytometry has become a highly specific and fully reproducible method, e.g., for the characterization of normal/reactive and tumor cells. For further coherence, the monoclonal antibodies designed against particular leukocyte antigens, also those formerly developed and already named, have been coded with so-called cluster of differentiation (CD) codes (Zola et al. 2007).

Flow cytometry indeed does not strictly belong to the molecular methods. However, for a broad and comprehensive view on the diagnostics and monitoring of hematological malignancies, this technique and its most relevant clinical applications have been discussed in this chapter. Flow cytometry, as a quick and relatively inexpensive technique, became a standard in contemporary hematological practice. The results of flow cytometric assays stand together with morphological and histochemical examination of bone marrow and other tissues, and complement well the information necessary to come up with the right diagnosis (Orfao et al. 2006).

The very first flow cytometers enabled merely the measurement of light scatter (two parameters) and one fluorescence signal (three parameters altogether). At present, flow cytometers most commonly used in clinical practice offer the simultaneous measurement of two parameters of light scatter and 3–6 different fluorescence signals (5–8 parameters altogether) (Herzenberg et al. 2002). The cytometers measuring 8–10 different fluorescence signals (10–12 parameters altogether) are becoming more and more popular, while 17–20 parameter cytometers are already being used in highly specialized research and development centers all over the world (Mahnke and Roederer 2007).

9.2 The Composition of a Flow Cytometer

A flow cytometer consists of three main systems, i.e., fluidics, optical and electronic systems, plus a computer and appropriate software. The main part of fluidics is an air pump, which produces and sustains the pressure—the driving force for all fluids flowing inside the cytometer. The streamed suspension of cells is injected or, less commonly, aspirated into a sheath buffer circuit. The cells are then focused hydrodynamically within the flow chamber (or flow cell) where they cross the laser beams. Particular physical properties of the sheath buffer, appropriate capillary diameter within the flow chamber and appropriate flow speed and character (laminar flow) guarantee a proper stream formation (10–100 μm in diameter), in which one properly aligned cell follows the other.

The main components of the optical system are the light sources, focusing lens, and collecting optics. In contemporary flow cytometers, the most commonly used light sources are gas lasers (based on e.g., argon (Ar), krypton (Kr), helium–neon (He–Ne)) and solid state lasers (based on crystals), emitting coherent, monochromatic, narrow light beam of high intensity and a specific wavelength. The collecting optics consists of wavelength specific optical filters (longpass filters, dichroic mirrors) which let through only the desired wavelengths to particular detectors, and deviate lower or higher wavelengths to be measured by other detectors.

The detectors of both scattered and fluorescence light belong to the electronic system of a flow cytometer. Contemporary flow cytometers employ digital systems without the need to convert the analog signals while passing through the detectors prior to their enhancement by logarithmic or linear photomultipliers, implemented in older instruments. In both situations, digital signals are processed in a computer, which is an integral part of the flow cytometer. After data acquisition into a digital format it is possible to analyze it and calculate the percentages of events matching the criteria desired in a given analysis (Radcliff and Jaroszeski 1998; Givan 2004; Maecker and Trotter 2006).

9.3 The Basics of a Flow Cytometric Assay

Flow cytometry allows for the analysis of any type of sample prepared as a single cell suspension like blood, bone marrow, cerebrospinal fluid, body cavity fluids, bronchoalveolar lavage fluid, and others. Moreover, it is possible to analyze biopsy material or solid tissues (e.g., lymph nodes) after homogenization and preparation of a single cell suspension. The biological material is stained with a mixture of highly specific fluorochrome-conjugated monoclonal antibodies. Each antibody in the mixture is typically conjugated with a different fluorochrome. Each fluorochrome has a specific spectrum of light emission (and absorption) covering a range of light wavelengths. The number of monoclonal antibodies that can be simultaneously used, as well as the selection of "compatible" fluorochromes, fully depends on the flow cytometer specifications. The recognition of a specific target antigen by a given fluorochrome-conjugated monoclonal antibody results in its visualization on a flow cytometric histogram or plot.

The entire image of the cells analyzed by flow cytometry is built based on the information about how they affect (scatter) the light beam while passing across the laser beams and what fluorescence is emitted by the excited antibody-bound fluorochromes. The scattered light is measured in two directions: along or under small 5–10° angle (forward scatter, FSC) and right angle to the laser beam direction (side scatter, SSC). The former depends on cell size and the refractory index of the cell, while the latter correlates with its internal complexity (granularity and nucleus shape) (Radcliff and Jaroszeski 1998; Givan 2004; Maecker and Trotter 2006). Besides the scatter characteristics, also the fluorescence is measured while the cells pass the flow chamber. The number of exciting lasers as well as the number of fluorescence detectors differs between distinct cytometers, but those most commonly used for routine practice are equipped with 2–3 lasers and 3–10 fluorescence detectors. This means that 3–10 different fluorochromes, which equal 3–10 different antigens, can be simultaneously investigated in a single cell. Given that the fluorescence signal derives from antibodies bound to antigens of different abundance and distribution, it is helpful to use a logarithmic scale to represent the fluorescence (Radcliff and Jaroszeski 1998; Givan 2004; Maecker and Trotter 2006). Thus, flow cytometric plots cover the scale of 4–5 log decades and enable visualization of signals differing in intensity by even two or three orders of magnitude, which is rather common in practice.

Flow cytometric fluorescence dot plots represent all cells in the sample, also those which did not bind any fluorochrome-conjugated antibody (see Figs. 9.1, 9.2, 9.3, 9.4). The cells typically have certain baseline autofluorescence levels (background level), and thus are visible on the plots around the beginning of the scale, although their spread can vary (depending on the cell type). The cells that bind fluorochrome-conjugated antibodies emit the fluorescence positively correlated to the number of recognized antigen–antibody complexes. The distinction between the background (i.e., negative) and positive signal is clear for highly expressed antigens, but requires the use of different types of controls when antigen expression is low and the positive signal overlaps with the background signal. There are several ways to describe and assign the fluorescence signal to the level of expression of an antigen. Frequently, the level of an antigen expression is measured as fluorescence intensity which positively correlates with the relative amount of the antigen. For example, highly expressed antigens can be assigned as "bright" or "high", while antigens of lower expression can be described as "dim", "weak", or "low". The expression of a given antigen in abnormal cells is also expressed in relation to the expression of the same antigen on the normal cellular counterparts of the altered (e.g., clonal) cells ("bright" also means higher intensity than the normal counterpart, or "dim" reflects dimmer fluorescence than that observed in the normal counterpart). Depending on the application, other characteristics of the antigen fluorescent profile of a given cell population can be used

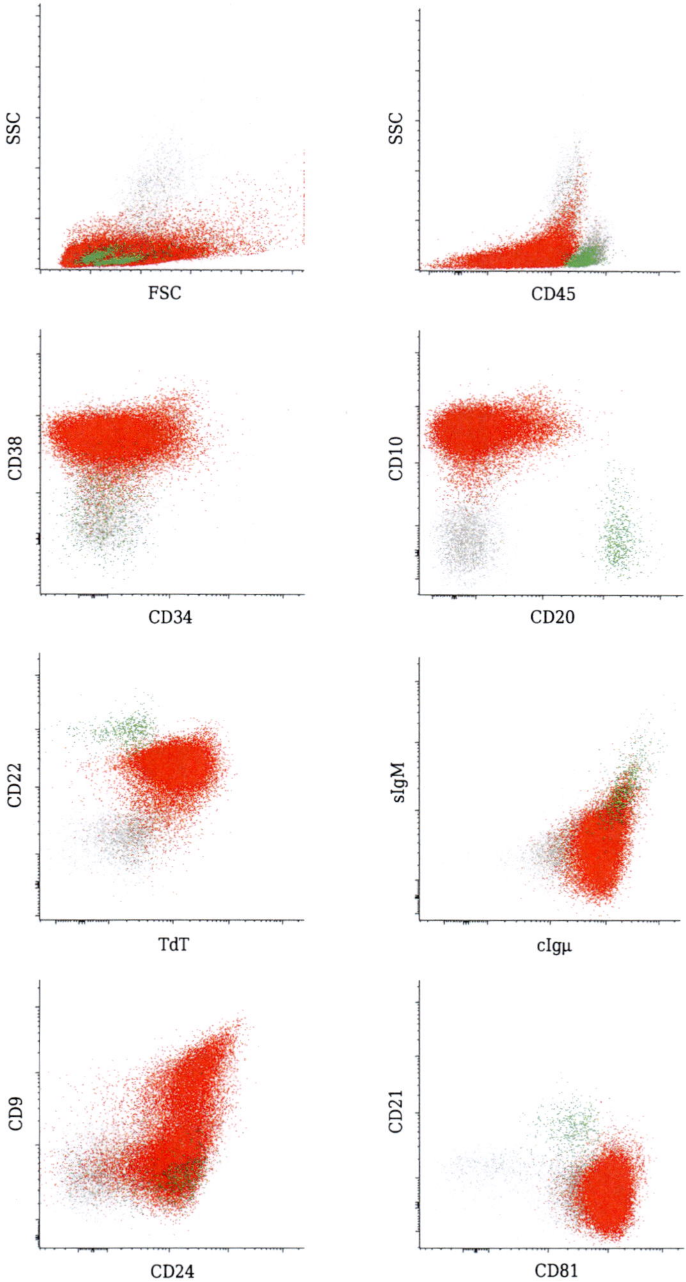

Fig. 9.1 Flow cytometric illustrative images of B-cell precursor acute lymphoblastic leukemia (BCP-ALL). The prevailing population in the bone marrow sample are leukemic blasts (depicted in *red*), which express the following antigens: CD45 (weak), CD19, CD22, CD10, nuclear TdT, CD24, CD81, CD9 (partially positive), CD38, and cytoplasmic Igμ. The blasts lack the expression of CD34, CD21, surface IgM and CD20 (asynchronous negativity). The overall phenotype of the blast population, classify this BCP-ALL as pre-B-ALL. The residual mature B lymphocytes are depicted in *green*, and other remaining cells populations in *gray*

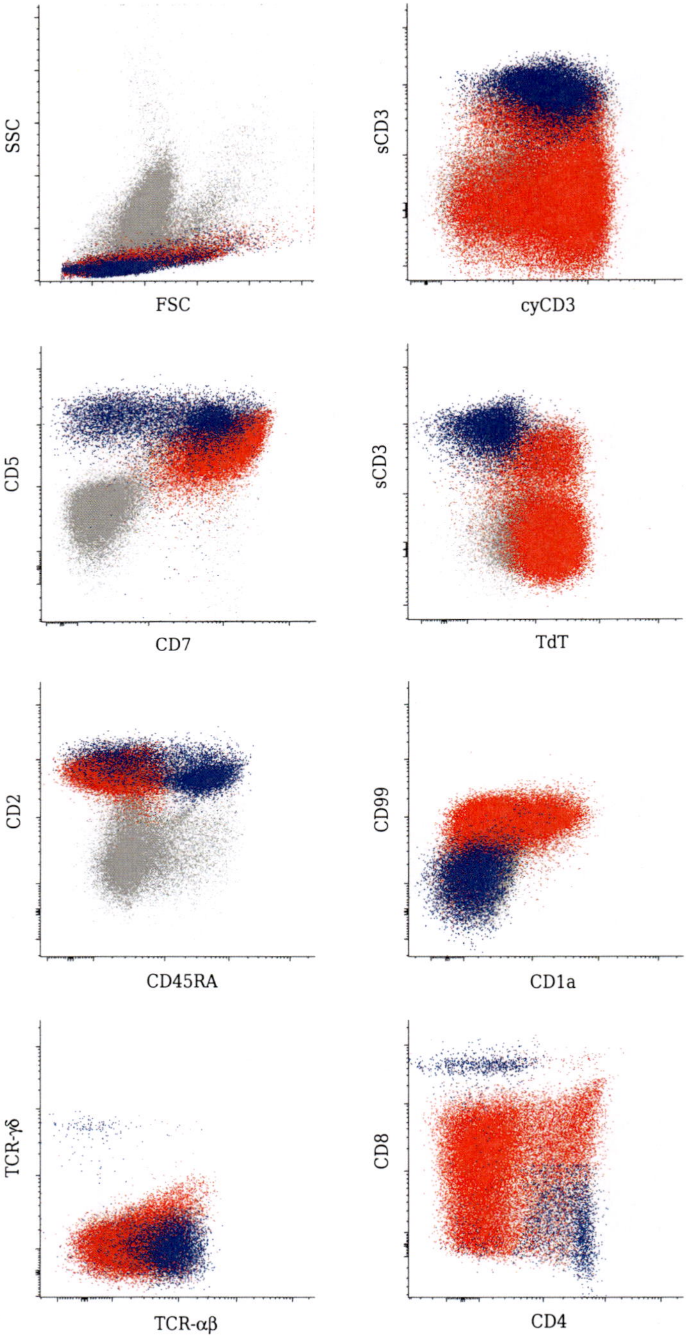

Fig. 9.2 Flow cytometric illustrative images of T-cell acute lymphoblastic leukemia (T-ALL). The leukemic blasts (depicted in *red*) express cytoplasmic CD3, CD7, CD2, CD5, nuclear TdT, CD99, and moreover, in part of the blasts CD8, CD1a, surface CD3, and TCR$\alpha\beta$. The overall phenotype of the blast population, classify this T-ALL as cortical thymocytic (common)-T-ALL CD3^{+}TCR^{+}. The residual mature T lymphocytes are depicted in *blue*, and other remaining cells in *gray*

and expressed as "heterogeneous", "partial", "bimodal" expression profile. Moreover, the expression level of a marker can be expressed as percentage of the population showing a particular level of fluorescence or being above a given cutoff level. Finally, to describe the intensity of antigen expression, symbols *****like "–", "–/+", "+", "++" are also used as for "negative", "partially positive", "positive" and "bright positive" antigen expression, respectively.

9.4 Immunophenotyping of Hematological Malignancies

Flow cytometric immunophenotyping plays a key role in hematological diagnostics. Cytometric assays, based on specific cell phenotypes, can precisely determine the lineage and maturation stage of transformed cells as well as patterns of aberrant marker expression (Szczepański et al. 2006).

There are many different strategies for appropriate antibody panel selection and many practical approaches to immunophenotyping of an unknown, abnormal cell population in a sample (van Wering et al. 2004). The most widely used is a two-step strategy. The first step is based on a fast and relatively reliable screening assay, designed to identify the suspected malignant cells and their lineage. In the second step, precise determination of their phenotype is made with a wider panel of antibodies directed against the "expected" antigens of the suspected malignant cell population. The latter also enables the determination of the leukemia-/lymphoma-specific phenotypes necessary for efficient detection of minimal residual disease during the course of therapy (Szczepański et al. 2001).

9.4.1 Immunophenotyping and Classification of Acute Lymphoblastic Leukemia

Diagnosis and classification of acute lymphoblastic leukemia (ALL) is currently based on flow cytometry immunophenotyping which overrides formerly introduced techniques (like cytomorphological examination). Taking into account the phenotypic features, two main types of ALL can be distinguished: B-cell precursor ALL (BCP-ALL; 80–85 % of ALL cases in children) and T-cell lineage ALL (T-ALL; 15–20 % of cases in children). The detailed immunophenotypic classification of ALL, originating from either B- or T-cell precursor cells was primarily proposed by Janossy and Greaves (Greaves et al. 1981) and reformulated by the EGIL group (European Group for the Immunological Characterization of Leukemias) (Bene et al. 1995).

Classification of BCP-ALL was based on the assumption that leukemic blasts are B-cell precursor cells, arrested at certain maturation stage, identifiable by immunophenotyping (Table 9.1). The current World Health Organization (WHO; Swerdlow et al. 2008) classification of BCP-ALL is in general concordant with the

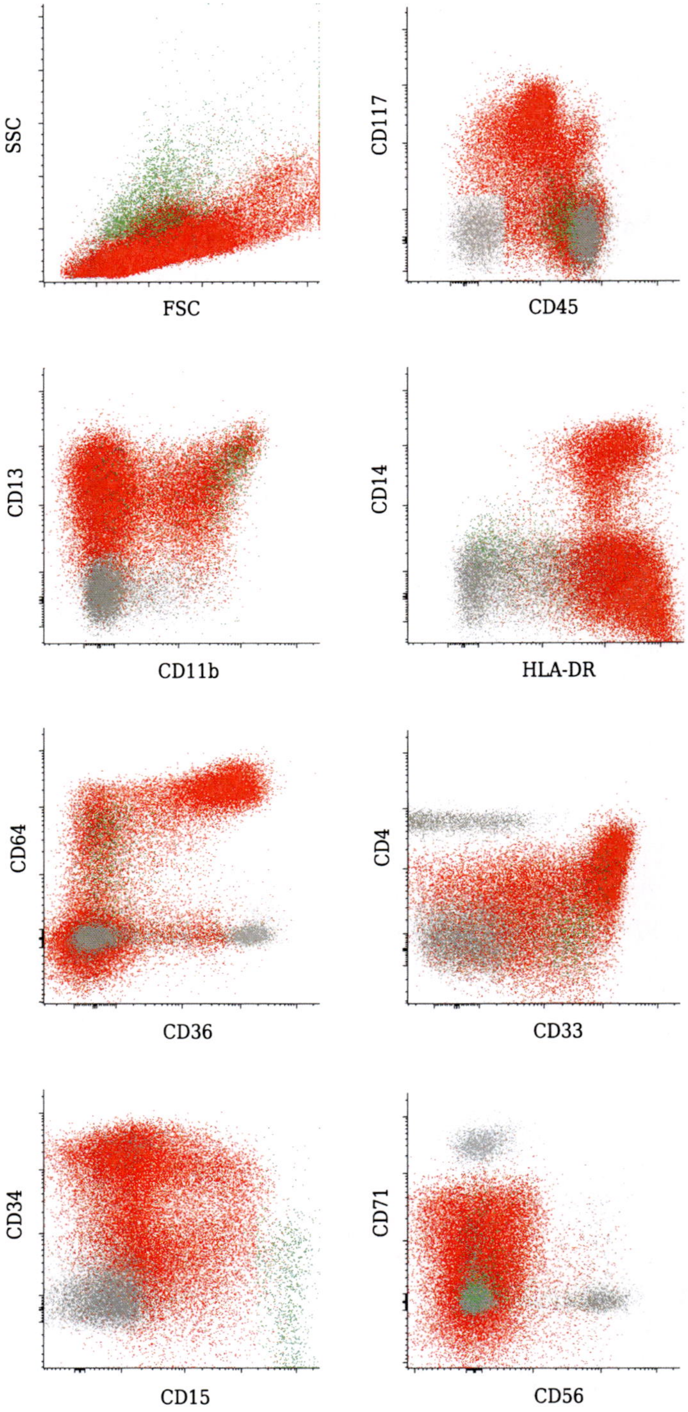
SSC
FSC
CD117
CD45
CD13
CD11b
CD14
HLA-DR
CD64
CD36
CD4
CD33
CD34
CD15
CD71
CD56

◀**Fig. 9.3** Flow cytometric illustrative images of acute myeloid leukemia (AML). The leukemic cells derive from myeloid and monocytic lineages (depicted in *red*) and form multiple populations in some of the dot plots, which is typical for AML-M5 subtype. The residual mature granulocytes are depicted in *green* and other remaining cells in *gray*

original EGIL classification, with the exclusion of mature B-ALL, currently regarded as a leukemic phase of Burkitt lymphoma (Szczepański et al. 2003; Vardiman et al. 2009). The main blast cell antigens that entitle to diagnose BCP-ALL are: intranucleic terminal deoxynucleotidyl transferase (TdT), cytoplasmic CD79a, surface CD19 and CD22. Other B-lineage antigens like CD10, CD20, cytoplasmic/surface immunoglobulin M (IgM) can distinguish between four subtypes of BCP-ALL. For example, CD10 is negative in pro-B-ALL and positive in the remaining three subtypes (common-ALL, pre-B-ALL, transitional-B-ALL) (Orfao et al. 2004; Jaffe 2009).

T-ALL was classified, based on EGIL criteria, into four subgroups: pro-T-ALL, pre-T-ALL, cortical thymocytic (common)-T-ALL, and mature-T-ALL (Table 9.2). In this classification, the most typical T-cell lineage marker is CD3, which can be detected only in the cytoplasm in the most immature T-ALL subtypes and/or on the cell surface in the more mature T-ALL subtypes. Other typical T-lineage markers that can be expressed in T-ALL are: CD1a, CD2, CD4, CD5, CD7, CD8 (Porwit-MacDonald et al. 2000). There are currently alternative criteria for T-ALL classification, of which the most important is the configuration of T-cell receptor encoding genes (germline or rearranged) and the pattern of their rearrangements (Asnafi et al. 2003).

The exemplary flow cytometric immunophenotyping results of ALL are shown in Figs. 9.1 and 9.2

9.4.2 Immunophenotyping and Classification of Acute Myeloid Leukemia

The classification of acute myeloid leukemia (AML), made by French–American–British Cooperative Group (FAB) is mainly based on cytomorphological and cytochemical examination and partly on assessment of maturation features (Bennett et al. 1985). AMLs are a heterogeneous group of hematological disorders, with eight subtypes identified by FAB, in which different myeloid lineages can be affected, i.e., neutrophilic lineage in AML-M1, AML-M2, AML-M3; neutrophilic and monocytic lineage in AML-M4 and AML-M5; erythroblastic lineage in AML-M6; megakaryoblastic lineage in AML-M7. Immunophenotyping assays can confirm the myeloid origin of blast cells in AML if certain myeloid lineage specific antigens are detected. The most typical myeloid lineage antigens expressed on blast cells in AML are CD13, CD33, CD117, CD15, CD64, lysozyme and/or cytoplasmic myeloperoxidase (MPO) (Szczepański et al. 2003) (Table 9.3). The

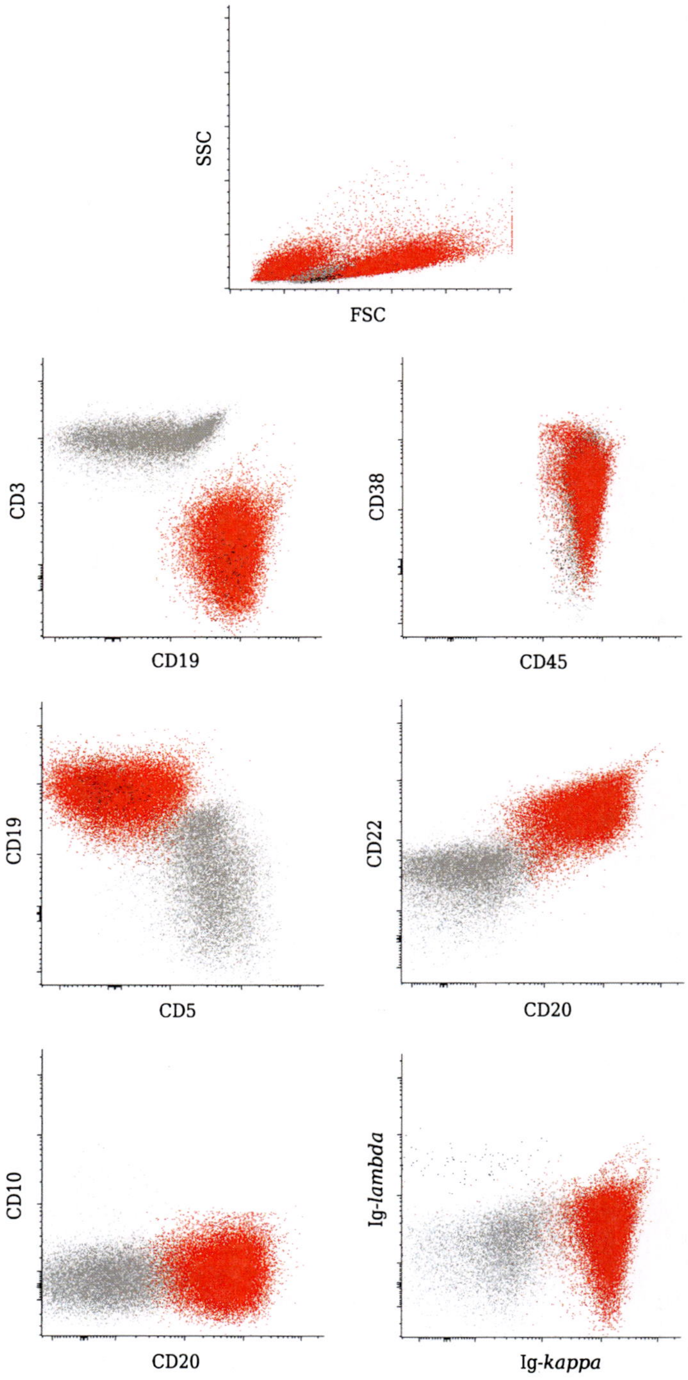
SSC
FSC
CD3
CD19
CD38
CD45
CD19
CD5
CD22
CD20
CD10
CD20
Ig-lambda
Ig-kappa

◀**Fig. 9.4** Flow cytometric illustrative images of B-cell non-Hodgkin lymphoma. The majority of the lymph node cells are lymphoid cells (depicted in *red*) having the phenotype of mature B lymphocytes: CD19$^+$, CD20$^+$, CD10$^-$, CD22$^+$, CD38$^+$. These cells are, however, clonal—only one type of surface immunoglobulin receptor light chains (Ig-kappa) is present. The residual lymphocytes of the lymph node are depicted in *gray*

leukemic cells in AML usually display a much more heterogeneous phenotype than in ALL, can express common antigens, and only the relative occurrence of certain antigens can be helpful in distinguishing between different morphological (FAB) subtypes (for example M1–M2 and M4–M5). The blast cells in AML-M6 and M7 typically bear antigens specific for their lineages, such as CD235a, CD71 and CD41, CD42, CD61, respectively (Table 9.3). On the other hand, the blast cells in most undifferentiated subtype of AML (AML-M0) can express very limited number of antigens, specific for myeloid lineage (e.g., CD117, CD13) but not necessarily (e.g., HLA-DR, CD34) (Wood 2007). In the most recent WHO classification, the main subtypes of AML are defined based on the genetic features of the blast cells (Vardiman et al. 2009); for example, a subgroup of AML with recurrent genetic abnormalities (e.g., translocations) resulting in the formation of fusion genes (e.g., *AML1-ETO* in AML with t(8;21), or *PML-RARA* with t(15;17) in acute promyelocytic leukemia—APL, a counterpart of AML-M3 FAB morphological subtype).

The exemplary flow cytometric immunophenotyping results of AML are shown in Fig. 9.3

9.4.3 Immnunophenotyping in Chronic Lymphoproliferative Disorders (Chronic Lymphoid Leukemias and Non-Hodgkin Lymphomas)

Optimal antibody combinations allow to precisely establish the cell origin of most chronic lymphoproliferative disorders (CLPD), including chronic lymphoid leukemias and non-Hodgkin lymphomas (NHL), particularly in cases where morphology and histopathology are inconclusive and in tissues with minimal disease dissemination (Swerdlow et al. 2008). Pan-B cell markers like CD19, in combination with CD20, CD22, CD37, and both surface membrane (sm) and cytoplasmic (cy) immunoglobulins (Ig) are routinely used to demonstrate the B-cell nature of the vast majority of CLPD (Fig. 9.4). Together with other T cell-associated antigens (e.g., smCD3, CD4, CD8, CD5 and/or CD7), these pan-B cell markers also contribute to the differential diagnosis between reactive/polyclonal lymphocytosis and enlarged lymphoid tissues versus clonal expansions of B- or T-cells (Barrena et al. 2011). The latter discrimination can be easily reached by means of using a rather simple staining for CD19 and the light chains (kappa and lambda) of surface membrane immunoglobulin receptor of B cells (smIgκ/smIgλ) (Fig. 9.4) and a panel of antibodies directed against distinct families of the T-cell receptor

Table 9.1 Immunophenotypic characteristics of BCP-ALL

	BCP-ALL subtype (WHO)	pro-B-ALL	Common ALL	pre-B-ALL	Transitional pre-B-ALL
	EGIL	B–I	B-II	B-III	–
Antigen					
CD19		+	+	+	+
nuTdT		+	+	+	+
CD10		–	+/++	+/++	+/++
cyCD79a		dim/+	+	+	+
CD34		–/+	–/+	–/+	–
CD22		dim/+	+	+	+
cyIgμ		–	–	+	+
CD20		–/+	–/+	+	+
V-pre-B/λ5		–	–	–	+
smIgM-CD79		–	–	–	+
smIgκ		–	–	–	–
smIgλ		–	–	–	–

sm surface membrane, *nu* nuclear, *cy* cytoplasmic, ++: highly positive, +: positive, –: negative, –/+: positive in part of the cases, *dim* weakly positive

Table 9.2 Immunophenotypic characteristics of T-ALL

	T-ALL subtype (WHO)	Imature		Common thymocytic (cortical) T-ALL		Mature T-ALL
		pro-T-ALL	pre-T-ALL	smCD3$^-$	smCD3$^+$	
	EGIL	T-I	T-II	T-III		T-IV
Antigen						
nuTdT		+	+	+	+	–/+
HLA-DR		+	–/+	–/+	–/+	–
CD34		+	–/+	–/+	–/+	–
CD1a		–	–/+	+	+	–/+
CD2		–/dim/+	dim/+	dim/+	dim/+	–/dim/+
cyCD3		+	+	+	+	+
CD5		–/dim/+	dim/+	dim/+	dim/+	dim/+
CD7		+	+	+	+	+
CD4$^-$/CD8$^-$		+	–/+	–/+	–/+	–/+
CD4$^+$/CD8$^-$		–/+	–	–/+	–/+	–/+
CD4$^-$/CD8$^+$		–	–/+	–/+	–/+	–/+
CD4$^+$/CD8$^+$		–	+	–/+	–/+	–/+
smCD3		–	–	–	+	++
TCR$\alpha\beta$		–	–	–	60–70 %	
TCR$\gamma\delta$		–	–	–	30–40 %	

sm surface membrane, *nu* nuclear, cy: cytoplasmic, ++: highly positive, +: positive, –: negative, –/+: positive in part of the cases, *dim* weakly positive

Table 9.3 Immunophenotypic characteristics of AML versus morphological profiles

FAB subtype	AML M0	AML M1/M2	AML M3	AML M4/M5	AML M6	AML M7
Antigen						
cyMPO	–	–/+	+	–/+	+	–
HLA-DR	+	+	–	+	–/+	+
CD34	+	–/+	–/+	–/+	+	+
CD117	+	+	+	–/+	+	+
CD33	+	+	+	+	–/+	+
CD13	–/+	+	+	+	–/+	+
CD11b	–	–/dim	–	+	–	–
CD15	–/+	dim/+	–/dim	–/+	–	–
CD64	–	–/dim	+	+	–	–
CD14	–	–	–	–/+	–	–
CD36	–	–	–	–/+	–/+	–/+
CD71	+	+	+	+	+/++	+
CD235a	–	–	–	–	+	–
CD41/CD42b/CD61	–	–	–	–	–	+

cy cytoplasmic, +: positive, –: negative, –/+: positive in part of the cases, *dim* weakly positive

(TCR) variable regions (beta and alpha or gamma and delta; TCRVβ and TCRVα or TCRV and TCRVδ), together with the identification of the so-called leukemia-associated phenotypes (LAP).

In addition, most WHO diagnostic subtypes of B-CLPD and T-CLPD show unique immunophenotypic profiles, enabling further subclassification of these entities (Swerdlow et al. 2008 and Zucchetto et al. 2006). As an example, B-chronic lymphocytic leukemia (B-CLL) is typically characterized by low expression of smIg, CD79b, CD22, and CD20 on cells that coexpress CD19, CD5, CD23, and CD200 in the absence of FMC7, and show variable expression of several markers associated to an adverse prognosis, e.g., cyZAP70, CD38, and CD49d (Orchard et al. 2004). Similarly, hairy cell leukemia (HCL) displays a unique CD103^{+}, CD25^{++}, CD11c^{++}, LAIR1/CD305^{++}, CD123^{++} phenotype. In turn, clonal plasma cells of both multiple myeloma (MM) and monoclonal gammopathy of undetermined significance (MGUS) express CD138^{+}, CD38^{++}, CD19^{-}, CD56$^{-/+}$. A summary of the most relevant immunophenotypic characteristics of these as well as other leukemic B-CLPD is shown in Table 9.4.

Regarding T-CLPD, distinct immunophenotypic profiles associated with unique diagnostic categories of the disease have also been reported (Gorczyca et al. 2002; Karube et al. 2008; Foss et al. 2011). Accordingly, T large granular lymphocyte leukemia (T-LGL) usually consists of T-cells displaying a smCD3^{+}/TCR$\alpha\beta^{+}$ or TCR$\gamma\delta^{+}$, CD8^{+}, CD57^{+}, cyPerforin^{+}, cyGranzyme^{+} cytotoxic phenotype, while T-cell prolymphocytic leukemia (T-PLL), Sézary syndrome (SS) and adult T cell leukemia/lymphoma (ATLL) show a CD4^{+} phenotype in association with a CD7$^{-/+}$/cyTCL1^{+}, CD7^{-}/CD26^{-} and CD25^{+} antigen profile, respectively (Swerdlow et al. 2008). In Table 9.5, a summary of the most relevant phenotypic

Table 9.4 Immunophenotypic characteristics of B-cell CLPD/non-Hodgkin lymphomas

Disease category	Markers									
	CD19	cyCD79b	CD22	CD20	CD5	CD10	CD23	smIg	cyIg	Other
From B-cell precursors										
Lymphoblastic lymphoma/leukemia	+	–	+	–/+	–	–/+	–	–	–/+	nuTdT^{+}; CD34$^{-/+}$
From peripheral B-cells										
SCLL/CLL	+	–/+	–/+	–/+	+	–	+	–/+	–	CD79b$^{-/+}$; CD11c$^{-/+}$; CD81$^{-/+}$; CD200^{+}; CD24^{+}; CD25^{+}, CD27^{+}; CD39^{+}, CD62L^{+}; CXCR5^{+}
PLL	+	+	+	+	–/+	–	–/+	+	–	CD25$^{-/+}$; CD11c$^{-/+}$; CD305$^{-/+}$
HCL	+	+	+	+	–	–	–	+	–	CD25^{++}; CD103^{+}; CD305^{++}; CD11c^{+}; CD24^{-}; CD123^{++}
MCL	+	+	+	+	+	–/+	–	+	–	CD200$^{-/+}$; CD43^{+}
FL	dim/+	+	+	+	–	–/+	–	+	–/+	cyBcl2^{++}; CD38^{+}; CD11c^{-}; CD43^{-}; CD305^{-}
DLBCL	+	+	+	+	–/+	–/+	–	–/+	–/+	CD200^{-}
BL	+	+	+	+	–	+	–	+	–	CD43^{+}; nuTdT$^{-/+}$; cyBcl2^{dim} CD38^{++}
SMZL	+	+	+	+	–	–	–	+	–/+	CD11c$^{-/+}$; CD103^{-}; CD25^{-}
MZL	+	+	+	+	–	–	–	+	–	
LPL	+	+	–/+	–/+	–	–	–	–/+	–/+	CD24^{+}; CD25^{+}; CD38^{+}

cy cytoplasmic; sm: surface membrane, *nu* nuclear, *SCLL* small cell lymphocytic leukemia, *CLL* chronic lymphocytic leukemia, *PLL* prolymphocytic leukemia, *HCL* hairy cell leukemia,*MCL*, mantle cell lymphoma, *FL* follicular lymphoma, *DLBCL* diffuse large B-cell lymphoma, *BL* Burkitt lymphoma, *SMZL* splenic marginal zone lymphoma, *MZL* marginal zone lymphoma, *LPL* lymphoplasmacytic lymphoma. ++: highly positive, +: positive, –: negative, –/+:positive in part of the cases, *dim* weakly positive

Table 9.5 Immunophenotypic characteristics of T/NK-cell CLPD/non Hodgkin lymphomas

Disease category	Markers							
	CD7	smCD3/ TCR	CD4	CD8	CD4/ CD8	CD2	CD5	Others
From T-cell precursors								
Lymphoblastic leukemia/lymphoma	+	–/+	–	–	–/+	–/+	–/+	nuTdT^{+}; CD1a$^{-/+}$; cyCD3^{+}
From peripheral T/NK-cells								
PLL	++	+	+	–	–	+	+	CD52^{+}; cyTCL1^{+}; CD45RA^{+}; CCR7^{+}; CD27^{+}; CD45RO^{-}; CD28^{+}
ATLL	–/	dim	–/+	+	–	–	+	+
CD25^{++}; CXCR4^{+}; CD57^{-}; CD56^{-}; CD11c^{-}								
T-LGL	+	+	–	+	–	+	+	CD56$^{-/+}$; CD57$^{-/+}$; CD16^{+}; CD11c$^{-/+}$; cyPerforin^{+}; cyGranzime^{+}
Mycosis fungoides/SS	–	dim	dim	–	–	dim	+	CD28^{+}; CD45RO^{+}; CD26^{-}
AITL	+	dim	+	–	–	+	+	CD10^{+}; CD279^{+}
Peripheral lymphomas "NOS"	–/+	–/+	–/+	–/+	–	–/+	–/+	
HSTL	+	+	–	–/+	–	+	–/+	TCR$\gamma\delta^{+}$
Extranodal NK/T-cell lymphoma nasal type	–/+	–	–/+	–/+	–	+	–/+	TIA^{+}; cyGranzime^{+}, cyPerforin^{+}; CD56^{+}
EATL	+	+	–	–/	dim	–	+	–
CD103^{+}, CD30$^{-/+}$								
ALCL ALK+	–/+	–/+	–/+	–/+	–	–/+	–/+	CD25$^{-/+}$; CD30^{+}; ALK^{+}
ALCL ALK–	–/+	–/+	–/+	–/+	–	–/+	–/+	CD25$^{-/+}$; CD30^{++}; ALK^{-}
CLPD-NK	+	–	–	–/+	–	–/+	–	cyGranzime^{+}; cyPerforin^{+}; CD56$^{-/+}$; CD16^{+};CD57$^{-/+}$
Aggressive NK-cell leukemia/ lymphoma	+	–	–	–/+	–	–	–	CD95^{+}; CD57^{-}

NK natural killer, *sm* surface membrane, *nu* nuclear, *PLL* prolymphocytic leukemia, *ATLL* adult T leukemia/lymhoma *LGL* large granular lymphoma, *SS* Sézary syndrome, *AITL* angioimmunoblastic T-cell lymphoma, *"NOS"* not otherwise specified, *HSTL* hepatosplenic T-cell lymphoma, *EATL* enteropathy-associated T-cell lymphoma, *ALCL* anaplastic large cell lymphoma, *ALK* anaplastic lymphoma kinase, *CLPD* chronic lymphoproliferative disorder. ++: highly positive, +: positive, –: negative, –/+: positive in part of the cases, *dim* weakly positive characteristics of the most frequent WHO diagnostic subtypes of leukemic T-cell CLPD have been presented.

The phenotype of NHL cells from lymphoid tissues has mostly been investigated by conventional immunocytochemical and immunohistochemical procedures. However, many recent studies on fine needle aspirate and biopsy specimens from distinct lymphoid and nonlymphoid tissues show that multiparameter flow cytometry immunophenotyping provides valuable complementary information (Barrena et al. 2011) over the more conventional approaches due to the unique immunophenotypic features of the distinct B and T/NK (natural killer)-NHL WHO subtypes. As an example, mantle cell lymphoma is typically associated with the accumulation of $CD5^{+}$ mature, clonal B-cells which in contrast to CLL, show lower expression of CD23 in the absence of CD200 (Palumbo et al. 2009). In turn, follicular lymphomas show coexpression of $CD10^{+}$, $CD38^{+}$, and $cyBcl2^{++}$, while Burkitt lymphoma cells are also $CD10^{+}$ and $CD38^{++}$ but $cyBcl2^{-/+}$. The most relevant immunophenotypic features of the most frequent subtypes of NHL are also summarized in Tables 9.4 and 9.5, and the exemplary flow cytometric immunophenotyping results of NHL are shown in Fig. 9.4.

9.5 Conclusions

Flow cytometry offers nowadays fast and reliable diagnostic support in clonal hematological conditions like acute leukemias and chronic lymphoproliferative disorders. The flow cytometric diagnostics is based on the identification of the immunophenotype of malignant cells. It aims at detection of aberrant antigen expression patterns and distinction from those observed in normal cells or under reactive conditions. Moreover, flow cytometric immunophenotyping can be used for precise determination of the lineage and maturation stage of malignant cells, thus enabling phenotype-based classification of different hematological disorders.

The accuracy of flow cytometric assay rises with the number of simultaneously used monoclonal antibodies, which is in turn dependent on the number of exciting lasers and fluorescence detectors of a flow cytometer. Flow cytometry is a constantly evolving technique, which helps to reveal phenotypic details of leukemias/lymphomas, contributing to their efficient diagnosis and classification.

References

Asnafi V, Beldjord K, Boulanger E, Comba B, Le Tutour P, Estienne MH, Davi F, Landman-Parker J, Quartier P, Buzyn A, Delabesse E, Valensi F, Macintyre E (2003) Analysis of TCR, pT alpha, and RAG-1 in T-acute lymphoblastic leukemias improves understanding of early human T-lymphoid lineage commitment. Blood 101:2693–2703

Barrena S, Almeida J, Del Carmen Garcia-Macias M, Lopez A, Rasillo A, Sayagues JM, Rivas RA, Gutierrez ML, Ciudad J, Flores T, Balanzategui A, Caballero MD, Orfao A (2011)

Flow cytometry immunophenotyping of fine-needle aspiration specimens: utility in the diagnosis and classification of non-Hodgkin lymphomas. Histopathology 58:906–918. doi:10.1111/j.1365-2559.2011.03804.x

Bene MC, Castoldi G, Knapp W, Ludwig WD, Matutes E, Orfao A, van't Veer MB (1995) Proposals for the immunological classification of acute leukemias. European Group for the Immunological Characterization of Leukemias (EGIL). Leukemia 9:1783–1786

Bennett JM, Catovsky D, Daniel MT, Flandrin G, Galton DA, Gralnick HR, Sultan C (1985) Proposed revised criteria for the classification of acute myeloid leukemia. A report of the French-American-British Cooperative Group. Ann Intern Med 103:620–625

Foss FM, Zinzani PL, Vose JM, Gascoyne RD, Rosen ST, Tobinai K (2011) Peripheral T-cell lymphoma. Blood 117:6756–6767

Givan AL (2004) Flow cytometry: an introduction. Methods Mol Biol 263:1–32

Gorczyca W, Weisberger J, Liu Z, Tsang P, Hossein M, Wu CD, Dong H, Wong JY, Tugulea S, Dee S, Melamed MR, Darzynkiewicz Z (2002) An approach to diagnosis of T-cell lymphoproliferative disorders by flow cytometry. Cytometry 50:177–190

Greaves MF, Janossy G, Peto J, Kay H (1981) Immunologically defined subclasses of acute lymphoblastic leukemia in children: their relationship to presentation features and prognosis. Br J Hematol 48:179–197

Herzenberg LA, Parks D, Sahaf B, Perez O, Roederer M, Herzenberg LA (2002) The history and future of the fluorescence activated cell sorter and flow cytometry: a view from Stanford. Clin Chem 48:1819–1827

Jaffe ES (2009) The 2008 WHO classification of lymphomas: implications for clinical practice and translational research. Hematol Am Soc Hematol Educ Program 113:523–531

Karube K, Aoki R, Nomura Y, Yamamoto K, Shimizu K, Yoshida S, Komatani H, Sugita Y, Ohshima K (2008) Usefulness of flow cytometry for differential diagnosis of precursor and peripheral T-cell and NK-cell lymphomas: analysis of 490 cases. Pathol Int 58:89–97

Maecker HT, Trotter J (2006) Flow cytometry controls, instrument setup, and the determination of positivity. Cytometry A 69:1037–1042

Mahnke YD, Roederer M (2007) Optimizing a multicolor immunophenotyping assay. Clin Lab Med 27:469–485

Orchard JA, Ibbotson RE, Davis Z, Wiestner A, Rosenwald A, Thomas PW, Hamblin TJ, Staudt LM, Oscier DG (2004) ZAP-70 expression and prognosis in chronic lymphocytic leukaemia. Lancet 363:105–111

Orfao A, Ortuño F, de Santiago M, Lopez A, San Miguel J (2004) Immunophenotyping of acute leukemias and myelodysplastic syndromes. Cytometry A 58:62–71

Orfao A, Lopez A, Flores J, Almeida J, Vidriales BM, Perez J, Kneba M, Macintyre E, Parreira A, Richards S, Szczepański T, Trka J, van der Velden VHJ, van Dongen JJM (2006) Diagnosis of haematological malignancies: new applications for flow cytometry. Hematology 5:6–13 (Education Program of the 11th Congress of the European Hematology Association, Amsterdam, The Netherlands June 15–18, 2006)

Palumbo GA, Parrinello N, Fargione G, Cardillo K, Chiarenza A, Berretta S, Conticello C, Villari L, Di Raimondo F (2009) CD200 expression may help in differential diagnosis between mantle cell lymphoma and B-cell chronic lymphocytic leukemia. Leuk Res 33:1212–1216

Porwit-MacDonald A, Björklund E, Lucio P, van Lochem EG, Mazur J, Parreira A, van den Beemd MW, van Wering ER, Baars E, Gaipa G, Biondi A, Ciudad J, van Dongen JJ, San Miguel JF, Orfao A (2000) BIOMED-1 concerted action report: flow cytometric characterization of CD7 + cell subsets in normal bone marrow as a basis for the diagnosis and follow-up of T cell acute lymphoblastic leukemia (T-ALL). Leukemia 14:816–825

Radcliff G, Jaroszeski MJ (1998) Basics of flow cytometry. Methods Mol Biol 91:1–24

Swerdlow SH, Campo E, Harris NL, Jaffe ES, Pileri SA, Stein H, Thiele J, Vardiman JW (2008) WHO classification of tumours of haematopoietic and lymphoid tissues (4th ed). IARC, Lyon, France

Szczepański T, Orfao A, van der Velden VHJ, San Miguel JF, van Dongen JJ (2001) Minimal residual disease in leukaemia patients. Lancet Oncol 2:409–417

Szczepański T, van der Velden VHJ, van Dongen JJM (2003) Classification systems for acute and chronic leukaemias. Best Pract Res Clin Haematol 16:561–582

Szczepański T, van der Velden VHJ, van Dongen JJM (2006) Flow-cytometric immunophenotyping of normal and malignant lymphocytes. Clin Chem Lab Med 44:775–796

Van Wering ER, van Lochem EG, Leenders M, van der Sluijs-Gelling AJ, Wind H, Gratama JW, Kraan J, Preijers FW (2004) Three-color flowcytometric analysis of mature and immature hematological malignancies. A guideline of the Dutch Foundation for Immunophenotyping of Hematological Malignancies (SIHON). J Biol Regul Homeost Agents 18:313–326

Vardiman JW, Thiele J, Arber DA, Brunning RD, Borowitz MJ, Porwit A, Harris NL, Le Beau MM, Hellström-Lindberg E, Tefferi A, Bloomfield CD (2009) The 2008 revision of the World Health Organization (WHO) classification of myeloid neoplasms and acute leukemia: rationale and important changes. Blood 114(5):937–951

Wood B (2007) Myeloid malignancies: myelodysplastic syndromes, myeloproliferative disorders, and acute myeloid leukemia. Clin Lab Med 27:551–575

Zola H, Swart B, Banham A, Barry S, Beare A, Bensussan A, Boumsell L, Buckley CD, Bühring HJ, Clark G, Engel P, Fox D, Jin BQ, Macardle PJ, Malavasi F, Mason D, Stockinger H, Yang X, Stockinger H, Yang X (2007) CD molecules 2006—human cell differentiation molecules. J Immunol Methods 319:1–5

Zucchetto A, Bomben R, Dal Bo M, Bulian P, Benedetti D, Nanni P, Del Poeta G, Degan M, Gattei V (2006) CD49d in B-cell chronic lymphocytic leukemia: correlated expression with CD38 and prognostic relevance. Leukemia 20:523–525

Chapter 10
Cytogenetics in Hematology

Olga Haus, Anna Poluha and Katarzyna Skonieczka

Abstract According to European LeukemiaNet—Workpackage Cytogenetics, cytogenetic analysis is mandatory to correctly diagnose and classify hematologic malignancies. Conventional cytogenetic analysis, which enables detection of both balanced and unbalanced chromosomal rearrangements, is still regarded as the gold standard of genetic diagnostics in hemato-oncology. However, a variety of rapidly developing state-of-the-art molecular and cyto-molecular techniques can now be applied, complementing the process of detection and analysis of recurrent genetic aberrations. Cytogenetics is currently recognized as an essential part of diagnostic process in hematologic malignancies. It helps to define specific disease entities, provides important prognostic and predictive information, influences therapy by setting the basis for individual treatment options that target cancer specific genetic abnormalities or their products, as well as helps to assess therapy effectiveness by indicating genetic remission or progression.

O. Haus (✉) · K. Skonieczka
Department of Clinical Genetics, Collegium Medicum in Bydgoszcz, Nicolaus Copernicus University in Toruń, Toruń, Poland
e-mail: haus@cm.umk.pl

K. Skonieczka
e-mail: k.skonka@wp.pl

O. Haus
Department of Hematology, Oncology, and Bone Marrow Transplantation, Medical University, Wrocław, Poland

A. Poluha
Department of Pediatric Hematology, Oncology and Transplantology, Children's University Hospital, Lublin, Poland
e-mail: poluha.anna@gmail.com

M. Witt et al. (eds.), *Molecular Aspects of Hematologic Malignancies*, Principles and Practice, DOI: 10.1007/978-3-642-29467-9_10,

10.1 Introduction

The recent WHO classification of tumors of hematopoietic and lymphoid tissue points to conventional cytogenetic analysis as a fundamental diagnostic tool for the detection of several recurrent genetic aberrations, recognized as mandatory to correctly diagnose particular types of leukemia. For example, detection of one of the aberrations typical for acute myeloid leukemia (AML) indicates the diagnosis of this disease entity, irrespective of the blast count (Swerdlow et al. 2008). Moreover, the identification of one of the recurrent aberrations enables prognostic risk stratification of patients, as well as the application of precisely targeted therapy, which increases treatment efficacy and decreases the risk of treatment related adverse effects. Favorable aberrations-bearing subtypes of AML which could be cured with a conventional chemotherapy with no need for allogeneic hematopoietic stem cell transplantation (allo-HSCT) are the example. On the contrary, the presence of aberrations listed below in childhood acute lymphoblastic leukemia (ALL), warrants the use of allo-HSCT (Szczepański et al. 2010):

- t(9;22)/*BCR-ABL* (*BCR*, breakpoint cluster region; *ABL*, Abelson murine leukemia viral oncogene homolog, encoding a tyrosine kinase),
- t(4;11)/*MLL-AF4* (*MLL* or *ALL1*, myeloid/lymphoid leukemia gene, human homolog of Drosophila trithorax gene; *AF4*, *ALL1*-fused gene from chromosome 4, protooncogene),
- hypodiploidy, especially near haploidy.

Among rapidly developing state-of-the-art molecular and cyto-molecular approaches to genetic evaluation, conventional (classical) cytogenetics (CC) is still regarded as the gold standard. However, not all of diagnostically or prognostically significant gene rearrangements or aberrant gene expressions are caused by chromosomal changes, detectable at the cytogenetic level (see also Chap. 2). Therefore, it is recommended to always complement CC analysis with molecular studies while evaluating patients with suspected or confirmed hematologic malignancy (Sandberg and Meloni-Ehrig 2010).

According to European LeukemiaNet (ELN)—Workpackage Cytogenetics, CC analysis is mandatory to correctly diagnose and classify hematologic malignancies. By revealing underlying chromosomal aberrations, both balanced and unbalanced, it provides clinicians with important prognostic information and, in many cases, sets the basis for the application of personalized therapy, targeted directly, or indirectly at cancer specific genetic changes (Haferlach et al. 2007a).

10.2 Technical Aspects

10.2.1 Cell Material

Bone marrow (BM) aspirate is regarded a reference source of viable cell material of diagnostic relevance to be studied in most hematologic malignancies, except for non-Hodgkin lymphoma (NHL), including chronic lymphocytic leukemia (CLL). Peripheral blood (PB) specimens could sometimes be used instead of BM, when the latter is impossible to obtain. PB seems to be a better choice in CLL and other NHL, especially for fluorescence in situ hybridization (FISH) studies, but it is of limited or no value in myelodysplastic syndromes (MDS) due to pancytopenia. In NHL cases the genetic analysis should be based on biopsied lymph node (LN) material, with occasional engagement of PB or BM for molecular or FISH studies, e.g. BM for verification of its involvement in malignancy.

A minimal volume of 2–3 ml of heparinized BM, 5–10 ml of heparinized PB or the biopsied LN, treated with sterile phosphate buffered saline (PBS) have to be transferred to the cytogenetic laboratory within 24 h, at room temperature. The diagnostic cytogenetic analyses are to be performed on the samples collected prior to any anticancer therapy. Even a single application of cytostatics or steroids can change the cytogenetic pattern of BM or PB cells (Gorczyca 2008; Haferlach et al. 2007a, b).

10.2.2 Cell Cultures

Creating optimal cell culture conditions is essential for the achievement of sufficient quality metaphases enabling detailed cytogenetic analysis. It is mandatory to carry out at least two cultures simultaneously: the reference unstimulated 24 h culture, and the stimulated culture supplemented with a mitogen or a cocktail of mitogens carefully designed for a suspected particular leukemia subtype.

If sufficient quantity of material is available, it is recommended to set several cultures varying in the culture time and in the mitogen type. Usually, cell cultures and CC analysis are not recommended and not necessary in routine CLL and other NHL diagnostics, because of the difficulties in obtaining sufficient number of analyzable metaphases. However, in case of CLL, the use of a special cocktail of interleukins (IL) and growth factors (GFs) or CpG-oligonucleotides alone or in combination with IL-2 allows to obtain good quality metaphases for G-banding using trypsin and Giemsa (GTG) analysis (Kotkowska et al. 2011).

Apart from the optimal culture conditions (such as appropriate culture medium, stable temperature of 37°C, and 5 % of CO_2) culture time is regarded the most important factor for successful CC analyses. In general, the parallel cultivation of at least two identical cultures varying only in culture time (direct: 30 min–2 h, 24 h, 48 h, and 96 h) is recommended. The 24 h cultures most reliably reflect the in vivo cytogenetic status of cells in the majority of hematological malignancies with rare exceptions, such as multiple myeloma, where longer incubation time (96 h) should be considered (Haferlach et al. 2007a; Hastings et al. 2012).

Harvesting of cultured cells is preceded by an exposure to colcemid for mitotic arrest and followed by hypotonic treatment and triple fixation of collected cell material in a mixture of methanol and acetic acid to assure optimal quality of metaphases. After preparation of sufficient number of slides, the remaining volume of harvested cell suspension in fixative should be stored in –20°C for further cytogenetic or molecular analyses.

The efforts of several networks and study groups working in the field of leukemia cytogenetics resulted in the creation of detailed standardized protocols for each procedure. According to Cytogenetic Guidelines and Quality Assurance, prepared by The Permanent Working Group "Cytogenetics and Society" of the European Cytogeneticists Association (ECA), the success rate for hematological chromosome analysis achieved by a given laboratory should approach 100 % (Hastings et al. 2012). However, it should be noted that the final rate of successful analyses in a particular laboratory highly correlates with its ability to adapt to possible changes in laboratory environment conditions (temperature, humidity, water quality). The same applies to banding and staining procedures (Gorczyca 2008).

10.3 Evaluation Methods

10.3.1 Conventional Cytogenetic Analysis

Conventional cytogenetic techniques, especially GTG-banding, have been introduced to diagnostic hematology nearly 40 years ago. Since then, besides the rapid development of new methods of chromosome analysis and classification, aided by state-of-the-art computer-assisted karyotype analysis, the fundamental principles of cytogenetic analysis still apply. Over the past decades, most of the laboratories furnished themselves with digital image processing systems equipped with complex software packages for capturing, processing, and archiving of the digitized chromosome images and, in some cases, with automatic metaphase finders and analyzers. However, CC analysis remains a highly demanding process with respect to workload and time and more importantly staff experience and expertise; therefore, it should always be performed by qualified cytogeneticists and in each case verified by at least one hematology cytogenetics specialist. It is recommended for all laboratories that at least 95 % of BM, PB or LN cytogenetic analyses should be effective, and the results of the analysis should be reported to referee no later than 21 days after receiving the sample (7 days for urgent BM cultures) (Hastings et al. 2012).

The aim of the chromosome study in hematologic malignancy is to find cytogenetically abnormal cell clone. As regards chromosome losses (e.g. monosomy), an abnormal clone is defined if three or more cells have lost the same chromosome, which excludes the possibility of reporting a random change. For structural abnormalities and chromosome gains, the presence of at least two cells with the same abnormality is sufficient (Frohling and Dohner 2008; Shaffer et al. 2009). Generally, the analysis of at least 20 metaphases is recommended to rule out the possibility of overlooking a small abnormal clone, but to obtain a reliable cytogenetic results in acute leukemias (AL) and MDS the detection of 10–20 metaphases with clonal abnormalities is completely sufficient (Haferlach et al. 2007a). However, in chronic myeloid leukemia (CML) the analysis of at least 30 metaphases is recommended by ELN in diagnostic as well as in control samples to assess the percentage of cells bearing Philadelphia (Ph) chromosome resulting from t(9;22), i.e. Ph(+) cells (Marin et al. 2008). As regards complex karyotype (the presence of at least three or, according to some authors, at least five recurrent aberrations per cell), it is recommended to generally enlarge the number of analyzed metaphases in order to maximize the likelihood of identifying a primary aberration as well as secondary ones (Mrózek et al. 2007; Shaffer et al. 2009).

The primary chromosome aberration, being frequently a primary genetic change in BM cell and leading to its malignant transformation, is defined by its presence in every abnormal metaphase. The primary aberrations give rise to malignant clones with unique biological characteristics (cytomorphology, immunophenotype) and clinical course of the underlying disease. Therefore, they serve as diagnostic as well as prognostic markers. The majority of aberrations recognized as primary leukemogenic events are balanced, that is without loss or gain of genetic material (e.g. inversions, balanced translocations). The unbalanced primary aberrations, associated with quantity changes of genetic material (e.g. deletions, isochromosomes, unbalanced translocations), are decidedly less frequent (Frohling and Dohner 2008).

Two main types of genetic changes arise as a result of reciprocal chromosomal translocations or chromosomal inversions. The first is a formation of a new fusion gene consisting of fragments of genes located at chromosomes breakpoints. One of the genes involved is usually a protooncogene or a tumor suppressor gene, the second is usually a gene taking part in cell cycle regulation, signal transduction, etc. The formation of a fusion gene results in the expression of a new, chimeric protein with altered activity. The classic examples of aberrations leading to the formation of a chimeric gene are:

- translocation t(9;22) associated with nearly all cases of CML, 5 % (in children) to 40 % (in adults) cases of ALL, and some cases of AML, causing formation of *BCR-ABL* fusion gene encoding a chimeric tyrosine kinase (Fig. 10.1),
- translocation t(15;17) associated with acute promyelocytic leukemia (APL), leading to *PML-RARA* fusion, which impairs *PML* suppressor gene function and changes the structure and function of a retinoid acid receptor α (RARA).

Unless included in the text, the names and function of the genes are presented in the legend to Table 10.1. This refers to the whole chapter.

The second type includes chromosomal changes leading to the altered expression of a structurally normal gene, usually a protooncogene, juxtaposing its coding sequence to strong promoters or enhancers of constantly active genes, or by removing its inhibitory elements. This mechanism could be exemplified by

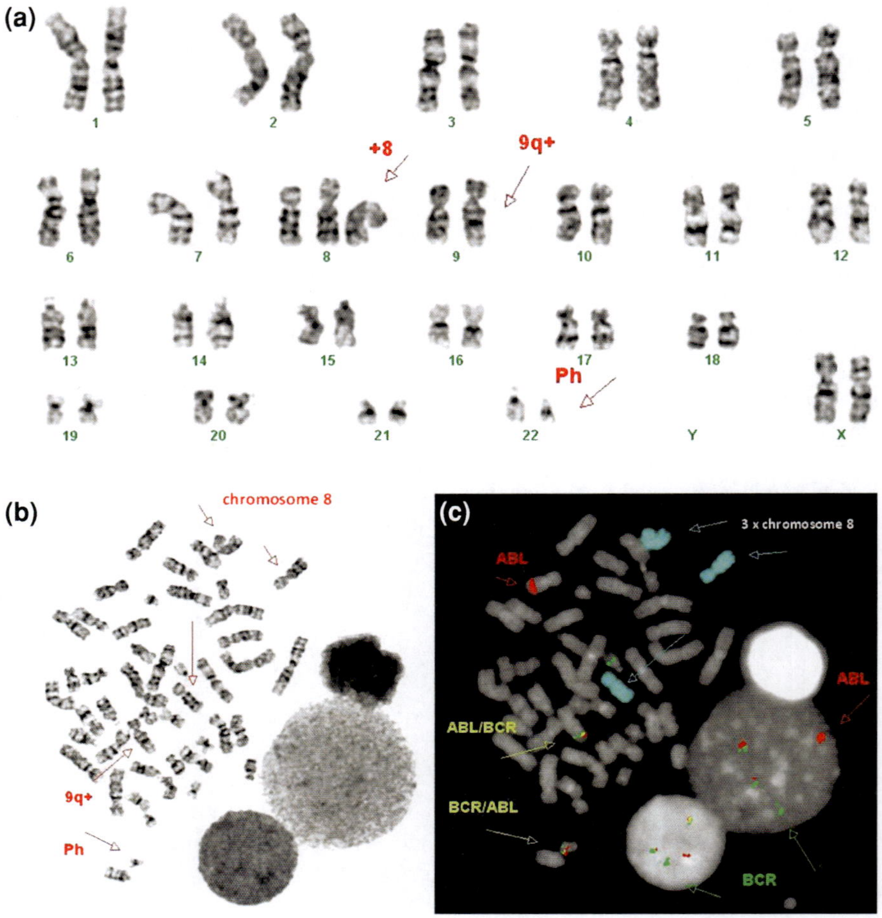

Fig. 10.1 Translocation, t(9;22)(q34;q11), and secondary aberration—trisomy 8 in a woman with chronic myeloid leukemia: a/GTG-banded karyotype: 47,XX,+8,t(9;22). The arrows show additional chromosome 8, derivative chromosome 9—der(9) and derivative chromosome 22—der(22) = Ph, b/GTG-banded metaphase (the basis for above presented karyotype): the arrows show abnormal chromosomes, c/FISH on the same metaphase, with whole chromosome painting (WCP) probes for chromosome 8 (*blue*), and specific probes for *ABL* (*red*) and *BCR* (*green*) genes. *Red arrow* shows *ABL* signal on normal chromosome 9, *green arrow*—*BCR* signal on normal chromosome 22, *yellow arrows*—mixed *red–green* fusion signals of *ABL-BCR* and *BCR-ABL* genes on derivative chromosomes 9 and 22 (Ph), respectively

aberrations involving juxtaposition of a coding sequence of *C-MYC* gene with the enhancer of immunoglobulin heavy chain gene *IGH* or immunoglobulin light chain genes, *IGK* and *IGL*, present in almost all cases of Burkitt lymphoma (Haferlach et al. 2007b; Huret 2008).

A range of recurring secondary chromosome aberrations have been described in hematologic malignancies. They appear during the course of disease and frequently precede or accompany its progression; therefore, they may emerge as

Table 10.1 Cytogenetic and molecular alterations in AML and their prognostic impact

Aberration	Genes involved	AML type	Prognosis	Comment	References
t(8;21)(q22;q22)	*RUNX1-RUNX1T1 (AML1-ETO)*	CBF-AML	favorable as compared to CN-AML	favorable only in *C-KIT*(-) cases	Gaidzik et al. (2011)
inv(16)(p13.1q22) t(16;16)(p13.1;q22)	*CBFB-MYH11*	CBF-AML	favorable as compared to CN-AML	–	Gaidzik et al. (2011)
t(3;21)(q26;q22)	*RUNX1-EVI1*	secondary AML	poor	constitutive *EVI1* overexpression also worsens prognosis independently of 3q26 alterations	Foran (2010)
t(15;17)(q22;q21) t(15;17)(q35;q21) t(11;17)(q12;q21) t(4;17)(q12;q21)	*PML-RARA* *NPM1-RARA* *NUMA1-RARA* *FIP1L1-RARA*	APL	favorable as compared to CN-AML	ATRA sensitive favorable only in *FLT3*-ITD(-) cases	Gulley et al. (2010); Licht and Sternberg (2005)
t(11;17)(q23;q21) interstitial dup(17)	*PLZF-RARA* *STAT5B-RARA*	APL	poor	ATRA resistant	Gulley et al. (2010); Licht and Sternberg (2005)
t(11;19)(q23;p13)	*MLL-MLLT1*	secondary AML	poor	–	Bacher et al. (2010)
t(9;11)(q23;q23)	*MLL-MLLT3*	secondary AML	intermediate	–	Bacher et al. (2010)
hsr, dmin, der(11)	*MLL* amplification		poor	–	Bacher et al. (2010)
hsr, dmin	*C-MYC* amplification		poor	–	Bacher et al. (2010)

CN-AML, cytogenetically normal AML *CBFB* core-binding factor beta subunit, *C-KIT* v-kit Hardy-Zuckerman 4 feline sarcoma viral oncogene homolog, protooncogene tyrosine-kinase Kit, *C-MYC* v-myc myelocytomatosis viral oncogene homolog (avian); *EVI1 MECOM*, *MDS1* and *EVI1* complex locus; *FIP1L1* FIP1 like 1 factor interacting with PAP; *FLT3* fms-related tyrosine kinase 3; *MLL* myeloid/lymphoid or mixed-lineage leukemia factor (trithorax homolog, Drosophila), *ALL1*; *MLLT1* myeloid/lymphoid or mixed-lineage leukemia factor (trithorax homolog, Drosophila), translocated to, 1; *ENL MLLT3* myeloid/lymphoid or mixed-lineage leukemia factor (trithorax homolog, Drosophila, translocated to, 3, *AF9*; *MYH11* myosin heavy chain 11, smooth muscle; *NPM1* nucleophosmin (nucleolar phosphoprotein B23); *NUMA1* nuclear mitotic apparatus protein 1; *PLZF* promyelocytic leukemia zinc finger; *PML* promyelocytic leukemia, probable transcription factor; *RARA* retinoic acid receptor alpha; *RUNX1 AML1* runt-related transcription factor 1, *CBFA2*; *RUNX1T1 ETO* runt-related transcription factor 1; *STAT5B* signal transducer and activator of transcription 5B prognostic markers. For example, an appearance of secondary aberrations, especially the isochromosome of chromosome 17 long arm, i(17)(q10), accompanied by the loss of one copy of *TP53* (p53 tumor suppressor) gene, in chronic phase of CML is considered an unfavorable prognostic factor, heralding progression into accelerated, or blastic phase. However, in AML subtypes characterized by the presence of one of the "low-risk" aberrations, the appearance of secondary aberrations generally does not alter the favorable outcome.

Secondary chromosomal abnormalities are usually unbalanced. Although some of them are identical with primary imbalancies (e.g. 5q−, 7q−, +8), they usually cannot serve diagnostic purposes due to their unspecific appearance in various diseases and their association with various primary abnormalities. One of the exceptions is trisomy 22 (+22). It is commonly recognized as a secondary change associated with pericentric inv(16)(p13q22), which is a "low-risk" primary aberration associated mainly with AML M4Eo, but is easy to overlook in GTG-banded karyotype (Fig. 10.2). The detection of +22 should warrant particularly thorough cytogenetic analysis or, preferably, FISH examination with a molecular probe specific for inv(16) (Grimwade et al. 2010; Mrózek et al. 2007).

CC analysis is a reference diagnostic tool in a range of hematologic malignancies. It enables genome-wide view of cytogenetic abnormalities present in malignant cells, either expected from the results of cytomorphologic evaluation or immunophenotyping, or completely unexpected. Moreover, cytogenetic studies are based on the analysis of population of cells with a high proliferating potential, therefore reflecting an in vivo characteristics of particular malignancy.

Genetic abnormalities, including cytogenetic aberrations, are primary tumorigenic events resulting in altered phenotype of malignantly transformed cells (e.g. abnormal morphology, aberrant expression of antigens). However, some of the phenotypic variations of populations of cells bearing the same genetic abnormality could be explained by the role of epigenetic factors, which generally do not influence the character of a specific malignant transformation. Therefore, more recently developed classification systems are based on specific recurring genomic aberrations (Harrison et al. 2010; Swerdlow et al. 2008).

10.3.2 Fluorescence In Situ Hybridization

Fluorescence in situ hybridization is a molecular cytogenetic technique routinely used in hematologic laboratories partly as excellent screening technique complementary to CC analysis or as a source of essential or additional information not available using standard cytogenetic analyses alone. It can be performed on various types of cytological samples, e.g. cultured cells, direct BM or PB smears, fresh, or processed tissue sections (formalin-fixed, frozen, or paraffin embedded). The major advantage of this technique over CC is that it enables the identification of chromosome aberrations without a need for cell culture and metaphase chromosome preparation. In order to estimate the percentage of cells with certain

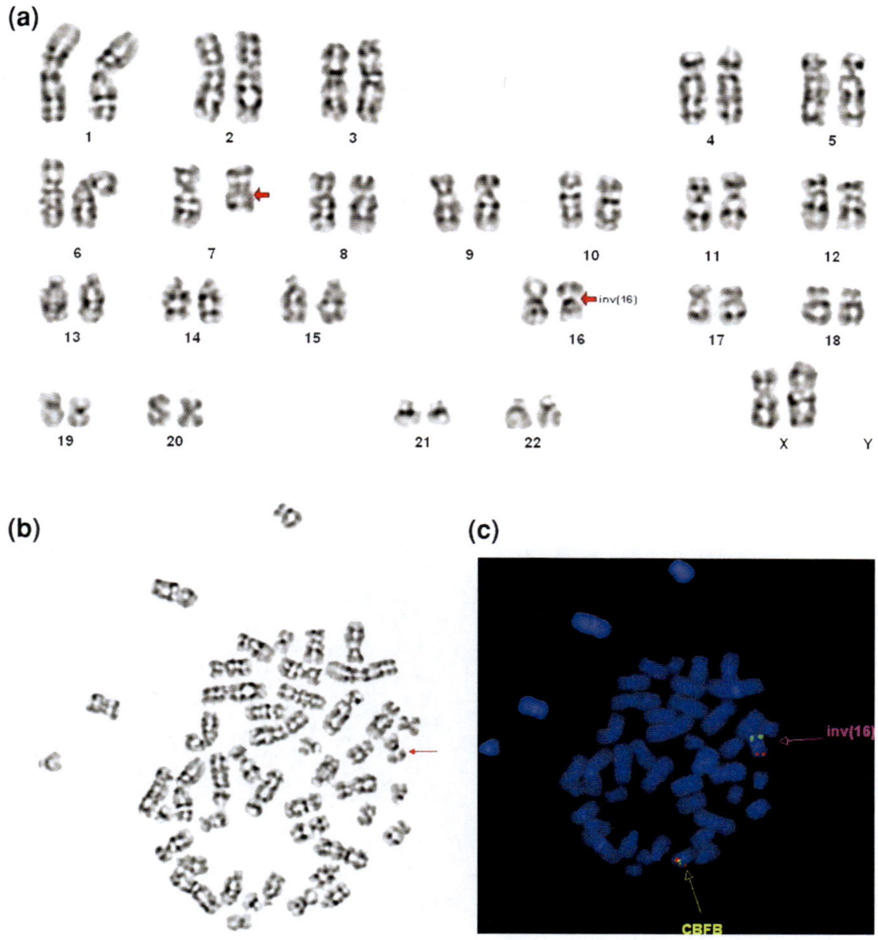

Fig. 10.2 Prognostically favorable inversion inv(16)(p11q22), with a secondary aberration—deletion of the long arm of chromosome 7 (7q-) in a woman with acute myeloid leukemia AML M4Eo: a/GTG-banded karyotype: 47,XX,del(7)(q22q35),inv(16)(p11q22). The *arrows* show abnormal chromosomes: 7q- and inv(16), b/GTG-banded metaphase (the basis for above presented karyotype): the *arrow* shows abnormal chromosome 16, c/FISH on the same metaphase, with the break-apart probe for *CBFB* gene: *yellow arrow* shows normal *red-green CBFB* signal, *violet arrow*—separation of *red* and *green* signals because of chromosome 16 inversion

abnormality, at least 100–200 cells, mainly interphase nuclei should be scored. However, efforts should be made, whenever possible, to include at least couple of metaphases into analysis to make the results more reliable, e.g. as to localization of unique DNA sequence signals (Hastings et al. 2012; Soszynska et al. 2008).

The essential component of FISH procedure is the molecular probe, i.e. DNA sequence, modified to incorporate fluorescent label, designed to hybridize to complementary target DNA sequence. There are four main types of probes that are commonly used for hemato-oncology FISH studies:

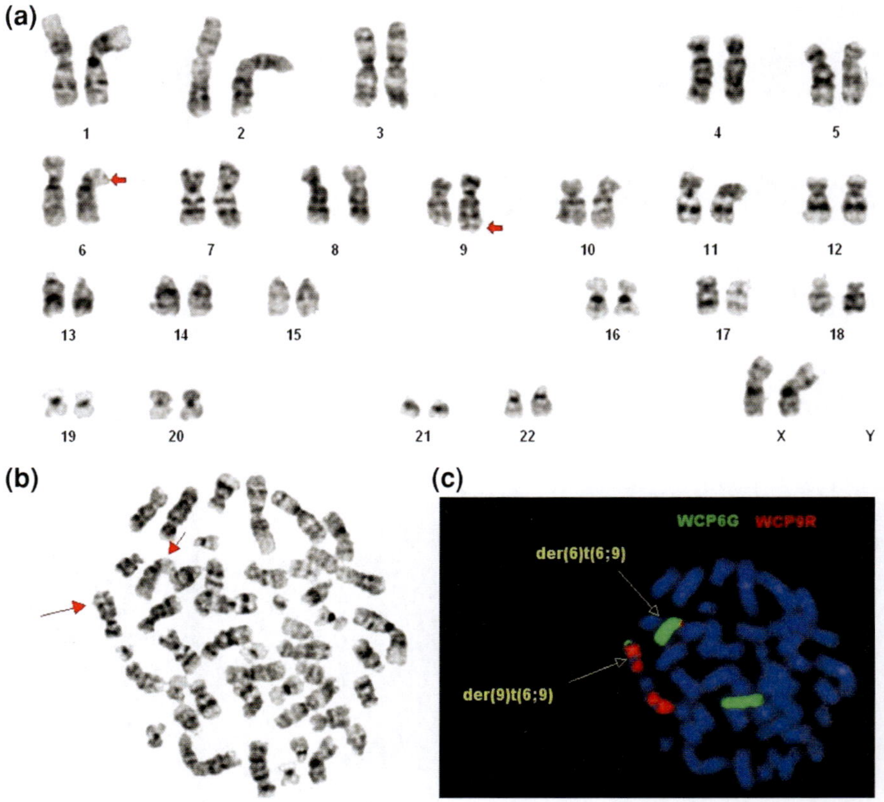

Fig. 10.3 Prognostically unfavorable translocation t(6;9) in a woman with acute myeloid leukemia with basophilia: a/GTG-banded karyotype: 46,XX,t(6;9)(p23;q34). The *arrows* show derivative chromosomes 6 and 9, b/GTG-banded metaphase (the basis for above presented karyotype): the *arrows* show abnormal chromosomes 6 and 9, c/FISH on the same metaphase, with WCP probes for chromosomes 6 (*green*), and 9 (*red*). The *arrows* show derivative chromosomes with mixed *green–red* [der(6)] and *red–green* signals [der(9)]

- Whole chromosome painting probes (WCP) and their variants—whole chromosome arm painting probes, used to identify large (>5Mbp) fragments of chromosomes, e.g. fragments translocated to nonhomologous chromosomes or nonhomologous arms. For diagnostic purposes WCP probes could only be applied on metaphase spreads (Fig. 10.3).
- Centromere-specific probes complementary to repetitive human α-satellite DNA sequences usually located near chromosome centromeres. Used mostly as an enumeration probe in metaphase preparations as well as interphase nuclei (Fig. 10.4).
- Telomere-specific probes complementary to DNA sequences localized in subtelomeric regions of chromosomes. Used to analyze the aberrations involving these regions, or to differentiate terminal and interstitial deletions.

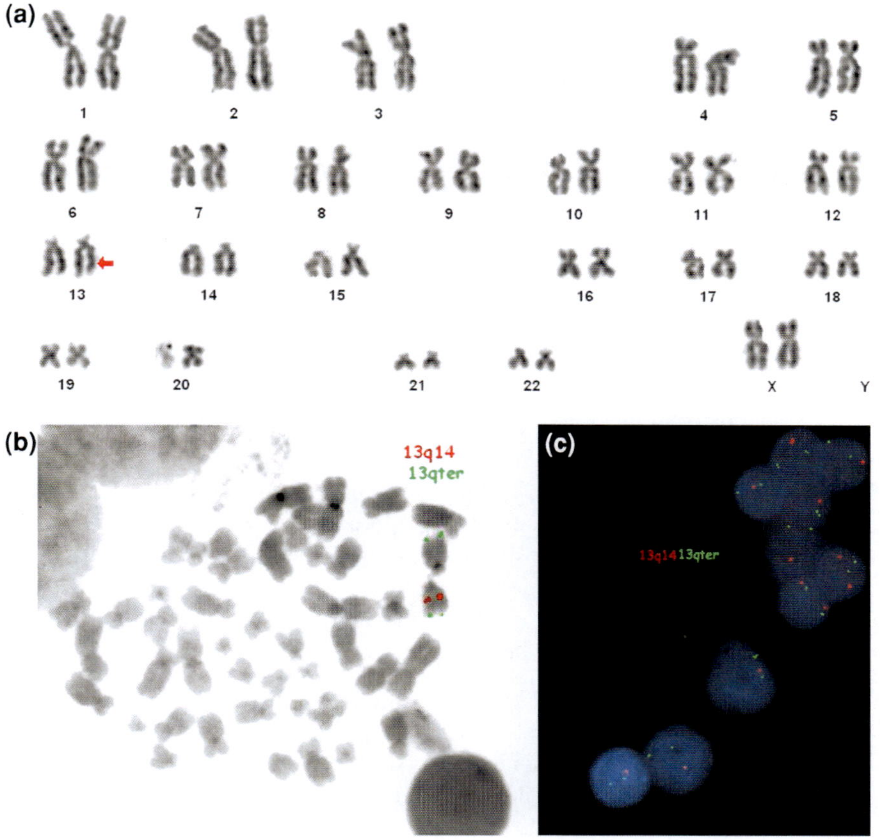

Fig. 10.4 Prognostically favorable deletion of 13q14 region in a woman with chronic lymphocytic leukemia B-CLL: a/GTG-banded karyotype: 46,XX. The *arrow* shows apparently normal chromosome 13, b/FISH on the same metaphase, with the probes for 13q14 region (*red*) and chromosome 13 subtelomeric region (*green*, control probe). Both chromosomes 13 have control *green* signals, but the upper one lost the signal of 13q14 region, c/Interphase FISH (nuc ish) showing single *red* 13q14 signals in majority of cells

- Unique sequence probes designed to detect a specific chromosome region, DNA sequence, or a gene. In hematological malignancies the most common types of these probes are:
  - Single or dual fusion translocation probes—a mixture of differently labeled, locus-specific probes, targeting the regions of chromosomes that fuse as a result of inter- or intrachromosomal structural aberration. There is a 5–10 % error threshold for single fusion probe (producing single fusion signal on one derivative chromosome) and 2.5–5 % for dual fusion probe (producing fusion signals on both derivative chromosomes). The most widely used dual fusion probe in hematologic malignancies is *BCR-ABL* translocation probe directed against translocation t(9;22) breakpoint regions. The interpretation of such

FISH assay results is based on the evaluation of hybridization signal pattern (relative localization of differently labeled probes). Overlapping signals usually reflect the fusion of *BCR* and *ABL* genes. Application of dual fusion probes also allows for detection of atypical localization, lack, or gain of signals, which can provide additional, potentially important information (Fig. 10.1). A novel type of fusion probes are tricolor differently labeled probes, designed to detect DNA sequences or genes localized on the same chromosome arm, and separated from each other by a distinctive sequence. The excision of this sequence by an interstitial deletion results in the juxtaposition of flanking genes, manifested as fusion of their signals in FISH examination, and disappearance of the interposed middle signal. This approach is used to detect microdeletions such as 4q12 microdeletion, resulting in *FIP1L1-PDGFRA* (*PDGFRA*, platelet-derived growth factor receptor alpha) fusion in hypereosinophilic syndrome (HES) (Fig. 10.5).

– Break-apart probes designed to detect DNA sequences located in opposite regions of targeted gene (5′ and 3′) that undergo separation in case of its rearrangement. They provide the best approach for rearrangements of genes coupling with multiple translocation partner genes, i.e. promiscuous genes, such as *MLL*, *TEL (ETV6*, ets variant 6), *CBFB*. Threshold error of this method is <2 % (Fink et al. 2009; Gorczyca 2008; Schaffer et al. 2009; Soszynska et al. 2008; van der Burg et al. 2004).

In many instances FISH is the best diagnostic and prognostic tool, better than CC or reverse-transcriptase polymerase chain reaction (RT-PCR), since it is largely independent of cell cultures, contamination or degradation of DNA/RNA, and capable of identifying aberrations impossible or difficult to diagnose by CC or RT-PCR.

10.3.3 Comparative Genomic Hybridization

Comparative genomic hybridization (CGH) is a method that enables genome-wide searching for chromosomal gains and losses. The technique is based on simultaneous hybridization of differently labeled DNA, the sample of interest and the control sample, to normal metaphase chromosomes. As a result, reference chromosomes appear uniformly stained, when there are neither gains nor losses of genetic material in the tested sample. In case of chromosomal imbalances, changes in the ratio of the intensities of the two fluorochromes, as compared to the expected one-to-one ratio seen in control sample, indicate regions of gain or loss of DNA sequences. Weaker staining of tested DNA indicates monosomy or partial deletion, while more intense staining points to additional copies of chromosomes or chromosomal sequences. The whole evaluation process is highly dependent on digital image capture systems equipped with the adequate software. Ultimate results are derived from digital chromosome profiles, created through the analysis of minimum 10 metaphases.

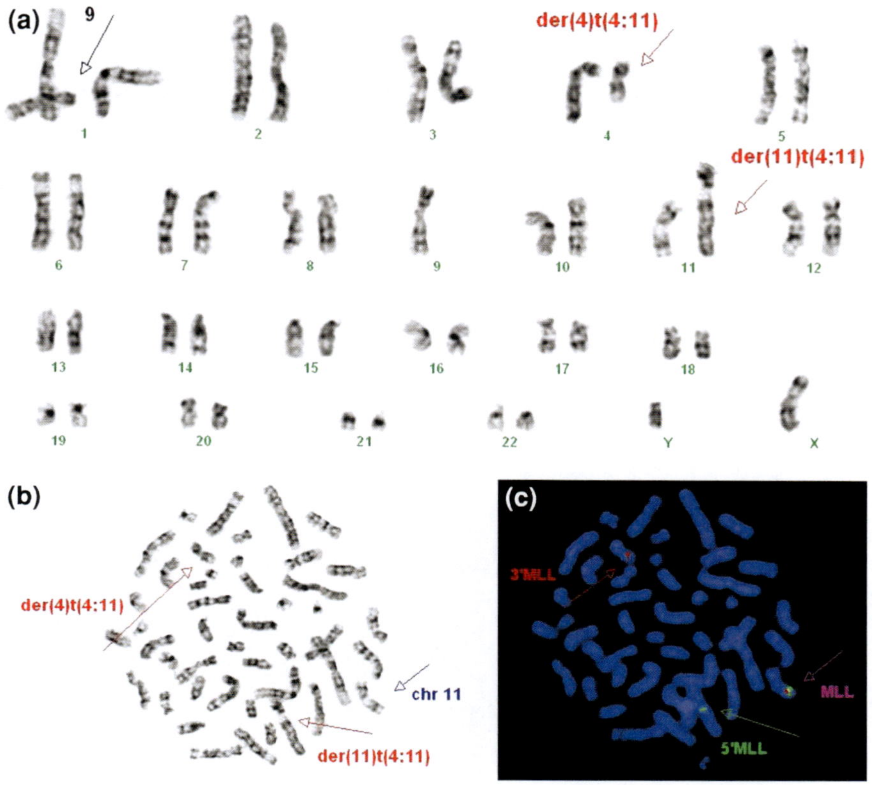

Fig. 10.5 Prognostically unfavorable translocation t(4;11) in a boy with acute lymphoblastic leukemia (B-ALL): a/GTG-banded karyotype: 46,XY,t(4;11)(q21;q23). *Red arrows* show derivative chromosomes 4 and 11. *Black arrow* shows normal chromosome 9 crossed with chromosome 1 on the metaphase spread, b/The same GTG-banded metaphase. *Red arrows* show derivative chromosomes 4 and 11, *black arrow*—normal chromosome 11, c/FISH on the same metaphase, with *MLL*-break-apart probe, showing splitting of signal between derivative chromosomes 4, and 11

CGH enables the detection of submicroscopic deletions spanning the region of 5–10 Mbp or amplifications exceeding 2–3 Mbp. It could be used as a complementary method to CC or FISH. The major disadvantage of this method is that it cannot identify balanced rearrangements, occurring in hematological malignancies as primary much more frequently than the unbalanced ones. Moreover, it does not allow to detect aberrations represented in minor clones, encompassing <40 % of cells in tested sample. Due to a relatively high frequency of false positive CGH results, each result should be confirmed in individual FISH experiments with probes targeting chromosomal regions suspected of loss or gain (Gorczyca 2008; Haferlach et al. 2007a).

10.3.4 Array CGH

Array CGH is a state-of-the-art molecular technique developed as a combination of two methods: CGH and DNA microarrays. It differs from CGH by the fact that labeled tested and control genomic DNA samples are hybridized to a set of (hundreds to thousands) reference genomic DNA sequences fixed or synthesized on silicon chips (microarrays) in place of metaphase preparations. Therefore, its resolution is much higher than achieved by conventional CGH, enabling detection of gains and losses of DNA sequences as small as 10 kbp. However, due to a relatively high costs of a single test, and the necessity of complicated bioinformatic analyses it is not yet routinely used as a diagnostic tool (Strefford et al. 2007).

10.4 Applications of Cytogenetics in Hematologic Malignancies

Cytogenetic studies are officially recognized as an essential part of the diagnostic process in hematologic malignancies. They provide important information of prognostic and predictive value, help to define specific disease entities, and influence therapy by setting the basis for treatment options that target specific genetic abnormalities.

10.4.1 Diagnosis

Genetic alterations are involved in the pathogenesis of hematologic malignancies as the early initiating events. Many of them help to define specific leukemia subsets. For example, the aforementioned t(15;17) is specific for APL, therefore its detection confirms the diagnosis of that unique type of leukemia even if the results of other diagnostic tests are inconclusive or suggestive of other entity (e.g. AML M2). Cytogenetics also plays a central role in differential diagnosis of myeloproliferative neoplasms (MPN). The presence of Ph chromosome indicates the diagnosis of CML, the only Ph(+) subtype of MPN. The lack of Ph and *BCR-ABL* points to other MPN. The detection of *FIP1L1-PDGFRA* in a myeloproliferation characterized by eosinophilia is highly suggestive of HES (Fink et al. 2009).

According to the current standards of cytogenetic evaluation in hemato-oncology a definitive diagnosis of specific disease entity based on CC findings could only be made when chromosomal alterations are visible in GTG-metaphases, e.g. t(8;21), t(9;22), large deletions, trisomies, monosomies. Nevertheless, additional FISH analysis, whenever applicable, should always accompany CC, in order to establish the percentage of cells with clonal aberration or to verify its type (e.g. standard, variant) (Atlas Genet Cytogenet Oncol Hematol 2011; Haferlach et al. 2007a).

Besides, FISH analysis is mandatory:

- in cases with failed cytogenetic study (absence or insufficient quality of metaphases),
- when clinical data are suggestive of disease entity characterized by submicroscopic aberration (e.g. *F1P1L1-PDGFRA*) or by abnormality known to be difficult to detect by CC analysis, e.g. t(15;17), inv(16),
- in case of a complex karyotype which could mask the presence of aberrations typical for the disease entity,
- when results of CC analysis are not definitive (e.g. identification of derivative chromosomes or markers),
- when cytogenetic analysis failed to reveal large chromosomal aberration expected on the basis of hematologic diagnosis, due to cryptic (masked) character of this aberration (lack of visible chromosome rearrangement, presence of underlying molecular change), e.g. masked Ph chromosome in Ph(−)*BCR-ABL*(+) CML
- when there is a discrepancy between the results of CC and RT-PCR,
- when a promiscuous gene is suspected to be rearranged (mainly *MLL*).

CC analysis accompanied by complementary FISH should be an obligatory part of diagnostic procedure in every case of hematologic malignancy. In entities characterized by diagnostically or prognostically important submicroscopic aberrations, such as *TP53* or 13q14 deletion in CLL (CLL, non-Hodgkin lymphomas, multiple myeloma) FISH should be a method of choice (Haferlach et al. 2007a, b; Hastings et al. 2012).

10.4.2 Prognosis

Genetic changes underlying malignant transformation determine biological characteristics of aberrant clone highly correlating with the course of a disease. Information on the prognostic significance (good, intermediate, poor) of recurring genetic abnormalities has been gathered from range of multivariate analyses of numerous groups of patients. Consequently, the result of cytogenetic analysis of malignant hematopoietic cells has been officially recognized as independent prognostic factor (Estey 2012; Giagounidis 2006; Haferlach et al. 2007b; Harrison et al. 2010; Palandri et al. 2008).

The prognostic significance of some of the aberrations depends on the disease entity. For example, in CML the presence of Ph chromosome and/or *BCR-ABL* fusion gene indicates better prognosis than its absence (atypical CML with poor prognosis), while in ALL it is always associated with very poor prognosis. Isolated deletion of 5q (5q-) is a factor of good prognosis in MDS but not in AML (Fig. 10.6). Such examples of inconsistent prognostic significance of genetic abnormalities are numerous and could be explained by the diversity of molecular changes underlying identical cytogenetic aberrations or by different prognostic impact of other biological features (e.g. other genomic alterations) coexisting with

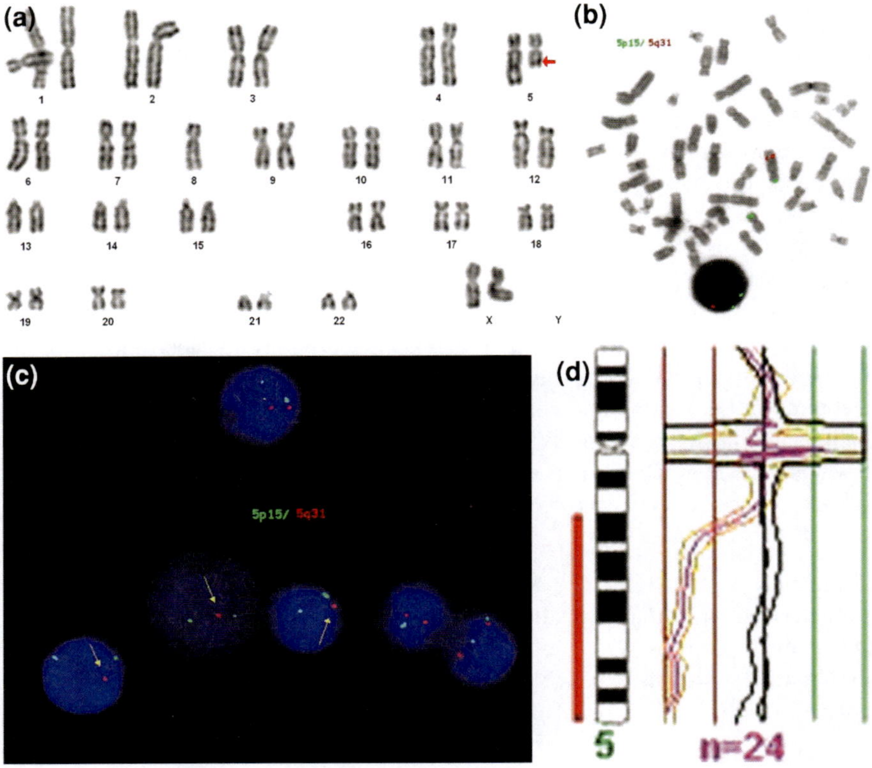

Fig. 10.6 Prognostically favorable isolated deletion of long arm of chromosome 5 (5q-) in a woman with myelodysplastic syndrome (MDS, 5q- syndrome): a/GTG-banded karyotype: 46,XX,del(5)(q13q33). The *red arrow* shows abnormal chromosome 5, b/FISH on the same metaphase, with the probes for 5q31 (*red*) and 5p15 (*green* control region), showing a lack of *red* signal on the lower chromosome 5, c/Interphase FISH showing lack of 5q31 *red* signal in one half of cells (*arrows*), d/CGH profile of deleted chromosome 5: the profile switch on the left, marked by *red* bar on the left side of chromosome 5 ideogram depicts a deletion of a part of long arm of this chromosome

a given aberration in various disease entities. What is more, the prognostic significance of some abnormalities varies even within the same subtype of hematological malignancy, depending on whether they are isolated or accompanied by other aberrations. The presence of translocation t(12;21)/*TEL-AML1* (*TEL*, translocation-Ets-leukemia; *AML1*, acute myeloid leukemia-1, both genes encoding for transcription factors) in childhood ALL is considered a good prognostic factor, but only when it appears as a sole cytogenetic abnormality and is detectable in the majority of analyzed cells. When it is present in small percentage of cells or is accompanied by other chromosome rearrangements it loses its prognostic significance (Soszynska et al. 2008). The example of consistent prognostic significance of a single aberration is the loss of one copy of *TP53* in FISH examination, which has a negative impact on prognosis mainly in CLL, but also in other leukemias, including CML, and AML (Grimwade et al. 2010).

Additional (secondary) chromosome aberrations are generally adverse prognostic factors (e.g. in CML), but may also have no prognostic impact (secondary changes in t(8;21)-positive or t(15;17)-positive AML) or presumably positive prognostic value (trisomy 22 in inv(16)-positive AML) (Dohner et al. 2010; Fabarius et al. 2011; Marin et al. 2008).

The identification of complex karyotype is linked to a significantly unfavorable prognosis in all malignancies, irrespective of how many favorable prognostic features it comprises (Dohner et al. 2010; Grimwade et al. 2010). Recently, a monosomal karyotype (the presence of at least two distinct autosomal monosomies or one monosomy and at least one structural autosome aberration) was indicated as the worst prognostic factor in AML. This finding was later confirmed for other blood malignancies, such as MDS, primary myelofibrosis, and others (Breems et al. 2008; Estey 2012; Patnaik et al. 2011).

The normal results of cytogenetic studies in hematologic malignancies may pose a challenge in terms of risk assessment. In some disease entities like MDS normal karyotype is associated with good prognosis, while in others it is only an intermediate prognostic factor due to the possibility of existence of gene rearrangements and mutations, e.g. *FLT3*-ITD (internal tandem duplication of *FLT3* gene), *CEBPA* (CCAAT/enhancer binding protein (C/EBP), alpha) double mutation, and others in AML, detectable only by molecular assays (see: Chap. 24). Those cytogenetically cryptic changes can also accompany visible chromosome aberrations, as described in AML, and the presence of some of them, e.g. *FLT3*-ITD in APL, *C-KIT* mutations in CBF-AML, i.e. AML with rearangements of *AML1(CBFA*, *RUNX1)* and/or *CBFB*, may be associated with reversal of prognostis (Dohner et al. 2010; Mrózek et al. 2007). In some entities normal karyotype or FISH result could be associated with poor prognosis, e.g. in HES, where better outcome is expected only when del(4)(q12)/*FIP1L1-PDGRFA* can be identified in FISH, or RT-PCR analysis (Fink et al. 2009).

Recurrent chromosome aberrations with respective gene rearrangements and other factors influencing the prognosis in AML, as an example of association of genetic changes and clinical and hematological data, are presented in Table 10.1.

10.4.3 Therapy

In most hematological malignancies cytogenetic aberrations play an important role in designing risk adapted therapies (treatment regimens). In leukemia characterized by favorable genetic changes standard treatment protocols could be used, whereas detection of adverse prognostic features calls for more intense regimens. Recent years have brought a range of genetically targeted therapeutic approaches. Some of them have become the treatment of choice in certain leukemia subsets leading to a long-term remission, e.g. the application of thyrosine kinase inhibitors (TKI) in therapeutic regimens for Ph(+) leukemias (see: Chap. 6) and HES with *FIP1L1-PDGFRA* fusion, as well as therapy with all-*trans* retinoic acid (ATRA) for t(15;17)-positive APL (see: Chap. 2) (Atlas Genet Cytogenet Oncol Haematol 2011; Fink et al. 2009; Haferlach et al. 2007b; Marin et al. 2008).

The development of new treatment protocols, improved to target certain genetic aberrations, leads to redefining the prognostic significance of those genetic markers. A chromosomal change previously recognized as high-risk factor could now be associated with standard prognosis if genetically tailored therapy is accessible, e.g. CML with a deletion within *ABL-BCR* gene on derivative chromosome 9 was associated with poorer prognosis than CML without this deletion in the era of interferon alpha (IFNα) treatment. Nowadays, with TKI treatment, the prognosis is equal in both disease entities (Marin et al. 2008; Palandri et al. 2008).

10.4.4 Monitoring of the Therapy

The adverse outcome of some hematological malignancies can be associated with progression of the disease, which is frequently preceded by the appearance of secondary genetic changes. Early detection of such aberrations in the context of worsening of patient's clinical status enables early recognition of disease progression and consequently immediate implementation of appropriate therapy (Frohling and Dohner 2008; Marin et al. 2008).

The goal of any therapeutic approach in hematologic malignancies should be the eradication of an aberrant neoplastic clone. If primary, cytogenetically visible abnormalities are detected in malignant cells at diagnosis, the monitoring of a disease status could be based on cytogenetic evaluation. Thus, lowering of a percentage of cells bearing the primary aberration in consecutive examinations is regarded the partial cytogenetic remission, while disappearance of cytogenetically abnormal clone is termed complete cytogenetic remission. Conventional karyotyping is recommended as a reference method to be used for the evaluation of cytogenetic remission, for example in CML, while FISH could be used as an additional approach enabling the screening of higher number of cells irrespective of their proliferative status (Haferlach et al. 2007a, b; Palandri et al. 2008). Additionally, FISH could play an important role in genetic monitoring of engraftment status in patients undergoing sex mismatched allogeneic hematopoietic stem cell transplantation, which fail to be evaluated with molecular methods (see: Chaps. 15 and 16).

10.4.5 Monitoring of Minimal Residual Disease

The monitoring of minimal residual disease is currently based mostly on standardized molecular methods (real-time-quantitative PCR, RQ-PCR). However, it is recommended for patients being in complete remission to undergo yearly cytogenetic evaluation. It enables the detection of disease relapse by identifying the reappearance of primarily diagnosed chromosome aberrations as well as the finding of new aberrations of yet unknown nature (e.g. aberrations in Ph-negative cells in TKI-treated CML). It also allows for an early diagnosis of secondary malignancy which is frequently preceded by the development of new clonal genetic abnormalities (Palandri et al. 2008).

10.5 Conclusions

Rapidly developing modern molecular cytogenetic methods, especially aCGH, are very much promising as diagnostic, prognostic, and predictive tools in hematologic malignancies. At present, however, they are too expensive and too sophisticated to be used in everyday clinical practice. Thus, conventional cytogenetics, supplemented with targeted fluorescence in situ hybridization or RT-PCR, is still the diagnostic method of choice in many hematologic entities, such as chronic myeloid leukemia, myelodysplastic syndromes, or acute leukemias. Cytogenetic examinations carried out and interpreted by experienced specialists, according to good laboratory practice and general rules of hemato-oncologic cytogenetics, may supply the information which allows for the stratification of patients to different risk groups and for the choice of the most efficient, genetically tailored therapy.

Acknowledgments The authors thank Ewa Duszeńko and Anna Jaśkowiec for their impressive cytogenetic work.

References

Atlas Genet Cytogenet Oncol Haematol (2011) http://atlasgeneticsoncology.org. Accessed 10 Sept 2011

Bacher U, Schnittger S, Haferlach T (2010) Molecular genetics in acute myeloidleukemia. Curr Opin Oncol 22:646–655

Breems DA, Van Putten WL, De Greef GE, Van Zelderen-Bhola SL, Gerssen-Schoorl KB, Mellink CH, Nieuwint A, Jotterand M, Hagemeijer A, Beverloo HB, Löwenberg B (2008) Monosomal karyotype in acute myeloid leukemia: a better indicator of poor prognosis than a complex karyotype. J Clin Oncol 26:4791–4797

Döhner H, Estey EH, Amadori S, Appelbaum FR, Büchner T, Burnett AK, Dombret H, Fenaux P, Grimwade D, Larson RA, Lo-Coco F, Naoe T, Niederwieser D, Ossenkoppele GJ, Sanz MA, Sierra J, Tallman MS, Löwenberg B, Bloomfield CD, European LeukemiaNet (2010) Diagnosis and management of acute myeloid leukemia in adults: recommendations from an international expert panel, on behalf of the European LeukemiaNet. Blood 115:453–474

Estey EH (2012) Acute myeloid leukemia: 2012 update on diagnosis, risk stratification, and management. Am J Hematol 87:90–99. doi:10.1002/ajh.22246

Fabarius A, Leitner A, Hochhaus A, Müller MC, Hanfstein B, Haferlach C, Göhring G, Schlegelberger B, Jotterand M, Reiter A, Jung-Munkwitz S, Proetel U, Schwaab J, Hofmann WK, Schubert J, Einsele H, Ho AD, Falge C, Kanz L, Neubauer A, Kneba M, Stegelmann F,

Pfreundschuh M, Waller CF, Spiekermann K, Baerlocher GM, Lauseker M, Pfirrmann M, Hasford J, Saussele S, Hehlmann R, Schweizerische Arbeitsgemeinschaft für Klinische Krebsforschung (SAKK) and the German CML Study Group (2011) Impact of additional cytogenetic aberrations at diagnosis on prognosis of CML: long-term observation of 1151 patients from the randomized CML Study IV. Blood 118:6760–6788

Fink SR, Belongie KJ, Paternoster SF, Smoley SA, Pardanani AD, Tefferi A, Van Dyke DL, Ketterling RP (2009) Validation of a new three-color fluorescence in situ hybridization (FISH) method to detect CHIC deletion, FIP1L1/PDGFRA fusion and PDGFRA translocations. Leukemia Res 33:843–846

Foran JM (2010) New prognostic markers in acute myeloid leukemia: perspectivefrom the clinic. Hematology Am Soc Hematol Educ Program 2010:47–55

Frohling S, Dohner H (2008) Chromosomal abnormalities in cancer. N Engl J Med 359:722–734

Gaidzik VI, Bullinger L, Schlenk RF, Zimmermann AS, Röck J, Paschka P,Corbacioglu A, Krauter J, Schlegelberger B, Ganser A, Späth D, Kündgen A,Schmidt-Wolf IG, Götze K, Nachbaur D, Pfreundschuh M, Horst HA, Döhner H,Döhner K (2011) RUNX1 mutations in acute myeloid leukemia: results from acomprehensive genetic and clinical analysis from the AML study group. J Clin Oncol 29:1364–1372

Giagounidis A (2006) Improving treatment outcomes by understanding cytogenetics in myelodysplastic syndromes. Haematol Rep 2:5–10

Gorczyca W (2008) Cytogenetics, FISH and molecular testing in hematologic malignancies. Informa Healthcare, UK

Grimwade D, Hills RK, Moorman AV, Walker H, Chatters S, Goldstone AH, Wheatley K, Harrison CJ, Burnett AK, on behalf of the National Cancer Research Institute Adult Leukaemia Working Group (2010) Refinement of cytogenetic classification in acute myeloid leukemia: determination of prognostic significance of rare recurring chromosomal abnormalities among 5876 younger adult patients treated in the United Kingdom Medical Research Council trials. Blood 116:354–365

Gulley ML, Shea TC, Fedoriw Y (2010) Genetic tests to evaluate prognosis andpredict therapeutic response in acute myeloid leukemia. J Mol Diagn 12:3–16

Haferlach C, Rieder H, Lillington DM, Dastugue N, Hagemeijer A, Harbott J, Stilgenbauer S, Knuutila S, Johansson B, Fonatsch C (2007a) Proposals for standardized protocols for cytogenetic analyses of acute leukemias, chronic lymphocytic leukemia, chronic myeloid leukemia, chronic myeloproliferative disorders, and myelodysplastic syndromes. Genes Chromosomes Cancer 46:494–499

Haferlach T, Bacher U, Kern W, Schnittger S, Haferlach C (2007b) Diagnostic pathways in acute leukemias: a proposal for a multimodal approach. Ann Hematol 86:311–327

Harrison CJ, Haas O, Harbott J, Biondi A, Stanulla M, Trka J, Izraeli S, Biology and Diagnosis Committee of International Berlin-Frankfürt-Münster study group (2010) Detection of prognostically relevant genetic abnormalities in childhood B-cell precursor acute lymphoblastic leukemia: recommendations from the Biology and Diagnosis Committee of the International Berlin-Frankfurt-Munster study group. Brit J Haematol 151:132–142. doi:10.1111/j.1365-2141.2010.08314.x

Hastings R, Howell R, Bricarelli FD, Kristoffersson U, Cavani S (2012) General guidelines and quality assurance for cytogenetics. A common European framework for quality assessment for constitutional, acquired and molecular cytogenetic investigations. E.C.A. permanent working group for cytogenetics and society. *E.C.A—European Cytogeneticists Association Newsletter* 29:7–25

Huret JL (2008) Chromosomes, leukemias, solid tumors, hereditary cancers. Atlas Genet Cytogenet Oncol Haematol. Available via http://AtlasGeneticsOncology.org/Educ/Hempat_e.html. Accessed 29 Oct 2011

Kotkowska A, Wawrzyniak E, Blonski JZ, Robak T, Korycka-Wolowiec A (2011) Chromosomal aberrations in chronic lymphocytic leukemia detected by conventional cytogenetics with DSP30 as a single agent. Leuk Res 35:1032–1038

Licht JD, Sternberg DW (2005) The molecular pathology of acute myeloid leukemia.Hematology Am Soc Hematol Educ Program 2005:137–142

Marin D, Milojkovic D, Olavarria E, Khorashad JS, de Lavallade H, Reid AG, Foroni L, Rezvani K, Bua M, Dazzi F, Pavlu J, Klammer M, Kaeda JS, Goldman JM, Apperley JF (2008) European LeukemiaNet criteria for failure or suboptimal response reliably identify patients with CML in early chronic phase treated with imatinib whose eventual outcome is poor. Blood 112:4437–4444

Mrózek K, Marcucci G, Paschka P, Whitman SP, Bloomfield CD (2007) Clinical relevance of mutations and gene-expression changes in adult acute myeloid leukemia with normal cytogenetics: are we ready for a prognostically prioritized molecular classification? Blood 109:431–448

Palandri F, Castagnetti F, Testoni N, Luatti S, Marzocchi G, Bassi S, Breccia M, Alimena G, Pungolino E, Rege-Cambrin G, Varaldo R, Miglino M, Specchia G, Zuffa E, Ferrara F, Bocchia M, Saglio G, Pane F, Alberti D, Martinelli G, Baccarani M, Rosti G, GIMEMA Working Party on Chronic Myeloid Leukemia (2008) Chronic myeloid leukemia in blast crisis treated with imatinib 600 mg: outcome of the patients alive after a 6 year follow-up. Haematol 93:1792–1796

Patnaik MM, Hanson CA, Hodnefield JM, Knudson R, Van Dyke DL, Tefferi A (2011) Monosomal karyotype in myelodysplastic syndromes, with or without monosomy 7 or 5, is prognostically worse than an otherwise complex karyotype. Leukemia 25:266–270

Sandberg AA, Meloni-Ehrig AM (2010) Cytogenetics and genetics of human cancer: methods and accomplishments. Cancer Genet Cytogenet 203:102–126

Shaffer LG, Slovak ML, Campbell LJ (2009) An international system for human cytogenetic nomenclature ISCN 2009. Karger, Basel

Soszynska K, Mucha B, Debski R, Skonieczka K, Duszenko E, Koltan A, Wysocki M, Haus O (2008) The application of conventional cytogenetics, FISH, and RT-PCR to detect genetic changes in 70 children with ALL. Ann Hematol 87:991–1002

Strefford JC, Worley H, Barber K, Wright S, Stewart AR, Robinson HM, Bettney G, van Delft FW, Atherton MG, Davies T, Griffiths M, Hing S, Ross FM, Talley P, Saha V, Moorman AV, Harrison CJ (2007) Genome complexity in acute lymphoblastic leukemia is revealed by array-based comparative genomic hybridization. Oncogene 26:4306–4318

Swerdlow SH, Campo E, Harris NL, Jaffe ES, Pileri SA, Stein H, Thiele J, Vardiman JW (eds) (2008) WHO classification of tumours of haematopoietic and lymphoid tissues. IARC, Lyon

Szczepański T, Harrison CJ, van Dongen JJ (2010) Genetic aberrations in paediatric acute leukaemias and implications for management of patients. Lancet Oncol 11:880–889

van der Burg M, Poulsen TS, Hunger SP, Beverloo HB, Smit EM, Vang-Nielsen K, Langerak AW, van Dongen JJ (2004) Split-signal FISH for detection of chromosome aberrations in acute lymphoblastic leukemia. Leukemia 18:895–908

Chapter 11
Monitoring of Minimal Residual Disease in Acute Lymphoblastic Leukemia

Tomasz Szczepański, Małgorzata Dawidowska and Katarzyna Derwich

Abstract In recent years, significant progress has been achieved in the monitoring of treatment effectiveness in hematological malignancies through the detection of so-called minimal residual disease (MRD). In this chapter, we present the methodological principles of MRD monitoring and its clinical application using acute lymphoblastic leukemia as a model disease. Detection of MRD kinetics during the first months of treatment has high prognostic value and it is currently employed for patient stratification in many treatment protocols. In high-risk patients and relapsed patients the MRD clearance is a prerequisite for effective stem cell transplantation. Therefore, MRD monitoring forms the basis for subsequent treatment intervention.

Tomasz Szczepański and Małgorzata Dawidowska contributed equally.

T. Szczepański (✉)
Department of Pediatric Hematology and Oncology,
Medical University of Silesia, 3 Maja 13/15, 41-800 Zabrze, Poland
e-mail: szczep57@poczta.onet.pl

M. Dawidowska
Department of Molecular and Clinical Genetics,
Institute of Human Genetics,
Polish Academy of Sciences, Strzeszyńska 32, 60-479 Poznań, Poland
e-mail: ma.dawidowska@wp.pl

K. Derwich
Department of Pediatric Oncology, Hematology and Transplantology,
Poznań University of Medical Sciences, Szpitalna 27/33, 60-572 Poznań, Poland
e-mail: kderwich@poczta.onet.pl

M. Witt et al. (eds.), *Molecular Aspects of Hematologic Malignancies*, Principles and Practice, DOI: 10.1007/978-3-642-29467-9_11,

11.1 Introduction

Using current treatment protocols, it is possible to achieve cure in a substantial group of acute lymphoblastic leukemia (ALL) patients, i.e. >80 % of children, and approximately 40 % of adult patients. Leukemia relapse still remains the most frequent cause of ALL treatment failure, affecting 20–30 % of childhood patients, and 45–65 % adults, respectively (Hoelzer et al. 2002). The relapse usually originates from small numbers of persistent malignant cells resistant to applied chemotherapy, defined as minimal residual disease (MRD) (Cave et al. 1998; Coustan-Smith et al. 2000; van Dongen et al. 1998; Szczepański 2007). Measuring MRD is the most reliable diagnostic tool to assess individual patient response to treatment (van Dongen et al. 1998). It is at least 100-fold more sensitive than standard cytomorphologic techniques applied for hematological remission assessment (light microscopy enables the detection of roughly one to five leukemic blasts among 100 normal cells; sensitivity of approximately 10^{-2}). Leukemia remission in bone marrow (assessed cytologically, defined as <5 % of lymphoblasts) is now achieved after 1 month of induction treatment in >95 % of children and >80 % of adult ALL patients. However, the application of more sensitive techniques such as multiparametric flow cytometry (FC) (sensitivity of approximately 10^{-4}) and particularly polymerase chain reaction (PCR)-based molecular methods (sensitivity of 10^{-4}–10^{-6}), allows the detection of persisting leukemic cells (MRD) in a subset of patients in hematological remission (Brisco et al. 1994; van Dongen et al. 1998; Coustan-Smith et al. 2000; Nyvold et al. 2002; Malec et al. 2004; Neale et al. 2004). This forms the basis for the application of MRD methodology into current treatment protocols.

11.2 Methods of MRD Monitoring

Current MRD methodology aims not only at the qualitative detection of persisting leukemic blasts but it should also allow their precise quantification. Therefore, reliable MRD techniques should be characterized by (Szczepański et al. 2001):

- possibility for precise quantitative analysis;
- the sensitivity of at least 10^{-3}, i.e. ability to detect one leukemic cell within the background of 1,000 normal cells (sensitivities of 10^{-4}–10^{-6} are preferable);
- leukemia specificity, i.e. reliable discrimination between normal and leukemic cells;
- the utilization of highly stable leukemia-specific markers, which are preserved throughout leukemia course;
- availability for the vast majority of patients;
- feasibility, high speed, and full reproducibility of the results, which enable intra- and inter-laboratory standardization of MRD methods and reliable application into clinical practice.

Currently, three techniques, using different types of leukemic cell markers, largely meet the above listed criteria for reliable MRD diagnostics.

11.2.1 Flow Cytometric Immunophenotyping for MRD Monitoring

Multiparameter FC, based on the detection of leukemia-specific immunophenotypes using different combinations of fluorochrome-labeled monoclonal antibodies, is the fastest, the cheapest, and the least labor intensive among all currently available MRD techniques (Brown and Wittwer 2000; Malec et al. 2004; Neale et al. 2004; Kerst et al. 2005; Dworzak and Panzer-Grumayer 2003; Lucio et al. 2001). A feature that allows the detection of persistent leukemic cells is the aberrant expression of cell-surface, cytoplasmic, and nuclear antigens, e.g. overexpression or the lack of expression of specific antigens, asynchronous expression of antigens (coexpression of antigens, which in normal cells do not occur simultaneously) or expression of antigens typical for T-lineage cells in B-lineage cells, and vice versa (cross-lineage expression). The basis for monitoring of MRD by FC is the identification of clone-specific immunophenotype, performed in each patient at the time of leukemia diagnosis, and then tracking the dynamics of MRD changes by quantitative detection of cells presenting the identified phenotype.

Flow cytometry is applicable in about 90–98 % of patients with ALL (Dworzak and Panzer-Grumayer 2003; Lucio et al. 2001; Kerst et al. 2005), but its sensitivity is lower (10^{-4}) as compared to methods based on real-time quantitative polymerase chain reaction (RQ-PCR; sensitivity of 10^{-4}–10^{-6}). Moreover, multicenter MRD monitoring by FC is much more difficult to standardize than that by RQ-PCR-based methodology. With the advent of novel multicolor (at least eight colors) FC and improved software, it is possible to make more precise multidimensional distinction between leukemic blasts and normal lymphocytic precursors (van Dongen et al. 2012). This modern approach gives also greatest possibilities for intra- and interlaboratory standardization (Kalina et al. 2012).

The results of research, published to date, aimed at comparison of MRD evaluation performed with the use of FC versus RQ-PCR with the use of immunoglobulin (Ig) and T-cell receptor (TCR) gene rearrangements as MRD markers (Ig/TCR-RQ-PCR), demonstrated high, though not complete convergence of MRD levels within the range of sensitivity of 10^{-4} (Kerst et al. 2005; Neale et al. 2004; Malec et al. 2004). The divergence of results is mainly due to the limited sensitivity of FC for the detection of the low levels of MRD ($<10^{-4}$) and due to the loss of MRD marker as a consequence of the evolution of leukemic clone. The risk of obtaining false negative results resulting from clonal evolution concerns MRD monitoring using both FC and Ig/TCR-RQ-PCR method (Malec et al. 2004). Due to the advantages and disadvantages of both techniques, it is currently assumed that the optimal regimen for monitoring MRD should provide the possibility to assess MRD by both methods, though in daily practice it is difficult to achieve, mainly for economy reasons (Kerst et al. 2005; Neale et al. 2004).

11.2.2 MRD Monitoring Using Fusion Gene Transcripts as RT-RQ-PCR Targets

Monitoring of MRD based on the detection of fusion gene transcripts typical for ALL is performed with the use of RT-RQ-PCR, a combination of reverse transcription (RT) with real-time quantitative polymerase chain reaction (Gabert et al. 2003; Braziel et al. 2003; van der Velden et al. 2003). After RT of mRNA into cDNA these markers are detected using specific pair of primers, located in exons of both translocation partner genes, so that to flank the breakpoint of the fusion transcript, and a TaqMan probe specific for the amplified region. The principle of the TaqMan technology is based on labeling the 5′ end of the probe with a reporter dye (fluorescent signal emitter) and with the so-called quencher dye at the 3′ end (absorption of the emitted fluorescence) (see also Chap. 20). The TaqMan technology exploits the 5′→3′exonuclease activity of DNA polymerase, causing the degradation of the probe during DNA synthesis (the elongation of primers). This results in the increase of the fluorescence, emitted by the reported dye dislocated from the quencher as a consequence of the probe degradation, and reflects the increase in the quantity of the PCR product. The crucial parameter in RQ-PCR analysis is a threshold cycle (*crossing point*, C_T) determined for each sample as the cycle number in which the fluorescence intensity exceeds the threshold (baseline determined based on the background fluorescence) for the first time. The C_T value is proportional to the amount of the target sequence (the lower the C_T, the higher the quantity of the amplified sequence) (van der Velden et al. 2003). Quantitative analysis of MRD is performed with the use of the C_T values of the samples and the standard curve, obtained by a serial dilution of the plasmid DNA, containing the cloned fusion gene of interest (Gabert et al. 2003).

The main advantage of this methodology is the stability of fusion gene transcripts in the course of the disease and high sensitivity of MRD determination (10^{-4}–10^{-6}) due to the lack of these aberrations in normal cells. The disadvantages of this technique include high susceptibility of RNA to degradation and the possibility of application in only subset of patients, due to the limited frequency of fusion genes. In childhood, B-cell precursor acute lymphoblastic leukemia (BCP-ALL) fusion genes are detected in approximately 45 % of patients; mostly *BCR-ABL* (*BCR*, breakpoint cluster region; *ABL1*, Abelson murine leukemia viral oncogene), *MLL-AF4* (*MLL*, mixed-lineage leukemia also named *ALL-1*; *ALL-1* fused gene from chromosomes 4), and *TEL-AML1* (*TEL*, translocation-Ets-leukemia; *AML1*, acute myeloid leukemia-1). In pediatric T-cell precursor ALL (T-ALL) fusion genes, mostly *SIL-TAL1* (*SIL*, *SCL/TAL1* interrupting locus; *TAL1*, T-cell acute lymphocytic leukemia 1) are present in approximately 15–25 % of patients (Szczepański et al. 2001) (See also Chap. 1). Moreover, fusion gene transcripts are leukemia specific, but not patient-specific markers, which increases the risk of obtaining false positive results as a consequence of cross-sample contamination, which might be difficult to identify. For some gene fusions, such as *SIL-TAL1* or various translocations involving *MLL* gene, it is possible to detect the fusion not only at the mRNA level, but also the DNA level, which due to the different locations of breakpoints at the DNA level, makes these markers specific for each patient (van der Velden et al. 2003; Meyer et al. 2009).

11.2.3 MRD Monitoring Using Clonal Immunoglobulin and T-cell Receptor Gene Rearrangements as RQ-PCR Targets

The most common current method of MRD monitoring is based on the detection of junctional region sequences of rearranged immunoglobulin and T-cell receptor encoding genes using RQ-PCR approach (Ig/TCR-RQ-PCR) (van der Velden et al. 2003; Szczepański et al. 2001, 2002; Pongers-Willemse et al. 1998; Jółkowska et al. 2007). This method is characterized by a sensitivity of 10^{-4}–10^{-5}, and the possibility to use in more than 95 % of patients with ALL (van der Velden et al. 2003).

Specific mechanism of V-(D)-J gene rearrangements (*V*, variable; *D*, diversity; *J*, joining), including random deletions and insertions of nucleotides in junctional regions, produces unique marker sequences specific to each leukemic clone (specific to each patient's leukemia). The basis for MRD analysis using this methodology is the identification of marker rearrangements in the material obtained at diagnosis of leukemia (before treatment), by PCR amplification of rearranged genes using standard combinations of primers (Pongers-Willemse et al. 1999; van Dongen et al. 2003; Kraszewska et al. 2012; Dawidowska et al. 2008). Clonality assessment, i.e. discrimination between amplicons derived from clonal leukemic cells and polyclonal PCR products derived from normal lymphocytes is performed with the use of heteroduplex analysis. The amplification products are subjected to denaturation and slow renaturation, leading to the formation of duplexes, which are separated by nondenaturating polyacrylamide gel electrophoresis (Langerak et al. 1997) (See also Chap. 23). Clonal Ig/TCR gene rearrangements are then identified by fluorescent sequencing followed by the analysis of homology with human germline sequences of V, D and J genes, available online in databases. This enables the design of patient-specific oligonucleotide primers (allele-specific oligonucleotides, ASO), which are subsequently used for RQ-PCR-based determination of MRD levels during follow-up. Quantification of MRD is performed with the use of previously described TaqMan technology, with ASO primers and germ-line primers and probes, specific to nonrearranged germ-line V, D, and J genes. MRD levels are determined based on the C_T values of the analyzed samples and a standard curve generated by serial dilution of DNA obtained before treatment (a reference sample—100 % blast cells) in the DNA of healthy donors (van der Velden et al. 2003; Pongers-Willemse et al. 1998).

Despite the relatively high costs and time consumption associated with a significant number of procedures, especially those concerning the identification of

Ig/TCR gene rearrangements and the design and testing of the ASO primers, this method is now recognized in Europe as the "gold standard" for MRD monitoring. This is, among others, due to a very advanced degree of standardization, concerning research protocols for the consecutive stages of the analysis, the guidelines on primers' and probes' design, as well as guidelines on the interpretation of quantitative data (Pongers-Willemse et al. 1999; van Dongen et al. 2003; van der Velden et al. 2007a). Extensive international standardization programs have ensured high reproducibility of MRD results between different centers, which have enabled the implementation of this methodology into treatment stratification in several clinical trials and modern therapeutic protocols, in both childhood, and adult ALL (van der Velden et al. 2007b; Flohr et al. 2008; Campana 2010; Bassan et al. 2009; Schmiegelow et al. 2010; Yamaji et al. 2010; Conter et al. 2010).

11.3 Clinical Aspects of MRD Monitoring in Childhood ALL

11.3.1 MRD During Induction and Consolidation Treatment

The results of numerous prospective studies revealed that monitoring of residual disease, particularly throughout the first months of treatment, provides valuable information on treatment effectiveness (patients response to therapy) and is highly predictive of leukemia relapse and treatment outcome (Cave et al. 1998; van Dongen et al. 1998; Dworzak et al. 2002; Nyvold et al. 2002; Biondi et al. 2000; Coustan-Smith et al. 1998; Panzer-Grumayer et al. 2000; Campana 2009, 2010; Yamaji et al. 2010; Conter et al. 2010). It has been proven that MRD assessment at specific time points during ALL treatment has significant prognostic value. The level of residual disease determined at the end of induction treatment has been documented to be independent prognostic factor in childhood ALL, superior to all previously recognized prognostic factors such as age at diagnosis, sex, initial white blood cell count, immunophenotype of leukemic cells, the presence of chromosomal aberrations, the time of remission, and steroid response as measured by the number of blast cells circulating in blood after 7 days of steroid administration (van Dongen et al. 1998; Cave et al. 1998; Conter et al. 2010). High clinical utility of MRD analysis has also been demonstrated in infant ALL, which constitutes a biologically distinct, more aggressive ALL subtype (Van der Velden et al. 2009).

The results of MRD quantification during the first 3 months of ALL therapy enable reliable risk group classification and further adjustment of treatment intensity. Undetectable or very low MRD levels at the end of induction has been correlated with favorable outcome, while high levels of residual cells are strongly predictive of leukemia relapse. In approximately 40–50 % of children negative MRD results are obtained after induction treatment, which corresponds to a percentage of patients obtaining long-term remission before the introduction of intensified multidrug ALL therapeutic protocols 40 years ago (van Dongen et al. 1998). The remaining children form a group of so-called 'MRD-positive patients', for whom the risk of relapse is dependent on the MRD level (Cave et al. 1998; Coustan-Smith et al. 1998; Goulden et al. 1998; van Dongen et al. 1998). Van Dongen et al. (1998) demonstrated that high MRD levels ($\geq 10^{-2}$), detected after induction of remission and before consolidation treatment are related to threefold increase of relapse incidence compared to low or undetectable MRD levels ($\leq 10^{-4}$). Similar results were obtained by Cave et al. (1998) who showed that MRD $\geq 10^{-2}$ at the end of induction and $\geq 10^{-3}$ at later time points is strongly associated with leukemia relapse.

The results of quantitative MRD analysis obtained at the end of induction treatment and before consolidation, are currently recognized as the most significant prognostic factors in childhood ALL (van Dongen et al. 1998; Biondi et al. 2000; Bene and Kaeda 2009; Campana 2009; Conter et al. 2010; Yamaji et al. 2010). Information on MRD levels at these two time points has already been implemented for risk group classification proposed by *International Berlin-Frankfurt-Münster Study Group* (I-BFM-SG) with low risk of relapse in patients MRD-negative at both time points, high risk of relapse in patients with MRD levels $\geq 10^{-3}$ at both time points and intermediate risk of relapse in the remaining patients (Biondi et al. 2000). Biondi et al. (2000) demonstrated significantly lower relapse free survival (RFS) for high-risk patients (4-year RFS: 44.7 %) as compared to intermediate and low-risk groups (RFS: 76.4 % and 97.7 %, respectively). It is noteworthy that MRD-based high-risk group is larger than the high-risk group determined with the use of classical risk factors (approximately 15 vs. 5 %, respectively) (van Dongen et al. 1998). Within the MRD-based low-risk group, half of the patients have already low ($\leq 10^{-4}$) or undetectable MRD levels after 2 weeks of treatment (Panzer-Grumayer et al. 2000). This group might particularly profit from treatment reduction.

Due to well documented clinical utility of quantitative monitoring of MRD, it has already been implemented into modern therapeutic protocols for childhood ALL (Flohr et al. 2008; Schmiegelow et al. 2010; Yamaji et al. 2010; Conter et al. 2010).

11.3.2 MRD in Relapsed ALL

Quantitative assessment of residual disease is also clinically valuable in the treatment of relapsed childhood ALL. It enables the evaluation of response to reinduction therapy and reliable assessment of the risk of subsequent relapse (Eckert et al. 2001; Coustan-Smith et al. 2004). The I-BFM-SG demonstrated that information on MRD levels, detected with the use of molecular techniques, on day 36 of reinduction treatment provides the basis for classification of patients into low-risk group (MRD $< 10^{-3}$) with event free survival (EFS) of 86 % and high-risk group (MRD $\geq 10^{-3}$) with 0 % EFS (Eckert et al. 2001). Similar results were obtained with the use of FC monitoring of MRD. Coustan-Smith et al. (2004)

showed that MRD levels $\geq 10^{-4}$ at the end of reinduction treatment strongly predispose to reemergence of leukemia relapse.

11.3.3 MRD in Management of Allogeneic Hematopoietic Stem Cell Transplantation

The assessment of MRD levels performed before and after allogeneic hematopoietic stem cell transplantation (allo-HSCT) has been documented to have high utility for clinical decision-making concerning conditioning regimen before HSCT as well as the management of posttransplant follow-up and treatment. Clinical significance of MRD monitoring in transplant settings was first reported by Knechtli et al. (Knechtli et al. 1998) and then confirmed in later studies (Bader et al. 2002, 2009; Uzunel et al. 2001; van der Velden et al. 2001; Pulsipher et al. 2009; Elorza et al. 2010; Lankester et al. 2010). In children subjected to HSCT, both in the first and in the second complete remission (I CR and II CR), the presence of residual disease prior to HSCT, particularly at high levels, strongly correlated with ALL relapse (Bader et al. 2002, 2009; Uzunel et al. 2001; van der Velden et al. 2001; Eckert et al. 2001; Knechtli et al. 1998; Lankester et al. 2010; Elorza et al. 2010). Also after HSCT, the monitoring of MRD enables early detection of emerging ALL relapse and preemptive immunomodulatory treatment (Pulsipher et al. 2009). More detailed information on MRD monitoring in the context of HSCT is included in Chap. 16.

11.4 MRD Monitoring in Adult ALL

Most data on clinical significance of MRD in ALL have been obtained in the studies of pediatric patients; however, its strong prognostic value has also been documented in adults with ALL (Brisco et al. 1996; Mortuza et al. 2002; Bruggemann et al. 2006; Holowiecki et al. 2008; Bassan et al. 2009; Kikuchi et al. 2010; Campana 2009). Different kinetics of MRD clearance, slower in adults and more rapid in children, have been demonstrated, which reflects greater resistance of leukemic blasts in case of childhood ALL than in adults (Bruggemann et al. 2006; Mortuza et al. 2002; Foroni and Hoffbrand 2002). Detectable MRD levels have been reported in 63 and 47 % of adults on day 24 and day 44 of treatment; respectively (Bruggemann et al. 2006), while in pediatric ALL MRD-positivity has been found in 25–58 % of patients within first 4–6 weeks of therapy (Cave et al. 1998; van Dongen et al. 1998; Nyvold et al. 2002). Greater percentage of MRD-positive results in adults than in children has also been reported at later time points.

Therefore, in adult ALL different time points for MRD detection and different proportion of patients in particular risk groups, compared to children, have been reported. In the study by Bruggemann et al. based on combined MRD results obtained at nine time points through the first year of treatment, three distinct risk groups have been identified: low risk [MRD $< 10^{-4}$ on day 11 and day 24; 3-year relapse rate (RR): 0 %], high risk (MRD $\geq 10^{-4}$ until week 16, 3-year RR: 94 %), and intermediate risk in the remaining patients (3-year RR: 47 %) (Bruggemann et al. 2006).

Similarly to childhood ALL, MRD results at the end of induction treatment have been documented to provide reliable prognostic information on the risk of leukemia relapse. MRD levels at this time point, in combination with conventional risk factors, enabled classification of adult patients into two groups: high-risk patients (MRD $\geq 10^{-3}$) and the remaining patients (MRD $< 10^{-3}$) with a 3-year RR: 9 and 71 %, respectively (Holowiecki et al. 2008). The prognostic value of MRD assessment during and after induction treatment in case of adult ALL has also been demonstrated by others (Mortuza et al. 2002; Brisco et al. 1996; Vidriales et al. 2003; Bassan et al. 2009; Kikuchi et al. 2010).

It has also been reported for adult patients that the conversion of negative MRD results into MRD-positivity enables early detection of leukemia relapse (molecular relapse) and prevention of overt hematological relapse through the modulation of therapy (Raff et al. 2007). These findings have already been implemented into some clinical protocols for adult ALL as the basis for the introduction of preventive treatment in patients with molecular relapse (Raff et al. 2007).

11.5 Conclusions

The clinical significance of quantitative assessment of MRD in ALL has been well documented by the results of many studies, performed both in childhood and adult patients, in de novo and relapsed ALL, as well as before and after allo-HSCT. The identification of specific time points for MRD quantification during ALL treatment, providing the most prognostically relevant information in the above-mentioned clinical situations, as well as the choice of the most reliable method for MRD monitoring have been the major goal of many research groups. International collaboration has resulted in extensive standardization of MRD diagnostics in ALL, which enabled its implementation into many clinical trials and modern therapeutic protocols. The level of MRD, assessed at relevant time points with the use of RQ-PCR or FC, is currently the most reliable prognostic factor in ALL, enabling the stratification of patients into risk groups, the adjustment of treatment intensity and relevant treatment modifications, including those in the management of HSCT. The main effort should now be focused on the optimization of MRD diagnostics through both broadening the panel of MRD targets as well as lowering the costs of MRD monitoring, to enable its application in even larger group of ALL patients.

Acknowledgments This chapter was partly supported by the Ministry of Science and Higher Education, grant N N407 311 839.

References

Bader P, Hancock J, Kreyenberg H, Goulden NJ, Niethammer D, Oakhill A, Steward CG, Handgretinger R, Beck JF, Klingebiel T (2002) Minimal residual disease (MRD) status prior to allogeneic stem cell transplantation is a powerful predictor for post-transplant outcome in children with ALL. Leukemia 16(9):1668–1672

Bader P, Kreyenberg H, Henze GH, Eckert C, Reising M, Willasch A, Barth A, Borkhardt A, Peters C, Handgretinger R, Sykora KW, Holter W, Kabisch H, Klingebiel T, von Stackelberg A (2009) Prognostic value of minimal residual disease quantification before allogeneic stem-cell transplantation in relapsed childhood acute lymphoblastic leukemia: the ALL-REZ BFM Study Group. J Clin Oncol 27(3):377–384. doi:10.1200/JCO.2008.17.6065, JCO.2008.17.6065[pii]

Bassan R, Spinelli O, Oldani E, Intermesoli T, Tosi M, Peruta B, Rossi G, Borlenghi E, Pogliani EM, Terruzzi E, Fabris P, Cassibba V, Lambertenghi-Deliliers G, Cortelezzi A, Bosi A, Gianfaldoni G, Ciceri F, Bernardi M, Gallamini A, Mattei D, Di Bona E, Romani C, Scattolin AM, Barbui T, Rambaldi A (2009) Improved risk classification for risk-specific therapy based on the molecular study of minimal residual disease (MRD) in adult acute lymphoblastic leukemia (ALL). Blood 113(18):4153–4162. doi:10.1182/blood-2008-11-185132, blood-2008-11-185132[pii]

Bene MC, Kaeda JS (2009) How and why minimal residual disease studies are necessary in leukemia: a review from WP10 and WP12 of the European LeukaemiaNet. Haematologica 94(8):1135–1150. doi:10.3324/haematol.2008.004267, haematol.2008.004267[pii]

Biondi A, Valsecchi MG, Seriu T, D'Aniello E, Willemse MJ, Fasching K, Pannunzio A, Gadner H, Schrappe M, Kamps WA, Bartram CR, van Dongen JJ, Panzer-Grumayer ER (2000) Molecular detection of minimal residual disease is a strong predictive factor of relapse in childhood B-lineage acute lymphoblastic leukemia with medium risk features. A case control study of the International BFM Study Group. Leukemia 14(11):1939–1943

Braziel RM, Shipp MA, Feldman AL, Espina V, Winters M, Jaffe ES, Petricoin EF, 3rd, Liotta LA (2003) Molecular diagnostics. Hematol Am Soc Hematol Educ Program 2003(1):279–293

Brisco J, Hughes E, Neoh SH, Sykes PJ, Bradstock K, Enno A, Szer J, McCaul K, Morley AA (1996) Relationship between minimal residual disease and outcome in adult acute lymphoblastic leukemia. Blood 87(12):5251–5256

Brisco MJ, Condon J, Hughes E, Neoh SH, Sykes PJ, Seshadri R, Toogood I, Waters K, Tauro G, Ekert H et al (1994) Outcome prediction in childhood acute lymphoblastic leukaemia by molecular quantification of residual disease at the end of induction. Lancet 343(8891): 196–200

Brown M, Wittwer C (2000) Flow cytometry: principles and clinical applications in hematology. Clin Chem 46(8 Pt 2):1221–1229

Bruggemann M, Raff T, Flohr T, Gokbuget N, Nakao M, Droese J, Luschen S, Pott C, Ritgen M, Scheuring U, Horst HA, Thiel E, Hoelzer D, Bartram CR, Kneba M (2006) Clinical significance of minimal residual disease quantification in adult patients with standard-risk acute lymphoblastic leukemia. Blood 107(3):1116–1123. doi:10.1182/blood-2005-07-2708, 2005-07-2708[pii]

Campana D (2009) Role of minimal residual disease monitoring in adult and pediatric acute lymphoblastic leukemia. Hematol Oncol Clin N Am 23(5):1083–1098, vii. doi:S0889-8588(09)00148-8, [pii] 10.1016/j.hoc.2009.07.010

Campana D (2010) Minimal residual disease in acute lymphoblastic leukemia. Hematol Am Soc Hematol Educ Program 2010:7–12. doi:10.1182/asheducation-2010.1.7, 2010/1/7[pii]

Cave H, van der Werff ten Bosch J, Suciu S, Guidal C, Waterkeyn C, Otten J, Bakkus M, Thielemans K, Grandchamp B, Vilmer E (1998) Clinical significance of minimal residual disease in childhood acute lymphoblastic leukemia. European Organization for Research and Treatment of Cancer–Childhood Leukemia Cooperative Group. N Engl J Med 339(9):591–598

Conter V, Bartram CR, Valsecchi MG, Schrauder A, Panzer-Grumayer R, Moricke A, Arico M, Zimmermann M, Mann G, De Rossi G, Stanulla M, Locatelli F, Basso G, Niggli F, Barisone E, Henze G, Ludwig WD, Haas OA, Cazzaniga G, Koehler R, Silvestri D, Bradtke J, Parasole R, Beier R, van Dongen JJ, Biondi A, Schrappe M (2010) Molecular response to treatment redefines all prognostic factors in children and adolescents with B-cell precursor acute lymphoblastic leukemia: results in 3184 patients of the AIEOP-BFM ALL 2000 study. Blood 115(16):3206–3214. doi:10.1182/blood-2009-10-248146, blood-2009-10-248146[pii]

Coustan-Smith E, Behm FG, Sanchez J, Boyett JM, Hancock ML, Raimondi SC, Rubnitz JE, Rivera GK, Sandlund JT, Pui CH, Campana D (1998) Immunological detection of minimal residual disease in children with acute lymphoblastic leukaemia. Lancet 351(9102):550–554. doi:10.1016/S0140-6736(97)10295-1, S0140-6736(97)10295-1[pii]

Coustan-Smith E, Gajjar A, Hijiya N, Razzouk BI, Ribeiro RC, Rivera GK, Rubnitz JE, Sandlund JT, Andreansky M, Hancock ML, Pui CH, Campana D (2004) Clinical significance of minimal residual disease in childhood acute lymphoblastic leukemia after first relapse. Leukemia 18(3):499–504

Coustan-Smith E, Sancho J, Hancock ML, Boyett JM, Behm FG, Raimondi SC, Sandlund JT, Rivera GK, Rubnitz JE, Ribeiro RC, Pui CH, Campana D (2000) Clinical importance of minimal residual disease in childhood acute lymphoblastic leukemia. Blood 96(8):2691–2696

Dawidowska M, Jolkowska J, Szczepanski T, Derwich K, Wachowiak J, Witt M (2008) Implementation of the standard strategy for identification of Ig/TCR targets for minimal residual disease diagnostics in B-cell precursor ALL pediatric patients: Polish experience. Arch Immunol Ther Exp (Warsz) 56(6):409–418. doi:10.1007/s00005-008-0045-y

Dworzak MN, Froschl G, Printz D, Mann G, Potschger U, Muhlegger N, Fritsch G, Gadner H (2002) Prognostic significance and modalities of flow cytometric minimal residual disease detection in childhood acute lymphoblastic leukemia. Blood 99(6):1952–1958

Dworzak MN, Panzer-Grumayer ER (2003) Flow cytometric detection of minimal residual disease in acute lymphoblastic leukemia. Leuk Lymphoma 44(9):1445–1455

Eckert C, Biondi A, Seeger K, Cazzaniga G, Hartmann R, Beyermann B, Pogodda M, Proba J, Henze G (2001) Prognostic value of minimal residual disease in relapsed childhood acute lymphoblastic leukaemia. Lancet 358(9289):1239–1241

Elorza I, Palacio C, Dapena JL, Gallur L, de Toledo JS, de Heredia CD (2010) Relationship between minimal residual disease measured by multiparametric flow cytometry prior to allogeneic hematopoietic stem cell transplantation and outcome in children with acute lymphoblastic leukemia. Haematologica 95(6):936–941. doi:10.3324/haematol.2009.010843, haematol.2009.010843[pii]

Flohr T, Schrauder A, Cazzaniga G, Panzer-Grumayer R, van der Velden V, Fischer S, Stanulla M, Basso G, Niggli FK, Schafer BW, Sutton R, Koehler R, Zimmermann M, Valsecchi MG, Gadner H, Masera G, Schrappe M, van Dongen JJ, Biondi A, Bartram CR (2008) Minimal residual disease-directed risk stratification using real-time quantitative PCR analysis of immunoglobulin and T-cell receptor gene rearrangements in the international multicenter trial AIEOP-BFM ALL 2000 for childhood acute lymphoblastic leukemia. Leukemia 22(4): 771–782

Foroni L, Hoffbrand AV (2002) Molecular analysis of minimal residual disease in adult acute lymphoblastic leukaemia. Best Pract Res Clin Haematol 15(1):71–90. doi: 10.1053/beha.2002.0186, S1521692602901866[pii]

Gabert J, Beillard E, van der Velden VH, Bi W, Grimwade D, Pallisgaard N, Barbany G, Cazzaniga G, Cayuela JM, Cave H, Pane F, Aerts JL, De Micheli D, Thirion X, Pradel V, Gonzalez M, Viehmann S, Malec M, Saglio G, van Dongen JJ (2003) Standardization and quality control studies of 'real-time' quantitative reverse transcriptase polymerase chain reaction of fusion gene transcripts for residual disease detection in leukemia—a Europe Against Cancer program. Leukemia 17(12):2318–2357

Goulden NJ, Knechtli CJ, Garland RJ, Langlands K, Hancock JP, Potter MN, Steward CG, Oakhill A (1998) Minimal residual disease analysis for the prediction of relapse in children with standard-risk acute lymphoblastic leukaemia. Br J Haematol 100(1):235–244

Hoelzer D, Gokbuget N, Ottmann O, Pui CH, Relling MV, Appelbaum FR, van Dongen JJ, Szczepanski T (2002) Acute lymphoblastic leukemia. Hematology Am Soc Hematol Educ Program :162–192

Holowiecki J, Krawczyk-Kulis M, Giebel S, Jagoda K, Stella-Holowiecka B, Piatkowska-Jakubas B, Paluszewska M, Seferynska I, Lewandowski K, Kielbinski M, Czyz A, Balana-Nowak A, Krol M, Skotnicki AB, Jedrzejczak WW, Warzocha K, Lange A, Hellmann A (2008) Status of minimal residual disease after induction predicts outcome in both standard and high-risk Ph-negative adult acute lymphoblastic leukaemia. The Polish Adult Leukemia Group ALL 4-2002 MRD Study. Br J Haematol. doi:10.1111/j.1365-2141.2008.07185.x, BJH7185 [pii]

Jółkowska J, Derwich K, Dawidowska M (2007) Methods of minimal residual disease (MRD) detection in childhood haematological malignancies. J Appl Genet 48(1):77–83

Kalina T, Flores-Montero J, van der Velden VHJ, Martin-Ayuso M, Böttcher S, Ritgen M, Almeida J, Lhermitte L, Asnafi V, Mendonça A, de Tute R, Cullen M, Sedek L, Vidriales MB, Pérez JJ, Mejstrikova E, Hrusak O, Szczepański T, van Dongen JJM, Orfao A (2012) EuroFlow standardization of flow cytometer instrument settings and immunophenotyping protocols. Leukemia (in press)

Kerst G, Kreyenberg H, Roth C, Well C, Dietz K, Coustan-Smith E, Campana D, Koscielniak E, Niemeyer C, Schlegel PG, Muller I, Niethammer D, Bader P (2005) Concurrent detection of minimal residual disease (MRD) in childhood acute lymphoblastic leukaemia by flow cytometry and real-time PCR. Br J Haematol 128(6):774–782. doi:10.1111/j.1365-2141.2005.05401.x, BJH5401[pii]

Kikuchi M, Tanaka J, Kondo T, Hashino S, Kasai M, Kurosawa M, Iwasaki H, Morioka M, Kawamura T, Masauzi N, Fukuhara T, Kakinoki Y, Kobayashi H, Noto S, Asaka M, Imamura M (2010) Clinical significance of minimal residual disease in adult acute lymphoblastic leukemia. Int J Hematol 92(3):481–489. doi:10.1007/s12185-010-0670-1

Knechtli CJ, Goulden NJ, Hancock JP, Grandage VL, Harris EL, Garland RJ, Jones CG, Rowbottom AW, Hunt LP, Green AF, Clarke E, Lankester AW, Cornish JM, Pamphilon DH, Steward CG, Oakhill A (1998) Minimal residual disease status before allogeneic bone marrow transplantation is an important determinant of successful outcome for children and adolescents with acute lymphoblastic leukemia. Blood 92(11):4072–4079

Kraszewska MD, Dawidowska M, Kosmalska M, Sedek L, Grzeszczak W, Szczepanski T, Witt M (2012) Immunoglobulin/T-cell receptor gene rearrangements in the diagnostic paradigm of pediatric T-cell acute lymphoblastic leukemia patients. Leuk Lymphoma. doi:10.3109/10428194.2011.654338

Langerak AW, Szczepanski T, van der Burg M, Wolvers-Tettero IL, van Dongen JJ (1997) Heteroduplex PCR analysis of rearranged T cell receptor genes for clonality assessment in suspect T cell proliferations. Leukemia 11(12):2192–2199

Lankester AC, Bierings MB, van Wering ER, Wijkhuijs AJ, de Weger RA, Wijnen JT, Vossen JM, Versluys B, Egeler RM, van Tol MJ, Putter H, Revesz T, van Dongen JJ, van der Velden VH, Schilham MW (2010) Preemptive alloimmune intervention in high-risk pediatric acute lymphoblastic leukemia patients guided by minimal residual disease level before stem cell transplantation. Leukemia 24(8):1462–1469. doi:10.1038/leu.2010.133, leu2010133[pii]

Lucio P, Gaipa G, van Lochem EG, van Wering ER, Porwit-MacDonald A, Faria T, Bjorklund E, Biondi A, van den Beemd MW, Baars E, Vidriales B, Parreira A, van Dongen JJ, San Miguel JF, Orfao A (2001) BIOMED-I concerted action report: flow cytometric immunophenotyping of precursor B-ALL with standardized triple-stainings. BIOMED-1 concerted action investigation of minimal residual disease in acute leukemia: International Standardization and Clinical Evaluation. Leukemia 15(8):1185–1192

Malec M, van der Velden VH, Bjorklund E, Wijkhuijs JM, Soderhall S, Mazur J, Bjorkholm M, Porwit-MacDonald A (2004) Analysis of minimal residual disease in childhood acute lymphoblastic leukemia: comparison between RQ-PCR analysis of Ig/TcR gene rearrangements and multicolor flow cytometric immunophenotyping. Leukemia 18(10):1630–1636

Meyer C, Kowarz E, Hofmann J, Renneville A, Zuna J, Trka J, Ben Abdelali R, Macintyre E, De Braekeleer E, De Braekeleer M, Delabesse E, de Oliveira MP, Cave H, Clappier E, van Dongen JJ, Balgobind BV, van den Heuvel-Eibrink MM, Beverloo HB, Panzer-Grumayer R, Teigler-Schlegel A, Harbott J, Kjeldsen E, Schnittger S, Koehl U, Gruhn B, Heidenreich O, Chan LC, Yip SF, Krzywinski M, Eckert C, Moricke A, Schrappe M, Alonso CN, Schafer BW, Krauter J, Lee DA, Zur Stadt U, Te Kronnie G, Sutton R, Izraeli S, Trakhtenbrot L, Lo Nigro L, Tsaur G, Fechina L, Szczepanski T, Strehl S, Ilencikova D, Molkentin M, Burmeister T, Dingermann T, Klingebiel T, Marschalek R (2009) New insights to the MLL recombinome of acute leukemias. Leukemia 23(8):1490–1499. doi:10.1038/leu.2009.33, leu200933[pii]

Mortuza FY, Papaioannou M, Moreira IM, Coyle LA, Gameiro P, Gandini D, Prentice HG, Goldstone A, Hoffbrand AV, Foroni L (2002) Minimal residual disease tests provide an independent predictor of clinical outcome in adult acute lymphoblastic leukemia. J Clin Oncol 20(4):1094–1104

Neale GA, Coustan-Smith E, Stow P, Pan Q, Chen X, Pui CH, Campana D (2004) Comparative analysis of flow cytometry and polymerase chain reaction for the detection of minimal residual disease in childhood acute lymphoblastic leukemia. Leukemia 18(5):934–938

Nyvold C, Madsen HO, Ryder LP, Seyfarth J, Svejgaard A, Clausen N, Wesenberg F, Jonsson OG, Forestier E, Schmiegelow K (2002) Precise quantification of minimal residual disease at day 29 allows identification of children with acute lymphoblastic leukemia and an excellent outcome. Blood 99(4):1253–1258

Panzer-Grumayer ER, Schneider M, Panzer S, Fasching K, Gadner H (2000) Rapid molecular response during early induction chemotherapy predicts a good outcome in childhood acute lymphoblastic leukemia. Blood 95(3):790–794

Pongers-Willemse MJ, Seriu T, Stolz F, d'Aniello E, Gameiro P, Pisa P, Gonzalez M, Bartram CR, Panzer-Grumayer ER, Biondi A, San Miguel JF, van Dongen JJ (1999) Primers and protocols for standardized detection of minimal residual disease in acute lymphoblastic leukemia using immunoglobulin and T cell receptor gene rearrangements and TAL1 deletions as PCR targets: report of the BIOMED-1 Concerted Action: investigation of minimal residual disease in acute leukemia. Leukemia 13(1):110–118

Pongers-Willemse MJ, Verhagen OJ, Tibbe GJ, Wijkhuijs AJ, de Haas V, Roovers E, van der Schoot CE, van Dongen JJ (1998) Real-time quantitative PCR for the detection of minimal residual disease in acute lymphoblastic leukemia using junctional region specific TaqMan probes. Leukemia 12(12):2006–2014

Pulsipher MA, Bader P, Klingebiel T, Cooper LJ (2009) Allogeneic transplantation for pediatric acute lymphoblastic leukemia: the emerging role of peritransplantation minimal residual disease/chimerism monitoring and novel chemotherapeutic, molecular, and immune approaches aimed at preventing relapse. Biol Blood Marrow Transplant 15(1 Suppl):62–71. doi:10.1016/j.bbmt.2008.11.009, S1083-8791(08)00489-8[pii]

Raff T, Gokbuget N, Luschen S, Reutzel R, Ritgen M, Irmer S, Bottcher S, Horst HA, Kneba M, Hoelzer D, Bruggemann M (2007) Molecular relapse in adult standard-risk ALL patients detected by prospective MRD monitoring during and after maintenance treatment: data from the GMALL 06/99 and 07/03 trials. Blood 109(3):910–915. doi:10.1182/blood-2006-07-037093, blood-2006-07-037093[pii]

Schmiegelow K, Forestier E, Hellebostad M, Heyman M, Kristinsson J, Soderhall S, Taskinen M (2010) Long-term results of NOPHO ALL-92 and ALL-2000 studies of childhood acute lymphoblastic leukemia. Leukemia 24(2):345–354. doi:10.1038/leu.2009.251, leu2009251[pii]

Szczepański T (2007) Why and how to quantify minimal residual disease in acute lymphoblastic leukemia? Leukemia 21(4):622–626

Szczepański T, Orfao A, van der Velden VH, San Miguel JF, van Dongen JJM (2001) Minimal residual disease in leukaemia patients. Lancet Oncol 2(7):409–417

Szczepański T, van der Velden VHJ, van Dongen JJM (2002) Real-time quantitative (RQ)-PCR for the detection of minimal residual disease in childhood acute lymphoblastic leukemia. Haematologica 87S1:183–191

Uzunel M, Mattsson J, Jaksch M, Remberger M, Ringden O (2001) The significance of graft-versus-host disease and pretransplantation minimal residual disease status to outcome after allogeneic stem cell transplantation in patients with acute lymphoblastic leukemia. Blood 98(6):1982–1984

van der Velden VH, Cazzaniga G, Schrauder A, Hancock J, Bader P, Panzer-Grumayer ER, Flohr T, Sutton R, Cave H, Madsen HO, Cayuela JM, Trka J, Eckert C, Foroni L, Zur Stadt U, Beldjord K, Raff T, van der Schoot CE, van Dongen JJ (2007a) Analysis of minimal residual disease by Ig/TCR gene rearrangements: guidelines for interpretation of real-time quantitative PCR data. Leukemia 21(4):604–611

Van der Velden VH, Corral L, Valsecchi MG, Jansen MW, De Lorenzo P, Cazzaniga G, Panzer-Grumayer ER, Schrappe M, Schrauder A, Meyer C, Marschalek R, Nigro LL, Metzler M, Basso G, Mann G, Den Boer ML, Biondi A, Pieters R, Van Dongen JJ (2009) Prognostic significance of minimal residual disease in infants with acute lymphoblastic leukemia treated within the Interfant-99 protocol. Leukemia 23(6):1073–1079. doi:10.1038/leu.2009.17, leu200917[pii]

van der Velden VH, Hochhaus A, Cazzaniga G, Szczepanski T, Gabert J, van Dongen JJ (2003) Detection of minimal residual disease in hematologic malignancies by real-time quantitative PCR: principles, approaches, and laboratory aspects. Leukemia 17(6):1013–1034

van der Velden VH, Joosten SA, Willemse MJ, van Wering ER, Lankester AW, van Dongen JJ, Hoogerbrugge PM (2001) Real-time quantitative PCR for detection of minimal residual disease before allogeneic stem cell transplantation predicts outcome in children with acute lymphoblastic leukemia. Leukemia 15(9):1485–1487

van der Velden VH, Panzer-Grumayer ER, Cazzaniga G, Flohr T, Sutton R, Schrauder A, Basso G, Schrappe M, Wijkhuijs JM, Konrad M, Bartram CR, Masera G, Biondi A, van Dongen JJ (2007b) Optimization of PCR-based minimal residual disease diagnostics for childhood acute lymphoblastic leukemia in a multi-center setting. Leukemia 21(4):706–713

van Dongen JJ, Langerak AW, Bruggemann M, Evans PA, Hummel M, Lavender FL, Delabesse E, Davi F, Schuuring E, Garcia-Sanz R, van Krieken JH, Droese J, Gonzalez D, Bastard C, White HE, Spaargaren M, Gonzalez M, Parreira A, Smith JL, Morgan GJ, Kneba M, Macintyre EA (2003) Design and standardization of PCR primers and protocols for detection of clonal immunoglobulin and T-cell receptor gene recombinations in suspect lymphoproliferations: report of the BIOMED-2 Concerted Action BMH4-CT98-3936. Leukemia 17(12): 2257–2317

van Dongen JJ, Seriu T, Panzer-Grumayer ER, Biondi A, Pongers-Willemse MJ, Corral L, Stolz F, Schrappe M, Masera G, Kamps WA, Gadner H, van Wering ER, Ludwig WD, Basso G, de Bruijn MA, Cazzaniga G, Hettinger K, van der Does-van den Berg A, Hop WC, Riehm H, Bartram CR (1998) Prognostic value of minimal residual disease in acute lymphoblastic leukaemia in childhood. Lancet 352(9142):1731–1738

van Dongen JJM, Lhermitte L, Böttcher S, Almeida J, van der Velden VHJ, Flores-Montero J, Rawstron A, Asnafi V, Lécrevisse Q, Lucio P, Mejstrikova E, Szczepański T, Kalina T, de Tute R, Brüggemann M, Sedek L, Cullen M, Langerak AW, Mendonça A, Macintyre E, Martin-Ayuso M, Hrusak O, Vidriales MB, Orfao A (2012) EuroFlow antibody panels for standardized n-dimensional flow cytometric immunophenotyping of normal, reactive and malignant leukocytes. Leukemia (in press)

Vidriales MB, Perez JJ, Lopez-Berges MC, Gutierrez N, Ciudad J, Lucio P, Vazquez L, Garcia-Sanz R, del Canizo MC, Fernandez-Calvo J, Ramos F, Rodriguez MJ, Calmuntia MJ, Porwith A, Orfao A, San-Miguel JF (2003) Minimal residual disease in adolescent (older than 14 years) and adult acute lymphoblastic leukemias: early immunophenotypic evaluation has high clinical value. Blood 101(12):4695–4700. doi:10.1182/blood-2002-08-2613, 2002-08-2613[pii]

Yamaji K, Okamoto T, Yokota S, Watanabe A, Horikoshi Y, Asami K, Kikuta A, Hyakuna N, Saikawa Y, Ueyama J, Watanabe T, Okada M, Taga T, Kanegane H, Kogawa K, Chin M, Iwai A, Matsushita T, Shimomura Y, Hori T, Tsurusawa M (2010) Minimal residual disease-based augmented therapy in childhood acute lymphoblastic leukemia: a report from the Japanese Childhood Cancer and Leukemia Study Group. Pediatr Blood Cancer 55(7):1287–1295. doi:10.1002/pbc.22620

Chapter 12
Gene Expression Profiling in Hematologic Malignancies

Przemysław Juszczyński, Bjoern Chapuy, Małgorzata Szczepaniak and Krzysztof Warzocha

Abstract The vast majority of hematologic malignancies are clinically, prognostically, and genetically complex diseases. High-throughput gene expression studies, coupled with analysis of copy number alterations, directed sequencing, and functional assays provided the "bird's eye view" on the tumor cell and its environment and greatly advanced the level of understanding of these tumors. In this chapter, we discuss the technical aspects of gene-expression profiling experiments, and review the results of major studies on lymphoid and myeloid leukemias and myelodysplastic syndromes that changed our understanding of these diseases. We also present translational and diagnostic implications of recent studies performed with the gene expression profiling platforms.

P. Juszczyński and B. Chapuy contributed equally

P. Juszczyński (✉) · K. Warzocha
Institute of Hematology and Transfusion Medicine,
Indiry Gandhi 14, 02-776 Warsaw, Poland
e-mail: pjuszczynski@ihit.waw.pl

B. Chapuy
Harvard Medical School, Dana-Farber Cancer Institute,
450 Brookline Avenue Mayer 515, Boston, MA 02215, USA

M. Szczepaniak
Department of Molecular and Clinical Genetics, Institute of Human Genetics,
Polish Academy of Sciences, Strzeszyńska 32, 60-479 Poznań, Poland

M. Szczepaniak
International Institute of Molecular and Cell Biology, Trojdena 4,
02-109 Warsaw, Poland

M. Witt et al. (eds.), *Molecular Aspects of Hematologic Malignancies*,
Principles and Practice, DOI: 10.1007/978-3-642-29467-9_12,

12.1 Introduction

The vast majority of hematologic malignancies are clinically, prognostically, and genetically complex diseases. Until the last decade of the twentieth century, analyses of molecular foundations of biologic heterogeneity of these tumors have focused on individual genes associated with treatment outcome, genes of known function in other tumors, or genes with known developmental role. Although these studies have provided important insights into the biology of hematologic malignancies and have led to identification and characterization of certain therapeutic targets, they have neither allowed for a comprehensive description of cellular functional status and pathogenetic mechanisms, nor for further subclassification of these diseases based on molecular features. Reaching these goals would not be possible without the technological milestone and high-throughput gene expression analyses.

In this chapter, we discuss the technical aspects of gene expression profiling experiments and issues concerning data analysis. Next, we review the results of major studies on lymphoid and myeloid leukemias and myelodysplastic syndromes that changed our understanding of these diseases (for information about gene expression profiling studies in lymphomas see Chap. 3).

12.2 Gene Expression Profiling: Brief Technical Overview

An experiment assessing the transcript abundance of thousands of genes in parallel is termed gene expression profiling (GEP). There are several different technologies that allow to simultaneously measure gene expression at medium to high throughput. Microarrays, representing high-throughput technology, are two-dimensional arrays of probes immobilized on a solid substrate, usually a glass slide or a silicon chip.

The first step of a GEP experiment requires preparation of biological material to be studied, typically RNA, and subsequent generation and labeling of cDNA. The prepared material is then hybridized to a microarray containing probes that capture complementary labeled nucleic acid under high-stringency hybridization conditions (Fig. 12.1).

In the second step of the experiment, after hybridization and scanning is completed, spot fluorescence intensities are matched to coordinates of probe/probe set grid locations and quantified. Microarrays are quality checked, adjusted for background noise, and normalized. These procedures eliminate nonbiological variation in microarrays and make signal intensities comparable between individual arrays. After preprocessing of the entire set of microarrays, expression data are obtained and used in further analyses to answer the biological questions behind the experiment. In general, these analyses can be performed in four specific approaches: differential analysis, class prediction (supervised learning), class discovery (unsupervised learning), and data mining/pathway analysis.

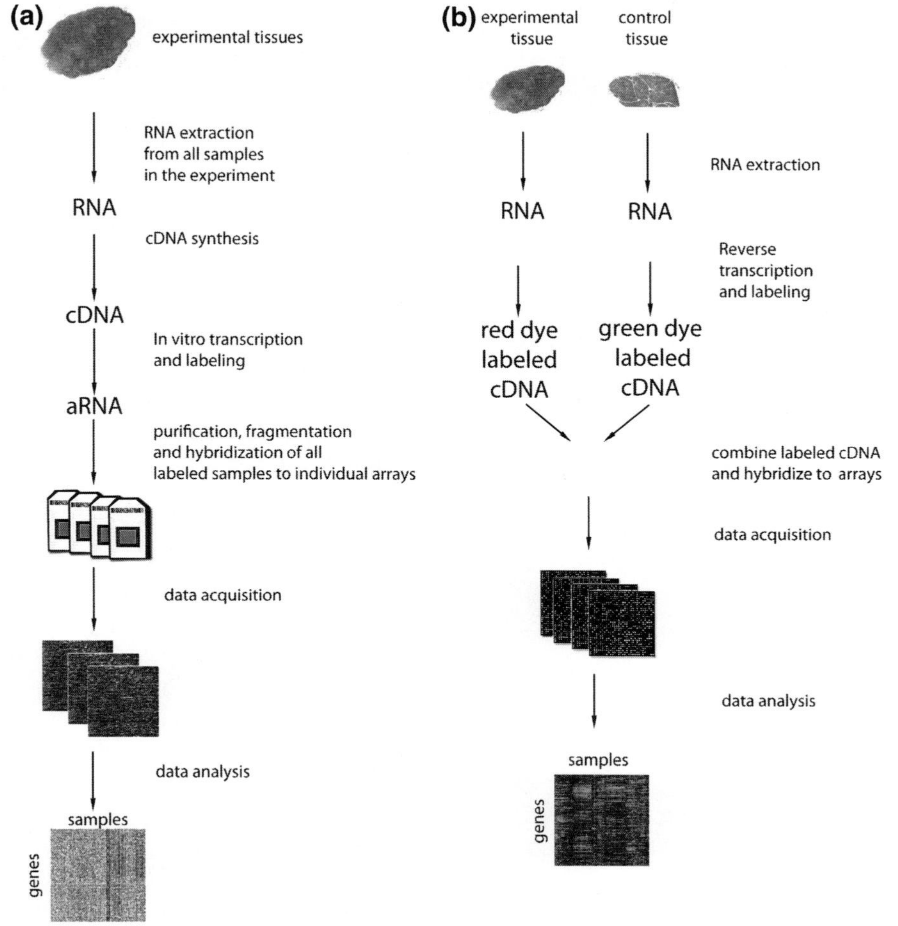

Fig. 12.1 Schematic representation of a microarray experiment. Microarray experiment begins with the extraction and labeling of RNA. Prepared, labeled, and purified material is then hybridized to microarrays. One channel microarrays (**a**) utilize only one detection channel and each chip can be hybridized with one sample. In two-channel microarrays (**b**), hybridization is performed with cDNA prepared from two samples to be compared (control vs. experimental, normal cells vs. malignant cells) that are labeled with two different fluorescent dyes (e.g., "*red*" and "*green*"). After labeling, cDNAs are mixed and hybridized to arrays. Upon hybridization and data acquisition, subsequent steps of data analysis are performed. *cDNA* complementary DNA, *aRNA* amplified RNA

In differential analysis (known also as marker selection), the sample classes (control vs. experimental) are determined a priori and the experiment is performed to identify the underlying transcriptional differences between these classes. Specific statistical tests, such as Student's *t*-test, ANOVA (Analysis of Variance), or SNR (signal to noise ratio) are used to assess whether gene expression levels are significantly different.

Class prediction (supervised learning) is an approach that searches for a gene expression signature that can predict an unknown sample class membership (e.g., to identify a type/subtype of leukemia). Supervised learning methods utilize not only expression data but also clinical or phenotypic labels to 'train' an algorithm on a set of clinically characterized samples with defined gene expression signatures. Subsequently, the obtained GEP-derived classifier is used to predict unknown sample identity based solely on its gene expression profile.

In contrast, class discovery (unsupervised learning) methods use solely the expression data to group samples that share similar features, with no prior phenotype knowledge. Obtained clusters (subgroups) represent an intrinsic and unbiased substructure within the cohort.

Data mining/pathway analyses in an exploratory way determine whether subgroups of genes in an identified transcriptional signature share similar characteristics, e.g., are regulated by the same transcription factor, represent a given signal transduction pathway, or are connected in some other biologically meaningful way. Identification of such connections can highlight the biological background of the gene expression profile of a studied subject.

As a high-throughput gene expression microarray can consist of >40,000 probes, such comparisons in fact test multiple (>40,000) hypotheses simultaneously. Since at a given α (critical threshold), the risk of incorrectly rejecting a null hypothesis (a type I error) increases as more hypotheses are tested, results of these analyses must be corrected for false positive calls. This problem in the first line should be avoided by preprocessing the data set to reduce the number of initial hypotheses (i.e., removing invariable or low expression transcripts to start with reduced number of genes). After reducing the complexity of the data set, the number of false positive calls can be further controlled by performing multiple hypothesis test adjustments, such as Bonferroni correction, family wise error rate (FWER), or false discovery rate procedure (FDR).

There are multiple tools that can be used to analyze microarray data, both open-access and commercial (Table 12.1). Many packages come in powerful suites that can perform all in silico analyses, are supported by very helpful user communities, are regularly updated, and come with a very extensive documentation (Baldi and Hatfield 2002; Mount 2004; Parmigiani 2003; Speed 2003; Gentleman 2005; Causton et al. 2003).

12.3 GEP in Acute Lymphoblastic Leukemia

12.3.1 Class Prediction in Acute Lymphoblastic Leukemia

Acute lymphoblastic leukemia (ALL) is the most common malignancy of childhood and a disease with a poor prognosis among adults. Although there are several cytogenetic abnormalities characteristic of ALL which determine the biology of

Table 12.1 Publicly available software packages for microarray data analysis and data mining

Software package	Description	URL
Genepattern	Comprehensive suite for most types of analyses; can be used to automate tasks and chain them in pipelines; programming environment	http://www.broadinstitute.org/cancer/software/genepattern/
D-chip	Probe-level and high-level analysis; allows analysis of SNP microarrays; intuitive graphical user interface	http://biosun1.harvard.edu/complab/dchip/
GSEA	Gene set enrichment analysis; determines whether a given set of genes shows concordant differences in expression between two biological states; useful for interpreting results of gene expression experiments	http://www.broadinstitute.org/cancer/software/gsea/index.jsp
R and Bioconductor	Programming environment; requires extensive knowledge of R syntax	http://www.r-project.org http://www.bioconductor.org
Oncomine	Microarray data repository with data mining interface	http://www.oncomine.org

the disease, impact prognosis, and guide therapy, they cannot account for the whole spectrum of the clinical heterogeneity of this disease, suggesting additional biological complexity (Faderl et al. 1998; Wetzler et al. 1999; Secker-Walker et al. 1997). The first milestone study attempting to refine the molecular taxonomy of ALL, performed over a decade ago, provided the proof of concept that gene expression signatures differ in ALL and AML (acute myeloid leukemia) and that the signature can further be used to accurately determine the type of new leukemia cases (Golub et al. 1999). These results demonstrated that cancer classification based solely on gene expression profile is feasible. Subsequent studies demonstrated that using only a single microarray platform and unsupervised learning algorithms, ALL samples can be classified into subtypes actually recapitulating known molecular categories characterized by specific genetic lesion: *BCR-ABL*, *E2A-PBX1*, *TEL-AML*, *MLL* rearrangements, hyperdiploid cases as well as T-lineage ALL (T-ALL); see also Chap. 1. In cross-validation experiments, obtained decision-treebased classifier achieved very high performance and allowed to accurately assign 96–97 % of cases (Ross et al. 2004; Yeoh et al. 2002). Observations that GEP classifiers recapitulate previously known, biologically and clinically defined ALL subclasses are not surprising, given the fact that these translocations deregulate major signaling cascades or transcriptional modulators.

The GEP studies, although proved to be very informative, did not provide the conclusive biologic insights into the genetic structure of ALL and pathomechanisms associated with the disease, especially in the case of normal karyotype ALL. Of note, even in the case of tumors carrying specific, hallmark chromosomal aberrations, the fusion genes in murine models fail to induce leukemia (with few exceptions, including *MLL-AF4* or *MLL-AF9* fusions) (Krivtsov et al. 2006, 2008). To identify cooperating oncogenic lesions, Mullighan et al. performed a genome-wide analysis of leukemic cells using high-resolution, single-nucleotide polymorphism (SNP) arrays, and targeted genomic DNA sequencing (Mullighan et al. 2008, 2009b). These studies revealed relatively low average number of DNA copy number alterations compared with many solid tumors—approximately six to eight lesions per case were present in B-lineage ALL (B-ALL) (Mullighan et al. 2007, 2008; Kuiper et al. 2007). Deletions, amplification, point mutations, or other structural rearrangements were present in 40 % of B-ALL cases. Structural abnormalities in B-ALL affect predominantly genes encoding principal regulators of B lymphocyte development and differentiation, including transcriptional regulators of lymphoid development (*PAX 5*-paired box 5, *IKZF1*-IKAROS family zinc finger 1,*EBF1*-early B-cell factor 1), cell cycle regulators, and tumor suppressor genes (*CDKN2A*-cyclin-dependent kinase inhibitor 2A, *CDKN2B*-cyclin-dependent kinase inhibitor 2B, *RB1*-retinoblastoma 1, and *PTEN*-phosphatase and tensin homolog) or key lymphoid signaling genes (*CD200, BTLA*–B, and T lymphocyte associated and *BLNK*-B-cell linker) (Mullighan et al. 2007, 2009b; Kuiper et al. 2007; Kawamata et al. 2008; Collins-Underwood and Mullighan 2010) and references therein). The *PAX5* gene was the most frequent target of somatic mutation, being altered in 31.7 % of cases, and *IKZF1* alterations were the second most frequent lesion (28.6 %) (Mullighan et al. 2009b). These mutations usually affect only a single copy of a gene (i.e., are haploinsufficient), result in loss of function in vitro, and accelerate the onset of ALL in murine leukemia models (Collins-Underwood and Mullighan 2010) and references therein).

These striking findings, demonstrating that B-cell differentiation factors are common targets of structural aberrations may suggest that the differentiation block is an important step in leukemogenesis. Such cells arrested in their development are more likely to acquire additional abnormalities and to maintain the progenitor cell self-renewal potential.

12.3.2 GEP Analyses of High-Risk B-ALL

Although recurrent cytogenetic and molecular abnormalities in B-ALL can predict increased risk of relapse, relapses in fact occur in all disease subtypes, including those with normal karyotype, suggesting additional biological mechanisms underlying the high-risk phenotype. This problem was addressed in numerous studies utilizing platform-based approaches to highlight the differences between low- and high-risk diseases. These studies indeed demonstrated the existence of transcriptional differences between B-ALL cases with poor and favorable outcomes (Holleman et al. 2004; Wei et al. 2006). In more recent studies, additional analyses of copy number alterations in B-ALL revealed that higher number of lesions inactivating B-cell differentiation genes is associated with poor outcome, suggesting the quantitative relationship between the degree of 'block' in B-cell differentiation, and treatment responsiveness (Mullighan et al. 2009b). The key abnormality with the prognostic impact on ALL outcome was inactivation of B-cell specific transcription factor, *IKZF1*. *IKZF1*-mutated B-ALLs exhibited the gene expression profile enriched in hematopoietic stem cell genes, suggesting that *IKZF1* inactivation influences the differentiation level of B-ALL cells (Mullighan et al. 2009b). Inactivating mutations and deletions of this transcription factor were associated with poor outcome of B-ALL, regardless of the associated cytogenetic abnormalities; in particular, inferior outcome of *IKZF1*-mutated cases was observed also in *BCR-ABL1* rearranged tumors. In Philadelphia chromosome-positive B-ALL, abnormalities of *IKZF1* gene were associated with near tripled risk of treatment failure (Mullighan et al. 2009b). Importantly, the gene expression profile of *BCR-ABL1*-negative but *IKZF1*-mutated cases was strikingly similar to that of *BCR-ABL1*–rearranged B-ALL, suggesting that similar clinical aggressiveness of tumors dependent on different pathogenetic mechanisms may be driven by similar transcriptional output (Mullighan et al. 2009b). The underlying molecular mechanism, responsible for similar gene expression profile of *IKZF1*-mutated and *BCR-ABL1*-rearranged cases can be at least partially explained by the presence of activated tyrosine kinase signaling within this leukemia subtype, triggered by activating mutations in the Janus kinases *JAK1, JAK2,* and *JAK3,* present in 10.7 % *BCR-ABL1*-negative, *IKZF1*-mutated, high-risk pediatric B-ALL cases (Mullighan et al. 2009c). In addition, these cases with very poor prognosis also exhibit rearrangements of cytokine receptor-like factor 2 (*CRLF2*), a lymphoid cytokine receptor that forms a heterodimer with interleukin 7 receptor alpha. Since overexpression of *CRLF2* and mutant *JAK* allele in murine interleukin-3-dependent pro-B cell line Ba/F3 results in cytokine-independent growth, these lesions likely represent novel transforming mechanisms in human ALL, associated with the aggressive clinical behavior of the disease (Mullighan et al. 2009a; Collins-Underwood and Mullighan 2010).

12.3.3 Translational Consequences of GEP in ALL

In addition to new clues refining our understanding of pathomechanisms in ALL, the platform-based studies in ALL also provide important practical consequences. The feasibility of gene expression-based classification of leukemias in clinical setting was demonstrated recently in a large study involving 3344 patients from centers in Europe, United States, and Asia (Haferlach et al. 2010). In this trial, gene expression-based classifier obtained in a retrospective analysis was further validated in a prospective study and reached 95.6 % sensitivity and 99.8 % specificity for standard subtypes of acute leukemias, including 8 subclasses of ALL. Of note, classification was performed in a highly objective manner, with a newly developed, fully customized chip, standardized laboratory procedures, and dedicated data processing algorithms.

Information gained from supervised analyses of defined disease subsets may also be utilized in the development of rapid diagnostic test. Supervised analyses comparing gene expression profile of mixed lineage leukemia (*MLL)*-rearranged B-ALLs and tumors with germline configuration of *MLL* revealed selective expression of the immunoregulatory protein, Galectin-1 (Gal-1) (Armstrong et al. 2002). Expression of the lectin was present regardless of the specific *MLL* translocation type and associated fusion partner (Juszczynski et al. 2010). Since Gal-1 can be evaluated in diagnostic ALL samples using intracellular flow cytometry or immunohistochemistry, these studies suggest that the analysis of Gal-1 expression may accelerate the diagnosis, and guide therapy and clinical trial enrollment of patients with *MLL*-rearranged B-ALL.

Results of GEP of high-risk ALL suggest that platform-based approaches identifying *IKZF1, JAK,* and *CRLF2* alterations might be clinically useful for personalized risk assessment, especially in patients with tumors without recurrent genetic abnormalities. Finally, GEP studies identify important rational therapeutic strategies in this disease (JAK inhibition in poor-risk *JAK*-mutated ALL) or guide the rational drug combinations.

12.4 GEP in Myeloid Neoplasia

12.4.1 GEP in Acute Myeloid Leukemia

Acute myeloid leukemia has been recognized as a genetically heterogeneous disorder that exhibits a maturation block and subsequent accumulation of myeloid progenitor cells (Marcucci et al. 2011; Estey and Dohner 2006; Lowenberg et al. 1999). Biology of this disease is largely, but not exclusively, determined by certain genetic alterations, as reflected in the current World Health Organization (WHO) classification. Numerous studies have demonstrated the ability of genome-wide gene expression platforms to predict AML cases with recurrent cytogenetic alterations, with an accuracy of almost 100 % (Schoch et al. 2002; Valk et al. 2004; Ross et al. 2004; Haferlach et al. 2005). Translocations involving the *MLL* gene (11q23) were predicted with 90 or 95 % in adult and childhood AML, respectively (Haferlach et al. 2005; Ross et al. 2004). Although these studies were performed in independent laboratories, with slightly different approaches, they were consistently able to determine robust gene signatures predicting cytogenetically defined subclasses. The diagnostic utility of GEP in distinguishing leukemias and myelodysplastic syndromes (MDS) has recently been proven in a European multi-center Microarray Innovations in Leukemia (MILE) study (Haferlach et al. 2005, 2010). Gene expression-based classifier built in this study achieved high accuracy and assigned tumors to correct diagnoses with sensitivity and specificity exceeding 95 %. Taken together, these results confirm the clinical utility of standardized GEP methodology for robust diagnosis of hematologic malignancies, but also highlight the biological differences of different leukemias harboring distinct cytogenetic abnormalities that underlie their unique gene expression profiles.

In addition to AMLs with recurrent cytogenetic abnormalities, a sizeable fraction of cytogenetically normal AMLs (CN-AML) exist. Certain molecular alterations like mutations in nucleophosmin 1 (*NPM1*), CCAAT/enhancer binding protein alpha (*CEBPA*), fms-related tyrosine kinase 3 (*FLT3*), or isocitrate dehydrogenase 1 (*IDH1/2*) have been identified in this group of AML, allowing for further subclassification of this disease. Strikingly, AMLs harboring mutations in *NPM1* and *CEBPA* feature a robust gene expression signature as reported recently by several multicenter trials (Haferlach et al. 2005, 2010; Kohlmann et al. 2010; Verhaak et al. 2009). The profile of *NPM1*-mutated AML was characterized by activation of distinct homeobox (*HOX*) cluster genes, and downregulation of meningioma 1 (*MN1*), brain and acute leukemia cytoplasmic (*BAALC*) and v-etserythroblastosis virus E26 oncogene homolog (*ERG*) genes (Becker et al. 2010; Verhaak et al. 2005). The highly unique gene expression profile, resulting in prediction accuracy exceeding 90 % in *NPM1*-mutated case, suggests that the *NPM1* mutation is a 'driver mutation' defining a biological entity and separate subclass in CN-AMLs (Kohlmann et al. 2010). Similar to *NPM1* mutations, leukemias with *CEBPA* mutations exhibit unique transcriptional profile, but the transcriptional output associated with these mutations depends on the type of mutation. Gene expression profile-based classifier is able to predict *CEBPA* mutations with 99 % specificity and 67 % sensitivity, but the relatively frequent biallelic mutations were called with highest accuracy and prediction errors were almost exclusively in monoallelic cases (Wouters et al. 2009). This dichotomy underscores the biologic differences between mono and biallelic mutations and suggests that monoallelic cases likely require additional lesions for leukemogenesis, while biallelic *CEBPA* mutations might represent an own subclass of CN-AML.

12.4.2 GEP in Myelodysplastic Syndromes

GEP studies in MDS have been challenged by the heterogeneous morphological and genetic background in MDS as well as by the technical limitations caused by the low numbers of neoplastic cells which yield low RNA levels. Despite these limitations, platform-based gene expression assays have been utilized to capture the different MDS subtypes, to distinguish MDS from AML, or to guide clinical therapeutic decisions. A predictor algorithm built on GEP data from 2143 patients, including 206 patients with MDS reached only 49 % prediction accuracy, reflecting the highly heterogeneous nature of this disease. The samples falsely not predicted to be MDS were either classified as AML or as default category 'none-of-the-targets'. Interestingly, the MDS classified as AML showed more rapid transformation to AML, while the 'none-of-the-targets' cases had more favorable prognosis (Mills et al. 2009). Based on these findings, the authors defined a prognostic classifier with higher predictive value, which has been confirmed on an independent data set using CD34 + enriched bone marrow of MDS patients (Sridhar et al. 2009). In addition to diagnostic implications, the MDS GEP data can provide important insight into the biologic characteristics of these tumors. Profiled CD34 + enriched bone marrow samples from MDS patients demonstrate similarities to interferon gamma (INFγ)-induced gene expression changes in physiological CD34 + hematopoietic progenitor cells, suggesting significant immune-driven component of MDS pathogenesis. Strikingly, differences in expression profiles could be correlated to MDS subtypes (Pellagatti et al. 2006). The same study highlighted increased abundance of mitochondrial genes, in particular of heme synthesis, in patients with a refractory anemia with ringed sideroblasts. The iron transporter ABCB7 [member 7 of sub-family B of ATP-binding cassette (ABC) transporters], was found to exhibit lower expression in patients with refractory anemia with ringed sideroblasts and correlated inversely with the number of sideroblasts in the marrow (Boultwood et al. 2008). Gene expression profiles in the early MDS stages present with abnormalities in apoptosis and chemokine signaling, whereas more advanced MDS stages were associated with impaired cell cycle control and DNA damage response (Pellagatti et al. 2010). In addition, different genetically defined MDS subtypes, including 5q-, trisomy 8, or -7/del(7q), exhibit different gene expression profile, suggesting that these lesions largely determine the biology of the disease (Pellagatti et al. 2010).

Platform analyses of gene expression in MDS can also be used to guide clinical decisions (Ebert et al. 2008). Lenalidomide, a drug highly effective in patients with a rare subtype of MDS harboring 5q deletion, exhibits clinical effectiveness also in approximately 25 % of non-5q-MDS patients. Since a priori prediction of response to lenalidomide in the absence of 5q deletion is not feasible with standard clinical tests, Ebert et al. established a 32-gene-based gene expression signature from pretreatment bone marrow samples of 16 patients, who responded to lenalidomide, and tested this classifier in a group of 26 independent patients (Ebert et al. 2008). The predicted responders were correct in 80 % of cases. Moreover, by analyzing the 32-gene- based signature, the authors reported a coordinated decrease of erythroid-specific genes in responders, suggesting that the mechanism of lenalidomide action might involve modulation of erythroid differentiation in this disease (Ebert et al. 2008). Gene expression signatures can also be used to a priori identify patients responding to combination of azacytidine and thalidomide (Raza et al. 2008). In this setting, higher expression of the gene sets reflecting cell cycle, DNA replication/repair, and genes associated with chromatin/spindle structure was associated with higher response rates.

12.4.3 GEP in Chronic Myeloid Leukemia

The pathogenesis of the chronic myeloid leukemia (CML) is driven by the reciprocal translocation between chromosomes 9 and 22, resulting in the presence of the Philadelphia chromosome, and the fusion protein BCR-ABL1. The constitutively active tyrosine kinase BCR-ABL1 drives the expansion of myeloid progenitor compartment in the bone marrow and ultimately gives rise to the accumulation of myeloid progenitors in the blood, resulting in the leukemic phenotype. The GEP can be used for CML diagnosis, discovery of biomarkers of the disease phase, and for predicting prognosis. Although not designed specifically for CML, the previously mentioned MILE study tested whether transcriptional profiles can be utilized to guide diagnosis of CML patients. In a group of over 2000 patients, 76 had a CML and expression profiles predicted the diagnosis of CML with sensitivity of 94.7 % and specificity of 99.9 %, underscoring the value of such unbiased procedure (Haferlach et al. 2010). However, the study did not include other myeloproliferative neoplasms, in case of which the differential diagnosis might be more challenging.

Gene expression studies in CML have also aimed at identifying signatures characteristic for the distinct clinical phases of CML and thus elucidate the mechanisms of transformation process from chronic to accelerated phase and finally to blast crisis. These studies defined a 3500 gene signature, differentially expressed between chronic phase CML and advanced CML (Radich et al. 2006). Of note, accelerated phase and blast crisis exhibited striking transcriptional similarity, suggesting that CML is rather a biphasic disease with chronic phase and advanced phase CML (Radich et al. 2006). Moreover, patients with gene expression profile closer to the advanced CML phase are less likely to respond to imatinib. The advanced CML was associated with deregulation of oncogenic pathways, including the WNT (wingless-type MMTV integration site family)/β-catenin and AP-1 (activator protein-1) pathway. A follow up in-depth analysis of this study builds a Bayesian model on six genes: *NOD1* (nucleotide-binding oligomerization domain containing 1), *DDX47* (DEAD (Asp-Glu-Ala-Asp) box polypeptide 47), *IGSF2* (member 2 of immunoglobulin superfamily), *LTB4R* (leukotriene B4 receptor), *SCARB1* (member 1 of scavenger receptor class B), and *SLC25A3* (member 3 of solute carrier family 25). This allowed to discriminate not only chronic phase from advanced phase, but also early chronic phase from late chronic phase with sensitivity of 77 % and specificity of 95 % (Oehler et al. 2009). These results are particularly interesting, given the fact that the distinction between early and late chronic phase is not possible with current clinically available tools other than time from diagnosis.

Several studies tried to predict an imatinib response signature from pretreatment gene expression profiles (Crossman et al. 2005). In a study that used unselected leukocytes from patients who failed previous INFγ therapy, a 128-gene signature predicting cytogenetic response at 12 months could be obtained. Of note, this signature was subsequently tested in three patients and successfully predicted response to imatinib (Frank et al. 2006). In a similar study, gene expression profiles obtained from CD34 + enriched samples were used for supervised comparison of patients with either complete cytogenetic response (CCyR) or without even a minor response at 12 months of imatinib. The resulting classifier predicted response rates with 86.9 % accuracy and outperformed the Sokal Score, the risk stratification system based on clinical variables (McWeeney et al. 2010). The genes included in the response classifier were in part regulated by WNT/β-catenin and significantly overlapped with the 'blast crisis signature' and the signature from the 'aggressive' disease, demonstrating that the biologically hardwired program of the disease progression and imatinib resistance are largely overlapping (Mitchell and Deininger 2011).

12.5 Conclusions

GEP technologies have provided extensive biologic information about human leukemias and related disorders, paving the way toward personalized therapy of ALL, AML, MDS, or CML patients. These platforms have been and will likely continue to be evaluated in studies of hematological malignancies with different aims. First, these technologies allow to improve diagnosis in morphologically overlapping entities or defined new "molecular" disease subclasses. Second, GEP data can provide important prognostic information and characterize the biologic foundation of a "poor risk" phenotype. Third, it can be successfully used to elucidate different biologic aspects of the defined disease subtypes. All these aims converge at the ultimate goal of identifying clinically useful diagnostic/prognostic markers and characterizing novel therapeutic targets.

The gene expression microarray technology has clearly demonstrated its value as a powerful tool answering exploratory research questions in specialized centers associated with clinical trials, but for different reasons it has not been widely adopted for clinical purposes. Microarrays have certain limitations hindering their clinical applications. In addition to relatively high cost, these techniques require highly specialized core laboratories, extensive bioinformatic processing, and at present lack standardized methodologies. For these reasons, this technology is unlikely to entirely replace widely used and established standard diagnostic and prognostic tools.

The genome-wide platforms continue to evolve and expand, extending into new areas and moving into more detailed and higher throughput technologies. For instance, it took almost 10 years to sequence entire human genome. Today, the same work can be done in a single center in a week or less, with a budget of a single laboratory. In fact, RNA sequencing and whole-genome or whole-exome sequencing technologies have become equally expensive as gene expression microarrays, with the advantage of having a broader resolution and the possibility of picking up additional genetic information, including mutations and translocations. This will likely lead to the substitution of gene expression platforms by these more comprehensive tools in the near future.

References

Armstrong SA, Staunton JE, Silverman LB, Pieters R, den Boer ML, Minden MD, Sallan SE, Lander ES, Golub TR, Korsmeyer SJ (2002) MLL translocations specify a distinct gene expression profile that distinguishes a unique leukemia. Nat Genet 30(1):41–47

Baldi P, Hatfield GW (2002) DNA microarrays and gene expression : from experiments to data analysis and modeling. Cambridge University Press, Cambridge

Becker H, Marcucci G, Maharry K, Radmacher MD, Mrozek K, Margeson D, Whitman SP, Wu YZ, Schwind S, Paschka P, Powell BL, Carter TH, Kolitz JE, Wetzler M, Carroll AJ, Baer MR, Caligiuri MA, Larson RA, Bloomfield CD (2010) Favorable prognostic impact of NPM1 mutations in older patients with cytogenetically normal de novo acute myeloid leukemia and associated gene- and microRNA-expression signatures: a Cancer and Leukemia Group B study. J Clin Oncol 28(4):596–604

Boultwood J, Pellagatti A, Nikpour M, Pushkaran B, Fidler C, Cattan H, Littlewood TJ, Malcovati L, Della Porta MG, Jadersten M, Killick S, Giagounidis A, Bowen D, Hellstrom-Lindberg E, Cazzola M, Wainscoat JS (2008) The role of the iron transporter ABCB7 in refractory anemia with ring sideroblasts. PLoS ONE 3(4):e1970

Causton HC, Quackenbush J, Brazma A (2003) Microarray gene expression data analysis: a beginner's guide. Blackwell, Malden

Collins-Underwood JR, Mullighan CG (2010) Genomic profiling of high-risk acute lymphoblastic leukemia. Leukemia 24(10):1676–1685

Crossman LC, Mori M, Hsieh YC, Lange T, Paschka P, Harrington CA, Krohn K, Niederwieser DW, Hehlmann R, Hochhaus A, Druker BJ, Deininger MW (2005) In chronic myeloid leukemia white cells from cytogenetic responders and non-responders to imatinib have very similar gene expression signatures. Haematol 90(4):459–464

Ebert BL, Galili N, Tamayo P, Bosco J, Mak R, Pretz J, Tanguturi S, Ladd-Acosta C, Stone R, Golub TR, Raza A (2008) An erythroid differentiation signature predicts response to lenalidomide in myelodysplastic syndrome. PLoS Med 5(2):e35

Estey E, Dohner H (2006) Acute myeloid leukaemia. Lancet 368(9550):1894–1907

Faderl S, Kantarjian HM, Talpaz M, Estrov Z (1998) Clinical significance of cytogenetic abnormalities in adult acute lymphoblastic leukemia. Blood 91(11):3995–4019

Frank O, Brors B, Fabarius A, Li L, Haak M, Merk S, Schwindel U, Zheng C, Muller MC, Gretz N, Hehlmann R, Hochhaus A, Seifarth W (2006) Gene expression signature of primary imatinib-resistant chronic myeloid leukemia patients. Leukemia 20(8):1400–1407

Gentleman R (2005) Bioinformatics and computational biology solutions using R and Bioconductor. Statistics for biology and health. Springer, New York

Golub TR, Slonim DK, Tamayo P, Huard C, Gaasenbeek M, Mesirov JP, Coller H, Loh ML, Downing JR, Caligiuri MA, Bloomfield CD, Lander ES (1999) Molecular classification of cancer: class discovery and class prediction by gene expression monitoring. Science 286(5439):531–537

Haferlach T, Kohlmann A, Schnittger S, Dugas M, Hiddemann W, Kern W, Schoch C (2005) Global approach to the diagnosis of leukemia using gene expression profiling. Blood 106(4):1189–1198

Haferlach T, Kohlmann A, Wieczorek L, Basso G, Kronnie GT, Bene MC, De Vos J, Hernandez JM, Hofmann WK, Mills KI, Gilkes A, Chiaretti S, Shurtleff SA, Kipps TJ, Rassenti LZ, Yeoh AE, Papenhausen PR, Liu WM, Williams PM, Foa R (2010) Clinical utility of microarray-based gene expression profiling in the diagnosis and subclassification of leukemia: report from the international microarray innovations in leukemia study group. J Clin Oncol 28(15):2529–2537

Holleman A, Cheok MH, den Boer ML, Yang W, Veerman AJ, Kazemier KM, Pei D, Cheng C, Pui CH, Relling MV, Janka-Schaub GE, Pieters R, Evans WE (2004) Gene-expression patterns in drug-resistant acute lymphoblastic leukemia cells and response to treatment. N Engl J Med 351(6):533–542

Juszczynski P, Rodig SJ, Ouyang J, O'Donnell E, Takeyama K, Mlynarski W, Mycko K, Szczepanski T, Gaworczyk A, Krivtsov A, Faber J, Sinha AU, Rabinovich GA, Armstrong SA, Kutok JL, Shipp MA (2010) MLL-rearranged B lymphoblastic leukemias selectively express the immunoregulatory carbohydrate-binding protein galectin-1. Clin Cancer Res 16(7):2122–2130

Kawamata N, Ogawa S, Zimmermann M, Kato M, Sanada M, Hemminki K, Yamatomo G, Nannya Y, Koehler R, Flohr T, Miller CW, Harbott J, Ludwig WD, Stanulla M, Schrappe M, Bartram CR, Koeffler HP (2008) Molecular allelokaryotyping of pediatric acute lymphoblastic leukemias by high-resolution single nucleotide polymorphism oligonucleotide genomic microarray. Blood 111(2):776–784

Kohlmann A, Bullinger L, Thiede C, Schaich M, Schnittger S, Dohner K, Dugas M, Klein HU, Dohner H, Ehninger G, Haferlach T (2010) Gene expression profiling in AML with normal karyotype can predict mutations for molecular markers and allows novel insights into perturbed biological pathways. Leukemia 24(6):1216–1220

Krivtsov AV, Twomey D, Feng Z, Stubbs MC, Wang Y, Faber J, Levine JE, Wang J, Hahn WC, Gilliland DG, Golub TR, Armstrong SA (2006) Transformation from committed progenitor to leukaemia stem cell initiated by MLL-AF9. Nature 442(7104):818–822

Krivtsov AV, Feng Z, Lemieux ME, Faber J, Vempati S, Sinha AU, Xia X, Jesneck J, Bracken AP, Silverman LB, Kutok JL, Kung AL, Armstrong SA (2008) H3K79 methylation profiles define murine and human MLL-AF4 leukemias. Cancer Cell 14(5):355–368

Kuiper RP, Schoenmakers EF, van Reijmersdal SV, Hehir-Kwa JY, van Kessel AG, van Leeuwen FN, Hoogerbrugge PM (2007) High-resolution genomic profiling of childhood ALL reveals novel recurrent genetic lesions affecting pathways involved in lymphocyte differentiation and cell cycle progression. Leukemia 21(6):1258–1266

Lowenberg B, Downing JR, Burnett A (1999) Acute myeloid leukemia. N Engl J Med 341(14):1051–1062

Marcucci G, Haferlach T, Dohner H (2011) Molecular genetics of adult acute myeloid leukemia: prognostic and therapeutic implications. J Clin Oncol 29(5):475–486

McWeeney SK, Pemberton LC, Loriaux MM, Vartanian K, Willis SG, Yochum G, Wilmot B, Turpaz Y, Pillai R, Druker BJ, Snead JL, MacPartlin M, O'Brien SG, Melo JV, Lange T, Harrington CA, Deininger MW (2010) A gene expression signature of CD34+ cells to predict major cytogenetic response in chronic-phase chronic myeloid leukemia patients treated with imatinib. Blood 115(2):315–325

Mills KI, Kohlmann A, Williams PM, Wieczorek L, Liu WM, Li R, Wei W, Bowen DT, Loeffler H, Hernandez JM, Hofmann WK, Haferlach T (2009) Microarray-based classifiers and prognosis models identify subgroups with distinct clinical outcomes and high risk of AML transformation of myelodysplastic syndrome. Blood 114(5):1063–1072

Mitchell B, Deininger M (2011) Techniques for risk stratification of newly diagnosed patients with chronic myeloid leukemia. Leuk Lymphoma 52(Suppl 1):4–11

Mount DW (2004) Bioinformatics: sequence and genome analysis, 2nd edn. Cold Spring Harbor Laboratory Press, Cold Spring Harbor

Mullighan CG, Goorha S, Radtke I, Miller CB, Coustan-Smith E, Dalton JD, Girtman K, Mathew S, Ma J, Pounds SB, Su X, Pui CH, Relling MV, Evans WE, Shurtleff SA, Downing JR (2007) Genome-wide analysis of genetic alterations in acute lymphoblastic leukaemia. Nature 446(7137):758–764

Mullighan CG, Miller CB, Radtke I, Phillips LA, Dalton J, Ma J, White D, Hughes TP, Le Beau MM, Pui CH, Relling MV, Shurtleff SA, Downing JR (2008) BCR-ABL1 lymphoblastic leukaemia is characterized by the deletion of Ikaros. Nature 453(7191):110–114

Mullighan CG, Collins-Underwood JR, Phillips LA, Loudin MG, Liu W, Zhang J, Ma J, Coustan-Smith E, Harvey RC, Willman CL, Mikhail FM, Meyer J, Carroll AJ, Williams RT, Cheng J, Heerema NA, Basso G, Pession A, Pui CH, Raimondi SC, Hunger SP, Downing JR, Carroll WL, Rabin KR (2009a) Rearrangement of CRLF2 in B-progenitor- and down syndrome-associated acute lymphoblastic leukemia. Nat Genet 41(11):1243–1246

Mullighan CG, Su X, Zhang J, Radtke I, Phillips LA, Miller CB, Ma J, Liu W, Cheng C, Schulman BA, Harvey RC, Chen IM, Clifford RJ, Carroll WL, Reaman G, Bowman WP, Devidas M, Gerhard DS, Yang W, Relling MV, Shurtleff SA, Campana D, Borowitz MJ, Pui CH, Smith M, Hunger SP, Willman CL, Downing JR (2009b) Deletion of IKZF1 and prognosis in acute lymphoblastic leukemia. N Engl J Med 360(5):470–480

Mullighan CG, Zhang J, Harvey RC, Collins-Underwood JR, Schulman BA, Phillips LA, Tasian SK, Loh ML, Su X, Liu W, Devidas M, Atlas SR, Chen IM, Clifford RJ, Gerhard DS, Carroll WL, Reaman GH, Smith M, Downing JR, Hunger SP, Willman CL (2009c) JAK mutations in high-risk childhood acute lymphoblastic leukemia. Proc Natl Acad Sci U S A 106(23):9414–9418

Oehler VG, Yeung KY, Choi YE, Bumgarner RE, Raftery AE, Radich JP (2009) The derivation of diagnostic markers of chronic myeloid leukemia progression from microarray data. Blood 114(15):3292–3298

Parmigiani G (2003) The analysis of gene expression data: methods and software Statistics for biology and health. Springer, New York

Pellagatti A, Cazzola M, Giagounidis AA, Malcovati L, Porta MG, Killick S, Campbell LJ, Wang L, Langford CF, Fidler C, Oscier D, Aul C, Wainscoat JS, Boultwood J (2006) Gene expression profiles of CD34+ cells in myelodysplastic syndromes: involvement of interferon-stimulated genes and correlation to FAB subtype and karyotype. Blood 108(1):337–345

Pellagatti A, Cazzola M, Giagounidis A, Perry J, Malcovati L, Della Porta MG, Jadersten M, Killick S, Verma A, Norbury CJ, Hellstrom-Lindberg E, Wainscoat JS, Boultwood J (2010) Deregulated gene expression pathways in myelodysplastic syndrome hematopoietic stem cells. Leukemia 24(4):756–764

Radich JP, Dai H, Mao M, Oehler V, Schelter J, Druker B, Sawyers C, Shah N, Stock W, Willman CL, Friend S, Linsley PS (2006) Gene expression changes associated with progression and response in chronic myeloid leukemia. Proc Natl Acad Sci U S A 103(8):2794–2799

Raza A, Mehdi M, Mumtaz M, Ali F, Lascher S, Galili N (2008) Combination of 5-azacytidine and thalidomide for the treatment of myelodysplastic syndromes and acute myeloid leukemia. Cancer 113(7):1596–1604

Ross ME, Mahfouz R, Onciu M, Liu HC, Zhou X, Song G, Shurtleff SA, Pounds S, Cheng C, Ma J, Ribeiro RC, Rubnitz JE, Girtman K, Williams WK, Raimondi SC, Liang DC, Shih LY, Pui CH, Downing JR (2004) Gene expression profiling of pediatric acute myelogenous leukemia. Blood 104(12):3679–3687

Schoch C, Kohlmann A, Schnittger S, Brors B, Dugas M, Mergenthaler S, Kern W, Hiddemann W, Eils R, Haferlach T (2002) Acute myeloid leukemias with reciprocal rearrangements can be distinguished by specific gene expression profiles. Proc Natl Acad Sci U S A 99(15):10008–10013

Secker-Walker LM, Prentice HG, Durrant J, Richards S, Hall E, Harrison G (1997) Cytogenetics adds independent prognostic information in adults with acute lymphoblastic leukaemia on MRC trial UKALL XA. MRC Adult Leukaemia Working Party. Br J Haematol 96(3):601–610

Speed TP ((2003)) Statistical analysis of gene expression microarray data. Interdisciplinary statistics. Chapman & Hall/CRC, Boca Raton

Sridhar K, Ross DT, Tibshirani R, Butte AJ, Greenberg PL (2009) Relationship of differential gene expression profiles in CD34+ myelodysplastic syndrome marrow cells to disease subtype and progression. Blood 114(23):4847–4858

Valk PJ, Verhaak RG, Beijen MA, Erpelinck CA, van Waalwijk Barjesteh, van Doorn-Khosrovani S, Boer JM, Beverloo HB, Moorhouse MJ, van der Spek PJ, Lowenberg B, Delwel R (2004) Prognostically useful gene-expression profiles in acute myeloid leukemia. N Engl J Med 350(16):1617–1628

Verhaak RG, Goudswaard CS, van Putten W, Bijl MA, Sanders MA, Hugens W, Uitterlinden AG, Erpelinck CA, Delwel R, Lowenberg B, Valk PJ (2005) Mutations in nucleophosmin (NPM1) in acute myeloid leukemia (AML): association with other gene abnormalities and previously established gene expression signatures and their favorable prognostic significance. Blood 106(12):3747–3754

Verhaak RG, Wouters BJ, Erpelinck CA, Abbas S, Beverloo HB, Lugthart S, Lowenberg B, Delwel R, Valk PJ (2009) Prediction of molecular subtypes in acute myeloid leukemia based on gene expression profiling. Haematol 94(1):131–134

Wei G, Twomey D, Lamb J, Schlis K, Agarwal J, Stam RW, Opferman JT, Sallan SE, den Boer ML, Pieters R, Golub TR, Armstrong SA (2006) Gene expression-based chemical genomics identifies rapamycin as a modulator of MCL1 and glucocorticoid resistance. Cancer Cell 10(4):331–342

Wetzler M, Dodge RK, Mrozek K, Carroll AJ, Tantravahi R, Block AW, Pettenati MJ, Le Beau MM, Frankel SR, Stewart CC, Szatrowski TP, Schiffer CA, Larson RA, Bloomfield CD (1999) Prospective karyotype analysis in adult acute lymphoblastic leukemia: the cancer and leukemia Group B experience. Blood 93(11):3983–3993

Wouters BJ, Lowenberg B, Erpelinck-Verschueren CA, van Putten WL, Valk PJ, Delwel R (2009) Double CEBPA mutations, but not single CEBPA mutations, define a subgroup of acute myeloid leukemia with a distinctive gene expression profile that is uniquely associated with a favorable outcome. Blood 113(13):3088–3091

Yeoh EJ, Ross ME, Shurtleff SA, Williams WK, Patel D, Mahfouz R, Behm FG, Raimondi SC, Relling MV, Patel A, Cheng C, Campana D, Wilkins D, Zhou X, Li J, Liu H, Pui CH, Evans WE, Naeve C, Wong L, Downing JR (2002) Classification, subtype discovery, and prediction of outcome in pediatric acute lymphoblastic leukemia by gene expression profiling. Cancer Cell 1(2):133–143

Part III
Molecular Procedures Involved in Hematopoietic Stem Cell Transplantation

Chapter 13
Allogeneic Transplantation of Hematopoietic Stem Cells

Jacek Wachowiak

Abstract Molecular and cytometric studies of human hematopoietic stem cells and its microenvironment have greatly contributed to a better understanding of their biology, including regulation of their function and mutual interaction. This has resulted in the improvements of the procedure of allogeneic hematopoietic stem cell transplantation (allo-HSCT) for hematological malignancies. In addition, molecular and cytometric studies enable better recognition of the pathology of toxic, immunological, and infectious complications related to allo-HSCT as well as better monitoring of post-transplant leukemia/lymphoma remission. Thereby, not only more effective prevention and early diagnosis of transplant-related complications, but also prompt diagnosis of imminent post-transplant leukemia/lymphoma relapse became possible. This, in turn, enables a preemptive treatment and precise evaluation of the response to the treatment. Finally, the long-term results of allo-HSCT for hematological malignancies systematically improve.

13.1 Introduction

Allogeneic hematopoietic stem cell transplantation (allo-HSCT) has nowadays become an important part of treatment for hematological malignancies. Its therapeutic potential results from the biology of the human hematopoietic stem cell (HSC) and from combined antileukemic effects of conditioning regimen (cytotoxic effect) along with graft-versus-leukemia reaction (immunotherapeutic effect).

J. Wachowiak (✉)
Department of Pediatric Oncology, Hematology and Transplantology,
Poznań University of Medical Sciences, Szpitalna 27/33, 60-572 Poznań, Poland
e-mail: jacek.wachowiak@plusnet.pl

M. Witt et al. (eds.), *Molecular Aspects of Hematologic Malignancies*, Principles and Practice, DOI: 10.1007/978-3-642-29467-9_13,

In addition, in a subset of patients allo-HSCT creates a platform for further therapeutic interventions. Due to the development of unrelated donors' registries, HLA allele-matched unrelated donor (MUD) can now be identified for 65–70 % of patients without HLA-matched sibling donor (MSD), thus enabling allo-HSCT in vast majority of patients with hematological malignancies and indication for transplantation.

After determination of indications for allo-HSCT, the next step concerns search for and selection of an optimal HSC donor. Then the optimal date for the procedure, the conditioning regimen, the source of hematopoietic stem cells, the required modifications of the transplant material, prophylaxis of immunological, toxic and infectious complications should be defined, as well as the principles for monitoring of the hematopoietic and immune system reconstitution, post-transplant complications, and the remission of the underlying disease.

In spite of the improving results of allo-HSCT for hematological malignancies, its efficacy is still limited due to the occurrence of post-transplant leukemia/ lymphoma relapse or life-threatening transplant-related complications, i.e., conditioning regimen-related organ toxicity, infectious complications, and immunological complications (non-engraftment/graft rejection, acute, and chronic graft versus host disease). Thus, there is still a need for such allo-HSCT procedure, which would assure still better total anti-malignancy effect along with lower risk of severe complications.

13.2 Molecular Aspects of Human Hematopoiesis in the Context of allo-HSCT

According to the definition proposed by the European Group for Blood and Marrow Transplantation (EBMT), HSCT refers to any procedure, during which hematopoietic stem cells of any donor type and any source are intravenously given to an appropriately prepared recipient in order to achieve total or partial repopulation and replacement of the hematopoietic system (Ljungman et al. 2010).

Human HSC is a multipotential somatic stem cell of mesenchymal origin with no typical cytomorphological features, but characterized by specific pattern of antigen expression: CD34+, CD133+, CD117+ (c-kit), CD135+ (flt3), and lack of expression of CD38 and Lin antigens (Wodnar-Filipowicz 2008). Moreover, the HSC demonstrates expression of CXCR4 receptor (C-X-C chemokine receptor type 4) for the stromal cell-derived factor-1 (SDF-1) and of numerous cell-adhesion molecules (CAMs), which are of primary importance for homing to marrow cavities, activating the function of transplanted HSCs, regulation of hematopoiesis, and mobilization of HSCs into peripheral blood (Majka and Ratajczak 2006; Rosu-Myles and Bhatia 2003).

Like all multipotent stem cells, the HSC demonstrates the ability to indefinitely divide and self-renew and to differentiate, under appropriate stimulation, into cells of a specific lineage (in this case toward progenitor cells of the erythroblast, myeloblast, megakaryoblast, and lymphoblast lineages) (Wodnar-Filipowicz 2008). These characteristics make the HSC capable of maintaining effective hematopoiesis throughout the entire human life, and of reconstituting a fully effective and sustained hematopoiesis after a HSC transplant.

Hematopoiesis, including its reconstitution after HSCT, results from interactions between HSCs and the bone marrow microenvironment, which beyond the period of fetal development is the only one to support sustained multilineage hematopoiesis in humans (Lam and Adams 2010). The bone marrow microenvironment consists of marrow stromal cells, creating a niche for HSCs, and of an extracellular matrix generated by the stromal cells.

It is currently believed that all stromal cells in the bone marrow (fibroblasts, adipocytes, endothelial cells, macrophages, osteoblasts, and progenitor mesenchymal cells) originate from a multipotent mesenchymal stromal cell (MSC). Experimental studies and clinical observations indicate that the administration of ex vivo expanded MSCs effectively supports engraftment of intravenously infused HSCs, especially if the dose of infused HSCs is suboptimal (Ball et al. 2008). Moreover, MSCs demonstrate immunomodulatory properties (they inhibit the function of T-lymphocytes and activate regulatory lymphocytes), which is of particular relevance in case of allo-HSCT from partially mismatched donors (Nauta and Fibbe 2007).

The extracellular matrix is composed of proteoglycans, elements of glycosaminoglycans, collagen, fibronectin, thrombospondin, laminin, sialoadhesin, hemonectin, and tenascin. It fills the space between hematopoietic stem cells and marrow stromal cells mediating communication between these cells.

Direct interactions between HSCs and bone marrow niche cells are facilitated by cell-adhesion molecules (CAMs), found on the surface of both hematopoietic and stromal cells, which enable anchoring of HSCs to stromal cells, including that following HSCT (Wodnar-Filipowicz 2008). Cell-adhesion molecules have been classified into six CAMs superfamilies: integrins, selectins, sialomucins, immunoglobulins, CD44 proteoglycans, and cadherins.

Three types of interactions between HSCs and the bone marrow microenvironment have been identified: (1) between HSCs and hematopoietic cytokines present in the extracellular matrix, (2) between HSCs and CAMs present on the surface of marrow stromal cells, and (3) between CAMs on the surface of HSCs and corresponding extracellular matrix ligands (Lam and Adams 2010).

In the bone marrow, the pool of quiescent HSCs and that of HSCs in the expansion phase remain in a dynamic balance, which is constantly regulated through internal and external mechanisms (Wodnar-Filipowicz 2008). The internal mechanisms include transcription and epigenetic regulation (through chromatin remodeling). The external mechanisms include: chemokines and hematopoietic cytokines released by marrow stromal cells, hormonal stimuli (parathyroid hormone), the influence of the sympathetic nervous system acting through osteoblasts, and oxidative conditions in bone marrow niches.

Chemokines constitute a family of small-molecule secreted proteins, which link to specific membrane receptors, and act not only as immune and inflammatory regulators, but also as regulators of hematopoiesis. The profiles of the receptors determine sensitivity to the chemotactic stimulus (Youn et al. 2000). There are four subfamilies of chemokines, distinguished on the basis of whether the first two cysteines are separated by a single amino acid residue (CXC) or three residues (CX3C) or they are adjacent (CC) or there is a single C. The previously mentioned SDF-1, belonging to CXC family (CXCL12) and its CXCR4 receptor on HSC, create an axis, which plays an important role in the regulation of hematopoiesis. The axis influences migration of HSCs to the bone marrow (in accordance with the SDF-1 gradient), homing to the bone marrow, reconstitution of hematopoiesis, differentiation, and survival of many cell types derived from both HSCs and hematopoietic progenitor cells (HPC) (Lam and Adams 2010; Majka and Ratajczak 2006).

Among hematopoietic cytokines released by the cells of the bone marrow niche some are of particular importance: the stem cell factor (SCF), Flt3 ligand (Flt3-L), angiopoietin-1 (ang-1), Notch ligands, Wnt (Wingless-type) ligands, Shh (Sonic Hedgehog) protein, and ligands from the TGF-beta (transforming growth factor-beta) family (Scadden 2006). These cytokines act synergistically and binding to specific receptors on the surface of a HSCs activate numerous signaling pathways (Blank et al. 2008). In this way, these locally released external factors control HSCs' proliferation (activate or inhibit, dependent on current needs), necessary for the maintenance of a stable HSCs pool, and differentiation of daughter cells resulting from the so-called 'asymmetric division' of a HSCs (Molofsky et al. 2006) (initially into a myeloid or lymphoid hematopoietic progenitor cell, and then into differentiated hematopoietic cells) (Wodnar-Filipowicz 2008).

Myeloid progenitor cells differentiate and mature toward cells of all specific hematopoietic lineages, i.e., erythrocytes, granulocytes (neutrophils, eosinophils, or basophils), monocytes, and megakaryocytes upon stimulation by hematopoietic growth factors; above all erythropoietin (EPO), thrombopoietin (TPO), granulocyte–macrophage and granulocyte colony-stimulating factors (GM-CSF, G-CSF), and by cytokines released by stromal cells, mainly interleukin-3 (IL-3), interleukin-4 (IL-4), and interleukin-5 (IL-5) (Akashi et al. 2000). At the same time lymphoid progenitor cells, stimulated by cytokines, develop from HSC and then differentiate and mature to become lymphocyte B, primarily under the influence of IL-3, IL-4, IL-5, and interleukin-7 (IL-7), or lymphocyte T, stimulated by IL-2, IL-4, IL-7, interleukin-9 (IL-9), and interleukin-10 (IL-10), or to become NK cells (Akashi et al. 1999). According to recent findings the bone marrow-derived plasmocytoid dendritic cells induce naive T lymphocytes to differentiate to become antigen-specific regulatory T lymphocytes, creating a milieu for the induction of transplantation tolerance (reciprocal donor/host) after allo-HSCT; however, its precise mechanism is still elusive (Cardenas et al. 2011).The rate of hematopoiesis is adjusted to match the current needs for these cell types and is regulated by numerous factors, including cytokines of the TGF-beta family, which either inhibit or stimulate proliferation, apoptosis, and/or differentiation of hematopoietic cells (Ruscetti et al. 2005). To sum up, allogeneic HSCs, intravenously infused into an appropriately conditioned recipient, upon interactions with the bone marrow microenvironment, are anchored to the bone marrow niches and undertake hematopoietic function, which is controlled by internal transcription factors, epigenetic factors, as well as chemokines, hematopoietic cytokines, and growth factors released by the bone marrow stromal cells. Thus, a fully functional and stable hematopoietic system and immune system are restored within several weeks and months, respectively, following the HSCT procedure. However, in allo-HSCT recipients, particularly after prior alloimmunization or in case of transplants from HLA mismatched donors, specific immunological complications may occur, i.e., nonengraftment/graft rejection, respectively, which make the reconstitution of hematopoiesis impossible, and/or acute and/or graft-versus-host disease (GvHD), which presents a significant disturbance to the hematopoiesis reconstitution process.

13.3 Allo-HSCT Procedure, Optimal Donor Selection and Transplant Management

13.3.1 Indications for HSCT in Malignant Diseases of the Hematopoietic System

Indications for allo-HSCT for hematological malignancies are determined in the context of the results of the conventional treatment, and the procedure is only justified if it significantly improves the chance of patient's complete recovery. Thus, allo-HSCT might be used as: (1) therapy of choice in malignant diseases of the hematopoietic system in which conventional therapies have completely failed, for instance in myelodysplastic syndrome (MDS) and juvenile myelo-monocytic leukemia (JMML); (2) consolidation of the first complete remission (CR1) of acute lymphoblastic leukemia (ALL) and acute myeloblastic leukemia (AML) with prognostic factors of high risk of relapse; (3)consolidation of the second or subsequent complete remission ($\geq$CR2) in patients with acute leukemia or lymphoma and high risk of subsequent relapse.

In the above-mentioned subsets of hematological malignancies, defined molecular markers, and the level of minimal residual disease (MRD) currently play a major role among prognostic factors being precise indication for allo-HSCT (see Chaps. 1, 2, and 11).

13.3.2 Selection of a HSC Donor

Upon determination of indications for allo-HSCT, the search for a suitable HSC donor procedure must immediately begin. The genetic basis and methods of the matching of the optimal HSC donor are discussed in details in Chaps. 14 and 21.

Unrelated HSC donor matching at the allele level with regard to A, B, Cw, DRB1, and DQB1 loci has resulted in a significant reduction of transplant-related mortality (TRM). According to the latest report by EBMT Pediatric Diseases Working Party (Miano et al. 2007), TRM up to day +100 after HSCT from MUD decreased from about 25 % in the early 1990s to about 15 % after the year 2000. Thus, in patients ≤18 years of age long-term results of MUD-HSCT have significantly improved and are now similar to those of HSCT from MSD, even if the unrelated donor matches the recipient in 9/10 allele (Miano et al. 2007). Thanks to the high resolution HLA typing, a similar improvement in MUD-HSCT effects has also been reported in adult patients (Hows et al. 2006).

13.3.3 Conditioning Regimen Prior to allo-HSCT

Each HSCT procedure is preceded by a conditioning regimen, whose aim depends on the type of transplant and the indication for the procedure (Gratwohl 2008; Vettenranta 2008). In allo-HSCT conventional conditioning regimen should be characterized by a complete myeloablative effect required for the total destruction of the patient's own "sick" bone marrow and the creation of the available space that could be populated by the transplanted allogeneic HSCs. Moreover, in order to avoid transplant rejection, the conditioning regimen should exert a desired immunosuppressive effect, which should be particularly strong in a transplant from unrelated donor (especially if mismatched) and from haploidentical donor. In recipients with hematologic malignancies, the conditioning regimen should also be characterized by a strong anti-leukemic effect. Apart from its myeloablative, immunosuppressive, and anti-leukemic effect, the conditioning regimen should be characterized with the lowest possible level of early and late organ toxicity.

With the exception of recipients with ALL aged above 2 years, in whom fractionated total body irradiation (FTBI)-based preparative regimen prior to allo-HSCT is recommended, all other patients with hematological malignancies (ALL ≤2 year of age, AML, chronic myelocytic leukemia, MDS, JMML) are usually conditioned with busulfan-based regimen. In case of a transplant from an unrelated donor, the immunosuppressive component of the conditioning regimen is strengthened by T-lymphocyte depletion in vivo, which consists of the intravenous administration of anti-thymocyte globulin (ATG) or suitable monoclonal antibodies (anti-CD52 or anti-CD3).

Although late consequences of busulfan at myeloablative doses are less pronounced for the developing organism of a child than those related to FTBI, early organ toxicity of busulfan, particularly its hepatotoxicity, represents a significant threat.

The risk of severe organ complications related to the toxicity of conventional myeloablative regimen (regimen related toxicity, RRT) is particularly high in older patients (above 65–70 years of age) and in recipients who, prior to allo-HSCT demonstrate an impaired organ function related to an underlying disease and/or a comorbidity. Therefore, since the late 1990s, the reduced intensity conditioning (RIC) is increasingly used in such patients to avoid severe RRT (Giralt 2005; Satwani et al. 2008). The primary objective of RIC is to achieve the level of immunosuppression which will prevent the rejection of the transplanted allogeneic HSCs. However, RIC does neither totally eliminate the recipient's hematopoietic system nor does it eliminate all the residual leukemic cells. The recipients conditioned with RIC receive a high dose of HSCs which, in combination with an intensive immunosuppressive treatment, is designed to initially guarantee a coexistence of the donor's and patient's hematopoietic systems, i.e., a development of a mixed chimerism (see Chap.15). Then, over subsequent weeks, in line with the reduction of the prophylactic immunosuppression, donor T-lymphocytes will gradually eliminate the recipient's own hematopoiesis and hopefully the residual leukemic cells. This should result in a state of complete donor chimerism and in a decreasing level of minimal residual disease (see Chap. 16). In order to reduce the time required to achieve complete chimerism, and to strengthen the GvL response, donor lymphocyte infusions (DLIs) are administered at defined time points under the quantitative control of hematopoietic chimersim and the level of minimal residual disease (MRD) (Giralt 2005).

In patients with high pretransplant MRD level, new components of a conditioning regimen should be applied in the future, such as a targeted therapy, which would significantly improve the antileukemic effect of the conditioning regimen, without increasing its toxicity (Bader et al. 2009; Pulsipher et al. 2008).

13.3.4 Sources, Collection, Processing, and Doses of Transplant Material

The CD34+ hematopoietic stem cells represent 1–3 % of the bone marrow mononuclear cells (BM-MNCs) and only 0.01–0.02 % of cells in the peripheral blood (PB). The HSC count in the umbilical cord blood (CB) is eight times higher than in the bone marrow, but the volume of cord blood and thus the number of CB-HSCs are limited (on average only 70–80 ml of CB can be collected). Nowadays, all the three above-mentioned sources of HSCs are used for allo-HSCT (Ljungman et al. 2010).

Bone marrow is the recommended HSC source in case of the HLA-identical sibling donor younger than 18 years and preferred source for nonmalignant disorders. The BM is harvested from the donor under general anesthesia by multiple aspiration from the crest of the ilium.

For successful allo-HSCT from a mismatched unrelated or haploidentical donor the peripheral blood is the source of HSCs, They are collected by leukapheresis using cell separators, after prior mobilization, i.e., after the administration for 4–5 days of the human recombinant granulocyte-colony stimulating factor (rHuG-CSF), which causes shift of CD34+ cells from the bone marrow to the peripheral blood and an increase of their concentration in the blood to >0.1 %.

The application of rHuG-CSF causes a decrease of the SDF-1level in the bone marrow, due to degradation by proteolytic enzymes secreted by neutrophiles, and an increase in SDF-1 concentration in peripheral blood (Hattori et al. 2001). On the other hand, rHuG-CSF causes decreased expression of the CXCR4 on CD34+ cells, which results in the mobilization of these cells into the peripheral blood (Petit et al. 2002). As demonstrated by Bogunia-Kubik et al. (2006b), differences in the number of CD34+ cells mobilized into the peripheral blood in healthy donors after a rHuG-CSF treatment depend on the polymorphism of the SDF-1 encoding gene (position 801 (G/A) of the 3′UTR region). The number of CD34+ cells in the product of leukapheresis is significantly higher in donors with the SDF-1-3′A allele, thus in donors with the SDF-1-3′GG genotype, a higher number of separations was necessary than in those with the SDF-1-3′A allele. Understanding of the HSC mobilization process has recently resulted in the application of a novel agent that disrupts the CXCR4-CXCL12 bond, the primary HSC anchor in the bone marrow, for mobilizing HSC for autologous transplantation in patients with non-Hodgkin's lymphoma and multiple myeloma (Kessans et al. 2010).

Further processing of the leukapheresis product is determined by the HSC donor type. In case of a mismatched or haploidentical donor the immunomagnetic positive selection of CD34+ or combined immunomagnetic depletion of CD3/CD19 lymphocytes should be performed (Lang and Handgretinger 2008). The optimum dose of transplanted nucleated cells (NC) and/or CD34+ cells, means a dose which ensures engraftment with the complete reconstitution of the hematopoietic and immune systems in shortest time period, along with nonincreased risk of GvHD and an appropriate GvL effect. In case of allo-HSCT, such dose depends on the source of HSC and the degree of class I and II HLA antigens compatibility at the allelic level between the donor and the recipient.

13.4 Reconstitution of the Hematopoiesis After Allogeneic Hematopoietic Stem Cell Transplantation and Molecular Indicators of Engraftment

The evidence of transplanted HSCs engraftment is provided by the absolute neutrophile count (ANC) of $\geq 0.5 \times 10^9$/l on 3 consecutive days and/or the blood platelet count of $\geq 20 \times 10^9$/l over at least 7 days without a transfusion of platelet concentrate. These counts are generally observed 2–3 weeks after a transplant from an HLA–matched sibling and about 3–4 weeks after a transplant from an unrelated donor, and usually are reached slightly faster if the transplanted CD34+ cells were obtained from the peripheral blood. Engraftment indicators occur at the latest after a cord blood transplant, especially from an unrelated donor, in which case the ANC of $\geq 0.5 \times 10^9$/l is achieved only about week 4, and the platelet count of $\geq 20 \times 10^9$/l only about week 5 after HSCT. If ANC fails to exceed the value of 0.5×10^9/l by day 28 after allo-HSCT, this qualifies as lack of engraftment. Graft rejection is diagnosed if ANC, despite prior indicators of engraftment, declines to the value of $<0.2 \times 10^9$/l, and remains at this level for at least 3 consecutive days.

The most precise assessment of engraftment is guaranteed by quantitative assays of posttransplant hematopoietic chimerism using the RQ-PCR method, making it possible to analyze chimerism at the sensitivity level of at least 10^{-3}, which may be increased by an assessment of lineage-specific chimerism (see Chap. 15). Evaluation of chimerism is of specific importance for those recipients who display a higher risk of graft failure by donor T-cells and NK cells, i.e., recipients after a transplant from partially mismatched and haploidentical donors, recipients who received nonmyeloablative conditioning regimen or who demonstrated signs of alloimmunization prior to allo-HSCT (Mattsson et al. 2008). Monitoring of chimerism is also useful in recipients with a hematopoietic malignancy and high risk of post-transplant recurrence of the disease who, due to a lack of specific markers, are not eligible to monitoring of minimal residual disease (Bader et al. 2008). In patients with suitable MRD markers, the most accurate assessment of residual disease, with the sensitivity of 10^{-4}–10^{-6}, is possible with the use of RQ-PCR, and with a slightly lower sensitivity, with the use of multiparameter flow cytometry (Bader et al. 2008; Szczepanski 2007) (see Chap. 16). The monitoring of post-transplant chimerism, ideally combined with the evaluation of the level of MRD, enables early identification and differentiation of an impending graft rejection or recurrence of leukemia. Thus, it is possible to undertake preemptive, and therefore more effective, immunointervention to prevent graft rejection (infusion of an additional dose of donor CD34+ cells and/or CD3 lymphocytes) (Mattsson et al. 2008), or a hematological relapse (cessation of GvHD prophylaxis and infusions of donor CD3 lymphocytes, if possible in combination with targeted therapy) (Kröger et al. 2010a, b; Pulsipher et al. 2008). Moreover, further monitoring of chimerism and MRD enables evaluation of the response to the intervention, and subsequently the optimal therapeutic decisions (Bader et al. 2008).

13.5 Complications of allo-HSCT and the Role of Non-HLA Gene Polymorphism

Despite continuous improvements in the allo-HSCT procedure, its efficacy remains limited due to transplant-related complications being the second most frequent cause of treatment failure, apart from the recurrence of the underlying disease in case of hematological malignancies (Carreras 2008; Cordonnier 2008; Devergie 2008). Therefore, the prophylaxis of these complications as well as their early diagnostics using molecular biology methods is of particular importance. The recipients of allogeneic HSC undergoing the conditioning regimen may experience not only toxic complications and infections but, first of all, specific immunological complications, such as nonengraftment or graft rejection, or an acute or chronic graft-versus-host disease (GvHD). The risk of both immunological and infectious complications is particularly high after the transplantations from the so-called 'alternative donors', i.e., from HLA-matched or mismatched unrelated donors and from haploidentical-related donors. Complications occurring up to day 100 after HSCT are termed 'early complications' and those occurring after that day–'late complications'.

Essential role in the etiopathogenesis and the course of allo-HSCT complications immunological, toxic, and infectious ones is played by cytokines released by immunocompetent cells of the recipient, during the conditioning regimen, and of the donor after transplantation (Choi et al. 2010; Coppell et al. 2003; Mehta 2005). Since in vitro studies showed significant differences in the level of cytokines released from peripheral blood cells of healthy donors as a result of mitogen stimulation, studies of the polymorphism of the cytokine-encoding genes and the impact of this polymorphism on the effects of allo-HSCT has been undertaken (Loefller et al. 2010). The results confirmed the existence of microsatellite and single nucleotide polymorphism (SNP) within cytokine-encoding genes, thus confirming the hypothesis on genetic predisposition to post-allo-HSCT complications, depending on diverse levels of cytokines production.

Attention has also been paid to predisposition to post-HSCT complications related to the polymorphism of other genes encoding: drug metabolizing enzymes (in the conditioning regimen and in GvHD prophylaxis), estrogenic receptor, vitamin D_3 receptor, receptor for Fcγ (FcγR) IIIb, myeloperoxidase (MPO), mannose-binding lectin (MBL), and receptors which activate antigen presenting cells responsible for the processes related to natural immunity (Bogunia-Kubik et al. 2006a; Dickinson 2008; Elhasid et al. 2010; Martin-Antonio et al. 2010; Mullighan and Petersdorf 2006).

The results of the studies on selected non-HLA polymorphisms in allogeneic HSC recipients and donors, provide an increasingly solid evidence that a pre-allo-HSCT evaluation of a genetic predisposition to toxic and infectious complications and, above all, to the occurrence of GvHD, may contribute to a better selection of an optimal conditioning regimen, GvHD prophylaxis, and anti-infection prophylaxis. This might result in further improvement in the outcomes of allo-HSCT by reduction in the risk of life-threatening complications of this procedure.

13.5.1 Early Toxic Complications of Conditioning Regimens

Early toxic complications of conditioning regimens are in majority similar to those observed after an intensive conventional chemotherapy (nausea, vomiting, lack of appetite, oral and gastrointestinal mucosa injury, hepatopathy, loss of hair, hemorrhagic cystitis). There are also similarities concerning prophylaxis and the principles of treatment if these complications occur. The hematologic toxicity of the conditioning regimens is not raised, since myeloablation is the objective of these regimens.

However, unlike the patients who undergo conventional chemotherapy, the recipients of allogeneic HSCs may experience dangerous and life-threatening complications resulting from the injury of vascular endothelium. The injury occurs under the simultaneous impact of several damaging factors, such as high-dose chemotherapy and FTBI used in the conditioning regimen, immunosuppressive drugs used in GvHD prophylaxis, and high concentration of proinflammatory cytokines, leukotrienes and thromboxanes released during the conditioning regimen, infection, and/or GvHD (Carreras 2008; Coppell et al. 2003). Endothelial injury leads to the activation of the coagulation cascade and the complement system, which may result in the development of hepatic venoocclusive disease (VOD), capillary leak syndrome, engraftment syndrome, diffuse alveolar haemorrhage (DAH), transplantation-associated microangiopathy (TAM), and idiopathic pneumonia syndrome. All these syndromes are related to a serious prognosis, with the risk of progression into multiorgan dysfunction syndrome (MODS), and by mortality rates of 18–97 % (Carreras 2008).

The increased risk of severe regimen-related toxic complications has been demonstrated to be linked with the polymorphism of tumor necrosis factor-alpha (TNF-alpha) (−308), tumor necrosis factor-beta (TNF-beta) (+1069), interleukin-10 (IL-10) (−1082, −819, −592), and interleukin-6 (IL-6) (−174) genes in the transplant recipients (Bogunia-Kubik et al. 2006a). Moreover, hepatotoxicity of high-dose busulfan-based conditioning regimens, used in the majority of HSC recipients, may be influenced by the polymorphism of the genes encoding isoenzymes of glutathione S-transferase (GST): *GSTA1*, *GSTM1*, and *GSTP1*, responsible for busulfan clearance (Elhasid et al. 2010; Ansari et al. 2010). Moreover, Pihusch et al. (2004) have found that the risk of VOD is also influenced by the polymorphism of the gene encoding plasminogen activator inhibitor-1 (PAI-1) (−675 4G/5G).

In turn, polymorphism associated with lower activity of methylenetetrahydrofolate reductase (MTHFR) have been correlated with liver toxicity (MTHFR-A128C) (Goekkurt et al. 2007), increased mucotoxic effect, and delayed reconstitution of megakaryopoiesis in HSCT recipients receiving methotrexate as GvHD prophylaxis (MTHFR-C677T) (Dickinson 2008).

13.5.2 Infectious Complications

All allo-HSCT recipients experience the breakdown of both systemic and local immune mechanisms due to combined cytotoxic and immunosuppressive effects of the conditioning regimen, GvHD prophylaxis and treatment and, in some recipients, also in vivo and/or ex vivo depletion of CD3 lymphocytes (Cordonnier 2008).

This is why, infectious complications of allo-HSCT remain the most frequent cause of failure in recipients with nonmalignant disease and the second most frequent (after relapse) cause of failure in recipients with malignancy, despite increasingly advanced methods of prevention, diagnosis, and treatment. The risk of infections after allo-HSCT is determined by many factors, including: prior infections of the recipient and the donor, the type of HSC donor, the type of conditioning regimen, the dose of CD3 lymphocytes, GvHD prophylaxis and—in case of GvHD occurence—its severity, duration, and therapy used.

Moreover, the risk of infectious complications following allo-HSCT is also influenced by the polymorphism of several genes. For instance, it has been postulated, that microsatellite polymorphism (CA repeats) at position 3 in the first intron of the interferon-gamma (INF-gamma) gene in the recipients of HSCs from an HLA-matched siblings may predispose to Epstein-Barr virus (EBV) infections, in relation to a decreased release of INF-gamma, as demonstrated in in vitro study (Dickinson 2008). Moreover, an increased risk of bacterial infection has been associated with MPO AG/AA, FcγR IIIb HNA-1a/HNA-1a donor genotypes, with FcγRIIa R-131 recipient genotype (Rocha et al. 2002), and MBL MBL2 donor and/or recipient genotype (Mullighan et al. 2002). The risk of infections is also influenced by the polymorphism of genes encoding the Toll-like receptors (TLR) of antigen-presenting cells, i.e., *TLR1* and *TLR6* polymorphism is linked to an increased post-allo-HSCT risk of fungal infections caused by *Aspergillus sp.*, while recipients with *TLR4* polymorphism have an increased risk of infections caused by Gram-negative bacteria (Napolitani et al. 2005; Schroder and Schumann 2005). Recently, Plantinga et al. (2009) demonstrated that an early stop codon Y238X polymorphism of a major beta-glucan receptor on macrophages (*DECTIN-1*) gene is associated with increased *Candida* colonization in HSC recipients, which is an important step toward improved predictive and preventive medicine for immunocompromised hosts, specifically toward individualized antifungal prevention in HSCT (Bochud and Calandra 2009).

The most important problem among the infectious complications after allo-HSCT, especially in recipients of HSCs from alternative donors and in the course of GvHD, is reactivation of herpesvirus-family and fungal infections. However, the implementation of molecular methods (PCR) in 1990s for early diagnosis of EBV, cytomegalovirus (CMV), adenovirus (ADV), BK virus (BKV), *Aspergillus sp.,* and *Candida sp.* infections enables application of preemptive therapy, i.e., therapy implemented on the basis of qualitative or quantitative results of molecular tests even before the occurrence of clinical symptoms of the disease (Cordonnier 2008). Moreover, a quantitative evaluation of viral DNA makes it possible to precisely assess the efficacy of the applied treatment, and presents an invaluable indication as to further therapy in terms of times and measures. The strategy of preemptive therapy has resulted in a significant improvement of the prognosis concerning infectious complications of allo-HSCT, which were previously diagnosed only at advanced, clinically evident stages.

13.5.3 Immunological Complications

The major immunological complications of allo-HSCT are nonengraftment/graft rejection, acute GvHD, and chronic GvHD.

13.5.3.1 Non-Engraftment/Graft Rejection

Lack of engraftment or rejection of the transplanted HSCs is a consequence of their destruction by the recipient's T-cells and/or NK cells which survived the conditioning regimen, or by antibodies (Mattsson et al. 2008). After a myeloablative conditioning regimen, this complication occurs in approximately 1 % of recipients after MSD-HSCT or MUD-HSCT and in approximately 5 % of recipients undergoing HSCT from a mismatched donor. Apart from the degree of donor-recipient HLA mismatches and the loci which these mismatches apply to, there are also other factors causing an increased risk of non-engraftment, i.e., ex vivo T-cells depletion from the transplant material, a low dose of transplanted hematopoietic stem cells, a nonmyeloablative conditioning regimen, a major AB0 incompatibility, and an alloimmunization of the recipient before allo-HSCT (Mattsson et al. 2008).

As previously mentioned, the most precise evaluation of engraftment or transplant rejection after allo-HSCT can be made with the help of quantitative testing of post-transplant hematopoietic chimerism, in particular—lineage-specific chimerism of T-cells, i.e., graft rejection effector cells, using the quantitative real-time PCR method (RQ-PCR) (see Chap. 15). If performed systematically and with a suitable frequency, chimerism monitoring make it possible to detect early the rejection process and to undertake early immunointervention (infusion of donor lymphocytes with or without an additional dose of CD34+ cells), thus providing a better chance of treatment success. It also enables to monitoring of the patient's response to intervention and therapeutic decision-making according to the results of successive assays of chimerism (Gorczyńska et al. 2004; Mattsson et al. 2008).

13.5.3.2 Graft-Versus-Host Disease (GvHD)

A fundamental and specific immunological complication of allo-HSCT is the graft-versus-host disease (GvHD), which is a complex of clinical symptoms manifested as a consequence of the interaction between donor's T-cells and HLA-presenting cells in the target organs and tissues of the recipient (Choi et al. 2010). GvHD is classified either as acute or chronic GvHD (up to day +100 and after day +100 after allo-HSCT, respectively). However, especially in patients conditioned for allo-HSCT with nonmyeloablative conditioning regimen who received an infusion of donor lymphocytes, the symptoms characteristic for an acute GvHD may occur beyond day +100 (persistent, recurrent, or late-onset acute GvHD) as well as overlaping syndromes of acute and chronic GvHD may appear (Filipovich et al. 2005). Depending on the expression of risk factors, acute GvHD occurs in about 10–30 % of recipients after MSD-HSCT and in about 30–60 % after MUD-HSCT, while chronic GvHD affects about 30–50 % of patients after MSD-HSCT and about 60–70 % after MUD-HSCT. As much as 15 % of complications-related deaths following MSD-HSCT and UD-HSCT are caused by either acute or chronic GvHD.

The development of acute GvHD is initiated by proinflammatory cytokines (TNF-alfa, IL-1, IL-6) released from macrophages and antigen presenting cells (APC) activated in consequence of the conditioning regimen tissue damage, including damage to gastrointestinal mucosa, which in addition facilitate the dislocation of bacterial endotoxins enhancing further release of proinflammatory cytokines (Choi et al. 2010; Devergie 2008). These cytokines augment the expression of HLA antigens and activate antigen presenting cells of the recipient. During antigen presentation, mature T-cells present in the transplant material recognize the MHC/peptide complex through a specific receptor (TCR). Class I HLA mismatches stimulate CD8+ lymphocytes, while class II mismatches stimulate CD4+ lymphocytes. The effect of antigen presentation and stimulation of the activation pathway is an increase in the concentration of calcium in the cytoplasm and activation of protein kinase C and tyrosine kinases. In turn, the transcription of genes for IL-2, INF-gamma, and their receptors is activated. These cytokines induce cytotoxic lymphocytes (CTL), NK cells, and the release of proinflammatory cytokines by monocytes and macrophages. As a result, there is a cumulative, direct action of cytotoxic lymphocytes, and NK cells against the host's target cells (cells in the basal layer of the epidermis, epithelial cells at the renewal zones of gastrointestinal mucosa, interlobular bile ducts epithelial cells and hepatocytes, and cells of the endothelium of the blood vessels), which leads to their damage and apoptosis. The severity of clinical manifestations of acute GvHD in the skin, gastrointestinal tract, and liver, as well as the overall deterioration of the clinical performance are graded according to a five-point scale, from 0 to IV (Devergie 2008).

Among the factors on the donor side which have the strongest impact on an increased risk of acute GvHD the major one is the degree of recipient-donor HLA antigens mismatches and the type of donor (MMD > MD > MSD) (Jacobsohn 2008). Other important factors are: the source of HSCs (peripheral blood > bone marrow > cord blood), the dose of CD3 lymphocytes in the transplant material, sex of the donor (F > M) (Jacobsohn 2008) and, after HLA-identical HSCT, also disparities in minor histocompatibility antigens, i.e., in polymorphic gene products differing in the recipient and the donor (Milosevic et al. 2010). On the recipient's side, the risk of acute GvHD increases with the recipient's age.

In addition, there is also a significant importance of the method used for donor-recipient HLA matching, as the incidence of severe acute GvHD has markedly decreased after the introduction of high-resolution DNA matching for unrelated-donor transplants (Giebel et al. 2003; Jacobsohn 2008).

In the majority of recipients, chronic GvHD develops as a sequence of acute GvHD (Devergie 2008). The most important role in its etiopathogenesis is played by the impaired ability of the thymus, damaged by the conditioning regimen and/or acute GvHD, to select autoreactive Th2 lymphocytes (Teshima et al. 2008). As a result, autoreactive Th2 lymphocytes, released from the thymus to peripheral tissues, promote the synthesis of antibodies by B lymphocytes. Target organs are: skin, oral and gastrointestinal mucosa, conjunctiva, lungs, muscles and joints, urogenital organs, liver, serous membrane, hematopoietic system, and immunological system. Clinical manifestations of chronic GvHD are similar to those of autoimmune diseases of the connective tissue (Filipovich et al. 2005).

Among the risk factors that contribute to an increased risk of chronic GvHD, the factor to be listed first is prior acute GvHD. Other risk factors are: donor-recipient HLA mismatch, transplant from an unrelated donor, older age of recipient and/or donor, donor-recipient sex mismatch (F > M), the use of peripheral blood as the source of transplanted CD34+ cells, and the use of donor lymphocyte infusion in the post-transplant period (Devergie 2008).

There is a growing evidence that the risk of acute and chronic GvHD is also influenced by polymorphisms of genes in donor and recipient, which regulate expression or biological activity of cytokines and chemokines like TNF-alpha, INF-gamma, IL-10, interleukin-6 (IL-6), chemokine (C–C motif) ligand 2 (CCL2), chemokine (C–C motif) ligand 5 (CCL5) known as RANTES (Regulated upon Activation, Normal T-cell Expressed, and Secreted), interleukin-1 receptor antagonist (IL-1Ra), interleukin-23 receptor (IL-23R), interleukin-7 receptor alpha (IL-7R alpha), interleukin-10 receptor beta (IL-10RB), and chemokine (C–C motif) receptor 9 (CCR9) (Bogunia-Kubik et al. 2006a; Dickinson 2008; Loeffler et al. 2010). However, definitive results concerning significance of polymorphism await future genome-wide studies of large multicenter HSC recipients cohorts (Hansen et al. 2010).

The identification of the genetic risk factors for acute and chronic GvHD, concerning both the donor and the recipient, should contribute to further optimization of GvHD prophylaxis and treatment, consequently, to improvement of the long-term allo-HSCT outcomes, which now are significantly and negatively influenced by GvHD.

13.6 Conclusions

There is a growing understanding of the molecular background of allo-HSCT procedure for hematological malignancies, posttransplant leukemia/lymphoma relapse, and transplant-related complications. Molecular methods are nowadays commonly used in allogeneic HSC recipients for monitoring and early diagnosis of leukemia/lymphoma relapse and immunological, infectious, or toxic complications after allo-HSCT. They are also used to evaluate response to undertaken therapeutic interventions.The growing use of molecular methods at all stages of the allo-HSCT procedure and posttransplant monitoring creates a perspective for further progress and the improvement of long-term results in recipients transplanted for hematological malignancies.

References

Akashi K, Traver D, Kondo M, Weissman IL (1999) Lymphoid development from hematopoietic stem cells. J Hematol 69:217–226

Akashi K, Traver D, Miyamoto T, Weissman IL (2000) A clonogenic common myeloid progenitor that gives rise to myeloid lineages. Nature 404:193–197

Ansari M, Lauzon-Joset JF, Vachon MF, Duval M, Theoret Y, Champagne MA, Krajinovic M (2010) Influence of GST gene polymorphisms on busulfan pharmacokinetics in children. Bone Marrow Transpl 45:262–267

Bader P, Kreyenberg H, Henze GH, Eckert C, Reising M, Willasch A, Borkhardt A, Peters C, Handgretinger R, Sykora KW, Holter W, Kabisch H, Klingebiel T, von Stackelberg A; ALL-REZ BFM Study Group (2009) Prognostic value of minimal residual disease quantification before allogeneic stem cell transplantation in relapsed childhood acute lymphoblastic leukemia: the ALL-REZ BFM Study Group. J Clin Oncol 27:377–384

Bader P, Willasch A, Klingebiel T (2008) Monitoring of post-transplant remission of childhood malignancies: is there a standard ? Bone Marrow Transpl 42(Suppl. 2):S31–S34

Ball LM, Bernardo ME, Locatelli F, Egeler RM (2008) Potential role of mesenchymal stromal cells in pediatric hematopoietic SCT. Bone Marrow Transpl 42:S60–S66

Blank U, Karlsson G, Karlsson S (2008) Signaling pathways governing stem-cell fate. Blood 111: 492–503

Bochud PY, Calandra T (2009) A new step toward individualized antifungal prevention in hematopoietic stem cell transplantation. Clin Infect Dis 49:733–735

Bogunia-Kubik K, Gieryng A, Dłubek D, Lange A (2006a) The presence of the SDF-1-3′A allele is associated with a higher field of CD34+ mobilization in healthy donors donated PBPC for allogeneic hematopoietic stem cell transplantation. Bone Marrow Transpl 37(Suppl. 1):S218

Bogunia-Kubik K, Wysoczanska B, Lange A (2006b) Non-HLA gene polymorphisms and the outcome of allogeneic hematopoietic stem cell transplantation. Curr Stem Cell Res Ther 1:239–253

Cardenas PA, Huang Y, Ildstad ST (2011) The role of pDC, recipient T_{reg} and donor T_{reg} in HSC engraftment. Mechanism of facilitation. Chimerism 2(3):65–70

Carreras E (2008) Early complications after HSCT. In: Apperley J, Carreras E, Gluckman E, Gratwohl A, Masszi T (eds) Haematopoietic stem cell transplantation. ESH & EBMT, Paris, pp 181–196

Choi SW, Levine JE, Ferrara JL (2010) Pathogenesis and management of graft-versus-host disease. Immunol Allergy Clin North Am 30:75–101

Coppell JA, Brown SA, Perry DJ (2003) Veno-occlusive disease: cytokines, genetics, and haemostasis. Blood Rev 17:63–70

Cordonnier C (2008) Infections after HSCT. In: Apperley J, Carreras E, Gluckman E, Gratwohl A, Masszi T (eds) Haematopoietic stem cell transplantation. ESH & EBMT, Paris, pp 199–217

Devergie A (2008) Graft versus host disease. In: Apperley J, Carreras E, Gluckman E, Gratwohl A, Masszi T (eds) Haematopoietic stem cell transplantation. ESH & EBMT, Paris, pp 219–234

Dickinson AM (2008) Non-HLA genetics and predicting outcome in HSCT. Int J Immunogenet 35:375–380

Elhasid R, Krivoy N, Rowe JM, Sprecher E, Adler L, Elkin H, Efrati E (2010) Influence of glutathione S-transferase A1, P1, M1, T1 polymorphisms on oral busulfan pharmacokinetics in children with congenital hemoglobinopathies undergoing hematopoietic stem cell transplantation. Pediatr Blood Cancer 55:1172–1179

Filipovich AH, Weisdorf D, Pavletic S, Socie G, Wingard JR, Lee SJ, Martin P, Chien J, Przepiorka D, Couriel D, Cowen EW, Dinndorf P, Farrell A, Hartzman R, Henslee-Downey J, Jacobsohn D, McDonald G, Mittleman B, Rizzo JD, Robinson M, Schubert M, Schultz K, Shulman H, Turner M, Vogelsang G, Flowers ME (2005) National institutes of health consensus development project on criteria for clinical trials in chronic graft-versus-host disease: I. Diagnosis and staging working group report. Biol Blood Marrow Transpl 11:945–956

Giebel S, Giorgiani G, Martinetti M, Zecca M, Maccario R, Salvaneschi L, Holowiecki J, Locatelli F (2003) Low incidence of severe acute graft-versus-host disease in children given hematopoietic stem cell transplantation from unrelated donors prospectively matched for HLA class I and II alleles with high-resolution molecular typing. Bone Marrow Transpl 31: 987–993

Giralt S (2005) Reduced-intensity conditioning regimens for hematologic malignancies: what have we learned over the last 10 years? Hematology Am Soc Hematol Educ Program 2005: 384–389

Goekkurt E, Stoehlmacher J, Stueber C, Wolschke C, Eiermann T, Iacobelli S, Zander AR, Ehninger G, Kröger N (2007) Pharmacogenetic analysis of liver toxicity after busulfan/ cyclophosphamide-based allogeneic hematopoietic stem cell transplantation. Anticancer Res 27:4377–4380

Gorczyńska A, Turkiewicz D, Toporski J, Kałwak K, Rybka R, Ryczan R, Sajewicz L, Chybicka A (2004) Prompt initiation of immunotherapy with an increasing number of autologous cells after allogeneic HCT can induce complete donor-type chimerism: a report of 14 children. Bone Marrow Transpl 33:211–217

Gratwohl A (2008) Principles of conditioning. In: Apperley J, Carreras E, Gluckman E, Gratwohl A, Masszi T (eds) Haematopoietic stem cell transplantation. ESH & EBMT, Paris, pp 129–144

Hansen JA, Chien JW, Warren EH, Zhao LP, Martin PJ (2010) Defining genetic risk for graft-versus-host disease and mortality following allogeneic stem cell transplantation. Curr Opin Hematol 17:483–492

Hattori K, Heissig B, Tashiro K, Honjo T, Tateno M, Shieh JM, Hackett NR, Quitoriano MS, Crystal RG, Rafii S, Moore MA (2001) Plasma elevation of stromal cell-derived factor-1 induces mobilization of mature and immature hematopoietic and stem cell. Blood 97:3354–3360

Hows JM, Passweg JR, Tichelli A, Locasciulli A, Szydlo R, Bacigalupo A, Jacobson N, Ljungman P, Cornish J, Nunn A, Bradley B, Socié G, IMUST Study Participating Centers; Late Effects Working Party of the European Group for Blood and Marrow Transplantation (EBMT) (2006) Comparison of long-term outcomes after allogeneic hematopoietic stem cell transplantation from matched sibling and unrelated donors. Bone Marrow Transpl 38:799–805

Jacobsohn DA (2008) Acute graft-versus host disease in children. Bone Marrow Transpl 41:215–221

Kessans MR, Gatesman ML, Kockler DR (2010) Plerixafor: a peripheral blood stem mobilizer. Pharmacotherapy 30:485–492

Kröger N, Bacher U, Bader P, Böttcher S, Borowitz MJ, Dreger P, Khouri I, Macapinlac HA, Olavarria E, Radich J, Stock W, Vose JM, Weisdorf D, Willasch A, Giralt S, Bishop MR, Wayne AS (2010a) NCI first international workshop on the biology, prevention, and treatment of relapse after allogeneic hematopoietic stem cell transplantation: report from the committee on disease-specific methods and strategies for monitoring relapse following allogeneic stem cell transplantation. part i: methods, acute leukemias, and myelodysplastic syndromes. Biol Blood Marrow Transpl 16:1187–1211

Kröger N, Bacher U, Bader P, Böttcher S, Borowitz MJ, Dreger P, Khouri I, Olavarria E, Radich J, Stock W, Vose JM, Weisdorf D, Willasch A, Giralt S, Bishop MR, Wayne AS (2010b) NCI first international workshop on the biology, prevention, and treatment of relapse after allogeneic hematopoietic stem cell transplantation: report from the committee on disease-specific methods and strategies for monitoring relapse following allogeneic stem cell transplantation. part ii: chronic leukemias, myeloproliferative neoplasms and lymphoid malignancies. Biol Blood Marrow Transpl 16:1325–1346

Lam BS, Adams GB (2010) Hematopoietic stem cell lodgment in the adult bone marrow stem cell niche. Int J Lab Hematol 32:551–558. doi:10.1111/j.1751-553X.2010.01250.x

Lang P, Handgretinger R (2008) Haploidentical SCT in children: an update and future perspectives. Bone Marrow Transpl 42(Suppl. 2):S54–S59

Ljungman P, Bregni M, Brune M, Cornelissen J, de Witte T, Dini G, Einsele H, Gaspar HB, Gratwohl A, Passweg J, Peters C, Rocha V, Saccardi R, Schouten H, Sureda A, Tichelli A, Velardi A, Niederwieser D, European Group for Blood and Marrow Transplantation (2010) Allogeneic and autologous transplantation for haematological diseases, solid tumors and immune disorders: current practice in Europe 2009. Bone Marrow Transpl 45:219–234

Loeffler J, Ok M, Morton OC, Mezger M, Einsele H (2010) Genetic polymorphisms in the cytokine and chemokine system: their possible importance in allogeneic stem cell transplantation. Curr Top Microbiol Immunol 341:83–96

Majka M, Ratajczak MZ (2006) Biological role of the CXCR4-SDF-1 axis in normal human hematopoietic cells. Methods Mol Biol 332:103–114

Martin-Antonio B, Granell M, Urbano-Ispizua A (2010) Genomic polymorphisms of the innate immune system and allogeneic stem cell transplantation. Expert Rev Hematol 3:411–427

Mattsson J, Ringdén O, Storb R (2008) Graft failure after allogeneic hematopoietic cell transplantation. Biol Blood Marrow Transpl 14(11):165–170

Mehta J (2005) Cytokines in hematopoietic stem cell transplantation. Cancer Treat Rev 126: 333–351

Miano M, Labopin M, HartmannO, Angelucci E, Cornish J, Gluckman E, Locatelli F, Fischer A, Egeler RM, Or R, Peters C, Ortega J, Veys P, Bordigoni P, Iori AP, Niethammer D, Rocha V, Dini G; Paediatric Diseases Working Party of the European Group for Blood and Marrow Transplantation (2007) Haematopoietic stem cell transplantation trends in children over the last three decades: a survey by the paediatric diseases working party of the European Group for Blood and Marrow Transplantation. Bone Marrow Transpl 39:89–99

Milosevic S, Bachnick B, Karim K, Bornkamm GW, Witter K, Gerbitz A, Mautner J, Behrends U (2010) Identification of MHC II-restricted minor histocompatibility antigens after HLA-identical stem-cell transplantation. Transplantation 90:1030–1035

Molofsky AV, Pardal R, Morisson SJ (2006) Diverse mechanism regulate stem cell self-reneval. Curr Opin Cell Biol 16:700–707

Mullighan CG (2006) Petersdorf EW (2006) Genomic polymorphism and allogeneic hematopoietic transplantation outcome. Biol Blood Marrow Transpl 12(1):19–27

Mullighan CG, Heatley S, Doherty K, Szabo F, Grigg A, Hughes TP, Schwarer AP, Szer J, Tait BD, Bik To L, Bardy PG (2002) Mannose-binding lectin gene polymorphisms are associated with major infection following allogeneic hemopoietic stem cell transplantation. Blood 99:3524–3529

Napolitani G, Rinaldi A, Bertoni F, Sallusto F, Lanzavecchia A (2005) Selected Toll-like receptor agonist combinations synergistically trigger a T helper type 1-polaryzing program in dendritic cells. Nat Immunol 6:769–776

Nauta AJ, Fibbe WE (2007) Immunomodulatory properties of mesenchymal stroma cells. Blood 110:3499–3506

Petit I, Szyper-Kravitz M, Nagler A, Lahav M, Peled A, Habler L, Ponomaryov T, Taichman RS, Arenzana-Seisdedos F, Fujii N, Sandbank J, Zipori D, Lapidot T (2002) G-CSF induces stem cell mobilization by decreasing bone marrow SDF-1 and up-regulating CXCR4. Nat Immunol 3:687–94

Pihusch M, Lohse P, Reitberger J, Hiller E, Andreesen R, Kolb HJ, Holler E, Pihusch R (2004) Impact of thrombophilic gene mutations and graft-versus-host disease on thromboembolic complications after allogeneic hematopoietic stem-cell transplantation. Transplantation 78: 911–918

Plantinga TS, van der Velden WJ, Ferwerda B, van Spriel AB, Adema G, Feuth T, Donnelly JP, Brown GD, Kullberg BJ, Blijlevens NM, Netea MG (2009) Early stop polymorphism in human DECTIN-1 is associated with increased candida colonization in hematopoietic stem cell transplant recipients. Clin Infect Dis 49:724–732

Pulsipher MA, Bader P, Klingebiel T, Cooper LJ (2008) Allogeneic transplantation for pediatric acute lymphoblastic leukemia: the emerging role of peritransplantation minimal residual disease/chimerism monitoring and novel chemotherapeutic, molecular, and immune approaches aimed at preventing relapse. Biol Blood Marrow Transpl 15(1):62–71

Rocha V, Franco RF, Porcher R, Bittencourt H, Silva WA Jr, Latouche A, Devergie A, Esperou H, Ribaud P, Socie G, Zago MA, Gluckman E (2002) Host defense and inflammatory gene polymorphisms are associated with outcomes after HLA-identical sibling bone marrow transplantation. Blood 100:3908–3918

Rosu-Myles M, Bhatia M (2003) SDF-1 enhances the expansion and maintenance of highly purified human hematopoietic progenitors. Hematol J 4:137–145

Ruscetti FW, Akel S, Bartelmez SH (2005) Autocrine transforming growth factor-beta regulation of hematopoiesis: many outcomes that depend on the context. Oncogene 24:5751–5763

Satwani P, Cooper N, Rao K, Veys P, Amrolia P (2008) Reduced intensity conditioning and allogeneic stem cell transplantation In childhood malignant and nonmalignant diseases. Bone Marrow Transpl 41:173–182

Scadden DT (2006) The stem-niche as an entity of action. Nature 441:1075–1079

Schroder NW, Schumann RR (2005) Single nucleotide polymorphisms of Toll-like receptors and susceptibility to infectious disease. Lancet Infect Dis 5:156–164

Szczepanski T (2007) Why and how to quantify minimal residual disease in acute lymphoblastic leukemia? Leukemia 21:622–626

Teshima T, Wynn TA, Soiffer RJ, Matsuoka K, Martin PJ (2008) Chronic graft-versus-host disease: How can we release Prometheus? Biol Blood Marrow Transpl 14:142–150

Vettenranta K, EBMT Paediatric Working Party (2008) Current European practice in pediatric myeloablative conditioning. Bone Marrow Transpl 41:S14–S17

Wodnar-Flipowicz A (2008) Biological properties of haematopoietic stem cells. In: Apperley J, Carreras E, Gluckman E, Gratwohl A, Masszi T (eds) red. Hematopoietic stem cell transplantation. ESH & EBMT, Paris 34–44

Youn BS, Mantel C, Broxmeyer HE (2000) Chemokines, chemokine receptors and hematopoiesis. Immunol Rev 177:150–174

Chapter 14
Genetic Basis of Donor–Recipient Matching in Allogeneic Transplantation of Hematopoietic Stem Cells

Jacek Nowak and Jacek Wachowiak

Abstract An extremely high genetic polymorphism of the human major histocompatibility complex (MHC; HLA) and profound involvement of its products in multidirectional immune pathways produce an enormous challenge for the hematopoietic stem cell transplantation (HSCT). In this chapter, the organization and polymorphisms of human MHC genetic loci have been summarized and the so far recognized immune pathways of allorecognition have been described. Joint cooperation of the MHC products with killer cell immunoglobulin-like receptors (KIR) and presentation of autologous and foreign peptides including minor histocompatibility antigens (mHA) have been characterized for their role in clinical stem cell transplantation. Sources of HSC for transplantation and basic principles of family, unrelated, and cord blood unit donor–recipient matching have been delineated. Finally, clinical significance of HLA, KIR, and mHA mismatches has been discussed in the context of recent data on pediatric and adult HSCT outcome.

14.1 Introduction

Immune response in the allogeneic transplant donor–recipient setting is mediated by multiple genes, i.e., cytokine, drug metabolism involved, Killer cell Immunoglobulin-like Receptor (KIR), and minor histocompatibility antigen (mHA) genes. However,

J. Nowak (✉)
Department of Immunogenetics, Institute of Hematology and Transfusion Medicine,
Indiry Gandhi 14, 02-776 Warsaw, Poland
e-mail: szpik@ihit.waw.pl

J. Wachowiak
Department of Pediatric Oncology, Hematology and Transplantology,
Poznań University of Medical Sciences, Szpitalna 27/33, 60-572 Poznań, Poland
e-mail: jacek.wachowiak@plusnet.pl

M. Witt et al. (eds.), *Molecular Aspects of Hematologic Malignancies*,
Principles and Practice, DOI: 10.1007/978-3-642-29467-9_14,

the major histocompatibility complex (MHC) genes form the most potent and the most polymorphic set of immune response genes. In humans, the MHC genes and their product protein molecules are called human leukocyte antigen (HLA) system.

14.2 Polymorphism of the Major Histocompatibility Complex Genes

In humans, several MHC loci are extremely polymorphic. Class I and class II loci associated alleles are being approved by the WHO (World Health Organization) Nomenclature Committee for factors of the HLA System. According to the international ImMunoGeneTics information system/HLA (IMGT/HLA) Database 3.4 (2011), for the HLA-B locus 2125 alleles and for A and C loci 1601 and 1102 alleles have been recognized, respectively. HLA class II loci are also highly polymorphic. Although the total number of approved alleles is extremely high (6058 specificities in 6 most polymorphic loci) only no more than 10 % of them are confirmed to be common and well-documented (CWD) alleles (626 specificities in 6 most polymorphic loci) (Cano et al. 2007). The CWD alleles are defined as those revealed at least three times in the representative worldwide population sample of 25,000 individuals. In local population of unique ethnic background the number of CWD specificities can be much lower, e.g., 160 specificities in 6 most polymorphic loci for European Polish population (Nowak et al. 2008b).

14.3 Organization of MHC Genetic Region and Cellular Expression of HLA Genes

Human MHC genes are located in the region of 4 Mb in length within the short arm of chromosome 6 (p21.3). In this area, 421 genes were defined including 252 expressed genes and 139 pseudogenes, thus composing one of the most genetically dense regions of the human genome. The whole MHC is traditionally divided into three classes of genes. Genes located in the region of MHC class I and II encode for HLA genes, while genes located in central MHC class III region encode for molecules that are structurally and functionally distinct from HLA molecules.

The classic HLA class I genes comprise loci A, B, and C. Their products (HLA molecules) are expressed on the surface of nearly all nucleated cells and platelet cells. The expression of nonclassic and HLA-related class I genes (HLA-E, F, G, H and MICA, -B, -C, -D, -E, -F, respectively) is restricted to the surface of certain types of cells or tissues. The classic and nonclassic HLA class I molecules are heterodimers of α and β polypeptide chains. They are composed of $\sim$44 kDa heavy chain (α chain, encoded by HLA gene) and apparently monomorphic 12 kDa light chain, β2-microglobulin (β2-M, encoded on chromosome 15).

An α chain creates the HLA class I molecule groove of α1 and α2 polymorphic domains and forms class I antigen recognition site (ARS). Foreign or self protein derived peptide epitope, is anchored in the groove and presented to the T-cell receptor (TCR) forming MHC-peptide-TCR complex.

HLA class II genes are organized in HLA-DR, -DQ, and -DP subregions, each of them composed of several polymorphic loci (DRB1, DRB2/6/7/8, DRB3/4/5, DRB9, DRA and DQA1, DQB1, DQB3, DQA2, DQB2 and DPA1, DPB1, DPA2, DPB2) that encode α or β polypeptide chains. All loci of the class II region remain in strong linkage disequilibrium. The characteristic feature of the DR subregion is the presence of a haplotype that belong to one of five types. The presence of particular DRB1 allele is regularly associated with the presence of one of three genes, DRB3, DRB4, or DRB5 or the absence of any of those genes, depending on the DR haplotype.

Cellular expression of HLA class II molecules is restricted to B-lymphocytes and antigen presenting cells (APC). Expressed HLA class II molecule typically consists of α (33 kDa) and β (29 kDa) polypeptide chains. Highly polymorphic $\beta 1$ domain of β chain together with $\alpha 1$ domain of α chain jointly create HLA class II ARS (HLA class II groove) presenting peptide epitope to TCR.

14.4 Killer Cell Immunoglobulin-Like Receptor System

KIR system includes a set of genes located on chromosome 19 (q13.4) within the leukocyte receptor cluster (LRC) subregion (Wende et al. 1999). The content of the KIR gene cluster depends on the haplotype (haplotypes of two types, A and B). KIR haplotypes are composed of 8–14 tightly linked genes including the so called framework genes, KIR3DL3, KIR2DL4, and KIR3DL2, common to all haplotypes. Type A haplotypes are additionally composed of KIR2DS4 activatory receptor gene and typically 6 inhibitory receptor genes and two pseudogenes. Type B haplotypes are composed of framework genes and 3–5 activatory receptor genes, 3–7 inhibitory receptor genes and 2 pseudogenes. Except for the haplotype arrangement, the variability of KIR system depends on considerable allelic polymorphism, normal or null expression and partial deletions or sequence variations of some genes.

KIR molecules have 2 (KIR2D) or 3 (KIR3D) extracellular protein domains and long (L) or short (S) cytoplasmic tail; KIR with L and S tail exhibit inhibitory and activatory functions, respectively. KIR-dependent mechanisms of donor–recipient immune recognition is based on the ligation of MHC class I molecule through KIR ligation site with KIR molecules expressed by the natural killer (NK)-cells and natural killer T (NKT)- cells (McQueen and Parham 2002). Depending on specific 77–84 amino acid residue sequence, the HLA-C molecules may contain C1 or C2 epitope and HLA-B molecules may contain either Bw4 or KIR nonligating Bw6 epitope. The binding specificity of HLA-C and B molecules is determined by the epitope. Thus, those KIR-ligating HLA molecules belong to C1, C2 or Bw4 supertypic groups. Upon challenge, these HLA molecules form supertypic KIR-ligand pairs, such as C1-KIR2DL2 or C1-KIR2DL3, C2-KIR2DL1, and Bw4-KIR3DL1 (Carrington and Norman 2003). The NK cells can lyse the HLA class I mismatched donor or recipient cells when inhibitory KIRs remain unbound by the missing group specific HLA class I molecule (KIR type HLA class I mismatch) or when activatory KIRs or other NK cell receptors (C-type lectin receptors) deliver a predominant activating signal (McQueen and Parham 2002). The allorecognition and lysis is fast, because it is performed by NK cells, which are immediately available in the circulation and tissues.

The expression of inhibitory KIRs on single NK cell is stochastic, but after thymic development it is restricted to only those KIRs that can be ligated by individual's own HLA class I molecules (Schonberg et al. 2011). This way some KIRs are not expressed even though relevant genes are present. In many cases, the KIR phenotype can not fully reflect the genotype.

14.5 Minor Histocompatibility Antigens

mHA are the oligopeptide fragments of self tissue-specific proteins that are presented in the context of HLA molecules, differing in amino acid sequence (usually by one residue) between stem cell donor and recipient, due to genetic polymorphism in the human genome. Potentially all proteins may be a source of mHA peptides but only those of amino acid sequence discrepant between the donor and the recipient can be immunologically recognized. Moreover, the presentation of mHA is MHC-restricted and the certain HLA, the so called 'restrictive element' is obligatory for the clinical effect of mHA mismatch. Mismatched mHA can stimulate immune recognition and T cell cytotoxicity and cause the graft versus host disease (GvHD) and graft versus leukemia (GvL) effect in certain configurations of mHA mismatch and their restrictive elements.

The expression of proteins that are the source of mHA can be ubiquitous or tissue-specific. The idea behind current laboratory and clinical trials is to stimulate GvL effect with hematopoietic tissue-specific mHAs.

14.6 Immune Recognition and MHC Restriction

In the hematopoietic stem cell transplant setting the main function of MHC molecules is the presentation of the self or foreign structure to TCR or KIR receptor giving rise to the allorecognition. The allorecognition can be of indirect, direct, and missing self-type, and in graft versus host or host versus graft (HvG) direction.

14.6.1 Indirect Allorecognition

Foreign or mutated peptides, including mHA peptides, are presented in the HLA molecule groove (ARS) and the nonself structure is detected by TCR of na T-cells. The detection induces the selection of T cell clones with TCR of high affinity to the self MHC-foreign peptide complex further inducing the proliferation and cytotoxic T-cell type response. The reaction is MHC-restricted since the foreign peptides are recognized by the T cells only in the context of own HLA molecule. The time necessary for mounting of the immune response after indirect immune recognition indicates that chronic GvHD can be induced in this mechanism.

14.6.2 Direct Allorecognition

Mismatched (foreign) HLA molecule is the trigger of T cell cytotoxicity independent of the presented peptide. About 10 % of circulating cytotoxic T-cells are immediately directed against foreign HLA molecules and can be promptly activated in allotransplantation settings. The emergency of the direct immune recognition can indicate its involvement in the acute GvHD.

14.6.3 Missing Self

KIR-type allorecognition is dependent on the ligation of KIR molecule on NK cell to a specific part of HLA class I molecule expressed on any cell (KIR ligation C1, C2, or Bw4 epitope on HLA molecule). This way the killer function of NK cell is inhibited by self HLA molecule and can be activated in the absence of self HLA molecule (missing self).

14.7 Methods of HLA/KIR/mHA Genotyping

Different DNA-based HLA typing methods are used for hematopoietic stem cell donor/recipient matching. The sequence-specific oligonucleotide (SSO) probe hybridization, sequence-specific primer (SSP) amplification, sequencing-based typing (SBT) and reference strand-based conformation analysis (RSCA) methods in several modifications, are most frequently used. Similar methods have been adapted for KIR and mHA genotyping. For the details on chosen methods used for HLA, KIR and mHA genotyping see Chap. 21.

14.8 Sources of Hematopoietic Stem Cells for Transplantation

14.8.1 Perfectly Matched Sibling Donors

The optimal donor of HSC from bone marrow or peripheral blood is a sibling of the patient that is identical in both alleles of each of HLA-A, B, C and DRB1 (and DQB1) loci (8/8 or 10/10 allele match, so called perfect match) since these alleles are the most polymorphic and have been evidenced to be the most clinically relevant (Lee et al. 2007; Bray et al. 2008). Such matched sibling donor (MSD) is available for 15–30 % of patients, depending on the number of children in families.

14.8.2 Matched Unrelated Donors

For those adult patients who have no family donor, the optimal option is a perfectly matched (8/8 or 10/10 HLA alleles) unrelated donor (MUD). Furthermore, the 9/10 allele-matched donor with one allele (but not antigen) mismatch in any locus but DRB1 is also considered compatible (MUD) by European Group for Blood and Marrow Transplantation (EBMT) (Ljungman et al. 2006). This kind of donor is available for 30–90 % of patients, depending on the commonness of the HLA genotype in the registry of donors and the ethnicity of the patient.

14.8.3 Alternative Donors

All remaining patients (5–50 %) in need of allogeneic hematopoietic stem cell transplantation (allo-HSCT) are dependent on the alternative donors, i.e., mismatched donors (MMD) with different degree of HLA disparity.

Three main subsets of alternative donors for adult patients are partly mismatched unrelated (MMUD) or partly mismatched family (MMFD) donors with 6-8/10 alleles matched, partially mismatched (or fully matched, in rare cases) unrelated cord blood units (4–6/6 antigens/alleles matched in A, B and DRB1 loci) and haplo-identical family donors with one haplotype shared with the patient (5/10 allele match). The haplo-identical donor, preferentially mother or father can rarely fall into MD group and more commonly it is MMFD (5–8/10 alleles matched).

14.9 Family, Unrelated and Cord Blood Unit Donor–Recipient Matching

14.9.1 Search for Optimal Family Donor

The search for the optimal, preferentially perfectly matched family donor starts with initial HLA typing (A, B, and DRB1 at low resolution level; see Chap. 21) in the patient and in all members of his/her immediate family (siblings and parents). When potentially matched sibling or, in rare cases—parent, is found the confirmatory typing in second blood sample is performed in patient and potentially matched family member(s). The retyping is expanded with HLA-C (and DQB1) low resolution typing and matched donor–recipient pair is reported to transplant center. Initial HLA typing indicating lack of potentially matched family donor enables the decision to initiate the search for matched unrelated stem cell donor if unrelated HSCT is recommended.

14.9.2 Search for Optimal Unrelated Donor

In unrelated donor search process, the high resolution genetic typing level (see Chap. 21) of both patient and donor is necessary and confirmation of the typing results is obligatory. For cord blood unit (CBU) matching in A and B loci the antigenic level and in DRB1 locus the allele-level is considered (Kamani et al. 2008).

For pediatric patients the criteria of matched and alternative donors are virtually the same. The matched CBU is defined with 6/6 and 5/6 antigen (in A and B loci) and allele (in DRB1 locus) match (Kamani et al. 2008). Mismatched CBU is defined as 4/6 (or less) antigen/allele matched and no more than two mismatches of six defined between patient and donor are recommended.

The unrelated search is one of the most challenging medical procedures involving coordination of international transfer of medical and immunogenetic information between many specialized centers such as transplant, search and donor centers, and national registries. It is coordinated by specialized search center having link to worldwide unrelated donor databases (Bone Marrow Donors Worldwide—BMDW and/or European Marrow Donor Information System—EMDIS). The search for the optimal unrelated donor starts with the initial website/Internet-integrated database survey of all worldwide unrelated donor registries in one procedure. The survey gives the information on the number and provisional HLA type (commonly of A, B and DRB1 type at low/intermediate resolution level) of potentially matched (6/6 antigens) or one antigen mismatched (5/6 antigens) donors and on the addresses of their registries. In the following steps of unrelated bone marrow donor search the collection of the blood sample of the donor, sample shipment, physical examinations, and laboratory tests are performed as well as further necessary HLA typing and confirmatory HLA retyping are performed. The desired result of this complex procedure is the selection of the MUD with acceptable biological features and medical status. The HLA of matched donor–recipient pair and medical data of the donor are submitted to the transplant physician for initial acceptance, followed by further detailed donor examinations and information session (so called 'donor clearance'), stem cells collection and transplantation. In case of the lack of MUD, the search for an alternative donor should be carried out, provided that alternative donor is also recommended as the source of HSCs in the given patient.

14.9.3 Degree of HLA Mismatching

Since HLA mismatches increase the risk of post-transplant complications and mortality the decision on transplantation from a mismatched donor or the choice of other therapeutic options should take these risks into account. Only the mismatched donors with permissible mismatches should be accepted by transplant physicians for HSCT;however, the definition of acceptability is a matter of a permanent debate. The adverse effect on the HSCT outcome depends on the total number of mismatched alleles, locus of the mismatch, and the resolution level of the mismatch (antigenic/low resolution or allelic/high resolution level). The transplant outcome may be further influenced by the location of the amino acid substitutions, especially by those located in ARS of the HLA molecule, since ARSs are the structures that directly bind peptide and T-cell receptor (TCR). The number of amino acid substitutions and even amino acids substituted in specific positions within the HLA molecule might be of a great importance. KIR-ligation diversity is suspected to influence the transplant outcome as well. Since KIR mismatches are thought to have beneficial clinical effect (Davies et al. 2002; Pérez -Martinez et al. 2009) it is postulated in HLA class I mismatched transplants to select the donor with HLA molecule belonging to the supertypic KIR ligation group (of C1, C2 or Bw4 epitope) alternative to that of the patient.

It has also been postulated that MHC haplotype match is important for the outcome of HSCT (Petersdorf et al. 2007b). All these types of HLA disparity, described as risk factors for the transplantation outcome, can be balanced to some extent with the modified transplant protocols and nontransplant therapeutic options available for the patient. The beneficial GvL effect also depends on HLA mismatch (Tiercy et al. 2007), but it is difficult to keep the balance between GvL and deleterious high-grade GvHD (see also Chaps. 13 and 15).

14.9.4 Cell Doses in HLA-Mismatched CBU

The CBU transplantations in adult patients and in those pediatric patients with higher body weight encounter the problem of insufficient cell dose in the unit for the reconstitution of the hematopoiesis. The frequency of graft failure in CBU transplantations is increased with decreased total nucleated cell count and CD34 positive cell dose used for the transplant. This quantitative factor is as important as HLA match and is boosted by the number of mismatches (Barker et al. 2010). To overcome the limited cell dose in CBU a double CBU transplantation is performed, in which only one CBU is finally engrafted and the role of the second one is assistance and aid (Rocha et al. 2010). The immune phenomena determining which one of the two transplanted CBUs become engrafted are not clear, so far (Scaradavou et al. 2010).

14.9.5 Non-inherited Maternal Antigens in HLA-Mismatched CBU

An interesting finding in CBU transplantation was a favorable outcome in cases where some of the mismatched HLA-A or B antigens or DRB1 alleles in the recipient belong to non-inherited maternal antigens (NIMA) of the transplanted CBU.

The donor exposure to NIMA during fetal life can improve survival in unrelated CBU transplantation and might particularly reduce the risk of relapse in case of recipients transplanted to cure malignancies, indicating that cord blood cells can generate an antileukemic effect (van Rood et al. 2009). The selection of a suitable CBU from the registry database is thus based on finding mismatched HLA alleles in maternal HLA genotype (the HLA type of the mother of CBU donor must additionally be known).

14.10 Clinical Significance of HLA Mismatches

14.10.1 Outcome of Matched Family and Matched Unrelated Transplantations

Since 1998, when advanced HLA typing methods replaced DNA fingerprinting, serology, and low resolution methods previously used for final donor matching, the overall survival (OS) of transplant patients has much improved (Viollier et al. 2008). However, new regimens used to prepare patients for transplantation and new strategies to prevent and treat GvHD, infectious and toxic complications or relapse, have also favorably affected the transplant outcome (Vicente et al. 2007). The comparison of related and unrelated transplant outcomes has shown that survival, mortality, relapse, and high-grade acute GvHD end points in patients after HSCT from precisely typed perfectly matched unrelated donors reach comparable levels to those observed in patients transplanted from classical MSD (Yakoub-Agha et al. 2006). These similarities of the outcome suggest that well-selected MUDs can perform as good as MSD (Yakoub-Agha et al. 2006) or even better in older patients with comparably older sibling donors having sometimes burdensome medical history.

14.10.2 Role of the Number of Disparate HLA

The number of HLA mismatches between the donor and the recipient greatly influence the outcome of unrelated donor HSCT (Nowak 2008). It was confirmed by a large multicenter analysis in 4796 patients after myeloablative HSCT that the OS was significantly worse (37 % vs. 44 %, $p < 0.0001$) when single allele/antigen mismatched (9/10) transplants have been used compared to perfectly matched (10/10) transplants (Petersdorf et al. 2007a). After HSCT from unrelated donors with three and more than three mismatches, the 5 year OS has shown further systematic deterioration compared to fully matched transplants (50 % vs. 29 % $p < 0.0001$) (Petersdorf et al. 2007a). However, the administration of anti-thymocyte globulin (ATG) combined with standard immunosuppression regimen may lead to similar acute GvHD incidence in patients transplanted from the donors with one A, B, DRB1, or DQB1 allele/antigen mismatched (7/8) compared to 8/8 allele match (Finke et al. 2003). In children with leukemia, the similar regimen produced acceptable event-free survival and OS after transplantations from 7 to 8/10 mismatched unrelated donors (Sedlacek et al. 2008a).

14.10.3 Role of HLA Haplotype Disparity

Strong linkage disequilibrium observed within the whole MHC genetic system (Nowak et al. 2008a) suggests the existence of an extensive haplotypic disparity between recipients and allele mismatched donors. HLA haplotypes are known to be ethnically specific to a wider extent than alleles (Middleton et al. 2003) and haplotypic mismatches exert adverse effects on stem cell transplant outcome (Petersdorf et al. 2007b).

14.10.4 Role of HLA DPB1 Disparity

As for DPB1 locus, the allelic mismatch has probably no adverse effect on OS, but conversely, DPB1 genotype match increases the frequency of leukemia relapse (Shaw et al. 2007). DPB1 alleles can be grouped according to the similarity of T-cell epitope (TCE) groups; DPB1 allele mismatch against similarity group shows weak adverse influence on both OS and leukemia relapse indicating the existence of permissive and non-permissive mismatched DPB1 allele combinations (Sizzano et al. 2010).

14.10.5 Level of HLA Disparity and Amino Acid Substitutions

The level of HLA disparity (antigenic or allele-level) affects the HSCT outcome (Greinix et al. 2005). It was coherently shown in case of transplantations from adult donor (Greinix et al. 2005) and CBU in pediatric patients (Liao et al. 2007) that no deleterious effect of a single allele-level mismatch exists. The linear increase of the number of amino acid substitutions in the disparate HLA molecule may cause the significant deleterious effect (Ferrara et al. 2001) or be irrelevant (Greinix et al. 2005) in HSCT.

The specific location of an amino acid substitution has been described to be effective, with special adverse role of the amino acid substitution in position 116 of HLA class I molecule heavy chain (Ferrara et al. 2001), which may be explained by the key role of this amino acid in HLA class I peptide binding motif.

14.10.6 Phase of Disease and HLA Disparity

The deleterious effect of a given HLA mismatch was more evident in the patients with low than high-risk disease (Petersdorf et al. 2007a). For patients without a perfectly matched donor, it is sometimes a better option to immediately accept partly mismatched or haploidentical HSCT donor than to extend the search beyond the optimal phase of the disease (Tiercy et al. 2007).

In clinical settings, the allo-HSCT from the MMD with <9 out of 10 identical HLA alleles is associated with higher risk of graft failure, GvHD, and transplant-related mortality (TRM). However, nowadays a T-cell depletion in vivo, with or without a graft engineering in vitro prior to MMD-HSCT, significantly improves the engraftment and reduces the risk of severe GvHD. Therefore, if MSD and MUD is not available, the recent treatment protocols recommend the MMD-HSCT for patients with very high risk or advanced hematological malignancies. Indications for such transplantation are precisely defined in current treatment protocols.

14.10.7 Hierarchy of Mismatched Donors

If more than one MMD is available, the hierarchy of a stem cell donor selection is recommended according to results of HLA typing, CMV-status, gender, age, body weight, and stem cell source. An allele mismatch is preferred over an antigen mismatch, and a mismatch within HLA class I is preferred over a mismatch within HLA class II. In HLA class I a mismatch in C locus is preferred, while in HLA class II a mismatch in DQB1 is preferred over that in DRB1.

14.10.8 In Vitro and In Vivo Graft Manipulation in Mismatched Transplantations

Peripheral blood stem cells (PBSC) are usually recommended as the hematopoietic stem cell source for the MMD-HSCT. This kind of transplant enables the collection of the appropriate megadose of nucleated cells for immunomagnetic positive selection of CD34 cells or for combined immunomagnetic depletion of CD3 and CD19 lymphocytes. Both procedures, along with high dose of CD34 cells ($>10 \times 10^6$/kg body weight) assure prompt engraftment with low incidence of GvHD. In addition, the later procedure effectively protects the recipient from post-transplant lymphoproliferative disease (PTLPD) which is attributed to the reactivation of Epstein-Barr virus (EBV). The source of the EBV in HSCT recipients is donor-derived B-lymphocytes (Lang and Handgretinger 2008). Moreover, antithymocyte globulin (ATG) is given prior to the transplantation for CD3 lymphocyte depletion in vivo. Admittedly, the HSCT with the megadose of CD34 cells along with T-cell depletion in vivo guarantee engraftment, whilst low dose of donor origin CD3 lymphocytes results in low risk of GvHD. After transplantation of positively selected CD34 cells, an immunological reconstitution is considerably delayed, which predisposes to occurrence of life-threatening infections and impairs the GvL effects. This consequently increases the risk of post-transplant malignancy relapse (Petersdorf 2007). To avoid these adverse events some authors recommend HSCT from mismatched family donors (MMFD) (Lu et al. 2006) and from mismatched unrelated donors (MMUD) (Sedlacek et al. 2008b) without any graft manipulation, exclusively after myeloablative conditioning regimen and in vivo CD3 lymphocyte depletion with cyclosporine A for GvHD prophylaxis, usually along with short-term methotrexate treatment. The rates of GvHD and TRM as well as probabilities of event free survival (pEFS) and overall survival (pOS) observed in studied patients after MMFD-HSCT and MMUD-HSCT were comparable to those observed after MSD-HSCT and MUD-HSCT, respectively. However, Sedlacek et al. (2008b) emphasizes that patients transplanted from MMUD should demonstrate no more than 3 mismatches out of 10 alleles and no more than one allele mismatch in A, B or DRB1 loci. The authors also state that transplantation using an alternative donor mismatched at any of the HLA loci is still a risky procedure. Therefore, it demands an appropriate experience of a transplant center and high level of medical care during and especially after transplantation.

14.11 Clinical Significance of KIR Disparity

As demonstrated in patients with acute myeloid leukemia, KIR ligand mismatches improve the outcomes of HLA haplotype-mismatched transplants by controlling leukemia relapse without causing GvHD (Ruggeri et al. 2007). Recently, Pérez-Martinez et al. (2009) observed beneficial graft-versus-tumor effect after haploidentical HSCT in the presence of inhibitory KIR-HLA mismatch in children with metastatic solid tumors. In unrelated donor transplant settings (Giebel et al. 2003) significantly better survival in patients with the KIR-ligand type HLA incompatible than in those with either fully HLA-matched or HLA-mismatched (those of matched KIR-ligand type HLA mismatch) transplant has been detected, but other studies did not confirm this finding (Bornhauser et al. 2004). Moreover, in clinical studies NK-cell alloreactivity implicated either beneficial or deleterious clinical outcome of allogeneic HSCT (Nguyen et al. 2011). The strong immune reactions provoked by the T-cell type recognition of incompatible HLA molecule can probably override the favorable effect of the simultaneous KIR-ligand mismatch recognition (Lowe et al. 2003). Since both KIR-binding epitope and TCR-binding site coexist on the same mismatched HLA molecule it is difficult to clearly show the advantage of the KIR-ligand mismatch. Simultaneously, the immunogenetic selection of an appropriate donor (HLA-matched and KIR-ligand-mismatched) is hampered.

Table 14.1 Names and source proteins of HLA class I and II restricted mHAs, according to Minor Histocompatibility Knowledge Database (2006)

mHA	Name	Source protein
HA-1	Minor histocompatibility antigen HA-1	Protein kinase C conserved region 1 (C1)
HA-2	Minor histocompatibility antigen HA-2	Myosin IG (MYO1G)
HA-3	Minor histocompatibility antigen HA-3	A-kinase anchor protein 13 (AKAP13)
HA-8	Minor histocompatibility antigen HA-8	Pumilio domain-containing protein
HB-1H	Minor histocompatibility antigen HB-1H	Unknown
HB-1Y	Minor histocompatibility antigen HB-1Y	Unknown
ACC-1	Minor histocompatibility antigen ACC-1	Bcl-2-related protein A1
ACC-2	Minor histocompatibility antigen ACC-2	Bcl-2-related protein A1
ACC-6	Minor histocompatibility antigen ACC-6	Human Serpin-like protein
SP110/HwA9	Minor histocompatibility antigen SP110 (HwA-9)	SP110 nuclear body protein
PANE1/HwA10	Minor histocompatibility antigen PANE1 (HwA10)	Proliferation associated nuclear element 1
UGT2B17	Minor histocompatibility antigen UGT2B17	Uridine diphosphoglucuronosyltransferase 2, polypeptide B17
LRH-1	Minor histocompatibility antigen LRH-1	Purinergic receptor P2X, ligand-gated ion channel, 5
LB-ECGF-1A	Minor histocompatibility antigen LB-ECGF-1A	Platelet-derived endothelial cell growth factor (ECGF1)
LB-ADIR-1F	Minor histocompatibility antigen LB-ADIR-1F	Torsin family 3, member A (TOR3A)
CTSH	Minor histocompatibility antigen CTSH	Catepsin H
LB-MR1-1R	Not submitted	MR1 (MHC, class I—related)
LB-PTK2B-1T	Not submitted	PTK2B (Protein tyrosine kinase 2 beta, variant 4)
LB-LY75-1K	Not submitted	LY75i (lymphocyte antigen 75)
LB-MTHFD1-1Q	Not submitted	MTHFD1 (methylene tetrahydrofolate dehydrogenase NADP dependent 1)

14.12 Clinical Significance of mHA Disparity

In HLA-matched stem cell transplant settings mismatched allele of mHA locus, called HA-1, predispose to acute GvHD (Goulmy et al. 1996). Clinical efficiency of favorable GvL effect can be higher when hematopoietic tissue-restricted mHA mismatch is the case (Marijt et al. 2003) and it depends probably on both class I and class II molecules restricted mHAs (Matte-Martone et al. 2008). Apparent GvL effect of HA-1, HA-8 and HY mHA mismatches in acute lymphoblastic leukemia and increased frequency of chronic GvHD has been recently confirmed (Markiewicz et al. 2009). In younger patients and children and in the male recipient–female donor transplant settings the effect of mHA mismatch seemed to be strengthened. The nomenclature of mHAs is not yet systematic and sometimes even source proteins are unknown (see Table 1). A number of other mHAs have been discovered so far with diverse ability to provoke GvHD and GvL effect, including class I restricted (e.g., HA-2, HA-3, HA-8, HB-1H, HB-1Y, ACC-1, ACC-2, ACC-6, SP110/HwA9, PANE1/HwA10, UGT2B17, LRH-1, LB-ECGF-1H, LB-ADIR-1F, CTSH) and class II restricted (e.g., LB-MR1-1R, LB-PTK2B-1T, LB-LY75-1K, LB-MTHFD1-1Q) mHA peptides (see Table 1). In the cohort of 730 patients transplanted between 1996 and 2003 Spellman et al. (2009) have shown no effect of incompatibility at a single HA-1, HA-2, HA-3, HA-8 or HB-1, and CD31 locus on the outcome of HLA-matched unrelated donor HSCT. Although MHC-restricted it seems likely that the multiple mHA disparity is common in allogeneic HSCT settings and the effect of a plethora of unknown mHAs overwhelms the effect of the individually tested mHA.

14.13 Conclusions

HLA-A, B, C, DRB1, and DQB1 allele match between HSC donor and recipient is crucial for the outcome of transplantation. However, many immune-related genes (HLA and non-HLA) remain nontested, creating a potential additional risk for the recipients. The search for HSC transplant donor is one of the most challenging medical procedures; therefore, close collaboration of the transplant physician with the stem cell donor search center and HLA typing laboratory is essential for the selection of the best available donor.

Acknowledgments This chapter was partly supported by the Ministry of Science and Higher Education, grant N N402 351138.

References

Barker JN, Scaradavou A, Stevens CE (2010) Combined effect of total nucleated cell dose and HLA match on transplantation outcome in 1061 cord blood recipients with hematologic malignancies. Blood 115:1843–1849

Bornhauser M, Schwerdtfeger R, Martin H, Frank K-H, Theuser C, Ehninger G (2004) Role of KIR ligand incompatibility in hematopoietic stem cell transplantation using unrelated donors. Blood 103:2860–2861

Bray RA, Hurley CK, Kamani NR, Woolfrey A, Muller C, Spellman S, Setterholm M, Confer DL (2008) National marrow donor program HLA matching guidelines for unrelated adult donor hematopoietic cell transplants. Biol Blood Marrow Transpl 14(9 Suppl):45–53

Cano P, Klitz W, Mack SJ, Maiers M, Marsh SG, Noreen H, Reed EF, Senitzer D, Setterholm M, Smith A, Fernández-Viña M (2007) Common and well-documented HLA alleles: report of the Ad-Hoc committee of the american society for histocompatiblity and immunogenetics. Hum Immunol 68:392–417

Carrington M, Norman P (2003) The KIR gene cluster. National center for biotechnology information, U.S. national library of medicine, National Institutes of Health, Bethesda

Davies SM, Ruggieri L, DeFor T, Wagner JE, Weisdorf DJ, Miller JS, Velardi A, Blazar BR (2002) Evaluation of KIR ligand incompatibility in mismatched unrelated donor hematopoietic transplants Killer immunoglobulin-like receptor. Blood 100:3825–3827

Ferrara GB, Bacigalupo A, Lamparelli T, Lanino E, Delfino L, Morabito A, Parodi AM, Pera C, Pozzi S, Sormani MP, Bruzzi P, Bordo D, Bolognesi M, Bandini G, Bontadini A, Barbanti M, Frumento G (2001) Bone marrow transplantation from unrelated donors: the impact of mismatches with substitutions at position 116 of the human leukocyte antigen class I heavy chain. Blood 98:3150–3155

Finke J, Schmoor C, Lang H, Potthoff K, Bertz H (2003) Matched and mismatched allogeneic stem-cell transplantation from unrelated donors using combined graft-versus-host disease prophylaxis including rabbit anti-T lymphocyte globulin. J Clin Oncol 21:506–513

Giebel S, Locatelli F, Lamparelli T, Velardi A, Davies S, Frumento G, Maccario R, Bonetti F, Wojnar J, Martinetti M, Frassoni F, Giorgiani G, Bacigalupo A, Holowiecki J (2003) Survival advantage with KIR ligand incompatibility in hematopoietic stem cell transplantation from unrelated donors. Blood 102:814–819

Goulmy E, Schipper R, Pool J, Blokland E, Falkenburg JH, Vossen J, Gratwohl A, Vogelsang GB, van Houwelingen HC, van Rood JJ (1996) Mismatches of minor histocompatibility antigens between HLA-identical donors and recipients and the development of graft-versus-host disease after bone marrow transplantation. N Engl J Med 334:281–285

Greinix HT, Fae I, Schneider B, Rosenmayr A, Mitterschiffthaler A, Pelzmann B, Kalhs P, Lechner K, Mayr WR, Fischer GF (2005) Impact of HLA class I high-resolution mismatches on chronic graft-versus-host disease and survival of patients given hematopoietic stem cell grafts from unrelated donors. Bone Marrow Transpl 35:57–62

ImMunoGeneTics information system/HLA Database 3.4 (2011) Anthony Nolan Research Institute, European Bioinformatics Institute, London, Cambridge. http://www.ebi.ac.uk/imgt/hla/docs/version_r340.html (Cited 30 Mar 2011)

Kamani N, Spellman S, Hurley CK, Barker JN, Smith FO, Oudshoorn M, Bray R, Smith A, Williams TM, Logan B, Eapen M, Anasetti C, Setterholm M, Confer DL, National Marrow Donor Program (2008) State of the art review: HLA matching and outcome of unrelated donor umbilical cord blood transplants. Biol Blood Marrow Transpl 14:1–6

Lang P, Handgretinger R (2008) Haploidentical SCT in children: an update and future perspectives. Bone Marrow Transpl 42(Suppl 2):S54–59

Lee SJ, Klein J, Haagenson M, Baxter-Lowe LA, Confer DL, Eapen M, Fernandez-Vina M, Flomenberg N, Horowitz M, Hurley CK, Noreen H, Oudshoorn M, Petersdorf E, Setterholm M, Spellman S, Weisdorf D, Williams TM, Anasetti C (2007) High-resolution donor-recipient HLA matching contributes to the success of unrelated donor marrow transplantation. Blood 110:4576–4583

Liao C, Wu JY, Xu ZP, Li Y, Yang X, Chen JS, Tang XW, Gu SL, Huang YN, Tang PH, Tsang KS (2007) Indiscernible benefit of high-resolution HLA typing in improving long-term clinical outcome of unrelated umbilical cord blood transplant. Bone Marrow Transpl 40:201–208

Ljungman P, Urbano-Ispizua A, Cavazzana-Calvo M, Demirer T, Dini G, Einsele H, Gratwohl A, Madrigal A, Niederwieser D, Passweg J, Rocha V, Saccardi R, Schouten H, Schmitz N, Socie G, Sureda A, Apperley J; European Group for Blood and Marrow (2006) Allogeneic and autologous transplantation for haematological diseases, solid tumours and immune disorders: definitions and current practice in Europe. Bone Marrow Transpl 37:439–449

Lowe EJ, Turner V, Handgretinger R, Horwitz EM, Benaim E, Hale GA, Woodard P, Leung W (2003) T-cell alloreactivity dominates natural killer cell alloreactivity in minimally T-cell-depleted HLA-non-identical paediatric bone marrow transplantation. Br J Haematol 123: 323–326

Lu DP, Dong L, Wu T, Huang XJ, Zhang MJ, Han W, Chen H, Liu DH, Gao ZY, Chen YH, Xu LP, Zhang YC, Ren HY, Li D, Liu KY (2006) Conditioning including antithymocyte globulin followed by unmanipulated HLA-mismatched/haploidentical blood and marrow transplantation can achieve comparable outcomes with HLA-identical sibling transplantation. Blood 107:3065–3073

Marijt WAE, Heemskerk MHM, Kloosterboer FM, Goulmy E, Kester MGD, van der Hoorn MAWG, van Luxemburg-Heys SAP, Hoogeboom M, Mutis T, Drijfhout JW, van Rood JJ, Willemze R, Falkenburg JH (2003) Hematopoiesis-restricted minor histocompatibility antigens HA-1- or HA-2-specific T cells can induce complete remissions of relapsed leukemia. Proc Natl Acad Sci USA 100:2742–2747

Markiewicz M, Siekiera U, Karolczyk A, Szymszal J, Helbig G, Wojnar J, Dzierzak-Mietla M, Kyrcz-Krzemien S (2009) Immunogenic disparities of 11 minor histocompatibility antigens (mHAs) in HLA-matched unrelated allogeneic hematopoietic SCTOrganization of the leukocyte receptor. Bone Marrow Transpl 43:293–300

Matte-Martone C, Liu J, Jain D, McNiff J, Shlomchik WD (2008) CD8+ but not CD4+ T cells require cognate interactions with target tissues to mediate GVHD across only minor H antigens, whereas both CD4 + and CD8 + T cells require direct leukemic contact to mediate GVL. Blood 111:3884–3892

McQueen KL, Parham P (2002) Variable receptors controlling activation and inhibition of NK cells. Curr Opin Immunol 14:615–621

Middleton D, Menchaca L, Rood H, Komerofsky R (2003) New allele frequency database: http://www.allelefrequencies.net. Tissue Antigens 61:403–407

Minor Histocompatibility Knowledge Database (2006) Leiden University Medical Center. http://www.lumc.nl/rep/cod/redirect/5033/dbminor. Accessed Feb 2012

Nguyen S, Beziat V, Roos-Weil D, Vieillard V (2011) Role of natural killer cells in hematopoietic stem cell transplantation: myth or reality? J Innate Immun 3:383–94

Nowak J (2008) Role of HLA in hematopoietic SCT. Bone Marrow Transpl 42(Suppl 2):S71–S76

Nowak J, Kalinka-Warzocha E, Juszczynski P, Mika-Witkowska R, Zajko M, Graczyk-Pol E, Coiffier B, Salles G, Warzocha K (2008a) Haplotype-specific pattern of association of human major histocompatibility complex with non-Hodgkin's lymphoma outcome. Tissue Antigens 71:16–26

Nowak J, Mika-Witkowska R, Polak M, Zajko M, Rogatko-Koros M, Graczyk-Pol E, Lange A (2008b) Allele and extended haplotype polymorphism of HLA-A, -C, -B, -DRB1 and -DQB1 loci in Polish population and genetic affinities to other populations. Tissue Antigens 71:193–205

Pérez -Martinez A, Leung W, Munoz E, Iyengar R, Ramirez M, Vicario JL, Lassaletta A, Sevilla J, Gonzalez-Vicent M, Madero L, Diaz-Perez MA (2009) KIR-HLA receptor-ligand mismatch associated with a graft-versus-tumor effect in haploidentical stem cell transplantation for pediatric metastatic solid tumors. Pediatr Blood Cancer 53:120–124

Petersdorf EW (2007) Risk assessment in haematopoietic stem cell transplantation: histocompatibility. Best Pract Res Clin Haematol 20:155–170

Petersdorf EW, Gooley T, Malkki M, Horowitz M (2007a) Clinical significance of donor-recipient HLA matching on survival after myeloablative hematopoietic cell transplantation from unrelated donors. Tissue Antigens 69(Suppl 1):25–30

Petersdorf EW, Malkki M, Gooley TA, Martin PJ, Guo Z (2007b) MHC haplotype matching for unrelated hematopoietic cell transplantation. PLoS Med 4:e8

Rocha V, Crotta A, Ruggeri A, Purtill D, Boudjedir K, Herr A-L, Ionescu I, Gluckman E (2010) Double cord blood transplantation: extending the use of unrelated umbilical cord blood cells for patients with hematological diseases. Best Pract Res Clin Haematol 23:223–229

Ruggeri L, Mancusi A, Capanni M, Urbani E, Carotti A, Aloisi T, Stern M, Pende D, Perruccio K, Burchielli E, Topini F, Bianchi E, Aversa F, Martelli MF, Velardi A (2007) Donor natural killer cell allorecognition of missing self in haploidentical hematopoietic transplantation for acute myeloid leukemia: challenging its predictive value. Blood 110:433–440

Scaradavou A, Smith KM, Hawke R, Schaible A, Abboud M, Kernan NA, Young JW, Barker JN (2010) Cord blood units with low CD34+ cell viability have a low probability of engraftment after double unit transplantation. Biol Blood Marrow Transpl 16:500–508

Schonberg K, Sribar M, Enczmann J, Fischer JC, Uhrberg M (2011) Analyses of HLA-C-specific KIR repertoires in donors with group A and B haplotypes suggest a ligand-instructed model of NK cell receptor acquisition. Blood 117:98–107

Sedlacek P, Formankova R, Mejstrikova E, Keslova P, Hubacek P, Dobrovolna M, Vrana M, Kupkova L, Pittrova H, Stary J (2008a) Allogeneic stem cell transplantation in children with leukemia using human leukocyte antigen-mismatched unrelated donors. Pediatr Transpl 12:24–31

Sedlacek P, Mejstrikova E, Formankova R, Keslova P, Dobrovolna M, Vrana M, Stary J (2008b) Allo-SCT in children with high-risk leukemia using unmanipulated grafts from alternative donors. Bone Marrow Transpl 42(Suppl 2):S10–15

Shaw BE, Gooley T, Madrigal JA, Malkki M, Marsh SG, Petersdorf EW (2007) Clinical importance of HLA-DPB1 in haematopoietic cell transplantation. Tissue Antigens 69(Suppl 1):36–41

Sizzano F, Zito L, Crivello P, Crocchiolo R, Vago L, Zino E, Fleischhauer K (2010) Significantly higher frequencies of alloreactive CD4 + T cells responding to nonpermissive than to permissive HLA-DPB1 T-cell epitope disparities. Blood 116:1991–1992

Spellman S, Warden MB, Haagenson M, Pietz BC, Goulmy E, Warren EH, Wang T, Ellis TM (2009) Effects of mismatching for minor histocompatibility antigens on clinical outcomes in HLA-matched, unrelated hematopoietic stem cell transplants. Biol Blood Marrow Transpl 15:856–863

Tiercy JM, Nicoloso G, Passweg J, Schanz U, Seger R, Chalandon Y, Heim D, Gungor T, Schneider P, Schwabe R, Gratwohl A (2007) The probability of identifying a 10/10 HLA allele-matched unrelated donor is highly predictable. Bone Marrow Transpl 40:515–522

van Rood JJ, Stevens CE, Smits J, Carrier C, Carpenter C, Scaradavou A (2009) Reexposure of cord blood to noninherited maternal HLA antigens improves transplant outcome in hematological malignancies. Proc Natl Acad Sci USA 106:19952–19957

Vicente D, Lamparelli T, Gualandi F, Occhini D, Raiola AM, Ibatici A, Van Lint MT, Gobbi M, Miglino M, Clavio M, Risso M, Frassoni F, Bacigalupo A (2007) Improved outcome in young adults with de novo acute myeloid leukemia in first remission, undergoing an allogeneic bone marrow transplant. Bone Marrow Transpl 40:349–354

Viollier R, Socie G, Tichelli A, Bacigalupo A, Korthof ET, Marsh J, Cornish J, Ljungman P, Oneto R, Bekassy AN, Fuehrer M, Maury S, Schrezenmeier H, van Lint MT, Wojcik D, Locasciulli A, Passweg JR (2008) Recent improvement in outcome of unrelated donor transplantation for aplastic anemia. Bone Marrow Transpl 41:45–50

Wende H, Colonna M, Ziegler A, Volz A (1999) Organization of the leukocyte receptor cluster (LRC) on human chromosome 19q13.4. Mamm Genome 10:154–160

Yakoub-Agha I, Mesnil F, Kuentz M, Boiron JM, Ifrah N, Milpied N, Chehata S, Esperou H, Vernant J-P, Michallet M, Buzyn A, Gratecos N, Cahn JY, Bourhis JH, Chir Z, Raffoux C, Socié G, Golmard JL, Jouet JP, French Society of Bone Marrow Transplantation and Cell Therapy (2006) Allogeneic marrow stem-cell transplantation from human leukocyte antigen-identical siblings versus human leukocyte antigen-allelic-matched unrelated donors (10/10) in patients with standard-risk hematologic malignancy: a prospective study from the French Society of Bone Marrow Transplantation and Cell Therapy. J Clin Oncol 24:5695–5702

Chapter 15
Chimerism Following Allogeneic Transplantation of Hematopoietic Stem Cells

Małgorzata Dawidowska, Katarzyna Guz, Ewa Brojer, Jacek Wachowiak and Michał Witt

Abstract Posttransplant hematopoietic chimerism is a condition caused by allogeneic hematopoietic stem cell transplantation. The chimerism is characterized by the presence of at least two genetically distinct cell populations in the body of the transplant recipient. Chimerism monitoring is a recognized tool for documentation of engraftment or graft failure, for assessment of the risk of graft rejection, occurrence of graft-versus-host disease, and the risk of relapse. Analysis of chimerism kinetics enables early identification of these adverse posttransplant events, as well as early intervention through adequate treatment and assessment of treatment effectiveness. This chapter presents essentials of chimerism classification and clinical significance

M. Dawidowska (✉) · M. Witt
Department of Molecular and Clinical Genetics, Institute of Human Genetics, Polish Academy of Sciences, Strzeszyńska 32, 60-479 Poznań, Poland
e-mail: ma.dawidowska@wp.pl

K. Guz · E. Brojer
Department of Immunohematology and Immunology of Transfusion Medicine, Institute of Hematology and Transfusion Medicine, Indiry Gandhi 14, 02-776 Warsaw, Poland
e-mail: kguz@ihit.waw.pl

E. Brojer
e-mail: ebrojer@ihit.waw.pl

J. Wachowiak
Department of Pediatric Oncology, Hematology and Transplantology, Poznań University of Medical Sciences, Szpitalna 27/33, 60-572 Poznań, Poland
e-mail: jacek.wachowiak@plusnet.pl

M. Witt
International Institute of Molecular and Cell Biology, Trojdena 4, 02-109 Warsaw, Poland
e-mail: wittmich@man.poznan.pl

M. Witt et al. (eds.), *Molecular Aspects of Hematologic Malignancies*, Principles and Practice, DOI: 10.1007/978-3-642-29467-9_15,

of chimerism monitoring. Routinely used approaches for chimerism analysis are also discussed: analysis of short tandem repeat polymorphism with the use of fluorescent polymerase chain reaction and analysis of *indel*, null, and single-nucleotide polymorphism markers by real-time polymerase chain reaction.

15.1 Introduction

Hematopoietic chimerism is a state created in the graft recipient by allogeneic hematopoietic stem cell transplantation (allo-HSCT), characterized by coexistence of cells of at least two different genotypes (donor-derived and recipient-derived cells). In case of cord blood transplants from multiple donors, the presence of more than two genetically different cell populations may be observed (Berglund et al. 2009). The term *chimerism* comes from Greek mythology, which describes the monstrous Chimera being a combination of a lion, a goat, and a snake. In biomedical sciences the term *chimera* refers to an organism, developed spontaneously or created artificially, whose body consists of cells derived from at least two genetically different organisms of usually the same (or rarely different) species. In hematology the term was introduced in the field of experimental transplantology in the 1950s. Ford et al. (1956) performed the first allo-HSCT in mice, and with the use of chromosomal markers they showed gradual appearance of donor-derived hematopoietic cells in the body of the recipient. The animals in which the phenomenon of posttransplant chimerism was demonstrated were called by those authors' *radiation-chimaeras* due to the use of irradiation as a myeloablative pretransplant conditioning. Successful allogeneic hematopoietic stem cell transplantations performed in humans initiated further interest in the phenomenon of chimerism and its clinical implications.

15.2 Types of Chimerism

Defining the type of chimerism in a transplant recipient after allo-HSCT is based on the identification of the genotype of the recipient's blood or bone marrow cells and thus tracing their origin to the donor's or to the recipient's hematopoietic stem cells. Identification of cells of donor origin exclusively indicates complete chimerism (CC), co-existence of cells of donor and recipient origin is termed mixed chimerism (MC), while identification of cells of the recipient origin exclusively is interpreted as autologous recovery (AR), i.e., total lack of chimerism. Monitoring of dynamic changes in chimerism in the posttransplant period enables definition of three subtypes of MC: transient mixed chimerism (TMC), stable mixed chimerism (SMC), and progressive mixed chimerism (PMC) (Bader et al. 2005; McCann et al. 2005). The types and subtypes of chimerism are defined in Table 15.1, and their clinical significance is described in Sect.15.4.

Table 15.1 Types and subtypes of posttransplant chimerism (Bader et al. 2005; McCann and Lawler 2004)

Chimerism type/subtype		Definition
Complete chimerism (CC)		Cells of donor origin exclusively
Mixed chimerism (MC)	Stable (SMC)	Cells of donor and recipient origin, co-existing in relatively stable proportions even long after transplantation
	Transient (TMC)	Cells of donor and recipient origin, co-existing for some time after transplantation, and then converting to CC
	Progressive (PMC)	Cells of donor and recipient origin, with an increasing percentage of recipient DNA (at least 5 % increase in subsequent time points after transplantation)

15.3 Methods for Chimerism Monitoring

The basis for chimerism monitoring is the selection of appropriate biological markers (immunological, biochemical, cytogenetic, or genetic) enabling discrimination between cells of donor and recipient origin. Qualitative methods, used in the past, limited chimerism monitoring to the detection of mixed or CC and AR. Quantitative techniques, currently the only ones of clinical utility, enable not only differential identification of the donor-derived and the recipient-derived cells, but also precise quantification of the percentage share of both cell types in the recipient's blood or bone marrow. The most widely used approaches exploit short tandem repeat (STR) polymorphism detected via polymerase chain reaction (the STR-PCR approach), single nucleotide polymorphism (SNP), and insertion/deletion polymorphism (*indel*) detected via real-time quantitative polymerase chain reaction (RQ-PCR) (Alizadeh et al. 2002; Thiede et al. 2001; Hochberg et al. 2003; Vignal et al. 2002; Wiedemann et al. 2010). In recent years, there have also been attempts to apply advanced molecular techniques of SNP genotyping for rapid and high-throughput chimerism analyses. These include pyrosequencing (also termed real-time sequencing) (Fakhrai-Rad et al. 2002; Hochberg et al. 2003; Wu et al. 2003) and minisequencing (referred to as single nucleotide primer extension, SnuPE) used for multiplexed genotyping and quantitative analysis of SNP alleles using microarrays (Syvanen 1999; Fredriksson et al. 2004). These methods are characterized by high efficiency of allele discrimination, high reproducibility, and the possibility to automate the procedures. However, in terms of sensitivity, these approaches are similar to STR-PCR (5×10^{-2} for pyrosequencing and 10^{-2} for minisequencing) and far less sensitive than RQ-PCR (10^{-3}–10^{-2} in case of SNP markers and 10^{-5}–10^{-4} in case of *indel* markers). Therefore, pyrosequencing and minisequencing have not been implemented into regular chimerism diagnostics so far, unlike RQ-PCR or PCR-STR, regarded as the gold standards in posttransplant monitoring.

15.3.1 Analysis of STR Polymorphism by Fluorescent PCR

Chimerism analysis based on polymorphism of microsatellite sequences (also referred to as STRs) utilizes identification of cells of donor and recipient origin based on differences in the length of the amplified region. Its length depends on the number of repeats of the basic nucleotide motif (2–6 nucleotides) in the selected polymorphic locus (Agrawal et al. 2004). Polymorphic sequences are amplified in separate, parallel reactions, using DNA of the donor, of the recipient before transplantation, and of the recipient in the analyzed posttransplant time points. One of the oligonucleotide primers used for the amplification of each STR sequence is fluorescently labeled, to generate fluorescently labeled amplicons to be detected electrophoretically in a plate sequencer or in a capillary sequencer with fluorescence excitation and detection system. The time of amplicon migration, relative to the migration of appropriate DNA size markers, enables determination of the length of the analyzed PCR products, and thus discrimination between STR alleles of the donor and of the recipient (qualitative analysis). Different alleles are represented graphically as separate peaks. Quantification of PCR products is based on the intensity of fluorescence emitted by amplicons, which is represented graphically as the area of the peaks. Since the intensity of fluorescence is proportional to the amount of each PCR product, and hence to the amount of cells of donor or recipient origin, these data are used for quantitative analysis, i.e., determination of proportions between the cells of different genotypes in the analyzed sample (Khan et al. 2004; Jółkowska et al. 2005).

The STR-PCR approach is characterized by nearly 100 % informativeness (discrimination between individuals is possible in virtually all analyzed donor/recipient pairs) and sensitivity of 5×10^{-2}, i.e., it enables detection of the less abundant cell population at the level of 5 % (Bader et al. 2005; Alizadeh et al. 2002; Thiede et al. 1999). The high informativeness, relative technical simplicity, and wide applicability of this method are its evident advantages. The main disadvantage of this approach lies in the competition between the alleles of the donor and of the recipient, amplified in the same reaction tube (posttransplant time point), with the use of the same oligonucleotide primers, and the fact that shorter fragments amplify more efficiently than longer ones, which might cause a shift in quantitative results (Alizadeh et al. 2002). Analysis of STR-PCR results might also be hampered by the presence of unspecific peaks. These include: polymerase slippage products (generating peaks termed as *stutter peaks*), products of template-independent nucleotide addition by terminal transferase activity of Taq polymerase (generating additional peaks, which in combination with specific peaks form double peaks), and unspecific fluorescence of the fluorochromes (generating dye-associated fluorescence peaks) (Schraml and Lion 2003).

Reliability of STR-PCR results might be improved by simultaneous analysis of several STR loci with the use of differentially labeled fluorescent primers in a multiplex setting (Thiede et al. 1999, 2001). Chimerism quantification is performed by calculation of the mean percentage of the donor/recipient cells obtained via amplification of multiple STR loci, which results in high reproducibility, and low inter-assay variability. The use of commercially available kits enables standardization and easy comparison of the results between different laboratories.

The STR-PCR approach, in either the singleplex or multiplex variant, is currently one of the most common approaches for chimerism analysis, due to a wide applicability, and relatively low cost of the analysis. Its clinical significance for the assessment of engraftment is well recognized. However, in case of relapse prediction (particularly early relapse prediction in acute leukemias, often characterized by a rapid progression) the sensitivity and specificity of this method is controversial. Therefore, more accurate and sensitive approaches for chimerism analysis have been searched for, including those based on RQ-PCR and polymorphic markers such as SNP or *indel.*

15.3.2 Analysis of Indel, Null, and SNP Markers by RQ-PCR

The real-time PCR is one of the most sensitive methods currently used for chimerism evaluation. Unlike in classical PCR, the amplification products are analyzed in the real time (not at the end of the reaction) so quantitative measurements can be made in the logarithmic phase of PCR, when a linear relationship between detection signal and the initial amount of the amplifiable DNA/RNA is observed (Alizadeh et al. 2002). Various techniques for fluorescent labeling of PCR products as well as thermal cyclers for fluorescence intensity readings are available. Fluorescent signal is read through the lid or tube walls, so the risk of cross contamination is reduced.

Most common is the TaqMan technology, based on dual-labeled TaqMan probes (Alizadeh et al. 2002; Maas et al. 2003; Koldehoff et al. 2006) with reporter dye at the 5′ end (e.g., FAM, VIC) and fluorescence-suppressing quencher at the 3′ end (e.g., TAMRA) or TaqMan MGB (minor groove binding)—shorter probes with unlabeled quencher at the 3′ end and a crescent-shaped molecule stabilizing the probe matrix duplex (Harries et al. 2005). Regardless of the probe type, its complete hybridization with the amplified sequence immediately prior to the elongation step of PCR is required for subsequent probe cleavage due to the 5′ exonuclease activity of Taq polymerase. As a result, the released reporter dye emits fluorescence, which becomes more intensive from cycle to cycle. Another variant of RQ-PCR is performed with a pair of hybridization probes (HybProbes): one labeled with fluorochrome at the 3′ end and the other with a different fluorochrome at the 5′ end (Jimenez-Velasco et al. 2005; Martínez-López et al. 2010). The probes are designed to hybridize with the PCR product in close proximity, leading to energy transfer, and light emission. At the primer extension phase, the two probes are removed from the complex and fluorescence disappears; fluorescence intensity at hybridization corresponds, therefore, to the number of copies of the target sequence at the end of the previous cycle. Nonspecific SYBR-Green dye labeling of amplification products has also been used for detection of hematopoietic chimerism (Bai et al. 2006).

In the RQ-PCR, the initial quantity of the amplified sequence is determined by the C_T value, i.e., the cycle in which the fluorescence level indicates entry of the reaction into the logarithmic increment phase (Alizadeh et al. 2002). RQ-PCR chimerism evaluation is based on the C_T analysis for the donor/recipient differentiation markers, which determines the proportion (i.e., percentage) of the donor and recipient cells in the tested material. Some authors simply refer the C_T values to the calibration curves prepared separately for recipient-specific and donor-specific markers via a series of positive DNA dilutions in the fixed amount of negative DNA (MC reconstruction) (Maas et al. 2003; Harries et al. 2005). Others prepare calibration curves to determine curve slopes, and perform a control gene co-amplification for "normalization" of the target signals and amplification of a "calibrator" DNA, which corresponds to the recipient or donor genotype. In this system, the C_T value of the donor/recipient marker and the control gene for DNA after transplantation refers to the C_T value of the "calibrator" DNA in the mathematical formulas ($\Delta\Delta C_T$, Pfaffl's model) (Alizadeh et al. 2002; Jimenez-Velasco et al. 2005). The source of positive and negative DNA for calibration curves and the "calibrator" DNA is usually the DNA of the donor and of the recipient prior to transplantation. However, this material is not always available; therefore, it seems more rational to use the DNA from volunteers with selected markers for the analysis of the donor/recipient pair (Willasch et al. 2007; Guz et al. 2010). The same calibrators and calibration curves can be used for different donor/recipient pairs with the same marker(s).

The selection of the donor and recipient informative markers is essential for chimerism monitoring by RQ-PCR. Such markers should be selected from biallelic polymorphisms with a high frequency of heterozygosity in a given population. In contrast to the STR-PCR method, markers usually originate from different loci, with the exception of rare cases when the donor, and recipient have the opposite homozygous polymorphism in the same locus. To ensure high informativeness of the RQ-PCR method, particularly in related donor/recipient pairs, a sufficiently large number of markers has to be analyzed. According to published data, it is possible to differentiate 80–98 % of donor/recipient pairs with the use of 16–25 polymorphisms from 8 to 15 loci (Alizadeh et al. 2002; Guz et al. 2010; Maas et al. 2003; Koldehoff et al. 2006; Willasch et al. 2007).

The precision of RQ-PCR for determining low copy numbers of amplifiable sequence is high. The method is excellent for detecting chimerism of <5 % (Willasch et al. 2007) as well as 10 % (Masmas et al. 2005) or even 30 % (Jimenez-Velasco et al. 2005). Its precision, however, is insufficient for the high proportion of the marker in the analyzed sample (Masmas et al. 2005; Willasch et al. 2007). Parallel analysis of a recipient-specific and donor-specific marker is, therefore, required. In the absence of a donor-specific marker, it is only possible to analyze a marker specific for the recipient, which should disappear after transplantation. It is not recommended to perform chimerism monitoring based solely on the analysis of a marker of the donor. The low RQ-PCR precision for large proportions of the donor genotype means that the decrease in the percentage of donor cells may be overlooked if the donor marker is not confronted with that of the recipient.

Selection of appropriate polymorphisms and proper design of primers and probes is essential for obtaining exclusively specific amplification products. The best markers are insertion/deletion (*indel*) polymorphisms, due to no background signal from negative DNA, in the vast majority of cases (Alizadeh et al. 2002; Masmas et al. 2005). The sensitivity for MC detection with *indel* markers is high: 0.01–0.001 % (10^{-4}–10^{-5}), i.e., one recipient cell can be detected in 10,000–100,000 donor cells (Jimenez-Velasco et al. 2005; Masmas et al. 2005; Koldehoff et al. 2006; Guz et al. 2010; Chen et al. 2011). In the reports published so far, one can find descriptions of shorter *indels* (at least 2 nucleotides) (Alizadeh et al. 2002; Bai et al. 2006) and longer *indels* (Lo et al. 2000; Legler et al. 2002; Jimenez-Velasco et al. 2005). It should be noted that, in some papers the short *indels* are erroneously classified as SNPs (Koldehoff et al. 2006; Willasch et al. 2007).

Another group of markers used for chimerism analysis are *null* alleles determined by gene deletion (Alizadeh et al. 2002; Jimenez-Velasco et al. 2005). Genes from the Y chromosome or the *RHD* (Rhesus blood group, D, antigen) gene are commonly used in chimerism diagnostics, due to their phenotypic manifestation (male gender, Rh-positive blood group).

Analysis of SNP markers with the use of RQ-PCR is more complicated, due to a lower specificity and sensitivity of detection, resulting from a nonspecific amplification of the alternative allele (Maas et al. 2003; Harries et al. 2005; Willasch et al. 2007). The nonspecific amplification threshold can be lowered by changing DNA concentration (Willasch et al. 2007) or with the use of TaqMan MGB probes instead of conventional TaqMan probes. MGB probes hybridize more efficiently when full complementarity with the SNP is assured (Harries et al. 2005). Another option is to design primers with different variants of the nucleotide substitutions within 2–3 nucleotides from the 3′ end (Maas et al. 2003), which lowers the threshold for nonspecific amplification. Generally, the sensitivity of such methods does not exceed 1–0.1 % MC (i.e. 10^{-2}–10^{-3}). Nevertheless, SNP analysis offers a better chance of finding markers differentiating the recipient and the donor cells than those previously described.

Results of numerous studies suggest a high clinical utility of chimerism determination with RQ-PCR, mainly for the prediction of relapse and disease-free survival (Koldehoff et al. 2006; Wiedemann et al. 2010; Liesveld and Rothberg 2008). The possibility of MC detection in cases of very low percentage of recipient cells (<1–5 %) is emphasized (Alizadeh et al. 2002; Jimenez-Velasco et al. 2005; Koldehoff et al. 2006). Such a level of chimerism is below the STR-PCR technique sensitivity. Jimenez-Velasco (2005) and Koldehoff (2006) point out the higher RQ-PCR efficiency in detection of MC as compared to STR-PCR, particularly at early stages of relapse (at the molecular level). The average reported interval between molecular relapse detection and the onset of clinical symptoms was 58 days for RQ-PCR versus 37.5 days for STR-PCR (Jimenez-Velasco et al. 2005) or 119.6 days for RQ-PCR versus 29.4 for STR-PCR (Koldehoff et al. 2006). Another potential RQ-PCR application is chimerism testing in case of low DNA concentration, such as early evaluation of chimerism in isolated cell subsets, e.g., CD3, CD13, CD14, CD15, CD19, CD56, CD138 (Maas et al. 2003; Kroger et al. 2006;

Willasch et al. 2010). The absolutely lowest amount of DNA necessary for credible quantification of lineage-specific chimerism was reported by Willasch (Willasch et al. 2010), as at least 0.5 ng of DNA in a RQ-PCR reaction mix.

In summary, the advantages of RQ-PCR chimerism analysis comprise: high sensitivity and specificity, performance within a closed system to minimize the risk of cross-contamination, and universality of the PCR conditions (possible simultaneous examination of different markers). The disadvantages include: difficulties with selection of donor/recipient differentiating markers, possibility of significant method error for high proportions of donor chimerism when recipient marker selection fails, time-consuming stage of the multiple PCR standardization, and high costs of the search for donor/recipient-specific markers. Moreover, no standardization of RQ-PCR procedures for chimerism analysis in a regular diagnostic setting has yet been elaborated.

15.4 Clinical Significance of Chimerism Analysis

Clinical significance of chimerism analysis has been studied in different aspects of hematopoietic stem cell transplantation: indication for transplantation (malignant vs. nonmalignant diseases), conditioning regimen for transplantation [myeloablative vs. reduced intensity conditioning (RIC)], origin of transplanted cells (bone marrow transplant vs. peripheral blood stem cell transplant vs. cord blood stem cell transplantation), dose of transplanted nucleated cells, and/or CD34 cells, preparation of transplanted material (nonmanipulated graft vs. immunomagnetic positive selection of CD34+ cells vs. immunomagnetic combined CD3/CD19 depletion vs. T-cell depletion in vivo/in vitro), the type of donor/recipient relation (family donor vs. unrelated donor; matched vs. mismatched vs. haploidentical donor), HLA match between HSC recipient and donor (number of mismatches, loci, resolution level) or dependent on the type of the analyzed biological material (whole vs. fractionated blood or bone marrow).

15.4.1 Myeloablative and Reduced Intensity Conditioning for HSCT

Monitoring of chimerism is routinely performed after HSCT preceded by a standard preparative regimen, i.e., myeloablative conditioning, in both malignant, and nonmalignant diseases. Recurrent detection of MC after the period of engraftment is an alarming condition in this type of transplantation, since it predisposes to an increased risk of graft failure, and in case of malignant diseases, to an increased risk of relapse. Clinical significance of MC is dependent on its subtype (i.e., SMC, TMC, and PMC). However, MC subtype identification is only possible based on regular analysis of dynamic chimerism changes throughout posttransplant follow-up.

Chimerism monitoring is of particular importance after RIC, whose role in specific transplantation situations is still increasing because of its much lower toxicity, as compared to the myeloablative regimen (Lange et al. 2010; Bashey et al. 2010; Gonzalez-Vicent et al. 2010). Due to incomplete elimination of the recipient's hematopoiesis, posttransplant MC is observed in all HSC graft recipients, as a result of immunological tolerance between cells of donor and recipient origin. Thus MC is an integral part of RIC transplantation. In case of nonmalignant indications for transplantation preceded with RIC, it is usually not necessary to reach CC. Even partial restoration of hematopoiesis from grafted cells (MC) is sufficient for the therapeutic effect of transplantation, e.g., correction of immunodeficiency or metabolic defect (Mielcarek and Storb 2003; Bader et al. 2005). In case of malignant diseases, the therapeutic effect of RIC transplant is based on the graft-versus-leukemia (GvL) mechanism and appropriate immunomodulatory treatment, focused on protection of the GvL effect (short term/less-intensive immunosuppression) or on intensification of this effect (donor lymphocyte infusion, DLI). In some diseases, RIC transplantation is combined with targeted therapy, e.g., tyrosine kinase inhibitors in chronic myelogenous leukemia with the expression of *BCR/ABL* (*BCR*, breakpoint cluster region; *ABL*, Abelson murine leukemia viral oncogene) fusion gene. Donor T-lymphocytes, responsible for the GvL effect, i.e., for the cytotoxic reaction against residual leukemic cells, are expected to eventually eliminate both malignant and nonmalignant recipient hematopoietic cells, which is manifested as CC. Chimerism monitoring after RIC transplantation enables evaluation of immunotherapy effectiveness, aimed at reaching the best GvL effect with the lowest possible risk of the health- or even life-threatening graft-versus-host disease (GvHD), complicating such immunotherapy.

The significance of the type of conditioning before HSCT as well as clinical utility of chimerism monitoring after both types of conditioning are described in more detail in Chap.13.

15.4.2 Documentation of Hematopoietic Reconstitution

The basic application of chimerism monitoring after HSCT with myeloablative conditioning, regardless of indication for transplantation, is an assessment of hematopoietic reconstitution from grafted donor cells, documenting engraftment, nonengraftment, or graft rejection. Transient MC might occur in the early posttransplant period (Dubovsky et al. 1999). Its conversion to CC proves engraftment and complete reconstitution of lympho- and hematopoiesis from donor-derived stem cells (Khan et al. 2004). In most successful HSCTs, CC is detected at early posttransplant time points, but it is dependent on individual characteristics of the patient, the time of initiation of chimerism monitoring, sensitivity of the chosen chimerism monitoring approach, and the type of biological material used for chimerism analysis (whole/fractionated blood or bone marrow). Exclusive detection of recipient-derived cells after HSCT (no chimerism) is the evidence for nonengraftment or graft rejection, if preceded by detection of CC. Detection of progressive MC suggests imminent graft rejection. In recipients with hematological malignancy, it may also indicate imminent relapse of the malignant process (Maury et al. 2001).

15.4.3 GvHD and Relapse Risk Assessment

Graft versus host disease is one of the most common and most serious complications of allo-HSCT, particularly in case of transplantations from nonrelated donors and mismatched donors. GvHD (accompanied by the GvL effect in patients transplanted for malignant diseases) is caused by an immune response of donor-derived immunocompetent cells against host tissues (Barrett and Le Blanc 2008; Couriel et al. 2004; Khan et al. 2004; Kolb 2008). The pathogenesis and symptoms of acute and chronic GvHD are described in more detail in Chap.13.

Immunosuppressive prophylaxis of GvHD decreases the efficiency of the therapeutic GvL effect, and hence increases the risk of relapse. Therefore, optimal GvHD management, aimed at simultaneous protection of the GvL effect, is a major challenge after allo-HSCT (Barrett and Le Blanc 2008). Occurrence of transient or stable MC, particularly in T-lymphocyte lineage, reflects immunological tolerance between cells of donor and recipient origin, and decreases the risk of both acute and chronic GvHD, but simultaneously increases the risk of relapse, due to reduction of the GvL effect (Ramirez et al. 1996; Mackinnon et al. 1994; Bader et al. 2008). Diagnostics and monitoring of GvHD is mainly based on clinical symptoms, while chimerism monitoring is applied for the assessment of the risk of GvHD, the effectiveness of GvHD prophylaxis, and for prediction/early detection of relapse, which might be induced by excessive GvHD prophylaxis (Sairafi et al. 2010).

15.4.4 Relapse

The possibility of an early detection of relapse after allo-HSCT performed in malignant diseases [acute lymphoblastic leukemia (ALL), acute myelogenous leukemia, chronic myelogenous leukemia, myelodysplastic syndrome] is one of the major, but also one of the most disputable, aspects of chimerism monitoring (Thiede et al. 2004; Bader et al. 1998, 2005; Gardiner et al. 1997; van Leeuwen et al. 1993; Ramirez et al. 1996; Wiedemann et al. 2010; Horky et al. 2011). It should be noted that, the effectiveness of early relapse detection is dependent on multiple factors, such as the underlying disease, pre-HSCT conditioning regimen, sensitivity of chimerism monitoring, and frequency and regularity of sample collection for chimerism analysis. Systematic monitoring of chimerism kinetics, performed in short time intervals with the use of highly sensitive methods, is particularly important in case of acute leukemias, often characterized by rapid relapse occurrence (Bader et al. 2004; Zeiser et al. 2005; Horky et al. 2011). For instance, in childhood ALL it is recommended to analyze chimerism in 1–2 week intervals, at least in an early posttransplant period (till day +100 posttransplant) but prolonged monitoring (until day +200) is suggested, followed by monitoring of chimerism once a month until month +18 posttransplant (Bader et al. 2005, 2008). The use of the highly sensitive approach (preferably RQ-PCR) enables detection of recipient-derived cells present at low levels (early detection of molecular relapse) as well as with the use of a low DNA concentration (the assessment of chimerism at early time points after HSCT) (Antin et al. 2001; Alizadeh et al. 2002; Horky et al. 2011; Wiedemann et al. 2010).

Before the introduction of quantitative methods into chimerism assessment, the sole fact of MC detection was regarded as a poor prognostic factor, predicting impending relapse. The implementation of quantitative techniques and gradual improvement of their sensitivity revealed that MC is often observed in patients who do not experience leukemia relapse. These usually low levels of recipient-derived cells, detected transiently or rarely stable after HSCT (TMC or SMC, respectively) constitute a population of residual nonmalignant host cells not eliminated through preHSCT conditioning. In contrast to progressive MC, transient and stable MC do not correlate with relapse (Serrano et al. 2000; Wiedemann et al. 2010). Progressive MC, identified by an increasing percentage of recipient-derived cells in subsequent chimerism analyses, reflects proliferation of malignant cells, which might initiate relapse if not eliminated by the GvL effect. Clinical significance of progressive MC as a prognostic factor for relapse has already been well documented (Bader et al. 1998, 2004; Ramirez et al. 1996; Serrano et al. 2000; Zeiser et al. 2005; Barrios et al. 2003; Horky et al. 2011). Identification of progressive MC, regarded as evidence for molecular relapse, is an indication for immunomodulatory treatment (DLI and/or reduction of immunosuppression) aimed at prevention of hematological and clinical relapse (Gorczynska et al. 2004; Formankova et al. 2003; Bader et al. 2004; Klingebiel and Bader 2008).

15.4.5 Lineage-Specific Chimerism

In recent years, there has been increasing interest in chimerism monitoring in specific cell subsets (lineage chimerism), separated from whole blood or bone marrow with the use of immunomagnetic or flow cytometric methods (Lion 2007). Monitoring of chimerism kinetics in selected cell lineages provides a more sensitive and specific tool for posttransplant assessment, as compared to analysis of unfractionated material. Hence it enables more adequate therapeutic decisions aimed at graft failure and relapse prevention (Lion 2007; Baron et al. 2004; Miura et al. 2006; Mattsson et al. 2001; Serrano et al. 2000; Maury et al. 2001; Antin et al. 2001; Sairafi et al. 2010; Bornhauser et al. 2009; Horn et al. 2009). The vast majority of literature data on lineage chimerism is focused on T lymphocytes (Childs et al. 1999; Baron et al. 2004; van Leeuwen et al. 1993; Serrano et al. 2000; Maury et al. 2001), B lymphocytes

(Zetterquist et al. 2000; Lion et al. 2001; Serrano et al. 2000; Maury et al. 2001), natural killer (NK) cells (Serrano et al. 2000; Maury et al. 2001; Baron et al. 2004), and CD34+ cells (Thiede et al. 2004; Lange et al. 2010; Bornhauser et al. 2009). Clinical significance of lineage-specific chimerism was studied in the context of the type of preHSCT conditioning (Serrano et al. 2000), the occurrence and treatment of GvHD and relapse (Zeiser et al. 2005; Mattsson et al. 2001), and graft failure (Lim et al. 2008; Baron et al. 2004; Maury et al. 2001).

The choice of an appropriate cell subset for chimerism monitoring determines its prognostic significance. Chimerism monitoring in cell lineage from which leukemia originated (leukemia lineage-specific chimerism) has been documented to have the highest clinical value for relapse prediction (Lion et al. 2001; Mattsson et al. 2001; van Leeuwen et al. 1993; Winiarski et al. 2000). Additionally, it has been suggested that, regardless of the type of malignancy, chimerism monitoring in the T-cell subset has particular clinical utility, due to their key role in the therapeutic GvL effect. According to this hypothesis, T-lineage MC increases the risk of relapse through immunological tolerance between cells of donor and recipient origin, which reduces the GvL effect (Mackinnon et al. 1994; Bader et al. 2005). However, there are also reports on a lack of correlation between T-lymphoid chimerism and relapse (Mattsson et al. 2001; van Leeuwen et al. 1993). Moreover, the role of NK-lineage chimerism in relapse prediction has been reported in case of childhood ALL, although not confirmed in adult patients (Guimond et al. 2000). Recently published reports indicate that chimerism monitoring with the use of RQ-PCR in selected cell subsets, particularly CD34+ cells, is highly predictive of relapse and yields results comparable to those of minimal residual disease (MRD) monitoring (Bacher et al. 2011; Lange et al. 2010; Wiedemann et al. 2010; Horky et al. 2011; Bornhauser et al. 2009). Therefore, this approach might be considered as an alternative to MRD testing, particularly in patients with no suitable markers for MRD analysis.

When lineage chimerism analysis is aimed at the assessment of the risk of graft failure and GvHD, then T-lymphocytes are of the greatest predictive value, due to their role in GvHD, and the GvL effect. Detection of T-lineage CC until day +100 postHSCT (Lim et al. 2008) or a high percentage of donor-derived T-lymphocytes early after transplantation (until day +28 postHSCT) (Baron et al. 2004) predisposes to acute GvHD. Additionally, T-lineage MC is regarded as the risk factor of graft rejection; the risk increases with progressive MC or with conversion from MC to AR, i.e., exclusive detection of recipient-derived cells (Dubovsky et al. 1999; Maury et al. 2001).

15.5 Chimerism and Minimal Residual Disease

Applicability of chimerism monitoring for detection and quantitative assessment of dynamic changes of residual disease is still disputable (Schilham et al. 2005; Khan et al. 2004; Bader et al. 2008; Horky et al. 2011). An effort has been made to address the question whether chimerism and MRD analyses might be used as alternative or complementary tools for posttransplant monitoring (Serrano et al. 2000; Zetterquist et al. 2000; Perez-Simon et al. 2002; Bornhauser et al. 2009). The vast majority of data on simultaneous analyses of chimerism and MRD comes from ALL studies. The basic difference between chimerism and MRD monitoring lies in the type of markers chosen for the analysis, which significantly influences specificity and sensitivity of the assays. Monitoring of MRD is aimed at a selective detection of residual leukemic cells, while in case of chimerism analysis; recipient-derived cells are detected without discrimination between residual malignant and normal cells. This is reflected by different sensitivities reached with currently available methods: 10^{-4}–10^{-6} in case of MRD quantification (van der Velden et al. 2003; Jółkowska et al. 2007) and 5×10^{-2}–10^{-4} in case of chimerism monitoring (Alizadeh et al. 2002), which might be increased to 10^{-3}–10^{-5} by analysis performed in cell subsets (Lion 2007; Bader et al. 2005).

However, there are also advantages of chimerism study over molecular post-transplant MRD monitoring. Diagnostic procedures are less complex (hence faster and more available) and most often exploit universal polymorphisms present in all patients, in contrast to molecular MRD analyses based on the detection of leukemia-specific or even patient-specific markers, limiting applicability of the approach (Stumph et al. 2008). Chimerism monitoring for relapse risk assessment seems to be of special value in case of acute myeloblastic leukemia, myeloblastic syndrome, and *BCR/ABL*-negative chronic myelogenous leukemia, i.e., in hematological malignancies without established, standardized, and sensitive methods of MRD monitoring. Moreover, all the abovementioned malignancies demonstrate a better response to early immune interventions than ALL. Thus an early diagnosis of imminent postHSCT relapse is of particular importance in all of them. Additionally, results of chimerism analyses with the use of bone marrow and blood are largely comparable, which is not the case in MRD diagnostics. The necessity of bone marrow aspiration is a major obstacle for the use of MRD in posttransplant assessment, particularly in case of acute leukemias, requiring intensive monitoring. Combination of chimerism analysis (particularly the leukemia-specific lineage chimerism) with posttransplant MRD monitoring offers the possibility to identify patients at risk of graft rejection and malignancy relapse, and enables the most adequate decisions on prevention and treatment of these adverse posttransplant events (Bader et al. 2008).

15.6 Conclusions

Chimerism analysis after allo-HSCT is a highly appreciated tool for the documentation of engraftment and the assessment of hematopoietic reconstitution. It is also useful for the assessment of the risk of GvHD and the risk of relapse, in case of hematological malignancies, enabling early intervention with the appropriate preventive treatment. However, the effectiveness of chimerism analysis for early detection of disease recurrence is still disputable. It is strongly dependent on the appropriate schedule of sample collection and the sensitivity of the approach chosen for chimerism monitoring. Analysis of STR polymorphism with the use of conventional PCR, still regarded as the basic tool for chimerism analysis, is currently being replaced by the highly sensitive RQ-PCR approach. The most recent data indicate that monitoring of posttransplant chimerism with this approach, particularly in selected cell subsets, is significantly informative of the risk of disease recurrence and yields highly concordant results with those of MRD monitoring. Therefore, RQ-PCR might be considered as an alternative to MRD testing, especially in case of hematological malignancies without standardized methods of MRD monitoring. RQ-PCR enables early identification of impending relapse, thus facilitating early, and potentially more successful preventive treatment. However, it should also be noted that current possibilities for therapeutic interventions in patients with impending postHSCT relapse are still of limited effectiveness. Therefore, chimerism testing might provide a sensitive tool for the evaluation of molecular response to novel therapeutic strategies.

Acknowledgments This chapter was partly supported by the Ministry of Science and Higher Education, grant N N407 311 839.

References

Agrawal S, Khan F, Talwar S, Nityanand S (2004) Short tandem repeat technology has diverse applications: individual identification, phylogenetic reconstruction and chimerism based post haematopoietic stem cell transplantation graft monitoring. Indian J Med Sci 58(7):297–304

Alizadeh M, Bernard M, Danic B, Dauriac C, Birebent B, Lapart C, Lamy T, Le Prise PY, Beauplet A, Bories D, Semana G, Quelvennec E (2002) Quantitative assessment of hematopoietic chimerism after bone marrow transplantation by real-time quantitative polymerase chain reaction. Blood 99(12):4618–4625

Antin JH, Childs R, Filipovich AH, Giralt S, Mackinnon S, Spitzer T, Weisdorf D (2001) Establishment of complete and mixed donor chimerism after allogeneic lymphohematopoietic transplantation: recommendations from a workshop at the 2001 Tandem Meetings of the International Bone Marrow Transplant Registry and the American Society of Blood and Marrow Transplantation. Biol Blood Marrow Transplant 7(9):473–485. doi:10.1053/bbmt.2001.v7.pm11669214, S1083-8791(01)50035-3X [pii]

Bacher U, Haferlach T, Fehse B, Schnittger S, Kroger N (2011) Minimal residual disease diagnostics and chimerism in the post-transplant period in acute myeloid leukemia. Sci World J 11:310–319. doi:10.1100/tsw.2011.16, 1704715 [pii]

Bader P, Beck J, Frey A, Schlegel PG, Hebarth H, Handgretinger R, Einsele H, Niemeyer C, Benda N, Faul C, Kanz L, Niethammer D, Klingebiel T (1998) Serial and quantitative analysis of mixed hematopoietic chimerism by PCR in patients with acute leukemias allows the prediction of relapse after allogeneic BMT. Bone Marrow Transplant 21(5):487–495

Bader P, Kreyenberg H, Hoelle W, Dueckers G, Handgretinger R, Lang P, Kremens B, Dilloo D, Sykora KW, Schrappe M, Niemeyer C, Von Stackelberg A, Gruhn B, Henze G, Greil J, Niethammer D, Dietz K, Beck JF, Klingebiel T (2004) Increasing mixed chimerism is an important prognostic factor for unfavorable outcome in children with acute lymphoblastic leukemia after allogeneic stem-cell transplantation: possible role for pre-emptive immunotherapy? J Clin Oncol 22(9):1696–1705

Bader P, Niethammer D, Willasch A, Kreyenberg H, Klingebiel T (2005) How and when should we monitor chimerism after allogeneic stem cell transplantation? Bone Marrow Transplant 35(2):107–119. doi:10.1038/sj.bmt.1704715, 1704715 [pii]

Bader P, Willasch A, Klingebiel T (2008) Monitoring of post-transplant remission of childhood malignancies: is there a standard? Bone Marrow Transplant 42(Suppl 2):S31–S34. doi:10.1038/bmt.2008.280, bmt2008280 [pii]

Bai L, Deng YM, Dodds AJ, Milliken S, Moore J, Ma DD (2006) A SYBR green-based real-time PCR method for detection of haemopoietic chimerism in allogeneic haemopoietic stem cell transplant recipients. Eur J Haematol 77(5):425–431. doi:10.1111/j.1600-0609.2006.00729.x, EJH729 [pii]

Baron F, Baker JE, Storb R, Gooley TA, Sandmaier BM, Maris MB, Maloney DG, Heimfeld S, Oparin D, Zellmer E, Radich JP, Grumet FC, Blume KG, Chauncey TR, Little MT (2004) Kinetics of engraftment in patients with hematologic malignancies given allogeneic hematopoietic cell transplantation after nonmyeloablative conditioning. Blood 104(8):2254–2262. doi:10.1182/blood-2004-04-1506, 2004-04-1506 [pii]

Barrett AJ, Le Blanc K (2008) Prophylaxis of acute GVHD: manipulate the graft or the environment? Best Pract Res Clin Haematol 21(2):165–176. doi:10.1016/j.beha.2008.02.004, S1521-6926(08)00005-4 [pii]

Barrios M, Jimenez-Velasco A, Roman-Gomez J, Madrigal ME, Castillejo JA, Torres A, Heiniger A (2003) Chimerism status is a useful predictor of relapse after allogeneic stem cell transplantation for acute leukemia. Haematologica 88(7):801–810

Bashey A, Owzar K, Johnson JL, Edwards PS, Kelly M, Baxter-Lowe LA, Devine S, Farag S, Hurd D, Ball E, McCarthy P, Lister J, Shea TC, Linker C (2010) Reduced-intensity conditioning allogeneic hematopoietic cell transplantation for patients with hematologic malignancies who relapse following autologous transplantation: a multi-institutional prospective study from the Cancer and Leukemia Group B (CALGB trial 100002). Biol Blood Marrow Transplant. doi: 10.1016/j.bbmt.2010.07.015, S1083-8791(10)00316-2 [pii]

Berglund S, Okas M, Gertow J, Uhlin M, Mattsson J (2009) Stable mixed donor–donor chimerism after double cord blood transplantation. Int J Hematol 90(4):526–531. doi:10.1007/s12185-009-0398-y , S1083-8791(10)00316-2 [pii]

Bornhauser M, Oelschlaegel U, Platzbecker U, Bug G, Lutterbeck K, Kiehl MG, Schetelig J, Kiani A, Illmer T, Schaich M, Theuser C, Mohr B, Brendel C, Fauser AA, Klein S, Martin H, Ehninger G, Thiede C (2009) Monitoring of donor chimerism in sorted CD34+ peripheral blood cells allows the sensitive detection of imminent relapse after allogeneic stem cell transplantation. Haematologica 94(11):1613–1617. doi:10.3324/haematol.2009.007765, 94/11/1613 [pii]

Chen DP, Tseng CP, Wang WT, Wang MC, Tsai SH, Sun CF (2011) Real-time biallelic polymorphism-polymerase chain reaction for chimerism monitoring of hematopoietic stem cell transplantation relapsed patients. Clin Chim Acta 412(7–8):625–630. doi:10.1016/j.cca.2010.12.018, S0009-8981(10)00769-2 [pii]

Childs R, Clave E, Contentin N, Jayasekera D, Hensel N, Leitman S, Read EJ, Carter C, Bahceci E, Young NS, Barrett AJ (1999) Engraftment kinetics after nonmyeloablative allogeneic peripheral blood stem cell transplantation: full donor T-cell chimerism precedes alloimmune responses. Blood 94(9):3234–3241

Couriel DR, Saliba RM, Giralt S, Khouri I, Andersson B, de Lima M, Hosing C, Anderlini P, Donato M, Cleary K, Gajewski J, Neumann J, Ippoliti C, Rondon G, Cohen A, Champlin R (2004) Acute and chronic graft-versus-host disease after ablative and nonmyeloablative conditioning for allogeneic hematopoietic transplantation. Biol Blood Marrow Transplant 10(3):178–185. doi:10.1016/j.bbmt.2003.10.006, S1083879103004191 [pii]

Dubovsky J, Daxberger H, Fritsch G, Printz D, Peters C, Matthes S, Gadner H, Lion T, Muller-Berat N (1999) Kinetics of chimerism during the early post-transplant period in pediatric patients with malignant and non-malignant hematologic disorders: implications for timely detection of engraftment, graft failure and rejection. Leukemia 13(12):2059, 2060

Fakhrai-Rad H, Pourmand N, Ronaghi M (2002) Pyrosequencing: an accurate detection platform for single nucleotide polymorphisms. Hum Mutat 19(5):479–485. doi:10.1002/humu.10078

Ford CE, Hamerton JL, Barnes DW, Loutit JF (1956) Cytological identification of radiation-chimaeras. Nature 177(4506):452–454

Formankova R, Sedlacek P, Krskova L, Rihova H, Sramkova L, Star J (2003) Chimerism-directed adoptive immunotherapy in prevention and treatment of post-transplant relapse of leukemia in childhood. Haematologica 88(1):117–118

Fredriksson M, Barbany G, Liljedahl U, Hermanson M, Kataja M, Syvanen AC (2004) Assessing hematopoietic chimerism after allogeneic stem cell transplantation by multiplexed SNP genotyping using microarrays and quantitative analysis of SNP alleles. Leukemia 18(2): 255–266. doi:10.1038/sj.leu.2403213, 2403213 [pii]

Gardiner N, Lawler M, O'Riordan J, De'Arce M, McCann SR (1997) Donor chimaerism is a strong indicator of disease free survival following bone marrow transplantation for chronic myeloid leukaemia. Leukemia 11(Suppl 3):512–515

Gonzalez-Vicent M, Perez A, Abad L, Sevilla J, Ramirez M, Diaz MA (2010) Graft manipulation and reduced-intensity conditioning for allogeneic hematopoietic stem cell transplantation from mismatched unrelated and mismatched/haploidentical related donors in pediatric leukemia patients. J Pediatr Hematol Oncol 32(3):e85–e90. doi:10.1097/MPH.0b013e3181cf813c

Gorczynska E, Turkiewicz D, Toporski J, Kalwak K, Rybka B, Ryczan R, Sajewicz L, Chybicka A (2004) Prompt initiation of immunotherapy in children with an increasing number of autologous cells after allogeneic HCT can induce complete donor-type chimerism: a report of 14 children. Bone Marrow Transplant 33(2):211–217. doi:10.1038/sj.bmt.1704321, 1704321 [pii]

Guimond M, Busque L, Baron C, Bonny Y, Belanger R, Mattioli J, Perreault C, Roy DC (2000) Relapse after bone marrow transplantation: evidence for distinct immunological mechanisms between adult and paediatric populations. Br J Haematol 109(1):130–137 bjh1961 [pii]

Guz K, Smolarczyk-Wodzyńska J, Dawidowska M, Jółkowska-Baraniak J, Orzinska A, Skulimowska J, Sawecka J, Kraszewska M, Tomaszewska A, Nasiłowska-Adamska B, Mariańska B, Wachowiak J, Witt M, Brojer E (2010) Evaluation of chimerism after allogeneic hematopoietic stem cell transplantation using the RQ-PCR method—its standardization and comparison with the STR-PCR method. Acta Haematol Pol 41(4):535–544

Harries LW, Wickham CL, Evans JC, Rule SA, Joyner MV, Ellard S (2005) Analysis of haematopoietic chimaerism by quantitative real-time polymerase chain reaction. Bone Marrow Transplant 35(3):283–290. doi:10.1038/sj.bmt.1704764, 1704764 [pii]

Hochberg EP, Miklos DB, Neuberg D, Eichner DA, McLaughlin SF, Mattes-Ritz A, Alyea EP, Antin JH, Soiffer RJ, Ritz J (2003) A novel rapid single nucleotide polymorphism (SNP)-based method for assessment of hematopoietic chimerism after allogeneic stem cell transplantation. Blood 101(1):363–369. doi:10.1182/blood-2002-05-1365, 2002-05-1365 [pii]

Horky O, Mayer J, Kablaskova L, Razga F, Krejci M, Kissova J, Borsky M, Jeziskova I, Dvorakova D (2011) Increasing hematopoietic microchimerism is a reliable indicator of incipient AML relapse. Int J Lab Hematol 33(1):57–66. doi:10.1111/j.1751-553X.2010.01249.x CLH1249 [pii]

Horn B, Soni S, Khan S, Petrovic A, Breslin N, Cowan M, Pelle-Day G, Cooperstein E, Baxter-Lowe LA (2009) Feasibility study of preemptive withdrawal of immunosuppression based on chimerism testing in children undergoing myeloablative allogeneic transplantation for hematologic malignancies. Bone Marrow Transplant 43(6):469–476. doi:10.1038/bmt.2008.339 bmt2008339 [pii]

Jimenez-Velasco A, Barrios M, Roman-Gomez J, Navarro G, Buno I, Castillejo JA, Rodriguez AI, Garcia-Gemar G, Torres A, Heiniger AI (2005) Reliable quantification of hematopoietic chimerism after allogeneic transplantation for acute leukemia using amplification by real-time PCR of null alleles and insertion/deletion polymorphisms. Leukemia 19(3):336–343. doi:10.1038/sj.leu.2403622 2403622 [pii]

Jółkowska J, Derwich K, Dawidowska M (2007) Methods of minimal residual disease (MRD) detection in childhood haematological malignancies. J Appl Genet 48(1):77–83

Jółkowska J, Pieczonka A, Strabel T, Boruczkowski D, Wachowiak J, Bader P, Witt M (2005) Hematopoietic chimerism after allogeneic stem cell transplantation: a comparison of quantitative analysis by automated DNA sizing and fluorescent in situ hybridization. BMC Blood Disord 5(1):1. doi:10.1186/1471-2326-5-1 1471-2326-5-1 [pii]

Khan F, Agarwal A, Agrawal S (2004) Significance of chimerism in hematopoietic stem cell transplantation: new variations on an old theme. Bone Marrow Transplant 34(1):1–12. doi:10.1038/sj.bmt.1704525 1704525 [pii]

Klingebiel T, Bader P (2008) Delayed lymphocyte infusion in children given SCT. Bone Marrow Transplant 41(Suppl 2):S23–S26. doi:10.1038/bmt.2008.49 bmt200849 [pii]

Kolb HJ (2008) Graft-versus-leukemia effects of transplantation and donor lymphocytes. Blood 112(12):4371–4383. doi:10.1182/blood-2008-03-077974 112/12/4371 [pii]

Koldehoff M, Steckel NK, Hlinka M, Beelen DW, Elmaagacli AH (2006) Quantitative analysis of chimerism after allogeneic stem cell transplantation by real-time polymerase chain reaction with single nucleotide polymorphisms, standard tandem repeats, and Y-chromosome-specific sequences. Am J Hematol 81(10):735–746. doi:10.1002/ajh.20693

Kroger N, Zagrivnaja M, Schwartz S, Badbaran A, Zabelina T, Lioznov M, Ayuk F, Zander A, Fehse B (2006) Kinetics of plasma-cell chimerism after allogeneic stem cell transplantation by highly sensitive real-time PCR based on sequence polymorphism and its value to quantify minimal residual disease in patients with multiple myeloma. Exp Hematol 34(5):688–694. doi:10.1016/j.exphem.2006.01.011 S0301-472X(06)00056-7 [pii]

Lange T, Hubmann M, Burkhardt R, Franke GN, Cross M, Scholz M, Leiblein S, Al-Ali HK, Edelmann J, Thiery J, Niederwieser D (2010) Monitoring of WT1 expression in PB and CD34(+) donor chimerism of BM predicts early relapse in AML and MDS patients after hematopoietic cell transplantation with reduced-intensity conditioning. Leukemia. doi:10.1038/leu.2010.283 leu2010283 [pii]

Legler TJ, Lynen R, Maas JH, Pindur G, Kulenkampff D, Suren A, Osmers R, Kohler M (2002) Prediction of fetal Rh D and Rh CcEe phenotype from maternal plasma with real-time polymerase chain reaction. Transfus Apher Sci 27(3):217–223. S1473-0502(02)00068-X [pii]

Liesveld JL, Rothberg PG (2008) Mixed chimerism in SCT: conflict or peaceful coexistence? Bone Marrow Transplant 42(5):297–310. doi:10.1038/bmt.2008.212 bmt2008212 [pii]

Lim ZY, Pearce L, Ingram W, Ho AY, Mufti GJ, Pagliuca A (2008) Chimerism does not predict for outcome after alemtuzumab-based conditioning: lineage-specific analysis of chimerism of specific diseases may be more informative. Bone Marrow Transplant 41(6):587–588. 1705937 [pii]

Lion T (2007) Detection of impending graft rejection and relapse by lineage-specific chimerism analysis. Methods Mol Med 134:197–216. 1-59745-223-8:197 [pii]

Lion T, Daxberger H, Dubovsky J, Filipcik P, Fritsch G, Printz D, Peters C, Matthes-Martin S, Lawitschka A, Gadner H (2001) Analysis of chimerism within specific leukocyte subsets for detection of residual or recurrent leukemia in pediatric patients after allogeneic stem cell transplantation. Leukemia 15(2):307–310

Lo YM, Lau TK, Chan LY, Leung TN, Chang AM (2000) Quantitative analysis of the bidirectional fetomaternal transfer of nucleated cells and plasma DNA. Clin Chem 46(9):1301–1309

Maas F, Schaap N, Kolen S, Zoetbrood A, Buno I, Dolstra H, de Witte T, Schattenberg A, van de Wiel-van Kemenade E (2003) Quantification of donor and recipient hemopoietic cells by real-time PCR of single nucleotide polymorphisms. Leukemia 17(3):630–633. doi:10.1038/sj.leu.2402857

Mackinnon S, Barnett L, Heller G, O'Reilly RJ (1994) Minimal residual disease is more common in patients who have mixed T-cell chimerism after bone marrow transplantation for chronic myelogenous leukemia. Blood 83(11):3409–3416

Martínez-López J, Crooke A, Grande S, Ayala R, Jiménez-Velasco A, Gamarra S, Meneu JC, Gilsanz F (2010) Real-time PCR quantification of haematopoietic chimerism after transplantation: a comparison between TaqMan and hybridization probes technologies. Int J Lab Hematol 32 (1 Ptq):e17–e25. doi:10.1111/j.1751-553X.2009.01166.x

Masmas TN, Madsen HO, Petersen SL, Ryder LP, Svejgaard A, Alizadeh M, Vindelov LL (2005) Evaluation and automation of hematopoietic chimerism analysis based on real-time quantitative polymerase chain reaction. Biol Blood Marrow Transplant 11(7):558–566. doi:10.1016/j.bbmt.2005.04.004 S1083879105002600 [pii]

Mattsson J, Uzunel M, Tammik L, Aschan J, Ringden O (2001) Leukemia lineage-specific chimerism analysis is a sensitive predictor of relapse in patients with acute myeloid leukemia and myelodysplastic syndrome after allogeneic stem cell transplantation. Leukemia 15(12): 1976–1985

Maury S, Jouault H, Kuentz M, Vernant JP, Tulliez M, Cordonnier C, Bories D (2001) Chimerism analysis by lineage-specific fluorescent polymerase chain reaction in secondary graft failure after allogeneic stem cell transplantation. Transplantation 71(3):374–380

McCann SR, Crampe M, Molloy K, Lawler M (2005) Hemopoietic chimerism following stem cell transplantation. Transfus Apher Sci 32(1):55–61. doi:10.1016/j.transci.2004.10.006 S1473-0502(04)00182-X [pii]

McCann SR, Lawler M (2004) Monitoring outcome: MRD, chimearism and relapse. In: Carreras E, Gluckman E, Gratwohl A, Masszi T, Apperlay J (eds) Haematopoietic stem cell transplantation. Forum Service Editore, Genoa, pp 197–212

Mielcarek M, Storb R (2003) Non-myeloablative hematopoietic cell transplantation as immunotherapy for hematologic malignancies. Cancer Treat Rev 29(4):283–290. S0305737203000045 [pii]

Miura Y, Tanaka J, Toubai T, Tsutsumi Y, Kato N, Hirate D, Kaji M, Sugita J, Shigematsu A, Iwao N, Ota S, Masauzi N, Fukuhara T, Kasai M, Asaka M, Imamura M (2006) Analysis of donor-type chimerism in lineage-specific cell populations after allogeneic myeloablative and non-myeloablative stem cell transplantation. Bone Marrow Transplant 37(9):837–843. doi:10.1038/sj.bmt.1705352 1705352 [pii]

Perez-Simon JA, Caballero D, Diez-Campelo M, Lopez-Perez R, Mateos G, Canizo C, Vazquez L, Vidriales B, Mateos MV, Gonzalez M, San Miguel JF (2002) Chimerism and minimal residual disease monitoring after reduced intensity conditioning (RIC) allogeneic transplantation. Leukemia 16(8):1423–1431

Ramirez M, Diaz MA, Garcia-Sanchez F, Velasco M, Casado F, Villa M, Vicario JL, Madero L (1996) Chimerism after allogeneic hematopoietic cell transplantation in childhood acute lymphoblastic leukemia. Bone Marrow Transplant 18(6):1161–1165

Sairafi D, Remberger M, Uhlin M, Ljungman P, Ringden O, Mattsson J (2010) Leukemia lineage-specific chimerism analysis and molecular monitoring improve outcome of donor lymphocyte infusions. Biol Blood Marrow Transplant 16(12):1728–1737. doi:10.1016/j.bbmt.2010.06.005 S1083-8791(10)00246-6 [pii]

Schilham MW, Balduzzi A, Bader P (2005) Is there a role for minimal residual disease levels in the treatment of ALL patients who receive allogeneic stem cells? Bone Marrow Transplant 35(Suppl 1):S49–S52

Schraml E, Lion T (2003) Interference of dye-associated fluorescence signals with quantitative analysis of chimerism by capillary electrophoresis. Leukemia 17(1):221–223. doi:10.1038/sj.leu.2402755

Serrano J, Roman J, Sanchez J, Jimenez A, Castillejo JA, Herrera C, Gonzalez MG, Reina L, Rodriguez MC, Alvarez MA, Maldonado J, Torres A (2000) Molecular analysis of lineage-specific chimerism and minimal residual disease by RT-PCR of p210(BCR-ABL) and p190(BCR-ABL) after allogeneic bone marrow transplantation for chronic myeloid leukemia: increasing mixed myeloid chimerism and p190(BCR-ABL) detection precede cytogenetic relapse. Blood 95(8):2659–2665

Stumph J, Vnencak-Jones CL, Koyama T, Frangoul H (2008) Comparison of peripheral blood and bone marrow samples for detection of post transplant mixed chimerism. Bone Marrow Transplant 41(6):589–590

Syvanen AC (1999) From gels to chips: "minisequencing" primer extension for analysis of point mutations and single nucleotide polymorphisms. Hum Mutat 13(1):1–10

Thiede C, Bornhauser M, Ehninger G (2004) Strategies and clinical implications of chimerism diagnostics after allogeneic hematopoietic stem cell transplantation. Acta Haematol 112(1–2): 16–23. doi:10.1159/000077555 AHA20041121_2016 [pii]

Thiede C, Bornhauser M, Oelschlagel U, Brendel C, Leo R, Daxberger H, Mohr B, Florek M, Kroschinsky F, Geissler G, Naumann R, Ritter M, Prange-Krex G, Lion T, Neubauer A,

Ehninger G (2001) Sequential monitoring of chimerism and detection of minimal residual disease after allogeneic blood stem cell transplantation (BSCT) using multiplex PCR amplification of short tandem repeat-markers. Leukemia 15(2):293–302

Thiede C, Florek M, Bornhauser M, Ritter M, Mohr B, Brendel C, Ehninger G, Neubauer A (1999) Rapid quantification of mixed chimerism using multiplex amplification of short tandem repeat markers and fluorescence detection. Bone Marrow Transplant 23(10):1055–1060. doi:10.1038/sj.bmt.1701779

van der Velden VH, Hochhaus A, Cazzaniga G, Szczepanski T, Gabert J, van Dongen JJ (2003) Detection of minimal residual disease in hematologic malignancies by real-time quantitative PCR: principles, approaches, and laboratory aspects. Leukemia 17(6):1013–1034

van Leeuwen JE, van Tol MJ, Joosten AM, Wijnen JT, Khan PM, Vossen JM (1993) Mixed T-lymphoid chimerism after allogeneic bone marrow transplantation for hematologic malignancies of children is not correlated with relapse. Blood 82(6):1921–1928

Vignal A, Milan D, SanCristobal M, Eggen A (2002) A review on SNP and other types of molecular markers and their use in animal genetics. Genet Sel Evol 34(3):275–305. doi:10.1051/gse:2002009

Wiedemann B, Klyuchnikov E, Kroger N, Zabelina T, Stahl T, Zeschke S, Badbaran A, Ayuk F, Alchalby H, Wolschke C, Bokemeyer C, Fehse B, Zander AR, Bacher U (2010) Chimerism studies with quantitative real-time PCR in stem cell recipients with acute myeloid leukemia. Exp Hematol 38(12):1261–1271. doi:10.1016/j.exphem.2010.08.006 S0301-472X(10)00370-X [pii]

Willasch A, Eing S, Weber G, Kuci S, Schneider G, Soerensen J, Jarisch A, Rettinger E, Koehl U, Klingebiel T, Kreyenberg H, Bader P (2010) Enrichment of cell subpopulations applying automated MACS technique: purity, recovery and applicability for PCR-based chimerism analysis. Bone Marrow Transplant 45(1):181–189. doi:10.1038/bmt.2009.89 bmt200989 [pii]

Willasch A, Schneider G, Reincke BS, Shayegi N, Kreyenberg H, Kuci S, Weber G, Van Der Reijden B, Niethammer D, Klingebiel T, Bader P (2007) Sequence polymorphism systems for quantitative real-time polymerase chain reaction to characterize hematopoietic chimerism-high informativity and sensitivity as well as excellent reproducibility and precision of measurement. Lab Hematol 13(3):73–84. doi:10.1532/LH96.07004 37054778R8633G01 [pii]

Winiarski J, Gustafsson A, Wester D, Dalianis T (2000) Follow-up of chimerism, including T- and B-lymphocytes and granulocytes in children more than one year after allogeneic bone marrow transplantation. Pediatr Transplant 4(2):132–139

Wu CJ, Hochberg EP, Rogers SA, Kutok JL, Biernacki M, Nascimento AF, Marks P, Bridges K, Ritz J (2003) Molecular assessment of erythroid lineage chimerism following nonmyeloablative allogeneic stem cell transplantation. Exp Hematol 31(10):924–933. S0301472X03002273 [pii]

Zeiser R, Spyridonidis A, Wasch R, Ihorst G, Grullich C, Bertz H, Finke J (2005) Evaluation of immunomodulatory treatment based on conventional and lineage-specific chimerism analysis in patients with myeloid malignancies after myeloablative allogeneic hematopoietic cell transplantation. Leukemia 19(5):814–821. doi:10.1038/sj.leu.2403719 2403719 [pii]

Zetterquist H, Mattsson J, Uzunel M, Nasman-Bjork I, Svenberg P, Tammik L, Bayat G, Winiarski J, Ringden O (2000) Mixed chimerism in the B cell lineage is a rapid and sensitive indicator of minimal residual disease in bone marrow transplant recipients with pre-B cell acute lymphoblastic leukemia. Bone Marrow Transplant 25(8):843–851. doi:10.1038/sj.bmt.1702337

Chapter 16
Peritransplantation Monitoring of Minimal Residual Disease in Acute Lymphoblastic Leukemia

Małgorzata Dawidowska, Katarzyna Derwich and Tomasz Szczepański

Abstract Minimal residual disease is currently the most powerful prognostic tool enabling prediction of the outcome in acute lymphoblastic leukemia (ALL). The monitoring of minimal residual disease during and after remission induction therapy has already been implemented into modern ALL therapeutic protocols for risk group stratification, thus influencing decisions on hematopoietic stem cell transplantation, which is a treatment option reserved for high-risk and relapsed ALL patients. Moreover, there is increasing evidence of the prognostic significance of residual disease assessment performed before and after transplantation. Peritransplantation assessment enables more adequate decisions concerning conditioning for transplantation, while post-transplant monitoring creates an opportunity for early intervention in case of an increased risk of ALL relapse. Peritransplantation monitoring of minimal residual disease might also be used to assess the effectiveness of treatment aimed at relapse prevention, as well as to evaluate novel treatment modalities, including those related or alternative to hematopoietic stem cell transplantation.

M. Dawidowska (✉)
Department of Molecular and Clinical Genetics, Institute of Human Genetics, Polish Academy of Sciences, Strzeszyńska 32, 60-479 Poznań, Poland
e-mail: ma.dawidowska@wp.pl

K. Derwich
Department of Pediatric Oncology, Hematology and Transplantology, Poznań University of Medical Sciences, Szpitalna 27/33, 60-572 Poznań, Poland

T. Szczepański
Department of Pediatric Hematology and Oncology, Medical University of Silesia, 3 Maja 13/15, 41-800 Zabrze, Poland
e-mail: szczep57@poczta.onet.pl

M. Witt et al. (eds.), *Molecular Aspects of Hematologic Malignancies*, Principles and Practice, DOI: 10.1007/978-3-642-29467-9_16,

16.1 Introduction

Minimal residual disease (MRD) assessment with the use of real-time quantitative polymerase chain reaction (RQ-PCR) or multiparametric flow cytometry immunophenotyping (FC) is currently the most reliable prognostic factor in the treatment of acute lymphoblastic leukemia (ALL) (Jółkowska et al. 2007). MRD monitoring provides valuable information on the effectiveness of treatment at different stages of ALL therapy (Campana 2009a, b, 2010a, b; van der Velden and van Dongen 2009; Bene and Kaeda 2009). The vast majority of data on the clinical significance of MRD, including peritransplantation analyses, i.e., performed before and after hematopoietic stem cell transplantation (HSCT), come from the study of childhood ALL and there is less data on HSCT-related MRD monitoring in adult ALL patients. Detailed information on the methodology of MRD testing and its clinical applicability is described in Chap. 11.

Because of the associated high risk of complications and significant cost, hematopoietic stem cell transplantation is a method of treatment reserved exclusively for high-risk and relapsed ALL patients (Goulden and Steward 2002; Jude and Chan 2010). The therapeutic effects of HSCT depend on three basic mechanisms: the elimination of leukemic blasts through intensive pretransplantation treatment (conditioning), hematopoietic reconstitution from donor-derived hematopoietic cells, and the antileukemic immunological reaction of T-lymphocytes against recipient cells (i.e. graft versus leukemia effect, GvL). Detailed information on HSCT is contained in Chap. 13. Minimal residual disease quantification prior to HSCT provides information on the clearance of residual disease, while post-transplant MRD monitoring enables the prediction of leukemia recurrence through the early detection of molecular relapse (Pulsipher et al. 2009; Bader et al. 2008, 2009; Lee et al. 2009). Therefore, HSCT-related MRD assessment is a valuable tool for making decisions on HSCT procedures as well as post-transplant treatment.

16.2 MRD in Risk Group Stratification

When discussing the significance of minimal residual disease in the context of hematopoietic stem cell transplantation, MRD assessment should be seen in a perspective broader than pre-HSCT testing and post-HSCT monitoring. The quantification of MRD levels at fixed time points during first-line chemotherapy has been documented to be a powerful predictor of the outcome in childhood ALL (Cave et al. 1998; Biondi et al. 2000; Bjorklund et al. 2003; van Dongen et al. 1998; Flohr et al. 2008). In modern ALL therapeutic protocols, the results of MRD testing during the first 3 months of therapy are the basis for stratifying patients into risk groups, which is followed by the choice of risk group-adjusted treatment (Zhou et al. 2007; Yamaji et al. 2010; Bassan et al. 2009; Flohr et al. 2008).

Given the current indications for HSCT in ALL, it should be emphasized that early MRD assessment during chemotherapy may determine further course of treatment, including any decisions concerning HSCT. For example, van Dongen and colleagues showed that the proportion of patients classified into the high-risk (HR) group on the basis of MRD results, is much larger (15 %) than the proportion of patients recruited for the HR group solely on the basis of traditional prognostic factors (5–10 %) (van Dongen et al. 1998). Thus, proper classification into the high-risk group by taking into account MRD results, followed by appropriately aggressive treatment (according to the HR protocol) allows the decision to perform HSCT before the occurrence of relapse, in the first complete remission (CR1). The effectiveness of the transplant is then the highest when compared to that of HSCT performed in the second or in subsequent remissions (≥CR2).

16.3 MRD Prior to Hematopoietic Stem Cell Transplantation

The appropriate reduction of the leukemic clone, which increases the effectiveness of pre-transplant conditioning and post-transplant GvL effect, is one of the factors determining the success of HSCT. The impact of pre-transplant leukemic burden on the outcome of HSCT is best demonstrated by the lower effectiveness of transplantations performed in patients who are not in complete hematological remission. The quantification of the level of MRD prior to HSCT enables a direct assessment of remission at the molecular level, and thus makes it possible to predict the risk of relapse after transplantation. The prognostic significance of the pretransplantation MRD status has been documented in numerous retrospective studies (van der Velden et al. 2001; Uzunel et al. 2001; Bader et al. 2002; Krejci et al. 2003; Knechtli et al. 1998a), and recently it was also confirmed in prospective trials (Sramkova et al. 2007; Elorza et al. 2010; Lankester et al. 2010). The clinical significance of MRD assessment prior to HSCT has been shown with the use of both semi-quantitative molecular approaches (Knechtli et al. 1998a; Uzunel et al. 2001; Bader et al. 2002) as well as quantitative methods (van der Velden et al. 2001; Krejci et al. 2003; Sramkova et al. 2007; Spinelli et al. 2007).

In contrast to the assessment of MRD during first-line ALL chemotherapy, there are still no uniform, widely accepted time-points of MRD monitoring before transplantation. Different time-points of pre-transplant MRD testing have been reported so far: 6–81 days before HSCT (Knechtli et al. 1998a), 0–30 days (Uzunel et al. 2001), 13–98 days (van der Velden et al. 2001), before consolidation (Bader et al. 2002; Sanchez et al. 2002; Spinelli et al. 2007; Sramkova et al. 2007). The vast majority of currently available data indicate that, for clinical utility, pre-HSCT MRD testing should be performed just before conditioning. A test at this time-point allows the clearance of residual leukemia through first-line chemotherapy to be determined, and thus is the most reliable assessment of the quality of remission. The status of molecular remission before HSCT is related to a much better prognosis than that of hematological remission with the evidence of residual leukemia in MRD analysis (Foster et al. 2011). Therefore, the assessment of minimal residual disease creates a possibility for the optimal planning of pre-HSCT conditioning and post-HSCT follow-up and treatment, dependent on the risk of relapse determined on the basis of pre-transplant MRD levels (Bader et al. 2008).

The clinical significance of pre-transplantation MRD assessment has been documented in numerous studies, using a variety of therapeutic protocols, different time-points of MRD testing, and different ways of reporting results (event-free survival, EFS; relapse-free survival, RFS; overall survival, OS). The probability of relapse after transplantation is significantly correlated with detectable MRD levels before HSCT (in particular, with high levels, usually $\geq 10^{-3}$), and is lower in patients with low ($<10^{-3}$) or undetectable levels of MRD. In the case of children with ALL, the EFS rate reported in patients with MRD-negative results before HSCT is between 70–80 %, whereas, in a group of MRD-positive patients EFS is only approximately 20–30 % (Knechtli et al. 1998a; Bader et al. 2002). In a prospective study by Bader et al. the EFS and the cumulative incidence of relapse (CIR) were 0.27 and 0.57, respectively, for patients with MRD $\geq 10^{-4}$ before HSCT, compared to 0.60 and 0.13 for patients with MRD $< 10^{-4}$. The study also demonstrated that MRD is the only independent prognostic factor predicting the outcome of HSCT in childhood ALL (Bader et al. 2009).

Moreover, pre-transplant MRD monitoring creates an opportunity to identify patients for whom transplant protocols other than the standard should be considered (Paganin et al. 2008). For patients at high risk of relapse, therapeutic procedures, both before and after transplantation, should aim at minimizing the risk of relapse after HSCT. In these patients, more intensive chemotherapy prior to HSCT, as well as the appropriate immunomodulatory post-transplant treatment (e.g. reducing the duration/intensity of immunosuppression and/or donor lymphocyte infusion, DLI) should be considered. Additionally, high pre-transplant MRD level provides an indication for a more intensive MRD monitoring after HSCT (Uzunel et al. 2001).

In the case of patients with low MRD levels prior to transplantation ($<5 \times 10^{-4}$), it is often possible to eliminate residual leukemic cells by properly conducted immunomodulatory therapy after HSCT, aimed at enhancing the GVL effect (van der Velden et al. 2001). Patients with MRD-negative pre-HSCT results, constitute a group with low risk of relapse, for whom, in the future, the application of novel ALL treatment protocols might be considered, with the modification or even the exclusion of the HSCT procedure.

16.4 MRD After Hematopoietic Stem Cell Transplantation

The monitoring of MRD levels after the transplantation of hematopoietic cells is focused on the early detection of leukemia relapse at the molecular level, enabling appropriate decisions on immunomodulatory treatment (i.e., DLI and/or reduction in the intensity and duration of immunosuppression), aimed at preventing relapse (Pulsipher et al. 2009). In addition, MRD monitoring after immunomodulatory treatment enables the assessment of the effectiveness of the treatment.

In contrast to MRD studies during first-line chemotherapy, and as in the case of MRD study before HSCT, the exact time-points for post-transplant MRD monitoring of the most predictive value have not yet been clearly established. In the reports published so far, MRD was monitored at different intervals: usually once a month during the first 3–6 months after transplantation, then at intervals of 2–3 months up to 12 months after transplantation and then at 18 and 24 months after HSCT (Knechtli et al. 1998b; Mortuza et al. 2002; Sanchez et al. 2002; Uzunel et al. 2003).

The vast majority of data on the clinical significance of post-transplant MRD monitoring were obtained in retrospective studies based on semi-quantitative molecular methods (Knechtli et al. 1998b; Mortuza et al. 2002; Uzunel et al. 2003). So far, there are few data obtained with the use of RQ-PCR approach (Spinelli et al. 2007). In all studies, concerning both children and adults, it has been shown that any detectable level of MRD at any time-point after transplantation, particularly a high level, is a risk factor for leukemia relapse (Spinelli et al. 2007; Knechtli et al. 1998b; Mortuza et al. 2002; Sanchez et al. 2002; Uzunel et al. 2003).

In a recent study, conducted with the use of RQ-PCR in adult ALL patients, it was demonstrated that MRD assessments of the highest prognostic value are those performed at day +100 after HSCT and not at earlier time-points, as previously suggested. The risk of leukemia recurrence is 80 % in patients with MRD-positive results at day +100 after HSCT, compared to 7 % in patients with MRD-negative results (Spinelli et al. 2007). However, these findings require confirmation in larger groups of both adult and pediatric patients, due to different kinetics of MRD changes observed in children and adults with ALL (Foroni and Hoffbrand 2002; Spinelli et al. 2007).

It should, however, be noted that a detectable level of MRD after HSCT does not always correlate with relapse. Low levels of MRD, particularly in the early post-transplant period, may be overcome by the therapeutic effect of transplantation through the mechanism of GvL. This is confirmed by observations of a low risk of recurrence in patients with initially low, and then undetectable levels of MRD after HSCT (Knechtli et al. 1998b). In addition, the GvL effect may be enhanced by immunomodulatory therapy (DLI and/or reduction of immunosuppression). However, the efficacy of immunotherapy in preventing leukemia relapse is greater, the sooner the treatment is undertaken. It is, therefore, necessary to perform MRD testing in an early period after the transplantation and at short time intervals. This, however, is highly challenging for logistical and financial reasons and, above all, it is a burden for patients due to the need for frequent bone marrow sampling. This refers particularly to B-cell precursor ALL (BCP-ALL) in which MRD levels detected in blood are up to 1,000 times lower than those observed in bone marrow, while T-ALL results of MRD quantification performed using peripheral blood and bone marrow are more comparable.

Due to the need for frequent bone marrow sampling, MRD monitoring after HSCT is often replaced or supplemented by the assessment of hematopoietic chimerism (Bader et al. 2008). Despite their lower specificity and usually lower sensitivity, chimerism tests are technically less complex and cheaper, compared to the methodology of RQ-PCR-based MRD monitoring, exploiting rearrangements of immunoglobulin and T-cell receptor genes as markers of residual leukemic cells. In addition, chimerism analyses are characterized by greater convergence of the results obtained from peripheral blood and bone marrow (Schilham et al. 2005; Stumph et al. 2008). The issue of chimerism monitoring has been discussed in detail in Chap. 15. So far, the most sensitive method of chimerism monitoring is the RQ-PCR approach using insertion/deletion (*indel*) polymorphism (Alizadeh et al. 2002). Sensitivity might further be increased by the assessment of lineage-specific chimerism, measured in the cell subset from which the leukemia originated (Winiarski et al. 2000; Lion 2007). Due to the greatest convergence of the results of lineage-specific chimerism monitoring with those of MRD testing, chimerism monitoring may provide a substitute for the analysis of residual disease if MRD assessment is not possible to perform (Bader et al. 2008).

16.5 Conclusions

MRD monitoring prior to and after hematopoietic stem cell transplantation is regarded to be a powerful predictor for post-transplant outcome in children with ALL. It offers opportunities to make more appropriate decisions on HSCT-related procedures (e.g. intensification of pre-transplant conditioning for the reduction of MRD), as well as post-transplant follow-up and treatment (e.g. relapse prevention through the introduction of immunomodulatory treatment and the assessment of its effectiveness). However, it should be emphasized that currently available methods for the prevention and treatment of ALL relapse are limited, and their effects are still unsatisfactory. Therefore, MRD monitoring may be the perfect tool to evaluate and compare the efficacy of novel therapeutic approaches (Schilham et al. 2005; Sramkova et al. 2007). A prospective evaluation of the significance of MRD monitoring in ALL, based on a standardized RQ-PCR methodology and uniform criteria for the interpretation of quantitative data, has become the subject of international multicenter trials (van Dongen et al. 2003; Sramkova et al. 2007; van der Velden et al. 2007a, b; Flohr et al. 2008). Within the next few years, the results of clinical trials are expected to address the question of whether the implementation of MRD monitoring into therapeutic protocols, including HSCT, significantly increases cure rates in ALL.

Acknowledgments This Chapter was partly supported by the Ministry of Science and Higher Education, Grant N N407 311 839.

References

Alizadeh M, Bernard M, Danic B, Dauriac C, Birebent B, Lapart C, Lamy T, Le Prise PY, Beauplet A, Bories D, Semana G, Quelvennec E (2002) Quantitative assessment of hematopoietic chimerism after bone marrow transplantation by real-time quantitative polymerase chain reaction. Blood 99(12):4618–4625

Bader P, Hancock J, Kreyenberg H, Goulden NJ, Niethammer D, Oakhill A, Steward CG, Handgretinger R, Beck JF, Klingebiel T (2002) Minimal residual disease (MRD) status prior to allogeneic stem cell transplantation is a powerful predictor for post-transplant outcome in children with ALL. Leukemia 16(9):1668–1672

Bader P, Kreyenberg H, Henze GH, Eckert C, Reising M, Willasch A, Barth A, Borkhardt A, Peters C, Handgretinger R, Sykora KW, Holter W, Kabisch H, Klingebiel T, von Stackelberg A (2009) Prognostic value of minimal residual disease quantification before allogeneic stem-cell transplantation in relapsed childhood acute lymphoblastic leukemia: the ALL-REZ BFM Study Group. J Clin Oncol 27(3):377–384. doi:10.1200/JCO.2008.17.6065 JCO.2008.17.6065 [pii]

Bader P, Willasch A, Klingebiel T (2008) Monitoring of post-transplant remission of childhood malignancies: is there a standard? Bone Marrow Transplant 42(Suppl 2):S31–S34. doi:10.1038/bmt.2008.280 bmt2008280 [pii]

Bassan R, Spinelli O, Oldani E, Intermesoli T, Tosi M, Peruta B, Rossi G, Borlenghi E, Pogliani EM, Terruzzi E, Fabris P, Cassibba V, Lambertenghi-Deliliers G, Cortelezzi A, Bosi A, Gianfaldoni G, Ciceri F, Bernardi M, Gallamini A, Mattei D, Di Bona E, Romani C, Scattolin AM, Barbui T, Rambaldi A (2009) Improved risk classification for risk-specific therapy based on the molecular study of minimal residual disease (MRD) in adult acute lymphoblastic leukemia (ALL). Blood 113(18):4153–4162. doi:10.1182/blood-2008-11-185132 blood-2008-11-185132 [pii]

Bene MC, Kaeda JS (2009) How and why minimal residual disease studies are necessary in leukemia: a review from WP10 and WP12 of the European LeukaemiaNet. Haematologica 94(8):1135–1150. doi:10.3324/haematol.2008.004267 haematol.2008.004267 [pii]

Biondi A, Valsecchi MG, Seriu T, D'Aniello E, Willemse MJ, Fasching K, Pannunzio A, Gadner H, Schrappe M, Kamps WA, Bartram CR, van Dongen JJ, Panzer-Grumayer ER (2000) Molecular detection of minimal residual disease is a strong predictive factor of relapse in childhood B-lineage acute lymphoblastic leukemia with medium risk features. A case control study of the International BFM study group. Leukemia 14(11):1939–1943

Bjorklund E, Mazur J, Soderhall S, Porwit-MacDonald A (2003) Flow cytometric follow-up of minimal residual disease in bone marrow gives prognostic information in children with acute lymphoblastic leukemia. Leukemia 17(1):138–148

Campana D (2009a) Minimal residual disease in acute lymphoblastic leukemia. Semin Hematol 46(1):100–106. doi:10.1053/j.seminhematol.2008.09.001 S0037-1963(08)00143-1 [pii]

Campana D (2009b) Role of minimal residual disease monitoring in adult and pediatric acute lymphoblastic leukemia. Hematol Oncol Clin North Am 23 (5):1083–1098, vii. doi:10.1016/j.hoc.2009.07.010 S0889-8588(09)00148-8 [pii]

Campana D (2010a) Minimal residual disease in acute lymphoblastic leukemia. Hematology Am Soc Hematol Educ Program 2010:7–12. doi:10.1182/asheducation-2010.1.7 2010/1/7 [pii]

Campana D (2010b) Progress of minimal residual disease studies in childhood acute leukemia. Curr Hematol Malig Rep 5(3):169–176. doi:10.1007/s11899-010-0056-8

Cave H, van der Werff ten Bosch J, Suciu S, Guidal C, Waterkeyn C, Otten J, Bakkus M, Thielemans K, Grandchamp B, Vilmer E (1998) Clinical significance of minimal residual disease in childhood acute lymphoblastic leukemia. European Organization for Research and Treatment of Cancer—Childhood Leukemia Cooperative Group. N Engl J Med 339 (9):591–598

Elorza I, Palacio C, Dapena JL, Gallur L, de Toledo JS, de Heredia CD (2010) Relationship between minimal residual disease measured by multiparametric flow cytometry prior to allogeneic hematopoietic stem cell transplantation and outcome in children with acute lymphoblastic leukemia. Haematologica 95(6):936–941. doi:10.3324/haematol.2009.010843 haematol.2009.010843 [pii]

Flohr T, Schrauder A, Cazzaniga G, Panzer-Grumayer R, van der Velden V, Fischer S, Stanulla M, Basso G, Niggli FK, Schafer BW, Sutton R, Koehler R, Zimmermann M, Valsecchi MG, Gadner H, Masera G, Schrappe M, van Dongen JJ, Biondi A, Bartram CR (2008) Minimal residual disease-directed risk stratification using real-time quantitative PCR analysis of immunoglobulin and T-cell receptor gene rearrangements in the international multicenter trial AIEOP-BFM ALL 2000 for childhood acute lymphoblastic leukemia. Leukemia 22(4):771–782. doi:10.1038/leu.2008.5 leu20085 [pii]

Foroni L, Hoffbrand AV (2002) Molecular analysis of minimal residual disease in adult acute lymphoblastic leukaemia. Best Pract Res Clin Haematol 15(1):71–90. doi:10.1053/beha.2002.0186

Foster JH, Hawkins DS, Loken MR, Wells DA (2011) Minimal residual disease detected prior to hematopoietic cell transplantation. Pediatr Blood Cancer 57(1):163–165. doi:10.1002/pbc.23079 B T

Goulden N, Steward C (2002) Clinical relevance of MRD in children undergoing allogeneic stem cell transplantation for ALL. Best Pract Res Clin Haematol 15(1):59–70. doi:10.1053/beha.2002.0185 S1521692602901854 [pii]

Jółkowska J, Derwich K, Dawidowska M (2007) Methods of minimal residual disease (MRD) detection in childhood haematological malignancies. J Appl Genet 48(1):77–83

Jude V, Chan KW (2010) Recent advances in hematopoietic stem cell transplantation for childhood acute lymphoblastic leukemia. Curr Hematol Malig Rep 5(3):129–134. doi:10.1007/s11899-010-0050-1

Knechtli CJ, Goulden NJ, Hancock JP, Grandage VL, Harris EL, Garland RJ, Jones CG, Rowbottom AW, Hunt LP, Green AF, Clarke E, Lankester AW, Cornish JM, Pamphilon DH, Steward CG, Oakhill A (1998a) Minimal residual disease status before allogeneic bone marrow transplantation is an important determinant of successful outcome for children and adolescents with acute lymphoblastic leukemia. Blood 92(11):4072–4079

Knechtli CJ, Goulden NJ, Hancock JP, Harris EL, Garland RJ, Jones CG, Grandage VL, Rowbottom AW, Green AF, Clarke E, Lankester AW, Potter MN, Cornish JM, Pamphilon DH, Steward CG, Oakhill A (1998b) Minimal residual disease status as a predictor of relapse after allogeneic bone marrow transplantation for children with acute lymphoblastic leukaemia. Br J Haematol 102(3):860–871

Krejci O, van der Velden VH, Bader P, Kreyenberg H, Goulden N, Hancock J, Schilham MW, Lankester A, Revesz T, Klingebiel T, van Dongen JJ (2003) Level of minimal residual disease prior to haematopoietic stem cell transplantation predicts prognosis in paediatric patients with acute lymphoblastic leukaemia: a report of the Pre-BMT MRD Study Group. Bone Marrow Transplant 32(8):849–851. doi:10.1038/sj.bmt.1704241 1704241 [pii]

Lankester AC, Bierings MB, van Wering ER, Wijkhuijs AJ, de Weger RA, Wijnen JT, Vossen JM, Versluys B, Egeler RM, van Tol MJ, Putter H, Revesz T, van Dongen JJ, van der Velden VH, Schilham MW (2010) Preemptive alloimmune intervention in high-risk pediatric acute lymphoblastic leukemia patients guided by minimal residual disease level before stem cell transplantation. Leukemia 24(8):1462–1469. doi:10.1038/leu.2010.133 leu2010133 [pii]

Lee S, Kim YJ, Chung NG, Lim J, Lee DG, Kim HJ, Min CK, Lee JW, Min WS, Kim CC (2009) The extent of minimal residual disease reduction after the first 4-week imatinib therapy determines outcome of allogeneic stem cell transplantation in adults with Philadelphia chromosome-positive acute lymphoblastic leukemia. Cancer 115(3):561–570. doi:10.1002/cncr.24026

Lion T (2007) Detection of impending graft rejection and relapse by lineage-specific chimerism analysis. Methods Mol Med 134:197–216 1-59745-223-8:197 [pii]

Mortuza FY, Papaioannou M, Moreira IM, Coyle LA, Gameiro P, Gandini D, Prentice HG, Goldstone A, Hoffbrand AV, Foroni L (2002) Minimal residual disease tests provide an independent predictor of clinical outcome in adult acute lymphoblastic leukemia. J Clin Oncol 20(4):1094–1104

Paganin M, Zecca M, Fabbri G, Polato K, Biondi A, Rizzari C, Locatelli F, Basso G (2008) Minimal residual disease is an important predictive factor of outcome in children with relapsed 'high-risk' acute lymphoblastic leukemia. Leukemia 22(12):2193–2200. doi:10.1038/leu.2008.227 leu2008227 [pii]

Pulsipher MA, Bader P, Klingebiel T, Cooper LJ (2009) Allogeneic transplantation for pediatric acute lymphoblastic leukemia: the emerging role of peritransplantation minimal residual disease/chimerism monitoring and novel chemotherapeutic, molecular, and immune approaches aimed at preventing relapse. Biol Blood Marrow Transplant 15(1 Suppl):62–71. doi: 10.1016/j.bbmt.2008.11.009 S1083-8791(08)00489-8 [pii]

Sanchez J, Serrano J, Gomez P, Martinez F, Martin C, Madero L, Herrera C, Garcia JM, Casano J, Torres A (2002) Clinical value of immunological monitoring of minimal residual disease in acute lymphoblastic leukaemia after allogeneic transplantation. Br J Haematol 116(3): 686–694 3311 [pii]

Schilham MW, Balduzzi A, Bader P (2005) Is there a role for minimal residual disease levels in the treatment of ALL patients who receive allogeneic stem cells? Bone Marrow Transplant 35(Suppl 1):S49–S52

Spinelli O, Peruta B, Tosi M, Guerini V, Salvi A, Zanotti MC, Oldani E, Grassi A, Intermesoli T, Mico C, Rossi G, Fabris P, Lambertenghi-Deliliers G, Angelucci E, Barbui T, Bassan R, Rambaldi A (2007) Clearance of minimal residual disease after allogeneic stem cell transplantation and the prediction of the clinical outcome of adult patients with high-risk acute lymphoblastic leukemia. Haematologica 92(5):612–618

Sramkova L, Muzikova K, Fronkova E, Krejci O, Sedlacek P, Formankova R, Mejstrikova E, Stary J, Trka J (2007) Detectable minimal residual disease before allogeneic hematopoietic stem cell transplantation predicts extremely poor prognosis in children with acute lymphoblastic leukemia. Pediatr Blood Cancer 48(1):93–100. doi:10.1002/pbc.20794

Stumph J, Vnencak-Jones CL, Koyama T, Frangoul H (2008) Comparison of peripheral blood and bone marrow samples for detection of post transplant mixed chimerism. Bone Marrow Transplant 41(6):589–590

Uzunel M, Jaksch M, Mattsson J, Ringden O (2003) Minimal residual disease detection after allogeneic stem cell transplantation is correlated to relapse in patients with acute lymphoblastic leukaemia. Br J Haematol 122(5):788–794 4495 [pii]

Uzunel M, Mattsson J, Jaksch M, Remberger M, Ringden O (2001) The significance of graft-versus-host disease and pretransplantation minimal residual disease status to outcome after allogeneic stem cell transplantation in patients with acute lymphoblastic leukemia. Blood 98(6):1982–1984

van der Velden VH, Cazzaniga G, Schrauder A, Hancock J, Bader P, Panzer-Grumayer ER, Flohr T, Sutton R, Cave H, Madsen HO, Cayuela JM, Trka J, Eckert C, Foroni L, Zur Stadt U, Beldjord K, Raff T, van der Schoot CE, van Dongen JJ (2007a) Analysis of minimal residual disease by Ig/TCR gene rearrangements: guidelines for interpretation of real-time quantitative PCR data. Leukemia 21(4):604–611

van der Velden VH, Panzer-Grumayer ER, Cazzaniga G, Flohr T, Sutton R, Schrauder A, Basso G, Schrappe M, Wijkhuijs JM, Konrad M, Bartram CR, Masera G, Biondi A, van Dongen JJ (2007b) Optimization of PCR-based minimal residual disease diagnostics for childhood acute lymphoblastic leukemia in a multi-center setting. Leukemia 21(4):706–713

van der Velden VH, Joosten SA, Willemse MJ, van Wering ER, Lankester AW, van Dongen JJ, Hoogerbrugge PM (2001) Real-time quantitative PCR for detection of minimal residual disease before allogeneic stem cell transplantation predicts outcome in children with acute lymphoblastic leukemia. Leukemia 15(9):1485–1487

van der Velden VH, van Dongen JJ (2009) MRD detection in acute lymphoblastic leukemia patients using Ig/TCR gene rearrangements as targets for real-time quantitative PCR. Methods Mol Biol 538:115–150. doi:10.1007/978-1-59745-418-6_7

van Dongen JJ, Langerak AW, Bruggemann M, Evans PA, Hummel M, Lavender FL, Delabesse E, Davi F, Schuuring E, Garcia-Sanz R, van Krieken JH, Droese J, Gonzalez D, Bastard C, White HE, Spaargaren M, Gonzalez M, Parreira A, Smith JL, Morgan GJ, Kneba M,

Macintyre EA (2003) Design and standardization of PCR primers and protocols for detection of clonal immunoglobulin and T-cell receptor gene recombinations in suspect lymphoproliferations: report of the BIOMED-2 Concerted Action BMH4-CT98-3936. Leukemia 17(12): 2257–2317

van Dongen JJ, Seriu T, Panzer-Grumayer ER, Biondi A, Pongers-Willemse MJ, Corral L, Stolz F, Schrappe M, Masera G, Kamps WA, Gadner H, van Wering ER, Ludwig WD, Basso G, de Bruijn MA, Cazzaniga G, Hettinger K, van der Does-van den Berg A, Hop WC, Riehm H, Bartram CR (1998) Prognostic value of minimal residual disease in acute lymphoblastic leukaemia in childhood. Lancet 352(9142):1731–1738

Winiarski J, Gustafsson A, Wester D, Dalianis T (2000) Follow-up of chimerism, including T- and B-lymphocytes and granulocytes in children more than one year after allogeneic bone marrow transplantation. Pediatr Transplant 4(2):132–139

Yamaji K, Okamoto T, Yokota S, Watanabe A, Horikoshi Y, Asami K, Kikuta A, Hyakuna N, Saikawa Y, Ueyama J, Watanabe T, Okada M, Taga T, Kanegane H, Kogawa K, Chin M, Iwai A, Matsushita T, Shimomura Y, Hori T, Tsurusawa M (2010) Minimal residual disease-based augmented therapy in childhood acute lymphoblastic leukemia: a report from the Japanese Childhood Cancer and Leukemia Study Group. Pediatr Blood Cancer 55(7): 1287–1295. doi:10.1002/pbc.22620

Zhou J, Goldwasser MA, Li A, Dahlberg SE, Neuberg D, Wang H, Dalton V, McBride KD, Sallan SE, Silverman LB, Gribben JG (2007) Quantitative analysis of minimal residual disease predicts relapse in children with B-lineage acute lymphoblastic leukemia in DFCI ALL Consortium Protocol 95-01. Blood 110(5):1607–1611 10.1182/blood-2006-09-045369 blood-2006-09-045369 [pii]

Chapter 17
Biobanks of Cellular Material

Wiesław Wiktor-Jędrzejczak and Elżbieta Urbanowska

Abstract Cellular material can be stored for a variety of purposes, including research, diagnostics, and therapy. Common requirements are the preservation of the identity of the donor of any material, the integrity of the particular material, and informed consent from the donor for its appropriate use. The technical procedures used differ depending on whether it is necessary to preserve cell viability. When cell viability is not required, for example in typical biobanking, the requirements for the conditions of storage are less demanding. In some situations, air-dried material is sufficient, whereas in others, the material must be processed appropriately and stored frozen. The latter also applies to the storage of cellular material for future transplantation. Such material can only be stored in specialized accredited tissue establishments that must conform to prescribed quality control measures to ensure that, after thawing, the material will resume proliferative activity when transplanted.

17.1 Introduction

Cellular material can be stored for a variety of purposes, from research to therapeutic applications. Storage for research purposes is collectively termed 'biobanking', and is carried out in facilities called 'biobanks'. Storage for therapeutic applications is now regulated tightly by appropriate Directives of the European Union (EU) and is

W. Wiktor-Jędrzejczak (✉) · E. Urbanowska
Department of Hematology, Oncology and Internal Diseases,
Medical University of Warsaw, Banacha 1a, 02-097 Warsaw, Poland
e-mail: wiktor@amwaw.edu.pl; wieslaw.jedrzejczak@wum.edu.pl

E. Urbanowska
e-mail: kropla@amwaw.edu.pl

M. Witt et al. (eds.), *Molecular Aspects of Hematologic Malignancies*,
Principles and Practice, DOI: 10.1007/978-3-642-29467-9_17,

carried out exclusively in accredited facilities called 'tissue establishments'. Moreover, cellular material is sometimes stored for diagnostic purposes, for the future performance of tests that are unavailable at the time of sample collection.

Biobanks and tissue establishments are both facilities in which designated (i.e., assigned to a particular individual) cellular material is stored under conditions that preserve the capacity for future use. A biobank can be created by almost any research laboratory for its own purposes, but it can also be a national effort to store material from as many individuals as possible. In fact, several countries have initiated national biobank programmes that in general are oriented toward collecting and storing genetic material from patients with various disorders for future collective analysis (Yuille et al. 2008). In contrast, tissue establishments are independent institutions (or parts of thereof) that perform all the necessary procedures to ensure that the function of cellular material is preserved after transplantation into patients. In the first part of this chapter, we describe biobanking and in the second part, storage for therapeutic use.

17.2 Biobanks

17.2.1 Definitions

The term biobank is not restricted to the storage of human-derived material and may refer to the storage of any primary material derived from all kinds of biological sources. There are specific institutions, such as the American Type Culture Collection (ATCC), that store established cell lines that have been derived from human, animal, or plant primary material (mainly neoplastic). Such secondary or tertiary material is used mainly for research on particular biological phenomena; it is not assigned to a particular individual donor. The storage of such material is not the subject of this chapter.

Biobanks are collections of biological samples whose primary characteristics include a precise description of the individuals from whom they have been collected, and the availability of consent from the donors for the use of this material for research purposes. Depending on the detailed purpose of a particular biobank, specific conditions may vary with respect to storage temperature (room to cryogenic temperatures), use of fixatives, and pre-storage isolation and purification procedures. Biobanks may range in size from a single drawer to large specialized institutions and commercial companies. They can be maintained by individual researchers or laboratories, hospitals, universities, and pharmaceutical companies.

The creation of a biobank requires detailed definition of the aim, types of samples being collected, the logistics of their collection, transportation and processing, and storage conditions. It also requires the preparation of consent forms and definition of the conditions under which the personal data of donors will be stored, secured, and retrieved.

Biobanks could be highly specialized and store collections of specific samples, such as hair, air-dried blood drops, air-dried semen drops or they can be designed for general storage of various types of material such as blood, urine, feces, and tissue specimens for investigations that are not even imagined at the time of storage. Frequently, biobanks are simply DNA banks and databases. Due to significant resistance of DNA to external conditions handling and storage of this material is relatively incomplicated, while other materials, including RNA, may require very sophisticated methods of processing and storage (Williams 2010).

17.2.2 Methodology

Nearly every researcher who investigates original material, i.e., obtained directly from individual donors, could benefit from the creation of his/her own biobank. It is particularly important for researchers who deal with very rare disorders, for which there is a paucity of patients and many investigations cannot be performed while the patient is available. If such biobanks are created within medical practice (and hence are associated with the medical records of primary donors), they may not require independent registration with the relevant agency for personal data protection; however, investigators are advised to consult their national laws and adhere to these regulations. Moreover, the creation and registration of a particular database should conform to the appropriate Directive 1995/46/EC on the protection of individuals. Such registration is usually necessary if the database is outside medical practice.

In general, specimens should be coded (preferentially bar-coded) to allow the blinding of researchers during analysis, and simultaneously to respect the privacy of the donors. Data files that contain personal and medical data that concern donors should be protected from unauthorized access and should be in both electronic and paper form to reduce the risk of accidental loss. Datasets for individuals should include all the necessary information that was defined in the original biobank proposal as well as a signed informed consent form from the donor. The consent form should also contain a statement that transfers the rights of ownership of the samples to the organization that runs the biobank, or permission to utilize these samples. Some countries have laws that automatically transfer the rights of the donor to the public domain, thus securing the right of the donor to anonymity. Proposals for standard consent forms for biobank donors are available in the literature (Beskow et al. 2010). For more information of informed consent see also Chap. 29.

Labels on specimens should be resistant to the conditions of storage, and the specimen inventory should allow for the rapid and precise retrieval of stored samples. If specimens are stored in mechanical freezers or liquid nitrogen tanks, it is important to store duplicates in different freezers or tanks in another location in case of power failure or the leak/vaporization of liquid nitrogen.

17.2.3 Organization

One of the best examples of national biobanking efforts is the UK Biobank (Elliott and Peakman 2008; Peakman and Elliott 2008). Its objective is to enable investigation of the role of genetic factors, exposure to environmental factors, and lifestyle in the etiology of major diseases of late and middle age, such as cardiovascular, neoplastic, and metabolic diseases. The goal is to collect material from 500,000 participants aged between 40 and 69 years and to process and store the material under conditions that allow as many assays to be performed as possible, and hence obtain maximum scientific return for the effort involved. For this purpose, participating centers collect approximately 45 ml of blood and 9 ml of urine for the UK Biobank from each of the recruited subjects. A complete blood count is performed and samples are then transported to a central laboratory, where they are aliquoted further and processed depending on the type of analysis for which they are being stored. The goal is to collect, process, and store 15 million samples; two-thirds at −80 °C and one-third at −196 °C. Several automated techniques are used to allow the rapid storage and retrieval of collected material (Elliott and Peakman 2008).

Similar efforts have been undertaken in many European countries. These efforts have led to the creation of the Biobanking and Biomolecular Resources Research Infrastructure (BBMRI), which was one of the first European Research Infrastructure projects funded by the European Commission (EC). The preparatory phase of this project ended in January 2011. A very large consortium was organized that includes 53 members and over 280 associated organizations. Practically, all European countries are represented, which might allow the creation of a pan-European biobank if member states of the European Union approve appropriate funding for this initiative. The declared intention is that the BBMRI would act as an intermediary between facilities that collect and store material and those that use it for medical research. To achieve this goal, it is proposed that the BBMRI would have an associated facility in each EU member state. The BBMRI would be part of a larger initiative called the European Research Infrastructure Consortium (ERIC), with headquarters in Graz, Austria.

17.3 Tissue Establishments (Banks of Cellular Material)

17.3.1 Definitions and Legal Requirements

Tissue establishments are separate institutions, or divisions of such institutions, that are devoted to the procurement, testing, processing, preservation, storage, and distribution of human tissues and cells that are intended for human applications, and of manufactured products that are derived from human tissues and cells and are intended for human applications. All their activities are collectively termed ‘banking’.

To ensure the maximal level of protection for human health, the EU has issued three directives (Directive 2004/23/EC; Commission Directive 2006/17/EC; and Commission Directive 2006/86/EC). The first of these directives sets standards of quality and safety for the donation, procurement, testing, processing, preservation, storage, and distribution of human tissues and cells. The remaining two are technical directives that implement the first with regard to: (i) certain technical requirements for the donation, procurement, and testing of human tissues and cells, (ii) traceability requirements, (iii) notification of serious adverse reactions and events, and (iv) certain technical requirements for the coding, processing, preservation, storage, and distribution of human tissues and cells. Together, they regulate the vast majority of activities that are concerned with cell banking for clinical use. In principle, they state that, in the EU, all activities associated with the clinical use of human tissues and cells must be carried out exclusively with the assistance of accredited tissue establishments. By this time, all three directives should have been implemented into the law of each member state.

Historically, the banking of cellular material for clinical use was pioneered by departments of embryology that carried out research on embryonic cells (Steinberger and Perloff 1965) and by experimental hematology laboratories that supported autologous bone marrow transplant programmes (Appelbaum et al. 1978). Nowadays, the cells that are stored most frequently for therapeutic purposes are those used in procedures of assisted reproduction and hematopoietic cells. Originally, these storage technologies were used only by the people who had developed them and were knowledgeable about all the technical details; the quality and dependability of the procedures depended on their expertise. Over time, the storage activities were employed on a much larger scale and were taken over by personnel who were trained specifically to perform certain procedures; hence, it became necessary to establish standard protocols of quality control and quality assurance. Moreover, it became necessary to introduce public regulations and the supervision of such activities.

Similarly to any other human biological material, cells can be collected only after informed consent has been obtained from the donor. This means that the banking of cellular material for clinical use is not only a logistic and technical challenge, but also an important legal and ethical issue. Moreover, the existence of a validated system for the precise identification of each banked portion of stored material is crucial for subsequent use of the material.

As already mentioned, the banking of cells for therapeutic purposes is permitted, at least in the EU, only in specialized institutions that are termed tissue establishments, which must meet specific requirements imposed by law. These establishments must also be accredited by specific authorized agencies for a particular country; for instance, in Poland, it is the National Center for Tissue and Cell Banking (Krajowe Centrum Bankowania Tkanek i Komórek). In general, accreditation is valid for 5 years, and must be renewed after this period; it can be withdrawn if the institution ceases to meet the requirements imposed by law to initiate a new tissue establishment, an institution must receive permission from the agency authorized by the government of the respective member state. The request for such permission must include information on the number, qualifications, and duties of the employed personnel, including the so-called 'responsible person', a position that was introduced by the Directive 2004/23/EU. Such a person should have higher qualifications in medicine or biology, at least 2 years professional experience, be independent of the facility director, and be responsible for fulfilling the requirements of quality assurance. The specific duties of the responsible person are listed in the aforementioned Directive. A list of appropriate equipment and details of the laboratory space are also required. The specifications for the latter are determined by country-specific sanitary regulations regarding such facilities, and are confirmed by a specific control agency. Furthermore, a precise description of the system of quality control is required, as well as a detailed description of the planned activities, including those that will be carried out directly by the facility and those that will be outsourced. In the latter case, it is necessary to provide written agreements, and if necessary, copies of documents that confirm that collaborating institutions are accredited to perform outsourced procedures.

The description of the quality assurance system must be related directly to the activities of a particular facility and must include standard operating procedures for all planned activities. Moreover, it should include all guidelines, instructions, forms, and a list of institutions that could use particular cells in the future.

After accreditation, the facility can initiate its activities. However, any relevant changes, in particular, a change in facility director or responsible person, should be reported to the accrediting institution. Thus, the creation of such a facility is a significant logistic undertaking and its functioning requires the fulfillment of several formal requirements.

17.3.2 Methodology

In this chapter, we describe hematopoietic cell banking as an example, although similar procedures can be applied to various cell types. Cell banking begins with the arrival at the tissue establishment of the cells to be stored. Cells should be collected in a sterile manner and transported in such a way as to preserve their viability, sterility, and identity, and they should be accompanied by an informed consent form signed by the donor or his/her legal representative. It is important to maintain an appropriate transport temperature, preferably around 4 °C if transportation takes several hours, although short-term transport (<1 h) can occur at room temperature (if it does not exceed 20 °C) (Antonenas et al. 2006; Jansen et al. 2009; Liozonov et al. 2008). Overheating of cellular material and freezing without the addition of freezing medium can cause cell death and prevent their further use.

The person who accepts the material upon its arrival in the tissue establishment should fill in a special form and assign a unique number to the material. This unique number should be used throughout all procedures carried out in the facility. The number should preferably be bar-coded and appear on all products derived from the material. The completed form should contain the personal data of the donor, place and conditions of cell collection, and details of transport. The collection and transportation of cellular material is a multistep procedure, and during each step, problems may occur, such as contamination with an infectious agent; detailed information about each step should help to identify the exact location of such a problem. The material is then processed using standard procedures that are specific for each type of material (Larghero et al. 2008; Wiktor-Jedrzejczak and Urbanowska 2002). These procedures include the performance of appropriate tests, the isolation or selection of cells in vitro, preparation for freezing, freezing, and placement in a freezer or liquid nitrogen container. The location of the material should be specified in detail, that is, the number of the freezer or liquid nitrogen container and the number of the drawer/box should be noted in the biobanking form and the electronic inventory of the particular facility. Information concerning the cellular material should include: cell number, viability, cellular composition, results of tests for bacterial and fungal contamination, and other information typical for the particular type of material, such as the number of cells with surface CD34 in the case of peripheral or cord blood.

In the simplest form, in vitro processing of cells includes the reduction of volume and the depletion or removal of red cells. However, processing may also include the use of more advanced methods such as the isolation of particular subsets of cells, treatment with various drugs, cell culture, or genetic modification of cells to correct inborn defects. Preparation for freezing includes mixing the cells with a cryoprotective medium and transferring the sample to a freezing bag (Bakken 2006; Rowley et al. 1994). The cryoprotective medium that is used most frequently is a mixture of 5–10 % dimethylsulfoxide (DMSO) and culture medium (e.g. Dulbecco's Modified Eagle's Medium). Freezing in special tubes called cryogenic or freezing vials is not recommended (although this is typical for research purposes) and is being replaced gradually by the use of special bags, although both approaches have advantages and disadvantages. The advantages of cryogenic tubes are their greater resistance to external damage than freezer bags and the fact that, given a single cell sample will be stored in many vials, the destruction of one or two of these vials does not significantly compromise the amount of material left for further use. However, one disadvantage is the need to use tens and sometimes hundreds of vials to freeze the material from a single donor, which is laborious. Even more important is the fact that the use of tubes leads to an open system, which is more vulnerable to contamination with infectious agents during processing than a closed system (Lazarus et al. 1991; Padley et al. 1996). Hence, the main advantage of freezing bags is that they provide a closed system. However, the major disadvantage is that, despite being made from special materials, bags are more vulnerable than tubes to external damage, which can lead to the destruction of the entire contents of the bag. The material used for the freezer bags should be resistant to changes in temperature in the range from +50 to −200 °C; many materials become extremely fragile at very low temperature and thus sensitive to mechanical damage (Valery and Pivacek 1996). In addition, the material must be biologically neutral. It is crucial to mark each bag (or tube) with the bar code of the donor in a manner that is also resistant to the conditions in which the bag or tube is processed and stored.

The samples should be frozen in a controlled way using special equipment that registers the required freezing rate of approximately 1 °C/min. However, in many processing facilities with equal effect a two-step method is used (Almici et al. 2003), which is much simpler and less time and labor consuming. The two-step method relies on putting the material to be frozen into a styrofoam box and placing the box in a −80 °C freezer. Such conditions approximate to a controlled rate freezing of approximately 1 °C/min until the final temperature of −80 °C is reached. On the next day, the frozen material can be transferred directly to liquid nitrogen. The two-step method can only be used in tissue establishments where it has been validated and compared with the programmed rate of freezing (Perez-Oteyza et al. 1998). An additional disadvantage of this method is the fact that no automatic recording of the freezing rate is made, and, therefore, cannot serve as part of quality control.

Human cells can be stored for intermediate periods (several months) in −80 °C freezers, but prolonged storage should be in liquid nitrogen (Ayello et al. 1998). It is also possible to use −140 °C mechanical freezers (Valery and Pivacek 1996). It is essential that mechanical freezers are equipped with backup systems in case of power failure and with a monitoring system that is connected to duty personnel who could intervene immediately and prevent an increase in temperature in the freezer. It is also necessary to have additional backup freezers available in case of complete freezer failure. Uncontrolled thawing of cells leads to their destruction. This is because the hyperosmotic solutions of DMSO that preserve cell viability, while frozen, are toxic to cells at temperatures above freezing and cause their death within 30–60 min. The most dangerous situation is when thawing and subsequent refreezing are not detected: the material might look the same but it will not produce the desired biological effect when used.

Storage in liquid nitrogen can be done in two ways: in either the vapor (temperature approximately −140 °C) or the liquid phase (−190 °C) (Wiktor-Jedrzejczak and Urbanowska 2002; Valery and Pivacek 1996). Both phases have advantages and disadvantages. Storage in the liquid phase prevents the unknown effects associated with the temperature changes that occur when the nitrogen tank is opened to insert or withdraw other bags. In general, the temperature remains within the range −60 °C to −180 °C, but these changes may occur many times over the years of storage because the liquid nitrogen tanks will contain hundreds or thousands of samples that are inserted and withdrawn periodically. The disadvantage of storage in the liquid phase is the danger of external contamination, because liquid nitrogen also preserves microorganisms. If the external surface of even one frozen sample is contaminated with infectious material from a donor, the entire tank might be contaminated. Such a risk is lower when the samples are stored in the vapor phase but the risk associated with temperature change during opening of the tank remains.

Storage requires careful supervision, mainly by electronic means. Hence, each freezer and liquid nitrogen tank must be connected to a system that monitors temperature constantly. In addition, each freezer and liquid nitrogen tank should have a log in which, at least once daily, authorized personnel confirm that the equipment has been inspected and record the temperature measured. Safety procedures for mechanical freezers have been outlined earlier, and liquid nitrogen storage tanks should be connected to larger tanks that constantly and automatically deliver liquid nitrogen to replace any gas that has vaporized. Cell storage facilities should possess additional backup tanks in case of leakage from one of the existing tanks. Rooms that contain many tanks should have an efficient ventilation system and a nitrogen-in-air concentration indicator to detect any increase in nitrogen concentration that could be potentially harmful to personnel.

After storage, frozen cells can be released to participate therapeutic establishments, such as transplant units, and might need to be transported long distances (e.g. to other countries). For such situations, tissue establishments should be equipped with special liquid nitrogen transportation tanks with electronic temperature registration. Such containers are sufficient to transport for several days and, after the end of transportation, the temperature can be verified finally by the facility that is going to use the material. The material can then be used immediately or stored for use at a later time.

In order to transplant stored frozen cellular material, it must first be thawed. Two methods are used for this purpose (Frey et al. 2006; Windrum et al. 2005). First, the material can be thawed in the laboratory, and the DMSO removed immediately (Rowley 1994). Then, the washed cells are suspended in an appropriate medium and infused into the patient. In the second approach, the cells are thawed at the bedside and then infused immediately into the patient together with the DMSO (Laroche et al. 2005; Preti et al. 1994). In the latter case, the DMSO is diluted in the patient's circulation and is then removed by the kidneys and by the lungs and rarely causes any serious side effects. As mentioned earlier, the key problem is the hyperosmosity of the DMSO solution and its harmful effects on thawed cells, which could lead to their destruction within a short time. However, there are also problems associated with removing the DMSO. To wash out the DMSO, the sample is diluted significantly, medium is added gradually to the thawed cell suspension, the diluted cell suspension is centrifuged, the supernatant containing DMSO is removed, and the cell pellet is reconstituted with DMSO-free medium. The danger associated with this procedure is related to the high number of neutrophils in preparations obtained by leukapheresis. Neutrophils are very fragile during the thawing procedure and may be destroyed during procedures to remove the DMSO, namely, centrifugation and resuspension. The disruption of neutrophils may lead to the release of large quantities of DNA, which is extremely sticky. If such a phenomenon occurs, the material cannot be used further. If this were the only transplantation material available for a particular patent, this might have tragic consequences. Owing to this problem, it is considered safer to thaw the material at the patient bedside and transfuse it immediately, and this approach is used routinely (Preti et al. 1994).

17.4 Conclusions

At present, the banking of cellular material for research or therapeutic use is a routine process. Banking for research purposes, which is called biobanking, is an undertaking that can range from the initiative of an individual researcher to national and international (pan-European) projects. The main goal of biobanking is to create a repository of material from as many individuals as possible to allow studies that can range from the investigation of rare disorders to population approaches. Banking for therapeutic use, mainly in transplantation, has to be carried out in accredited facilities, where the main goals are to preserve the identity of individuals and to maintain the sterility and viability of cells after thawing to enable successful transplantation. Extreme attention is paid to quality control as a measure to ensure the safety of the entire procedure. Whereas biobanking is supposed to provide material for the development of solutions to many unsolved medical problems, cell banking for therapeutic use is aimed at resolving the particular health problems of many individuals. Thus, the two approaches complement each other.

References

Almici C, Ferremi P, Lanfranchi A, Ferrari E, Verardi R, Marini M, Rossi G (2003) Uncontrolled-rate freezing of peripheral blood progenitor cells allows successful engraftment by sparing primitive and committed hematopoietic progenitors. Haematologica 88:1390–1395

Antonenas V, Garlin F, Webb M, Santor M, Bradstock KT, Gottlieb D (2006) Fresh PBSC harvests, but not BM, show temperature-related loss of CD34 viability during storage and transport. Cytotherapy 8:158–165

Appelbaum FR, Herzig GP, Ziegler JL, Graw RG, Levine AS, Deisseroth AB (1978) Successful engraftment of cryopreserved autologous bone marrow in patients with malignant lymphoma. Blood 52:85–95

Ayello J, Semidei-Pomales M, Preti R, Hesdorffer C, Reiss RF (1998) Effects of long-term storage at −90 degrees C of bone marrow and PBSC on cells recovery, viability, and clonogenic potential. J Hematother 7:385–390

Bakken AM (2006) Cryopreserving human peripheral blood progenitor cells. Curr Stem Cell Res Ther 1:47–54

Beskow LM, Friedman JY, Hardy NC, Lin L, Weinfurt KP (2010) Developing a simplified consent form for biobanking. PLoS ONE 5(10):e13302

Commission Directive 2006/17/EC of 8 February 2006 implementing Directive 2004/23/EC of the European Parliament and of the Council as regards certain technical requirements for the donation, procurement and testing of human tissues and cells

Commission Directive 2006/86/EC of 24 October 2006 implementing Directive 2004/23/EC of the European Parliament and of the Council as regards traceability requirements, notification of serious adverse reactions and events and certain technical requirements for the coding, processing, preservation, storage and distribution of human tissues and cells

Directive 2004/23/EC of the European Parliament and of the Council of 31 March 2004 on setting standards of quality and safety for the donation, procurement, testing, processing, preservation, storage and distribution of human tissues and cells

Directive 95/46/EC of the European Parliament and of the Council of 24 October 1995 on the protection of individuals with regard to the processing of personal data and on the free movement of such data

Elliott P, Peakman TC (2008) The UK Biobank sample handling and storage protocol for the collection, processing and archiving of human blood and urine. Int J Epidemiol 37:234–244 on behalf of UK Biobank

Frey NV, Lazarus HM, Goldstein SC (2006) Has allogeneic stem cell cryopreservation been given the ‘cold shoulder’? An analysis of the pros and cons of using frozen versus fresh stem cell products in allogeneic stem cell transplantation. Bone Marrow Transplant 38:399–405

Jansen J, Nolan PL, Reeves MI, Akard LP, Thompson JM, Dugan MJ, Hanks SG (2009) Transportation of peripheral blood progenitor cell products: effects of time, temperature and cell concentration. Cytotherapy 11:79–85

Larghero J, Garcia J, Gluckman E (2008) Sources and stem cell procurement. In: Apperley J, Carreras E, Gluckman E, Gratwohl A, Masszi T (eds) Haematopoietic stem cell transplantation, The EBMT handbook, 2008 Rev edn. Forum Service Editore, Genoa pp 112–127

Laroche V, McKenna DH, Moroff G, Schierman T, Kadidlo D, McCullough J (2005) Cell loss and recovery in umbilical cord blood processing: a comparison of postthaw and postwash samples. Transfusion 45:1909–1916

Lazarus HM, Magalhaes-Silverman M, Fox RM, Creger RJ, Jacobs M (1991) Contamination during in vitro processing of bone marrow for transplantation: clinical significance. Bone Marrow Transplant 7:241–246

Liozonov M, Dellbrugger C, Sputtek A, Fehse B, Kroger N, Zander AR (2008) Transportation and cryopreservation may impair haematopoietic stem cell function and engraftment of allogeneic PBSCs, but not BM. Bone Marrow Transplant 42:121–128

Padley D, Koontz F, Trigg ME, Gingrich R, Strauss RG (1996) Bacterial contamination rates following processing of bone marrow and peripheral blood progenitor cell preparations. Transfusion 36:53–56

Peakman TC, Elliott P (2008) The UK Biobank sample handling and storage validation studies. Int J Epidemiol 37(Suppl 1):i2–i6

Perez-Oteyza J, Bornstein R, Corral M, Hermosa V, Alegre A, Torrabadella M, Ramos P, Garcia J, Odriozola J, Navarro JL (1998) Controlled-rate versus uncontrolled-rate cryopreservation of peripheral blood progenitor cells: a prospective multicenter study. Group for Cryobiology and Biology of Bone Marrow Transplantation (CBTMO). Spain. Haematologica 83:1001–1005

Preti RA, Razis E, Ciavarella D, Fan Y, Kuhns RE, Cook P, Wong G, Wuest DL, Ahmed T (1994) Clinical and laboratory study of refrigerated and cryopreserved bone marrow for transplantation. Bone Marrow Transplant 13:253–260

Rowley SD, Bensinger WI, Gooley TA, Buckner CD (1994) Effect of cell concentration on bone marrow and peripheral blood stem cell cryopreservation. Blood 83:2731–2736

Steinberger E, Perloff WH (1965) Preliminary experience with a human sperm bank. Am J Obstet Gynecol 92:577–579

Williams MA (2010) Stabilizing the code-methods to preserve RNA prove their worth. Biomark Insights 5:139–143

Wiktor-Jedrzejczak WW, Urbanowska E (2002) Isolation and cryopreservation of haematopoietic stem and progenitor cells from peripheral blood and cord blood. In: Phillips GO (ed) Advances in Tissue Banking. World Scientific Publishing, Singapore, pp 201–231

Windrum P, Morris TC, Drake MB, Niederwieser D, Ruutu T (2005) Variation in dimethyl sulfoxide use in stem cell transplantation: a survey of EBMT centres. Bone Marrow Transplant 36:601–603 EBMT Chronic Leukaemia Working Party Complications Subcommittee

Valery CR, Pivacek LE (1996) Effect of the temperature, the duration of frozen storage and the freezing container on in vitro measurements in human peripheral blood mononuclear cells. Transfusion 36:303–308

Yuille M, van Ommen GJ, Bréchot C, Cambon-Thomsen A, Dagher G, Landegren U, Litton JE, Pasterk M, Peltonen L, Taussig M, Wichmann HE, Zatloukal K (2008) Biobanking for Europe. Brief Bioinform 9:14–24

Part IV
Molecular Diagnostic Protocols

Chapter 18
Biobanking of Cellular Material

Anna Poluha and Elżbieta Urbanowska

Abstract Research biobank are well-organized resources developed for the purpose of collecting, processing, storing, and distributing biological samples, accompanied by associated relevant clinical data, to make them accessible to further scientific investigation. In order to be efficient and reliable, genetic biobanks must implement specific guidelines. The detailed protocols for each step of the biobanking process strictly depend on the type and the aims of particular institution. However, some general policies should be followed, regarding key components of the banking process: obtaining informed initial consent to participate, proper collection of biological material, handling and transport of samples, freezing, storage, and retrieval of collected tissue as well as collection, protection, and sharing of relevant data.

18.1 Introduction

The key components of the banking process are obtaining informed initial consent to participate, proper collection of biological material, handling and transport of samples, freezing, storage, and retrieval of collected tissue, collection, protection, and sharing of relevant data.

A. Poluha (✉)
Department of Pediatric Hematology, Oncology and Transplantology,
Children's University Hospital, Chodźki 2, 20-093 Lublin, Poland
e-mail: poluha.anna@gmail.com

E. Urbanowska
Department of Hematology, Oncology and Internal Diseases,
Medical University of Warsaw, Banacha 1a, 02-097 Warsaw, Poland
e-mail: kropla@amwaw.edu.pl

M. Witt et al. (eds.), *Molecular Aspects of Hematologic Malignancies*,
Principles and Practice, DOI: 10.1007/978-3-642-29467-9_18,

18.2 Consent Procedure

Preliminary issue that needs to be considered in the biobanking process is the protection of rights of those who submit biological samples and information. This is achieved by obtaining and documenting initial information and voluntary consent to participate. In the research banking model, where samples of potential interest are collected and stored until needed, a prospective and possibly broad type of consent is applicable, as it is not possible, at the time of consent procedure, to predict all the future applications with the use of collected biological material. A consent should be obtained by qualified biobank personnel and/or clinical staff after providing patient or his/her legal representative with relevant information about the implications of their decision to participate. It is to be documented by signing a written and dated consent form. It is particularly important to emphasize that participation is voluntary and the decision to withdraw from the study will not affect the standard of care the patient is receiving or will receive. For more information on informed consent see Chap. 29.

18.3 Material Collection

Samples (blood, bone marrow, lymph node tissue) are collected from consented participants either as a surplus to the clinical needs (e.g. collecting material for initial diagnosis or for standard laboratory tests) or are gathered specifically for research purposes.

18.3.1 Blood Collection

5–10 ml is the minimum volume recommended for most applications

- draw blood into an appropriately labeled evacuated collection tubes containing anticoagulant (the recommended anticoagulant for further molecular studies is EDTA (ethylenediaminetetraacetate)
- mix blood with anticoagulant by inverting tubes gently 6–8 times.

18.3.2 Bone Marrow Aspiration

2–4 ml is the recommended minimum volume although any amount of bone marrow aspirate, that is surplus to the diagnostic needs, should be considered a valuable sample. An excessive suction is to be avoided during aspiration as it may cause dilution of bone marrow aspirate with peripheral blood. Therefore, syringes of a maximum volume of 5 ml should be used for the aspiration. The vacuum collecting systems are not recommended.

- Collect bone marrow aspirated during routine diagnostic procedure into an appropriately labeled collection tubes containing anticoagulant (EDTA).
- Mix bone marrow aspirate with anticoagulant by inverting tubes gently 6–8 times.

18.3.3 Lymph Node Biopsy

25 mg of the unprocessed tissue is the recommended amount. For satisfactory sampling, it is essential that the material prepared for banking contains cross sections of a lymph node that represent its complete architecture. A formalin fixation should be avoided.

- Place sample in the appropriate container (e.g. Petri dish) and submit fresh to the bank without a delay.
- If delay is unavoidable, lymph node samples can be transported or stored for short periods at 4 °C in tissue culture medium or normal saline.

18.4 Freezing the Samples

For protocol of isolation of mononuclear cells (MCs) from blood and bone marrow—see Chap. 19.

18.4.1 Freezing Mononuclear Cells with Preservation of Their Viability

This procedure of freezing is used for banking MCs to be used for transplantation. Addition of cryoprotectant dimethylsufoxide (DMSO) to cryopreserving solution plays an important role in maintaining cell viability. It should be emphasized that processing of cell suspension mixed with DMSO has to be carried fast, since DMSO is considerably cytotoxic in temperatures above 0 °C.

- Prepare cryopreserving solution: 40 % RPMI-1640 medium (Roswell Park Memorial Institute medium), 40 % FCS (fetal calf serum), 20 % DMSO.
- Place container with cryopreserving solution in a styrofoam box filled with mixture of ice and water (ice bath) to lower its temperature.
- Mix cell suspension with liquid protective–nutritious medium (60 % RPMI- 1640, 40 % FCS) to reach the concentration of 1×10^7 cells per 1 ml of final solution.
- Place prepared cell suspension in a refrigerator to cool it down to 4–8 °C.
- Divide cell suspension into 0.5 ml aliquots and pipette them into required amount of properly labeled cryovials placed in the ice bath.
- Gradually add 0.5 ml of cooled cryopreserving solution to each cryovial while mixing gently.

- Transfer cryovials to the freezer storage box and place the box immediately in the freezer equipped with a software for programed freezing. If such a device is inaccessible, the freezer storage box can be placed in a container filled with isopropyl alcohol (which helps maintain the uniform cooling rate) and then transferred to –80 °C freezer and subsequently to liquid nitrogen.

18.4.2 Snap Freezing of Mononuclear Cells

Snap frozen cells are suitable for extraction of DNA and RNA for further molecular research and for isolation of proteins for enzymatic studies.

- Mix cell suspension with liquid protective–nutritious medium (60 % RPMI 1640, 40 % FCS) to reach the concentration of 1×10^7 cells per 1 ml of final solution.
- Divide cell suspension into 0.5 ml aliquots and pipette them into required amount of properly labeled cryovials.
- Centrifuge at $500 \times g$ for 5 min, 4 °C.
- Discard the supernatant.
- Gently tap the vials to loosen cell pellet.
- Close the cryovials and immediately submerge them into liquid nitrogen.

18.4.3 Snap Freezing of Lymph Nodes

Snap frozen lymph node tissue is suitable for the same analyses as snap frozen MCs.

- Place representative cross-sections of lymph node in properly labeled cryovials.
- Close the cryovials and immediately submerge them into liquid nitrogen.

18.5 Sample Retrieval

18.5.1 Retrieval of Cells in Viable State

- Prepare cell washing solution (90 % RPMI-1640, 10 % FCS) and cool it down in an ice bath.
- Transfer cryovial containing desired material directly from liquid nitrogen into 37 °C water bath minimizing exposure to ambient temperature.
- Gently agitate until disappearance of ice crystals.
- Transfer cell suspension to 10 ml tube and gradually add 5 ml of cell washing solution, while mixing gently.
- Centrifuge at $100 \times g$, 5 min, 4 °C.
- Discard the supernatant.
- Gently tap the vials to loosen cell pellet.
- Add 1 ml of cell washing solution.

18.5.2 Retrieval of Snap Frozen Cells and Lymph Node Tissue

- Retrieve frozen vials containing desired material from a storage container and place them into prechilled metal racks, while minimizing exposure of the storage container to ambient temperature.
- Transfer retrieved samples to the container appropriately labeled for further purposes (transport, storage).

18.6 Transportation of Banked Material in a Frozen State

The correct handling of the sample during transportation is crucial to further successful application of the material. Frozen cells or tissues should be transported in liquid nitrogen in a proper transporting container equipped with the temperature monitoring and registering system. Once placed in liquid nitrogen, samples should be kept in these conditions until analysis. They must not be transferred to mechanical freezers (e.g. –80 °C freezer), even for short time storage.

18.7 Data Collection and Protection

Collection of relevant clinical and sample associated information accompanying banked material is an integral part of cell banking process. The range of collected data strictly depends on the type of the repository and the needs of further research (if known). However, some general policies should be followed in each bank regarding protection of data and personal information as well as their use, in accordance with terms of the consent given by the participant and as regulated by the appropriate Research Ethics Board. Each bank should establish their own or be granted an access to an existing computer based sample associated data collection system with customizable interface (web-based) possibly compatible with other relevant databases. The access to clinical and sample data should be strictly controlled within each institution, limited to authorized personnel only. For more information on data collection and protection see Chaps. 17 and 29.

18.8 Conclusions

Biobanks are fundamental in advancing biomedical research, especially in the area of cancer research. The increasing number of human biological samples, accompanied by extensive clinical data are being stored in numerous biorepositories worldwide. It is generally understood that only collaborative actions focusing on high-quality biobanking can pave the way toward highly efficient, large scale, high-throughput studies, leading to improved understanding of pathomechanisms of various diseases, that could later be translated into safe and effective therapies.

Further Reading

Hewitt RE (2011) Biobanking: the foundation of personalized medicine. Curr Opin Oncol 23:112–119

International Society for Biological and Environmental Repositories (ISBER) (2008) Collection, storage, retrieval and distribution of biological materials for research. Cell Preserv Technol 6:3–58. doi:10.1089/cpt.2008.9997

Kauffmann F, Cambon-Thomsen A (2008) Tracing biological collections: between books and clinical trials. JAMA 299:2316–2318

Sak J, Pawlikowski J, Goniewicz M, Witt M (2012) Population biobanking in selected European countries and proposed model for a polish national DNA bank. J Appl Genetics (in press). doi 10.1007/s13353-012-0082-4

Végvári A, Welinder C, Lindberg H, Fehniger TE, Marko-Varga G (2011) Biobank resources for future patient care: developments, principles and concepts. J Clin Bioinforma 1:24. doi:10.1186/2043-9113-1-24

Yuille M, Illig T, Hveem K, Schmitz G, Hansen J, Neumaier M, Tybring G, Wichmann E, Ollier B (2010) Laboratory management of samples in biobanks: european consensus expert group report. Biopreserv Biobank 8:65–69. doi:10.1089/bio.2010.8102

Chapter 19
Isolation of Mononuclear Cells from Human Blood and Bone Marrow by Density Gradient Centrifugation

Małgorzata Dawidowska

Abstract Isolation of mononuclear cells (MNC) does not belong to the set of molecular procedures, however, it is the first step of isolation of nucleic acids from peripheral blood or bone marrow in many protocols used for molecular analyses in hemato-oncological diseases. In this chapter, the protocol for isolation of MNCs by density gradient centrifugation is presented. This basic protocol might be subjected to modifications, depending on the specific needs of particular applications.

19.1 Introduction

The isolation of mononuclear cells (MNC), although does not belong to the set of molecular procedures, is the first step of cell sample processing used in many molecular diagnostic protocols in hemato-oncology. The separation of mononuclear cells (lymphocytes and monocytes) from other components of blood/bone marrow (basically granulocytes, erythrocytes, plasma) is often performed prior to nucleic acid extraction or before the separation of specific cell subsets to increase the yield and purity of these procedures. There are several commercially available density gradient centrifugation media for MNCs' isolation, characterized by density of 1.077 g/ml at 20 °C, enabling separation of highly purified, viable MNCs suitable for further applications. The basic protocol presented in this chapter is based on the method developed by Bøyum (1968a, b; 1976) but it might be subjected to modifications, including the use of centrifugation media of different densities, depending on the specific needs of particular applications.

M. Dawidowska (✉)
Department of Molecular and Clinical Genetics, Institute of Human Genetics,
Polish Academy of Sciences, Strzeszyńska 32, 60-479 Poznań, Poland
e-mail: ma.dawidowska@wp.pl

M. Witt et al. (eds.), *Molecular Aspects of Hematologic Malignancies*,
Principles and Practice, DOI: 10.1007/978-3-642-29467-9_19,

19.2 Biological Material

Bone marrow or peripheral blood should be collected into anticoagulant (e.g. EDTA) containing tubes, and mixed well to prevent clot formation. The material should optimally be subjected to further procedures as soon as possible, not later than within 24 h from collection. If RNA is to be isolated from the MNC fraction, MNC isolation, followed by RNA extraction should preferably be performed immediately after blood/bone marrow aspiration.

The isolation of the MNC fraction might be the first step in seperating selected cell subsets of blood/bone marrow (e.g. CD3 lymphocyte subset) by immunomagnetic or flow cytometric method. In this case, the isolation of MNCs should be performed at a time which allows the isolation of cell subsets within a maximum of 8 h after blood/bone marrow collection. Blood/bone marrow samples which are to be subjected to fractionation (isolation of MNC/isolation of cell subsets) must not be frozen.

19.3 Protocol for MNC Isolation by Density Gradient Centrifugation

Materials required:

- Commercially available gradient medium for isolation of MNCs (density 1.077 g/ml), stored in dark at 4 °C, brought to room temperature (18–20 °C) prior to isolation
- PBS buffer (phosphate buffered saline) (137 mM NaCl, 2.7 mM KCl, 8 mM Na_2HPO_4, 1.46 mM KH_2PO_4; pH 7.4), brought to room temperature prior to isolation
- Erythrocyte lysis buffer (0.15 M NH_4 Cl, 0.01 M $KHCO_3$, 0.37 g/l EDTA).

Protocol:

1. Determine white blood cells count (WBC) in the blood/bone marrow sample.
2. Dilute the sample in PBS buffer to obtain a final WBC of 10×10^6/ml or dilute the sample twofold and threefold in case of blood and bone marrow sample, respectively. The dilution of blood/bone marrow prevents MNCs being trapped by aggregates of erythrocytes.
3. Prepare 10–15 ml of gradient medium in a 50 ml tube.
4. Carefully apply up to 35 ml of diluted blood/bone marrow sample, slowly down the side of the tube (avoid intermixing) to form a layer over the aliquot of the gradient medium.
5. Centrifuge at $400 \times g$ for 30 min at 18 °C using a swinging bucket rotor. Allow to decelerate without braking.
6. After centrifugation four layers can be distinguished:

- erythrocytes and granulocytes (at the bottom)
- aliquot of the density gradient medium (over the bottom layer)
- mononuclear cells and platelets (thin layer over the gradient medium layer)
- plasma fraction (upper layer).

7. Carefully aspirate and discard the upper plasma layer, taking care not to disturb the mononuclear layer at the plasma/gradient medium interface.
8. Collect the MNCs from the interface and transfer into a fresh 50 ml tube. The harvested MNC fraction is further purified from platelets, plasma, and density gradient medium through subsequent steps of washing and centrifugation.
9. Add 10 ml of PBS buffer and wash MNCs by gentle mixing using a vortex and/or by thorough pipetting. Centrifuge at $400 \times g$ for 10 min at 4 °C and discard the supernatant.
10. In case of erythrocyte contamination of the MNC fraction, add 2 ml of erythrocyte lysis buffer, incubate for 5 min at room temp and centrifuge at $400 \times g$ for 5 min at 4 °C. Discard the supernatant. If no erythrocyte contamination is visible, proceed directly to step 11.
11. Wash the MNC fraction twice by resuspending the cells in PBS buffer (by gentle vortexing and/or pipetting), and centrifuging at $400 \times g$ for 5 min at 4 °C. Discard the supernatant.
12. Resuspend the cells in PBS buffer (to 10×10^6/ml) and transfer into a fresh 1.5 ml tube. Centrifuge at $250 \times g$ for 5 min at 4 °C and discard the supernatant.
13. The MNC fraction might be used directly for further applications, stored overnight at 4 °C (suspended in PBS buffer) or stored at −80 °C for later use (as a cell pellet). For a subsequent RNA isolation, it is recommended to store MNC at −80 °C with a cryoprotectant.

19.4 Conclusions

Since its development in 1968, the method for MNC isolation by density gradient centrifugation, described by Bøyum has been widely used in the field of immunological and molecular research and diagnostics. Although the method itself does not belong to molecular procedures, it was included in this part of the book to provide a basic protocol for the separation of the cells used for further molecular diagnostic procedures in hematological malignancies. This basic protocol might be subjected to modifications, depending on the specific requirements of further applications.

Acknowledgements This chapter was partly supported by the Ministry of Science and Higher Education, grant N N407 311 839.

References

Bøyum A (1968a) Isolation of mononuclear cells and granulocytes from human blood. Isolation of monuclear cells by one centrifugation, and of granulocytes by combining centrifugation and sedimentation at 1 g. Scand J Clin Lab Invest Suppl 97:77–89

Bøyum A (1968b) Isolation of leucocytes from human blood. Further observations. Methylcellulose, dextran, and ficoll as erythrocyteaggregating agents. Scand J Clin Lab Invest Suppl 97:31–50

Bøyum A (1976) Isolation of lymphocytes, granulocytes and macrophages. Scand J Immunol Suppl 5:9–15

Chapter 20
Molecular Techniques Commonly Used in Hemato-oncology

Monika D. Kraszewska and Ewa Ziętkiewicz

Abstract Molecular studies in hematological malignancies are based on nucleic acid analysis. The choice of molecular methods depends on molecular changes that are expected. The techniques described in this chapter include: methods of tissue collection, DNA and RNA extraction, DNA and RNA storage recommendations, DNA and RNA amplification (PCR, reverse transcription and real time quantitative PCR), electrophoretic analysis of the length of amplified fragments, DNA sequencing, analysis of DNA methylation, and analysis of large genomic deletions.

20.1 Introduction

The majority of molecular studies in hematological malignancies is based on nucleic acid analysis. DNA aberrations in malignant cells may range from point mutations (nucleotide substitutions or small insertions and deletions—indels), through deletions, duplications, or inversions of larger subchromosomal regions, to duplications, losses, or translocations of the whole chromosomes; they can even affect the entire cell genome (mono- or poliploidy). While some of these mutations may be heritable, usually aberrant DNA in clonal populations of malignant cells differs from that present in the unaffected somatic cells. Moreover, DNA in malignant cells can undergo epigenetic changes (aberrant methylation patterns).

M. D. Kraszewska · E. Ziętkiewicz (✉)
Institute of Human Genetics, Polish Academy of Sciences,
Strzeszyńska 32, 60-479 Poznań, Poland
e-mail: zietkiee@man.poznan.pl

M. D. Kraszewska
e-mail: m.kraszewska@gmail.com

M. Witt et al. (eds.), *Molecular Aspects of Hematologic Malignancies*,
Principles and Practice, DOI: 10.1007/978-3-642-29467-9_20,

All these alterations can be studied using a variety of molecular biology methods. The effects of DNA aberrations can also be observed at the level of RNA. However, analysis of RNA expression is more complicated, since, in contrast to DNA sequence, transcriptome profile depends on the tissue/cell type, and—within a given cell type—it changes with time (age), and in response to the environmental factors (lifestyle, diet, medication).

The information encoded in nucleic acids can aid diagnosis of hemato-oncologic malignancies and allow stratification of patients into risk groups that may be subjected to different therapeutic regimes. Depending on the detected aberrations and their molecular consequences, appropriate therapies can be applied and their effects monitored. Moreover, since polymorphisms in various genes might influence drug metabolism, their impact on the drug response can be predicted and therapeutic strategy can be accordingly adjusted. Therefore, collecting biological material for nucleic acids' analyses should be regarded a crucial procedure in all hemato-oncology centers.

20.2 Biological Material for DNA-Based Molecular Analyses

20.2.1 Tissue Collection

Blood or bone marrow obtained for DNA-based molecular analyses should be collected into tubes containing EDTA (ethylenediamine tetra-acetic acid) salts as anticoagulant. Using heparin is also possible; however, since heparin is known to contribute to polymerase chain reaction (PCR) inhibition, DNA extraction from such samples should be preceded by isolation of mononuclear cells by density gradient centrifugation (see Chap. 19) (Bruggemann et al. 2010). The amount of blood required for isolation is 2–10 ml; in case of bone marrow, 1–2 ml should be sufficient for a good yield of DNA. Blood or bone marrow should be delivered to the laboratory for further processing within 24 h and, if possible, kept at 4 °C. If longer storage is expected, it should be frozen in −20 °C; however, frozen material cannot be used for mononuclear cell isolation.

Solid tissue fragments should be placed in sterile plastic containers, suitable for tissue storage, and should be positioned on sterile cotton swabs soaked with PBS buffer (phosphate buffered saline). Lymph nodes should be obtained from patients in the amount of at least 25 g. Tissue fragments should be stored and transported at 4 °C and should reach the laboratory within 24 h from collection. If longer storage is necessary, the tissue should be frozen at −20 °C, or if possible, at −80 °C.

Material collected for cytogenetic analyses can be preserved in the cytogenetic fixative solution (3:1 mixture of methanol and glacial acetic acid). However, as a consequence of such treatment, proteins are denatured and lipids are removed from the cells, leaving the DNA exposed and prone to damage during storage of cell suspension.

20.2.2 Tissue Preparation

DNA isolation from frozen samples does not differ from isolation using fresh material, except that lower DNA yields should be expected. If DNA is to be isolated from archival tissues preserved in formalin and embedded in paraffin blocks, it is necessary to perform extra steps to ensure efficient DNA extraction. In the process of formaldehyde fixing, DNA in samples is not damaged directly. However, the fixative cross-links with the DNA-associated proteins contributes to shredding DNA into small pieces, which leads to lower efficiency of DNA amplification in PCR. In order to obtain better yields, DNA extraction can be preceded by removal of paraffin by xylene and alcohol washes (Goelz et al. 1985; Wickham et al. 2000; Coura et al. 2005) or direct microwave melting (Banerjee et al. 1995); heating up samples might also remove some cross-linking caused by formalin (Shi et al. 1991).

DNA isolation from material fixed for cytogenetic analyses is possible, but it has to be preceded by removal of a fixative solution. This can be done by: centrifugation at $400\times g$, 5 min, 4 °C; cell washing with 70 % ethanol; centrifugation at $400\times g$, 5 min, 4 °C; and final resuspension at 4 °C PBS; to ensure maximum removal of the fixative solution, cell washing in PBS can be repeated several times.

20.2.3 DNA Isolation

It is recommended that DNA isolation is executed in a dedicated lab space. It is best if a separate room can be devoted just to DNA isolation. If this is not feasible, at least a laminar flow cabinet should be used. The use of a laminar flow cabinet has two main purposes: it prevents infectious agents possibly present in patients' material from spreading through the air, and what is equally important, it prevents DNA samples from cross contamination in case of spillage or aerosol forming. For the same reason, tips with filters are recommended. Although DNA is generally robust to degradation, using a nuclease-free workspace is suggested.

Four main methods of DNA isolation are widely applied: phenol–chloroform approach, salt precipitation method, silica-membrane-based DNA purification, and a technique based on the use of magnetic beads. This latter method additionally can be automated when large amounts of samples have to be processed in a short time. The silica-membrane-based method is usually recommended in the hemato-oncology setting. It allows extraction from small volumes of blood or bone marrow as well as pellets of mononuclear cells, it is time efficient, and yields DNA of high quality. DNA isolated with the use of this method can be directly applied to PCR, but DNA concentration after isolation should be adjusted before amplification.

Many silica-membrane-based nucleic acid purification sets are commercially available on the market. Generally, cell pellet is first treated with proteinase K and lysis buffer, and then incubated for 15 min in 56 °C. DNA is then precipitated with 96 % ethanol, and the mixture is transferred onto DNA isolation columns to allow binding to silica membrane. Columns are washed, and DNA is eluted from the column using buffer or twice autoclaved MiliQ water. DNA concentration and purity should be assessed by measuring absorbance at 260 and 280 nm on a spectrophotometer.

Silica-membrane-based nucleic acid purification sets are suitable for DNA isolation from all types of biological materials, including blood, bone marrow, mononuclear cells, and cells isolated from bodily fluids, but also from solid tissues and archival formalin- and paraffin-fixed material. Isolation of DNA from larger fragments of tissues or paraffin blocks requires an additional, initial step of mechanic and enzymatic homogenization (with addition of proteinase K).

20.2.4 DNA Storage

Once isolated, DNA should be stored in conditions that prevent it from being degraded by nucleases. In general, the quality of DNA stored at high concentrations remains good for longer periods and is generally better than that of DNA stored at low concentrations. Hence, DNA eluted from isolation columns should be dissolved in relatively low amounts of buffer (or water) and treated as a stock solution, used to prepare working solutions when necessary. If longer DNA storage is expected, elution from the columns should be performed with a suitable elution buffer instead of water. Such buffers contain chelating agents (most often EDTA), scavenging divalent cations that are necessary for nuclease performance. DNA can be stored at 4 °C or −20 °C for periods of up to 3 months; when longer periods are required, storage at −80 °C is recommended. Of note, multiple freezing−thawing steps contribute more to DNA degradation than longer storage at 4 °C. Hence, DNA should be frozen only when its use is not frequent. Multiple freezing−thawing of the stock DNA can be avoided by aliquoting it into several tubes; this would prevent degradation of the whole stock in case of nuclease contamination or cross contamination of the whole material in case of inattentive pipetting.

20.3 Biological Material for RNA-Based Molecular Analyses

20.3.1 Tissue Collection

RNA undergoes degradation within minutes from collection of the samples, while still in cells. Collecting biological material for RNA isolation therefore requires special care to avoid unnecessary RNA degradation. Blood or bone marrow samples should be delivered to the laboratory within 24 h, but much shorter delivery times are strongly recommended. If possible, samples should be kept at 4 °C. It is extremely important that they are neither frozen nor stored in temperatures higher than 37 °C, as such extreme temperatures lead to cell membrane disruption, intracellular nuclease spillage, and in consequence, RNA degradation. If longer transport is expected, or a very good RNA quality is required (e.g. for quantitative analyses), additional RNA stabilizing reagents should be added to the blood and bone marrow samples at the time of collection. These stabilizing reagents are available commercially from many manufacturers and allow material storage in room temperature for up to several weeks. Prior to RNA extraction, blood and bone marrow samples should be subjected to mononuclear cell isolation (see Chap. 19) or, at least, to erythrocyte lysis.

20.3.2 Tissue Preparation

Erythrocyte lysis is performed by incubation of blood/bone marrow samples in hypotonic solution (0.15 M NH_4Cl; 0.01 $KHCO_3$; 0.37 g/L EDTA) for 5 min at room temperature, followed by centrifugation 400×*g*, 4 °C) and two PBS washes using the same centrifugation parameters. In case of solid tissue samples, they should be cut into smaller pieces and either placed in liquid nitrogen, or suspended in RNA stabilizing solution. Fragmentation of the samples is important, because the stabilizing solution has limited capability to penetrate tissues. An additional homogenization step has to be added prior to RNA isolation.

RNA isolation from frozen samples (stored at least at −80 °C) is possible but not recommended, due to low stability of RNA. Technically, the method does not differ from isolation using fresh material. It is also possible to isolate RNA from formalin fixed and paraffin embedded samples, or from samples banked in the cytogenetic fixative solution. RNA isolation procedure (like in the case of DNA isolation) has to be preceded by removing fixatives and tissue hydration, followed by the standard RNA extraction procedure (Stanta et al. 1998). However, extensive RNA degradation should be expected. Molecular analyses performed on RNA extracted from frozen or archival samples should be interpreted with caution.

20.3.3 RNA Isolation

The main types of RNA used for molecular analyses in hemato-oncology are: mRNA (messenger RNA), containing information transcribed from DNA, and miRNA (micro RNA)/siRNA (small interfering RNA), responsible for RNA interference and gene silencing (Xu and Li 2007).

During the process of isolation, RNA becomes exposed to nucleases ubiquitously present in laboratories, therefore, strict clean-work rules have to be implemented. RNA isolation should be performed in dedicated cabinets providing spatial separation of the isolation process from the rest of the laboratory. A dedicated pipette set, and freshly sterilized filtered pipette tips should be used. Prolonged handling of the extracted RNA has to be avoided. RNases denatured by heating or freezing can easily renature at room temperature. To protect RNA from degradation, RNases have to be inactivated by using 0.1 % v/v diethyldicarbonate (DEPC) solutions or one of many other commercially available RNase inactivating agents.

RNA isolation usually includes: initial extraction (protein denaturation), precipitation, and reprecipitation in isopropanol, wash with ethanol, and suspension of RNA. Three main methods of RNA isolation are currently used: the acid-guanidinum-phenol-chloroform (AGPC) method (Chomczynski and Sacchi 1987); its modification with the use of Trizol or other commercially available reagents during the first step; and silica-membrane-based RNA purification. The first two methods allow RNA purification from various amounts of starting material and further suspension of isolated nucleic acid in appropriate amount of buffer. Silica-membrane methods are limited by the amount of cells which can be processed; the usual yield of RNA does not exceed 3–6 μg. However, membrane binding stabilizes RNA, which ensures consistent nucleic acid quality.

For the purpose of hemato-oncological diagnostics, application of silica membrane-based methods is usually recommended. According to the manufacturer's protocol, lysis buffer and sodium acetate is added to 500 μl of whole blood/bone marrow/MNC pellet and vortexed. Phenol and chloroform solutions are added and the sample is centrifuged. Nucleic acids are precipitated with 96 % ethanol and placed on the silica membrane column. The column is washed with washing buffers containing ethanol. RNA is then eluted twice with the elution buffer.

To avoid contamination with traces of DNA, which is the main reason for false positive results in RNA analysis, extracted RNA should be subjected to a DNase digestion step.

RNA quality is assessed by 2 % agarose gel electrophoresis. The presence of 28 and 18S rRNA (5034 and 1870 nucleotide bands respectively) indicates RNA integrity. RNA concentration and purity is also assessed by measuring absorbance at 260/280 nm.

20.3.4 RNA Storage

RNA should be stored at −80 °C or, preferably, in liquid nitrogen. Buffers used to store RNA should contain 1 mM EDTA (pH 8) or 0.5 % SDS, both of which act as RNase inhibitors. It is important that all reagents used for suspending RNA are DEPC treated. Isolated RNA should be aliquoted into several tubes, to prevent repeated freeze and thaw cycles. To stabilize RNA for longer periods, suspension in isopropanol or ethanol is recommended. Alternatively, RNA can be reverse transcribed into cDNA straight after isolation. For cDNA storage, the basic DNA storage rules apply (see Sect. 20.2.4).

20.4 Polymerase Chain Reaction

Polymerase chain reaction, a basic method of specific DNA fragments amplification, relies on enzymatic replication of the DNA using thermostable DNA polymerase (*Taq* polymerase, originating from *Thermus aquaticus*) and target-specific primers. The amplification is performed in thermal cyclers—appliances that can be programmed to user-defined temperature profiles. DNA template sequence is exponentially copied in a number of repeated cycles of heating and cooling, allowing DNA denaturation, annealing of the primers, and their elongation by the *Taq* polymerase. The DNA generated in each cycle is itself used as a template for replication, such that the amount of a target sequence (amplicon) is doubled with every cycle (theoretically, after n cycles there should be 2^n copies of the original template). In practice, this exponential increase is attenuated by the polymerase exhaustion, reagents' depletion, and accumulation of products; the reaction finally reaches a plateau after 20–40 cycles.

A standard PCR must contain template DNA and reagents: *Taq* polymerase, a buffer containing Mg^{2+}, a set of four deoxyribonucleotidetriphosphates (dNTPs), specific forward and reverse primers flanking the region of interest. Exemplary PCR components and their final concentrations are listed in Table 20.1. The volume of a typical PCR depends on the individual user needs, but usually should not be lower than 10 µl, because of the problems related to water evaporation (salt concentration changes can easily inhibit the PCR).The upper limit of PCR volume depends on the type of thermal cycler, but usually does not exceed 100 µl. The PCR conditions vary depending on the type of DNA template. In case of difficult targets (e.g. high GC content, repetitive sequences, etc.), higher Mg^{2+} concentration, addition of dimethylsulfoxide (DMSO) or of urea may be beneficial. Amplification of each target requires small adjustments of reagent concentrations or temperature settings (especially primer annealing temperature). The standard primer annealing temperature in PCR reaction is 55 °C.

The recommended PCR conditions are as follows. Annealing temperature should be adjusted to individual target DNA fragments:

95 °C	7 min	
94 °C	30 s	30-40 x
52-60 °C	45 s	30-40 x
72 °C	90 s	30-40 x
72 °C	10 min	

Primer design is crucial for a successful DNA amplification. Primers should be complementary to DNA sequences flanking the region of interest (forward—complementary to the sense strand and reverse to the antisense strand). They should not contain long mononucleotide repeats (especially cytosine and guanine residues—C and G) and should be at least 18 nucleotides long to prevent unspecific annealing. Primers should contain no more than 50 % of CG pairs and should not contain sequences promoting formation of hairpins. Complementary sequences

Table 20.1 Recommended composition of PCR reaction mix

Component	Starting	Volume/ reaction (μl)	Final
PCR buffer	10 x	2.5	1 x
$MgCl_2$	15 mM	2.5	1.5 mM
Four dNTPs	20 mM, each	0.25	200 μM
Primer F	10 μM	0.5	0.2 μM
Primer R	10 μM	0.5	0.2 μM
Taq DNA polymerase	5 U/μl	0.1	0.5 U
Template DNA	20 ng/μl	2	40 ng
MiliQ water		16.65	
Total volume		25	

in forward and reverse primers should be also avoided to prevent formation of primer dimers. There are many computer programs available for primer design, including free tools available online (e.g. Primer3 available at http://frodo.wi.mit.edu/ (Rozen and Skaletsky 2000).

The yield and specificity of a PCR can be assessed electrophoretically in agarose gels; the amplicon should be examined for its size and the presence of undesired PCR products (smears or additional bands). Moreover, agarose electrophoresis may be sufficient to complete some molecular analyses, such as detection of fusion genes or internal tandem duplications. PCR is often a start point for various mutation analysis methods.

20.5 Reverse Transcription

In reverse transcription (RT), two different types of primers can be used: random primers (Fritz et al. 1991) or oligo (dT) (Myers and Gelfand 1991) primers. Oligo (dT) primers are more often used when forming cDNA libraries, as they prime reverse transcription from polyA tails of mRNA. Random oligonucleotides allow better efficiency of RT reaction, which might be important in cases when limited starting amount of RNA is available. In addition, only random oligonucleotide primers are suitable if siRNA is to be analyzed.

Two enzymes are most often applied in RT: Moloney Murine Leukemia Virus (M-MLV) and Avian Myeloblastoma Virus (AMV), both capable of using RNA as well as RNA:DNA hybrids as templates for reverse transcription. Reverse transcription has to be performed in the presence of RNase inhibitors and (*2S,3S*)-1,4-*Bis*-sulfanylbutane-2,3-diol (DTT), which acts as a reverse transcriptase stabilizing agent.

Reverse transcription commercial sets are widely available. Most often, RT reaction is conducted at 44 °C for 1 h, followed by reverse transcriptase thermal inactivation (92 °C, 10 min). Standard protocols recommend using 1–2 μg of RNA template, and are designed to obtain roughly similar amounts of cDNA.

The quality of cDNA is typically assessed by PCR specific toward housekeeping genes: *S15* (small ribosome subunit protein 15) or *ALB* (albumin).

PCR analysis of RNA can be performed in a one-step or a two-step process of reverse transcription (RT). One-step process is based on performing RT and PCR in one tube, with gene-of-interest specific PCR primers. Such an approach minimizes the contamination risk by limiting the handling of a sample, but it narrows the analysis to only one gene at a time. In addition, reverse transcription buffer lowers the PCR efficiency. The two-step approach is based on first performing RT to obtain cDNA, and further using cDNA as a template in various separate PCR reactions. In this approach, cDNA can be stored easily and used whenever needed.

20.6 Real-Time Quantitative PCR

Real-time quantitative PCR (RQ-PCR) is a method allowing quantification of specific DNA or RNA sequences. Applied to cDNA template, it is used for assessing the expression levels of genes. Applied to genomic DNA it is used for assessing the number of cellular copies of the template; one of its applications is a detection of minimal residual disease (MRD).

The method is based on the general PCR methodology; however, in RQ-PCR the amount of amplification product is measured in real time, during the exponential stages of the PCR. There are two main approaches used in RQ-PCR, which allow fluorophore-based, accurate detection of the amount of DNA template. The first approach uses a fluorescent dye (i.e. SYBR Green), which specifically binds to double stranded DNA (dsDNA), measuring the increase in amplified template throughout each cycle. The shortcoming of this approach is that the dye would bind to all dsDNA PCR products, including nonspecific PCR products. The second, more sensitive approach, recommended in hemato-oncological analyses (see Chap. 23), is based on the use of TaqMan® probes. A probe, complementary to the target sequence, is labeled with a fluorochrome on one end and a quencher on the other end; PCR primers flank the segment targeted by the probe. As the template is amplified, the $5' \rightarrow 3'$ exonuclease activity of Taq polymerase cleaves the probe. In effect, fluorochrome becomes separated from the quencher and, excited by the light source, emits a light signal which due to separation is no longer quenched. This is measured by the detection system of the RQ-PCR thermal cycling device.

20.7 DNA Sequencing

DNA sequencing is now one of the most basic techniques applied in hemato-oncology. It is used for detection of mutation and remains necessary for the design of patient-specific targets used for minimal residual disease monitoring. Sequencing techniques presently used for diagnostic purposes rely on the principle of dideoxy chain-termination (Sanger method). In the PCR-based dideoxy sequencing, elongation of a specific primer annealed to a thermally denatured template (typically, a PCR product) is terminated by the incorporation of dideoxynucleotides, which are added at low concentration to the mixture of normal dNTPs. A set of DNA fragments of varying lengths is then denatured and separated by size by electrophoresis in high-resolution acrylamide sequencing gels or columns (capilars). A variety of technical approaches used for the detection of DNA fragments is beyond the scope of this chapter. In the most widely used automated sequencing machines, detection of DNA fragments is based on using ddNTPs labeled with different fluorescent dyes (dye-terminator sequencing); the data output has a form of fluorescent peak trace chromatograms. Most of the currently used sequencers allow efficient reading of sequences that are 300–1000 bp long; the quality of the read is poor in the first 15–40 bases of the sequence and deteriorates after 700–900 bases.

Pyrosequencing is an alternative method of DNA sequencing based on the "sequencing by synthesis" principle. Sequencing of a single strand of DNA is done by synthesizing its complementary strand, and simultaneously detecting, which base was added at each step. Detection of each dNTP incorporation is based on a series of stoichiometric enzymatic reactions, which generate visible light detected in real time (Pareek et al. 2011). In the classical settings, the method allows reading DNA sequence of 300–500 nucleotides.

The template DNA used in sequencing reactions should not be contaminated with reagents coming from the amplification step preceding sequencing (polymerase, primers, nucleotides, and buffers). The sequencing template can be purified using silica-membrane-based methods; columns are available commercially for purification of PCR products or DNA fragments excised from agarose gels. DNA from bands excised from polyacrylamide gels can be eluted by overnight incubation in sterile MilliQ water and used directly for sequencing. PCR product can also be purified enzymatically, with the use of exonucleases or shrimp alkaline phosphatase (SAP). The quality and amount of a purified PCR amplification product should be additionally checked by performing an agarose gel electrophoresis and its quantity should be assessed spectrophotometricaly. If the PCR amplification is well balanced, it is possible to sequence the PCR product directly, with no need for purification.

Many commercial laboratories offer performing sequencing for a moderate price and using such services becomes a common practice. The results are delivered to the user in the form of chromatograms. If a sequencing reaction is to be performed in-house, it is usually prepared with the use of a commercially available sequencing reagent set, which contains all the reagents necessary for sequencing; sequencing reaction has to be prepared and performed according to the manufacturer's guidelines.

A number of commercial and non-commercial software packages available for reading and editing chromatograms are available. Many of them automatically trim low quality DNA traces. Such chromatograms should always be read manually by the user in order to assess their quality. This is especially important in hematological aplications, where it is essential to ensure that weaker signals coming from mutated neoplastic subclones are not mistakenly interpreted by the sequence analysis program. The results of sequencing can also be aligned with publicly available genome databases to facilitate localization of mutated or rearranged sequences.

20.8 DNA Methylation Analysis

It has been clearly established that aberrant DNA hypermethylation contributes to the development of cancer. Several methods are now available for DNA methylation studies, all based on PCR amplification of sodium bisulfite treated DNA (Herman et al. 1996). Bisulfite treatment of DNA allows discrimination of methylated and unmethylated cytosines. The key is a high rate of cytosine conversion to uracil under conditions where 5-methylcytosine remains unconverted, while DNA is protected against degradation. The converted DNA sequence is then amplified by PCR with primers specific for bisulfite-modified DNA.

In a typical sodium bisulfite conversion procedure using commercially available kits, DNA is mixed with sodium bisulfite in the presence of DNA protecting buffer, and incubated for several hours in thermal conditions recommended by the manufacturer (60 and 95 °C). Bisulfite-converted DNA is then applied onto silica membrane columns. After desulphonation and washing, purified converted DNA is eluted from the column. According to manufacturers' estimations, the DNA yield after conversion should be similar to the amount used for conversion.

Bisulfite-converted DNA is amplified by methylation-specific PCR (MS-PCR). Two sets of primers targeting analyzed CpG island are used for each gene: methylated DNA-specific (MDS) primers and unmethylated DNA-specific (UDS) primers. Amplification with MDS primers indicates that the analyzed CpG island is methylated, while amplification with UDS primers indicates the unmethylated status of the CpG island. Amplification of DNA template with both primer sets indicates the presence of two populations of cells, one with methylated and the other with unmethylated CpG island. A schematic representation of MS-PCR method is pictured in Fig. 20.1.

Correct primer design is the key step for a successful MS-PCR assay. The primers must be placed in a way that their 3′ end fall within a CpG dinucleotide. Preferentially, only one or two CpG dinucleotides should be included in a primer sequence. Several computer programs, including free online tools, are available for designing MS-PCR primers (Li and Dahiya 2002). To confirm the specificity of the designed primers, control cross-reactions should be performed (MDS primers with converted unmethylated DNA and UDS primers with converted methylated DNA; no amplification should occur using both primer sets with normal, unconverted DNA).

It is worth noting that MS-PCR is a very sensitive method, capable of detecting hypermethylation levels, which are not yet influencing the cell functioning. For a more accurate methylation level assessment, MethyLight method should be applied.

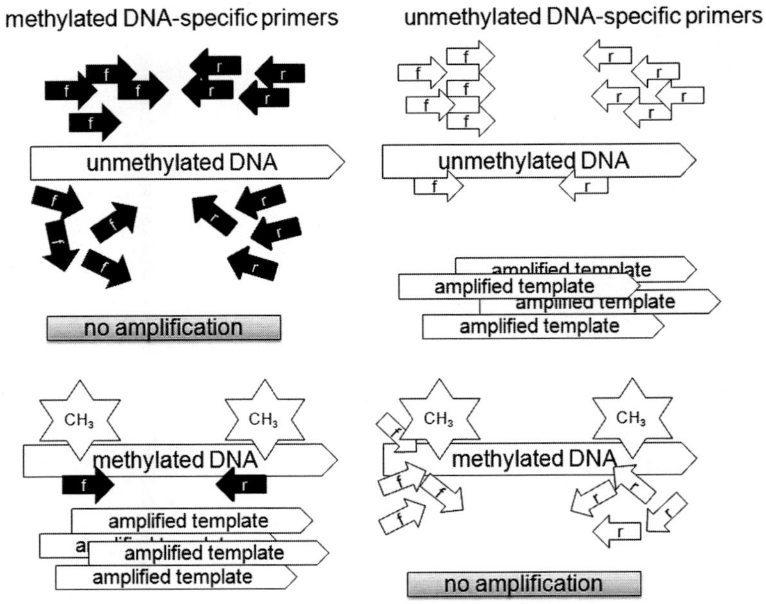

Fig. 20.1 Schematic representation of MS-PCR method. Two primer sets are designed for each analyzed region—methylated DNA-specific, MDS primers (*black arrows*) and unmethylated DNA-specific, UDS primers (*white arrows*). MDS primers allow amplification of methylated template, while UDS primers allow amplification of only unmethylated template. Performing both reactions separately on the same template provides information about the methylation status of tested DNA: all DNA methylated—only MDS amplification occurs, mix of methylated and unmethylated DNA—both reactions show amplification, and unmethylated DNA—only UDS amplification occurs

It is based on the real-time quantitative PCR approach and uses both methylation-specific primes and methylation-specific probes (Fraga and Esteller 2002).

MS-PCR approach to DNA hypermethylation studies is a fast and straightforward method; however, it has its pitfalls. The main problem is that CpG dinucleotides within one CpG island can be differentially methylated. The MS-PCR analysis only provides information about the methylation status of these particular CG dinucleotides that are incorporated into the primer or probe sequence; no further conclusions about the methylation status of flanking CG dinucleotides can be drawn.

20.9 Multiplex Ligation-Dependent Probe Amplification

This modification of PCR allows simultaneous analysis of sequence changes in up to 40 different genomic regions. The multiplex ligation-dependent probe amplification (MLPA) reaction consists of a set of probe pairs specific for genomic sequences of interest. One of the probes in each pair contains a fragment

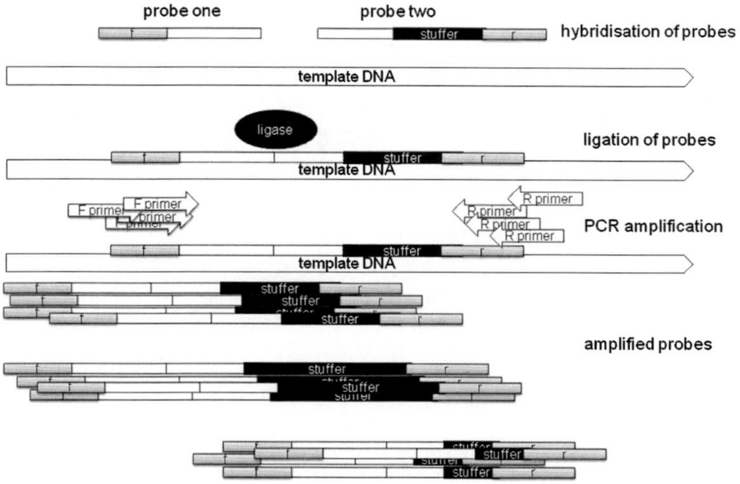

Fig. 20.2 Schematic representation of MLPA method. Each region of interest is assessed by the use of a pair of probes complementary to it. Probe one consists of a DNA fragment, complementary to the region of interest and an F primer fragment at its 5′ end. Probe two from this same pair consists of a DNA fragment compleimentary to template DNA immediately placed next to the hybridizing fragment of probe one, stuffer sequence, and a cR primer sequence at its 3′ end. After hybridization, both probes are ligated and then amplified. If there is a change introduced in the template DNA falling at the spot of ligation of probe one and probe two, no amplification is observed. Stuffer sequence length is different for each probe set allowing analysis of up to 40 regions at once

complementary to the analyzed template, and the universal primer F sequence at its 5′ end. The other probe contains a specific sequence complementary to the template immediately adjacent to the fragment recognized by the first probe, a stuffer sequence of unique size distinguishing it from other probe sets and a sequence complementary to the universal primer R at its 3′ end. Probes of each pair anneal to the complementary DNA template in a head-to-tail way; if both match the target sequence, they become ligated by the ligase present in the reaction mixture. Ligated probes form a single-stranded DNA template, which can be amplified using fluorescence-labeled universal primers and Taq polymerase. Multiple probe assessment in one reaction is possible because each probe pair has an individual length dependent on the stuffer sequence (130–480 nt, increments of 4–10 nt). Amplification products are further analyzed by capillary electrophoresis. The efficiency of the amplification (the height of a peak) is proportional to the number of copies in the original template. The results are analyzed by comparing the peaks' height with the results for the control samples. A schematic representation of MLPA method is pictured in Fig. 20.2.

MLPA is most commonly used for identification of large genomic deletions or duplications, simple sequence changes, as well as DNA methylation status within sequences covered by the probes. Commercially available sets of probes and reagents allow easy analysis of a large number of genes and genomic regions.

20.10 Conclusions

Molecular studies in hematological malignancies are based on nucleic acid analysis. Most techniques developed many years ago are still used as golden standards in the diagnostic and research laboratories. On the other hand, the standard molecular methodology is being constantly innovated and it is likely that in a few years, molecular hematology laboratories will be mostly automated and equipped with high throughput devices, while the analyses will be based on DNA chip approach and next generation sequencing. Nevertheless, high-tech laboratory settings will require well-trained staff with expertise and experience in basic molecular methods.

References

Banerjee SK, Makdisi WF, Weston AP, Mitchell SM, Campbell DR (1995) Microwave-based DNA extraction from paraffin-embedded tissue for PCR amplification. Biotechniques 18(5):768–770, 772–763

Bruggemann M, Schrauder A, Raff T, Pfeifer H, Dworzak M, Ottmann OG, Asnafi V, Baruchel A, Bassan R, Benoit Y, Biondi A, Cave H, Dombret H, Fielding AK, Foa R, Gokbuget N, Goldstone AH, Goulden N, Henze G, Hoelzer D, Janka-Schaub GE, Macintyre EA, Pieters R, Rambaldi A, Ribera JM, Schmiegelow K, Spinelli O, Stary J, von Stackelberg A, Kneba M, Schrappe M (2008) Standardized MRD quantification in European ALL trials: proceedings of the second international symposium on MRD assessment in Kiel, Germany, 18–20 September 2008. Leukemia 24(3):521–535. doi:10.1038/leu.2009.268, leu2009268 [pii]

Chomczynski P, Sacchi N (1987) Single-step method of RNA isolation by acid guanidinium thiocyanate-phenol-chloroform extraction. Anal Biochem 162(1):156–159. doi:10.1006/abio.1987.9999, 0003-2697(87)90021-2 [pii]

Coura R, Prolla JC, Meurer L, Ashton-Prolla P (2005) An alternative protocol for DNA extraction from formalin fixed and paraffin wax embedded tissue. J Clin Pathol 58(8):894–895. doi:10.1136/jcp.2004.021352, 58/8/894 [pii]

Fraga MF, Esteller M (2002) DNA methylation: a profile of methods and applications. Biotechniques 33(3):632, 634, 636–649

Fritz JD, Greaser ML, Wolff JA (1991) A novel 3′ extension technique using random primers in RNA-PCR. Nucleic Acids Res 19(13):3747

Goelz SE, Hamilton SR, Vogelstein B (1985) Purification of DNA from formaldehyde fixed and paraffin embedded human tissue. Biochem Biophys Res Commun 130(1):118–126. 0006-291X(85)90390-0 [pii]

Herman JG, Graff JR, Myohanen S, Nelkin BD, Baylin SB (1996) Methylation-specific PCR: a novel PCR assay for methylation status of CpG islands. Proc Natl Acad Sci U S A 93(18):9821–9826

Li LC, Dahiya R (2002) MethPrimer: designing primers for methylation PCRs. Bioinformatics 18(11):1427–1431

Myers TW, Gelfand DH (1991) Reverse transcription and DNA amplification by a Thermus thermophilus DNA polymerase. Biochemistry 30(31):7661–7666

Pareek CS, Smoczynski R, Tretyn A (2011) Sequencing technologies and genome sequencing. J Appl Genet 52(4):413–435. doi:10.1007/s13353-011-0057-x

Rozen S, Skaletsky H (2000) Primer3 on the WWW for general users and for biologist programmers. Methods Mol Biol 132:365–386

Shi SR, Key ME, Kalra KL (1991) Antigen retrieval in formalin-fixed, paraffin-embedded tissues: an enhancement method for immunohistochemical staining based on microwave oven heating of tissue sections. J Histochem Cytochem 39(6):741–748
Stanta G, Bonin S, Perin R (1998) RNA extraction from formalin-fixed and paraffin-embedded tissues. Methods Mol Biol 86:23–26. doi:10.1385/0-89603-494-1:23
Wickham CL, Boyce M, Joyner MV, Sarsfield P, Wilkins BS, Jones DB, Ellard S (2000) Amplification of PCR products in excess of 600 base pairs using DNA extracted from decalcified, paraffin wax embedded bone marrow trephine biopsies. Mol Pathol 53(1):19–23
Xu W, Li J-y (2007) MicroRNA gene expression in malignant lymphoproliferative disorders. Chin Med J 120(11):996–999

Chapter 21
Genetic Methods of HLA Typing

Jacek Nowak, Renata Mika-Witkowska and Elżbieta Graczyk-Pol

Abstract Several molecular techniques have been adapted for the human leukocyte antigen (HLA) typing with their advantages and drawbacks, which greatly improved the feasibility and precision of HLA typing as compared to previously used methods. Molecular techniques enabled more accurate analyses of the influence of HLA disparities on hematopoietic stem cell (HSC) transplant outcome. The principles of the new 2010 HLA nomenclature, the HLA genotype assignment, both with accurate and ambiguous results generated using most common techniques, have been presented in this chapter. Basic features, such as throughput and resolution of the methods, have been outlined. Detailed exemplary protocols of polymerase chain reaction (PCR)-based procedures of HLA-typing using sequence specific primer (SSP), sequence specific oligonucleotide probes (SSO), and sequencing-based typing (SBT) techniques have been described. There is currently an increasing interest in the typing of different nonHLA genetic polymorphisms that are involved in transplantation immunity pathways. Among them, the protocols of killer immunoglobulin-like receptor (KIR) and minor histocompatibility antigen (mHA) PCR-SSP typing have been presented in detail.

J. Nowak (✉) · R. Mika-Witkowska · E. Graczyk-Pol
Department of Immunogenetics, Institute of Hematology and Transfusion Medicine, Indiry Gandhi 14
02-776 Warsaw, Poland
e-mail: szpik@ihit.waw.pl

R. Mika-Witkowska
e-mail: renatamika@ihit.waw.pl

E. Graczyk-Pol
e-mail: dobory@ihit.waw.pl

M. Witt et al. (eds.), *Molecular Aspects of Hematologic Malignancies*, Principles and Practice, DOI: 10.1007/978-3-642-29467-9_21,

21.1 Introduction

With the application of new molecular techniques to HLA typing, posttransplant outcome has greatly improved (Viollier et al. 2008). The most commonly used genetic methods of human leukocyte antigen (HLA), killer immunoglobulin-like receptor (KIR), and minor histocompatibility antigen (mHA) typing are based on the sequence-specific primer (SSP) amplification of genomic DNA (PCR-SSP methods) or sequence-specific oligonucleotide probe reverse hybridization (PCR-SSO methods). Sequencing-based typing (SBT) method come into use with increasing frequency for HLA typing purpose. Since HLA represents a system of many genetic loci associated with highly polymorphic alleles (Robinson et al. 2011), the high level of similarity of alleles (Holdsworth et al. 2009) causes difficulties in resolving some ambiguous HLA typings.

According to the 2010 HLA nomenclature provided by the World Health Organization (WHO) Nomenclature Committee for Factors of the HLA System (http://www.ebi.ac.uk/imgt/hla/stats.html), the assignment of the allele consists of the name of the HLA locus followed by asterisk and 2–4 sets of numerical digits (or sometimes letters) separated by a colon, e.g. A*02:01, A*02:01:01:02L. Two first sets assign for a family of similar alleles and the consecutive number of allele exonic sequence, respectively. Third and fourth sets assign for the silent exonic nucleotide substitution(s) leading to synonymous coding for an amino acid and the intronic nucleotide substitution(s), respectively. The polymorphisms assigned by the difference in the set 3 and 4 seem not to have direct biological significance in hematopoietic stem cell (HSC) transplantation, although the donor-recipient mismatch within the set 3 or 4 can indicate broader haplotypic disparity. The letter at the end of the allele name may assign for N—null allele, L—an allele with low expression on the cell surface, S—an allele encoding a protein which is expressed as a secreted molecule only or Q—an allele with unconfirmed (questionable) expression.

DNA-based tests dedicated for HLA typing may give results at low (antigenic) or high (allelic) resolution level, that apply when first set of digits or two first sets of digits are resolved, respectively (e.g. A*02 or A*02:05). However, most commonly, HLA typing tests generate results at intermediate resolution level, with allelic ambiguities where several similar alleles are not excluded, e.g. A*02:01 or A*02:01:01:02L or A*02:05 or A*02:06. The intermediate resolution result can be noted using long or short HLA notation or using brief 2–4 letter National Marrow Donor Program (NMDP) code, e.g. A*02:01/02:01:01:02L/02:05/02:06, A*02:01/05/06 or A*02:GS, respectively. NMDP codes can be easily expanded to the allele scope (and vice versa) using NMDP web page DNA Type Lookup Tool (http://bioinformatics.nmdp.org). Generic SSP, and SSO (see Sect. 21.2) tests give low or intermediate level resolution results. SSP tests, the so-called "high resolution" (HR) tests and SSO "high definition" (HD) tests give more frequently (still not always) HR results. The common difficulty with HR level achievement is caused by the sequence similarity of different families of HLA alleles (allelic ambiguities) combined with diploid structure of human genotypes producing a "heterozygous ambiguities cis/trans". SBT tests are also not free from ambiguous results. Ambiguities at the allele level are commonly caused by an incomplete knowledge about sequence of some alleles, extremely high homology of heterozygous alleles, and intronic location of polymorphic sites. A “heterozygous ambiguity cis/trans” can be sometimes resolved by using additional typing(s) with new specific primers for SSP or new probes including haplotype-specific specialty probes in SSO method. Sequencing of additional exons/introns or separate retyping of alleles after separating of the diploid samples into their haploid components by haplotype-specific DNA extraction can be also used to resolve some specific ambiguities (Nagy et al. 2007).

For quality control the HLA typing laboratories participate in external quality control workshops (at least ten blind samples per year for each HLA locus and level of resolution). Internal quality control of entitled laboratory staff (typing of at least four blind samples per year for adapted methods) is required. All new lots of commercial HLA typing kits should be controlled by retyping of known, previously typed samples with the new kit of certain specificity.

For the selection of HLA matched HSC sibling donor (family donor) the HLA-typing at the scope of A, B, C, and DRB1 loci (and DQB1, recommended by some but not all specialists) at the low resolution level is sufficient (see also Chap. 14). HR HLA-typing of donor and recipient in A, B, C, and DRB1 loci (and DQB1, recommended by European Group for Blood and Marrow Transplantation, but not by NMDP) is required as a minimum for HLA matching of unrelated donor. For the final selection of the donor-recipient pair the typing should be confirmed with duplicate typing performed in second samples drawn independently to show the reproducibility of the results (i.e. the absence of technical and clerical errors).

There are various commercially available kits for HLA-SSP, SSO, and SBT typing. The SSP technique is flexible and is adapted for both low and HR tests, but it is usually recommended for low scale typing. The SSO techniques are well adapted for intermediate/high-throughput laboratories. SBT techniques give the definitive forward and reverse nucleotide sequences of amplified gene fragments, thus providing the highest possible resolution of the results, and allowing for the identification of all known polymorphisms and any novel polymorphisms. Like SSO, the SBT methods are highly laborious, but they are basically performed in a manual mode. However, it is possible to adapt some prePCR SBT steps to bio-robotic stations that greatly improve the throughput rate of the SBT. Here we describe examples of detailed typing procedures for these three most widely used techniques of HLA typing.

21.2 HLA Genotyping

21.2.1 Polymerase Chain Reaction-Based Sequence-Specific Primers Method

Matched oligonucleotide primers, without 3′-end mismatches, are more efficiently used by thermo-stable DNA polymerase in the PCR reaction than mismatched primers (Schaffer and Olerup 2001). Primer pairs are designed to hybridize to single alleles or families of similar alleles. With precisely controlled PCR conditions, matched primer pairs allow to amplify the sequence in stake. After the PCR, the amplified DNA fragments are size-separated by agarose gel electrophoresis, visualized by staining with ethidium bromide or SYBR green and exposure to ultraviolet light, documented by photography and interpreted. Interpretation of PCR-SSP results is based on the presence or absence of specific PCR products in reaction tubes with primers of known allele specificity. An internal positive control primer pair is included in each PCR. The internal positive control primer pair matches conserved regions of the human growth hormone or β-globin gene, which are present in all human DNA samples. Due to extensive polymorphism of HLA loci, the PCR-SSP kits are only provided commercially in the format of PCR microtube sets with predeposited specific primers of precisely described allelic specificity and microtube location (HLA SSP typing trays).

21.2.1.1 PCR-SSP, Stepwise Procedure

1. Place in the room temperature (19–25 °C): DNA samples, appropriate primers (in commercially prepared primer tray), PCR buffer, and Taq DNA polymerase (5 units/μl).
2. Mix DNA sample briefly by vortexing.
3. Place the primer tray in a PCR tray rack.
4. Vortex the PCR buffer.
5. Prepare the reaction mix in a 1.5 ml tube by adding volumes of the following reagents, expanded by the number of primer wells: PCR buffer (4 μl per well), Taq DNA polymerase (0.1 μl per well), and molecular grade sterile water (6 μl per well).
6. Vortex for 5 s. Pulse-spin the tube in a microcentrifuge to bring all liquid down from sides of the tube.
7. Add 8 μl of the reaction mix and 2 μl of water into the negative control well.
8. Add the DNA sample (2.2 μl per well) to the remaining reaction mix.
9. Vortex for 5 s and pulse-spin the tube. Place the primer tray in PCR cooler rack.
10. Aliquot 10 μl of the sample reaction mixture into each well, except for the negative control well, of the primer tray.
11. Seal the primer tray with the adhesive PCR seal. Check that all reaction wells are completely covered to prevent evaporative loss during PCR cycling.
12. Place the primer tray in the thermal cycler and perform PCR according to PCR cycling parameters, as indicated below. Do not allow more than 5 min delay between PCR setup and thermal cycling.
13. Remove the primer tray from the thermal cycler and inspect the PCR tray to make sure that there is approximately the same volume of fluid in each PCR well.
14. Detect and analyze PCR products by agarose gel electrophoresis (see below).

15. Interpret the typing results with the lot specific interpretation worksheet or dedicated computer interpretation software.

PCR cycling parameters

94 °C	2 min	
94 °C	10 s	10 cycles
65 °C	1 min	
94 °C	10 s	20 cycles
61 °C	50 s	
72 °C	30 s	
4 °C	hold	

Agarose gel electrophoresis

1. Prepare the 2 % (w/v) agarose gel, with ethidium bromide (EtBr) in a final concentration 0.5 μg/ml, (e.g. 2 μl of 10 mg/ml concentrated EtBr per 40 ml of gel solution).
2. Load the PCR products to the 2 % agarose gel slots.
3. Load a DNA size marker in one well per row.
4. Perform electrophoresis in 1X TBE buffer:

- voltage 140–150 V
- current 60 mA
- time 3–5 min

21.2.1.2 Evaluation and Interpretation of Results

The detected PCR product band patterns are composed of HLA allele or allele group specific amplicons and, for example, human growth hormone amplicons of the internal control. Inspect gel photograph for positive and negative reactions and transfer the results in appropriate positions of interpretation table or computer software. In positive HLA-specific reactions, the internal control band may be suppressed because of competitive amplification of specific and control sequences. Evaluation is aimed at checking for HLA-specific amplifications. The constellation of bands in the gel photograph and those manually entered in the interpretation table or computer software must be checked twice and resultant HLA genotype must be analyzed by two members of a laboratory staff authorized for HLA typing using PCR-SSP method. Specific amplicons must have expected lengths, specified in the interpretation table, and be clearly visible. In most cases, specific PCR products are smaller (85–315 bp) than the products of the internal control (430 or 800 bp). Apparent homozygosity should be confirmed with broad locus-specific test and a family data on haplotype segregation, if available. The presence of bands in a negative control well indicate contamination of the reaction mix with foreign DNA. If any specific annotations on nonuniform interpretation of the band patterns are made by the manufacturer of the HLA genotyping kit, they should be considered during evaluation and interpretation of the results.

21.2.2 Polymerase Chain Reaction-Based Sequence-Specific Oligonucleotide Probe Method

21.2.2.1 PCR-SSO, Principle of the Method

There are several commercial kits available for the HLA typing with the use of PCR-SSO method (Dalva and Beksac 2007). Since these HLA typing kits are locus specific, the target DNA is PCR-amplified using a locus/exon 2-specific or locus/exon 2- and 3-specific primer mixes for class II and class I genotyping, respectively. The PCR product is biotinylated enabling its detection with the use of R-phycoerythrin-conjugate of strepavidin (SAPE). The PCR product is denatured and hybridized to different complementary DNA probes conjugated each to one of 100 types of polystyrene beads stained with certain proportions of infrared and red trademarked fluorophores. A flow analyzer is used to identify the fluorescence intensity of the microspheres passing through a red laser, which excites the internal dyes to distinguish the microsphere set and then through a green laser, which excites the R-phycoerythrin on the reporter molecule. The assignment of HLA genotype is based on the reaction pattern compared to patterns associated with published HLA gene sequences. The most common results of the SSO method involve low to intermediate resolution results with frequent allelic and heterozygous cis/trans ambiguities. The expansion of the method to HD procedure is based on using additional, so-called specialty, probes. These specialty probes represent two or three specific probes linked by short nonhybridizing spacers and are able to hybridize to one DNA strand located polymorphisms only. This way a portion of allele and heterozygous cis/trans ambiguities can be resolved and thus the resolution of the HD typing is greatly improved.

21.2.2.2 PCR-SSO, Stepwise Procedure

Amplification

1. Prepare 20 ng/μl dilutions of DNA to be tested.
2. Thaw DNA, oligonucleotide primers, and D-mix provided with commercial kit and keep cool until use.
3. Vortex D-mix and the primers for 15 s; centrifuge for 3–5 s.
4. Prepare the amplification mixture (reaction volumes are 20 μl). Add indicated volumes of reagents expanded by the number of reactions: D-mix (13.8 μl) primers (4 μl) into a sterile tube. Vortex 15 s, and place in a PCR-cooler rack.
5. Pipette 2 μl of DNA into the bottom of a PCR tube/well. Avoid evaporation and contamination of the DNA.
6. Immediately before use add Taq DNA polymerase (0.2 μl per reaction) to the amplification mixture prepared in step 4.
7. Vortex, spin down.

8. Aliquot 18 μl of amplification mixture into each tube/well containing DNA, avoiding cross-contamination.
9. Seal the tubes/wells tightly.
10. Perform the PCR, according to thermal cycling profile, as indicated below.
11. It is recommended to use 2–5 μl of resulting PCR products for analysis by agarose gel electrophoresis aimed at confirmation of good quality of amplicons prior to hybridization assay. Amplified DNA is then hybridized and tested according to the procedure described by the manufacturer of the kit (see below).

PCR cycling parameters

96 °C	3 min	
96 °C	20 s	5 cycles
60 °C	20 s	
72 °C	20 s	
96 °C	10 s	30 cycles
60 °C	15 s	
72 °C	20 s	
72 °C	10 min	
4 °C	hold	

Hybridization procedure

1. Denaturation/Neutralization

   (a) Transfer 5 μl of each amplified DNA sample into a well of a 96-well PCR tray or 0,2 ml PCR tubes. Make sure sample location and IDs are noted.
   (b) Add 2.5 μl denaturation buffer. Mix thoroughly and incubate at room temp., 10 min.
   (c) Add 5 μl neutralization buffer and mix. Note the color change to clear or pale yellow.
   (d) Place PCR tray with neutralized PCR product on a PCR cooler rack.

2. Hybridization
   Make sure that the thermal cycler has been turned on and the 60 °C program has been started to warm the thermal block and the lid.

   (a) Combine appropriate volumes of bead mixture (4 μl per reaction) and hybridization buffer (34 μl per reaction) to prepare hybridization mixture.
   (b) Add 38 μl hybridization mixture to each well.
   (c) Cover tray with a seal, place it in a tray holder, and vortex thoroughly at low speed.
   (d) Remove the PCR tray from a holder and place into the prewarmed thermal cycler (60 °C).
   (e) Incubate 15 min.
   (f) Place tray in the holder and remove the seal.
   (g) Quickly add 100 μl of wash buffer to each well. Cover the tray with a tray seal. Centrifuge 5 min, 1,000–1,300 × g. Remove the wash buffer with one energetic motion of the PCR tray.

(h) Repeat step g) two times for a total of three wash steps. Prepare 1X SAPE solution during third centrifugation.

3. Labeling

(a) Place the tray in the tray holder. Add 50 μl of 1X SAPE solution to each well. Seal the tray and vortex thoroughly at low speed. Place the tray in the preheated thermal cycler (60 °C) and incubate 5 min.
(b) Place the tray in the tray holder. Remove the seal and quickly add 100 μl of the wash buffer to each well.
(c) Seal the tray and centrifuge tray 5 min, 1,000–1,300 × g, discard the supernatant.
(d) Add 70 μl of the wash buffer to each well, mix. Transfer all mixes to the reading microtiter plate. Final volume should be at least 80 μl.
(e) Cover the microtiter plate with the seal and aluminum foil. Keep the plate in the dark at 4 °C until placed in flow analyzer for data acquisition.
(f) For the best results, read samples as soon as possible. Prolonged storage of samples (more than 4 h) may result in the loss of signals. If the samples cannot be read immediately store sealed samples overnight at 4 °C in the dark. Thoroughly mix the samples immediately before reading.

4. Data Acquisition

(a) Turn on the flow analyzer and set up the system for calibration and sample acquisition.
(b) Choose a template according to the product catalog ID and lot number.
(c) Create a new file for the samples to be analyzed.
(d) Enter the sample IDs.
(e) Check all the template settings and IDs twice.
(f) Load the reading microtitre plate onto the XY platform of the analyzer and fill the reservoir with sheath fluid.
(g) Start data acquisition.
(h) Analyze collected data using dedicated HLA software.

21.2.2.3 Evaluation and Data Interpretation

The total number of analyzed beads should exceed 100 for each bead color-coded type. A significant reduction in the bead count may suggest bead loss during assay and can void test results. The fluorescent signal of the sequence-specific reporter probes should clearly contrast for positively and negatively assigned probes (see Fig. 21.1). Control fluorescent signal (MFI, mean fluorescent intensity) from amplified exons should be higher than 1,200 arbitrary units (AU) and negative (background) control MFI shall not exceed 20 AU. Resultant genotypes composed of allelic specificities that do not belong to common and well documented alleles (nonCWD alleles, see also Chap. 14) or unusual HLA allele(s) as for ethnical

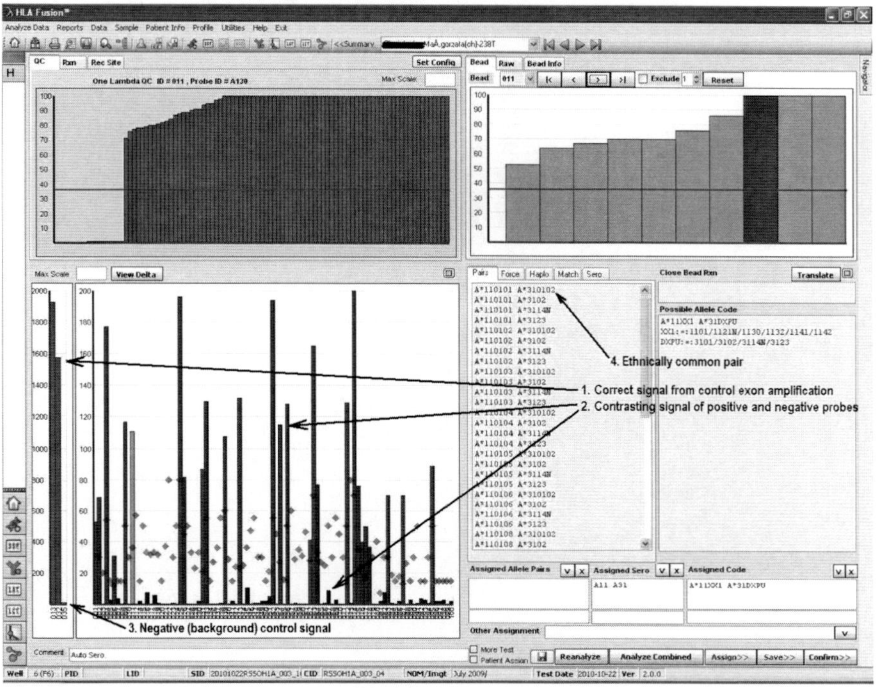

Fig. 21.1 Analysis of the row data in PCR-SSO genotyping of HLA-A locus in a flow analyzer. An ambiguous genotype at the allelic level has not been resolved in the patient—HLA-A*11:XX, 31:DXPU. The evaluation of the results shows *1* correct signal of amplified exons 2 and 3; *2* contrasting signal of positive and negative probes; *3* correct low negative (*background*) control; and *4* one pair of alleles common in the patient and ethnically matched control group, i.e. A*11:01:01, 31:01:02, assigned as "ethnically common pair"

background of typed individual should be confirmed by retyping, preferably using new DNA isolate. The final results of genotyping generated by the interpretation software must be verified by two members of laboratory staff authorized for HLA typing using PCR-SSO method and the given flow analyzer.

21.2.3 Sequencing-Based Typing

21.2.3.1 SBT, Principle of the Method

Exons 2–4 of the HLA genes show the highest level of polymorphism among other gene fragments. In SBT they are commonly amplified using locus/exon-specific primer mixes. Sequencing is subsequently performed using locus/exon-specific primers and PCR-based color-coded dideoxy nucleotide chain-termination Sanger method (Sanger and Coulson 1975) (see also Chap. 20).

21.2.3.2 SBT, Stepwise Procedure

1. Primary PCR amplification—exons 2–4 of HLA gene
   (a) Using commercially available kit prepare a PCR reaction mix. Add volumes: PCR buffer (16 μl per well), Taq DNA polymerase (0.3 μl per well) into a 1.5 ml tube and vortex.
   (b) Aliquot the mix into PCR tubes, containing respective exon-specific primer pairs,
   (c) Add 4 μl of genomic DNA (20 ng/μl).
   (d) Perform the PCR, according to the following cycling profile:

95 °C	10 min	
96 °C	20 s	36 cycles
60 °C	30 s	
72 °C	3 min	
4 °C	hold	

2. Primary PCR product—verification and purification
   (a) Analyze 3 μl of the PCR products in 2 % w/v agarose gel electrophoresis (30 min, 8–10 V/cm). Weak amplification bands suggest new DNA isolate should be used and/or primary amplification to be repeated.
   (b) Purification of the primary PCR product.
      - Add 3 μl of endonuclease/alkaline phosphatase solution to the PCR product, mix, and pulse spin down.
      - Incubate: 37 °C, 15 min; 80 °C, 15 min.
3. Secondary PCR sequencing amplification—forward and reverse primers
   Exons 2–4 of each purified primary PCR product are amplified in six separate reactions using ready to use sequencing mixes, each containing one of the six forward or reverse primers (2F, 2R, 3F, 3R, 4F, 4R).
   (a) Aliquot 8 μl of sequencing mixes with forward or reverse primer to six different PCR tubes per each sample.
   (b) Add 2 μl of purified primary PCR product (diluted 1:1 with molecular grade sterile water) to each of six primer sequencing mixes, mix well, and spin down.
4. Sequencing PCR amplification
   Perform the sequencing PCR, according to cycling profile as follows:

96 °C	20 s	
50 °C	30 s	25 cycles
60 °C	2 min	
4 °C	hold	

5. Purification of the sequencing products—precipitation
   (a) Add 2 μl of NaOAc/EDTA to each of 1.5 ml tube (one tube per each secondary PCR product.
   (b) Transfer the secondary PCR products to the respective tubes, mix, spin down.
   (c) Add 25 μl of absolute ethanol, vortex.
   (d) Centrifuge 30 min, 2,000 × g, discard the supernatant.
   (e) Add 50 μl of 80 % ethanol.
   (f) Leave the pellets to dry.
6. Sequencing electrophoresis
   (a) Add 15 μl of formamide to dried sequencing products.
   (b) Incubate 2 min, 95 °C.
   (c) Apply denaturated samples at the capillary start point.
   (d) Perform sequencing electrophoresis with the use of the appropriate program of the sequencer.

21.2.3.3 Evaluation and Interpretation of Results

The sequencer software executes collection of the sequence data while the analysis of SBT-HLA genotyping is performed with the use of a software dedicated for the alignment of current library of HLA alleles and the resultant sequence along with template (see Fig. 21.2). The nucleotide sequences including polymorphic sites are identified by the analysis of fluorescent signal peaks of consecutive bases in the sequence. Reliability of the resultant sequence is first verified by comparison of the peaks of all bases and polymorphic sites with template for forward and reverse sequence, simultaneously. The height of peaks can be biased by technical problems and it normally become lower as PCR substrates are consumed when the sequencing amplification progresses. The height of the peaks and their differences comparing to the background signal present in the form of frilly peaks is considered in verification. When the difference between peaks and the background is too small the SBT typing results are nonreliable and the typing should be repeated. The second step of verification is the analysis of polymorphic sites indicating heterozygous genotype. After the analysis is completed the software generates the proposed resultant alleles of the genotype. The final software generated genotype interpretation must be verified by two members of laboratory staff authorized for HLA typing using PCR-SBT method. In case of cis/trans ambiguous result additional typing(s) using supplementary SBT tests, PCR-SSP or PCR-SSO HD might be performed, if necessary. The final result of SBT must fall in the scope of generic and supplementary SSP and SSO typing results, if done in parallel.

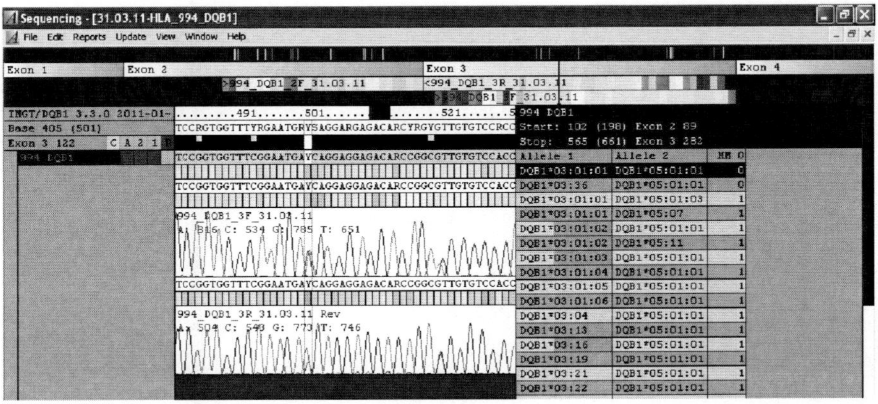

Fig. 21.2 Analysis of the row data in sequencing-based typing of HLA-DQB1 locus. A heterozygous ambiguity cis/trans result has been achieved with either HLA-DQB1*03:01:01, 05:01:01 or DQB1*03:36, 05:01:01 alternative genotypes. Several additional proposed genotypes are less probable and need at least one mismatched (MM) nucleotide modification to be justified. The sequence exhibits the T/C unambiguous nucleotide polymorphism at the position 501, assigned as Y position

21.3 *KIR* Genotyping

21.3.1 KIR-SSP Method

The primer sets amplify specific fragments (Gomez-Lozano and Vilches 2002) of the human KIR sequences deposited in centralized KIR database, provided by the European Bioinformatics Institute, (http://www.ebi.ac.uk/ipd/kir/). Primer pairs are designed to be matched with locus-specific KIR genes or their variant subtypes. Due to extensive polymorphism of KIR loci and haplotypes, the PCR-SSP kits are only provided commercially in the format of PCR microtube sets with predeposited specific primers of precisely described allelic specificity and microtube location (KIR SSP typing trays).

21.3.2 KIR-SSP, Stepwise Procedure

1. For the 24 tube formatted KIR SSP typing tray prepare the PCR reaction mix consisting of 168 μl of molecular grade sterile water, 84 μl of PCR buffer and 2.2 μl of Taq DNA polymerase (5 U/μl) and mix well.
2. For a negative control pipette 10 μl of the reaction mix into the empty PCR tube.

3. Pipette 27 μl of sample DNA into the reaction mix, mix well, and dispense 10 μl aliquots into the remaining 23 primer cocktail containing tubes of the KIR SSP typing tray.
4. Perform the PCR, according to the following cycling profile:

96 °C	2 min	
96 °C	15 s	10 cycles
65 °C	1 min	
96 °C	15 s	20 cycles
61 °C	50 s	
72 °C	30 s	
4 °C	hold	

5. Run 2 % agarose gel in 1X TBE buffer for 3–5 min,
6. Perform evaluation of the results under ultraviolet light with the enclosed evaluation sheet.

21.3.3 Evaluation and Interpretation of Results

The detected PCR product band patterns are composed of KIR gene-specific amplicons and human growth hormone amplicons as the internal control. In positive KIR-specific reactions, the internal control band may be suppressed because of competitive amplification. Evaluation is based on checking for KIR-specific amplicons which are smaller (85–315 bp) than the products of the internal control (430 or 800 bp). The pattern of the specific bands is entered in the enclosed evaluation sheet or computer interpretation software and the typing result is analyzed with the help of the interpretation chart or dedicated software. The presence of bands in a negative control well indicate contamination of the reaction mix with foreign DNA. The constellation of the bands in the gel photograph and those manually entered in the interpretation table or computer software must be checked twice for concordance and final KIR genotype must be interpreted by two members of laboratory staff authorized for KIR typing using PCR-SSP-typing method.

21.4 mHA Genotyping

The primer sets in PCR-SSP format amplify specific fragments of ten different autosomal (HA-1, HA-2, HA-3, HA-8, HB-1, ACC-1, ACC-2, HwA-9(SP110), HwA-10(PANE1), UGT2B17) and one male sex-specific HY minor histocompatibility antigen genes (Spierings et al. 2006) described in a minor histocompatibility dbMinor database (http://www.lumc.nl/dbminor).

21.4.1 mHA-SSP, Stepwise Procedure

1. Using commercially available SSP-mHA kit prepare the PCR reaction mix for 40 reactions, consisting of 450 μl of mHA PCR buffer, and 4.5 μl of Taq DNA polymerase (5 U/μl).
2. For a negative control pipette 10 μl of PCR reaction mix into the empty PCR tube.
3. Pipette 107 μl of sample DNA (50 ng/μl) into the mHA PCR reaction mix.
4. Dispense 10 μl aliquots into the 38 typing wells with primer cocktail contained in the kit.
5. Perform PCR, according to the cycling profile:

94 °C	2 min	
94 °C	10 s	10 cycles
65 °C	1 min	
94 °C	10 s	20 cycles
61 °C	50 s	
72 °C	30 s	
4 °C	hold	

6. Run 2 % agarose gel with 1X TBE buffer for 10 min.
7. Perform evaluation of the results under ultraviolet light with the enclosed evaluation sheet.

21.4.2 Evaluation and Interpretation of Results

The detected PCR product band patterns are composed of mHA gene-specific amplicons. The internal control band of HLA-DRA invariant chain gene fragment (1,009 bp) should be visible. The internal control band is weaker in the presence of a mHA gene amplicon. The constellation of the bands in the gel photograph and those manually entered in the interpretation table or computer software must be checked twice for concordance and final genotype must be interpreted by two members of laboratory staff authorized for mHA typing using PCR-SSP method. The dbMinor database can be screened for the HLA restriction of the immunogenic mHA alleles and for putative immune reactivity in the specific HLA-typed and mHA-typed donor-recipient combination.

21.5 Conclusions

The typing of HLA and other immune-related gene polymorphisms using appropriate and well controlled molecular-based methods is a crucial component of HSC donor-recipient matching. The reliability, the level of resolution, and feasibility of the typing methods used must be considered in the process of donor-recipient matching. Since ambiguous results can not always be resolved the appropriate understanding of ambiguities is of particular importance for the HSC outcome.

Acknowledgments This chapter was partly supported by the Ministry of Science and Higher Education, Grant No. N N402 351138.

References

Dalva K, Beksac M (2007) HLA typing with sequence-specific oligonucleotide primed PCR (PCR-SSO) and use of the Luminex technology. Methods Mol Med 134:61–69

Gomez-Lozano N, Vilches C (2002) Genotyping of human killer-cell immunoglobulin-like receptor genes by polymerase chain reaction with sequence-specific primers: an update. Tissue Antigens 59:184–193

Holdsworth R, Hurley CK, Marsh SG, Lau M, Noreen HJ, Kempenich JH, Setterholm M, Maiers M (2009) The HLA dictionary 2008: a summary of HLA-A, -B, -C, -DRB1/3/4/5, and -DQB1 alleles and their association with serologically defined HLA-A, -B, -C, -DR, and -DQ antigens. Tissue Antigens 73:95–170

Nagy M, Entz P, Otremba P, Schoenemann C, Murphy N, Dapprich J (2007) Haplotype-specific extraction: a universal method to resolve ambiguous genotypes and detect new alleles—demonstrated on HLA-B. Tissue Antigens 69:176–180

Robinson J, Mistry K, McWilliam H, Lopez R, Parham P, Marsh SG (2011) The IMGT/HLA database. Nucleic Acids Res 39:D1171–D1176

Sanger F, Coulson AR (1975) A rapid method for determining sequences in DNA by primed synthesis with DNA polymerase. J Mol Biol 94:441–448

Schaffer M, Olerup O (2001) HLA-AB typing by polymerase-chain reaction with sequence-specific primers: more accurate, less errors, and increased resolution compared to serological typing. Tissue Antigens 58:299–307

Spierings E, Drabbels J, Hendriks M, Pool J, Spruyt-Gerritse M, Claas F, Goulmy E (2006) A uniform genomic minor histocompatibility antigen typing methodology and database designed to facilitate clinical applications. PLoS ONE 1:e42

Viollier R, Socie G, Tichelli A, Bacigalupo A, Korthof ET, Marsh J, Cornish J, Ljungman P, Oneto R, Bekassy AN, Fuehrer M, Maury S, Schrezenmeier H, van Lint MT, Wojcik D, Locasciulli A, Passweg JR (2008) Recent improvement in outcome of unrelated donor transplantation for aplastic anemia. Bone Marrow Transplant 41:45–50

Chapter 22
Post-Transplant Chimerism Analysis Through STR-PCR and RQ-PCR

Małgorzata Dawidowska, Katarzyna Guz, Agnieszka Orzińska, Justyna Smolarczyk-Wodzyńska, Monika D. Kraszewska and Michał Witt

Abstract The analysis of chimerism following allogeneic hematopoietic stem cell transplantation is a valuable tool for the documentation of engraftment, for the assessment of the risk of graft versus host disease, the risk of graft rejection, and in case of malignancies, the risk of relapse. The monitoring of post-transplant chimerism is aimed at discrimination among complete chimerism, mixed chimerism, and autologous recovery (no chimerism), which in case of mixed chimerism identification is followed by quantitative analysis for the determination of percentage share between donor-derived and recipient-derived cells. These goals might be achieved by different approaches. Protocols for chimerism analysis with

M. Dawidowska (✉) · M. D. Kraszewska · M. Witt
Department of Molecular and Clinical Genetics, Institute of Human Genetics, Polish Academy of Sciences, Strzeszyńska 32, 60-479 Poznań, Poland
e-mail: ma.dawidowska@wp.pl

M. D. Kraszewska
e-mail: m.kraszewska@gmail.com

M. Witt
e-mail: wittmich@man.poznan.pl

K. Guz · A. Orzińska · J. Smolarczyk-Wodzyńska
Department of Immunohematology and Immunology of Transfusion Medicine, Institute of Hematology and Transfusion Medicine, Indiry Gandhi 14, 02-776 Warsaw, Poland
e-mail: kguz@ihit.waw.pl

A. Orzińska
e-mail: orzinska@ihit.waw.pl

J. Smolarczyk-Wodzyńska
e-mail: jsmolarczyk@ihit.waw.pl

M. Witt
International Institute of Molecular and Cell Biology, Trojdena 4, 02-109 Warsaw, Poland

M. Witt et al. (eds.), *Molecular Aspects of Hematologic Malignancies*, Principles and Practice, DOI: 10.1007/978-3-642-29467-9_22,

the use of two currently most widely used methods have been described in this chapter: STR-PCR approach, i.e., polymerase chain reaction for the analysis of microsatellite polymorphism and RQ-PCR approach exploiting real-time quantitative PCR for the analysis of *indel* and null polymorphism.

22.1 Introduction

Since the implementation of molecular methods into the monitoring of chimerism after allogeneic hematopoietic stem cell transplantation (allo-HSCT), numerous approaches have been developed and tested for their utility in clinical practice. The basic requirements for the methods of chimerism analysis include:

- the possibility to discriminate between donor-derived and recipient-derived cells,
- the possibility to identify *complete chimerism* (detection of donor-derived cells, exclusively; CC), *mixed chimerism* (detection of both donor-derived and recipient-derived cells; MC), and *autologous recovery*, i.e., no chimerism (detection of recipient-derived cells, exclusively),
- quantitative analysis enabling determination of percentage share between the cells of the donor and the recipient, in case of the identification of mixed chimerism.

Moreover, optimal approaches for chimerism diagnostics should be characterised by:

- sufficient sensitivity (at least 5×10^{-2}, though sensitivities of 10^{-3}–10^{-4} or higher are preferred) enabling not only the documentation of engraftment but also early detection of relapse or graft failure,
- maximum informativeness (approximately 100 %) enabling wide applicability in all donor-recipient pairs,
- high intra-assay and inter-assay reproducibility,
- possibility for standardization,
- cost-effectiveness and relatively easy procedures, facilitating wide applicability in a regular diagnostic setting.

It is difficult to meet all these requirements with a single method. However, these criteria are most adequately addressed by two approaches, currently most widely used for chimerism monitoring, i.e., (1) the analysis of microsatellite polymorphism via polymerase chain reaction with fluorescently labeled primers (usually termed STR-PCR approach) and (2) real-time quantitative polymerase chain reaction for the analysis of *indel* (insertion/deletion) and null polymorphism (Thiede et al. 1999; Thiede et al. 2004; Alizadeh et al. 2002; Masmas et al. 2005). The principles of application of these methods for chimerism analysis have been discussed in details in Chap. 15.

22.2 Cell Sample Processing for Chimerism Analysis

The following type of biological material might be used for chimerism analysis:

- blood,
- bone marrow,
- mononuclear cells (MNC) isolated from blood or bone marrow,
- cell subsets (e.g., CD3 cells) isolated from blood or bone marrow.

Blood (10 ml) or bone marrow (3–5 ml) samples should be collected into tubes containing EDTA (ethylenediamine tetra acetic acid) salts as anticoagulant, transported and stored at room temperature or at 4 °C. If MNC fraction is to be isolated from blood/bone marrow for chimerism analysis, the samples should be processed no longer than within 24 h from collection. If particular cell fraction (e.g., CD3) is to be isolated, blood/bone marrow should preferably be fractionated within 8 h. If the samples are to be fractionated (MNCs or cell subset isolation), they should not be frozen. If chimerism analysis is to be performed using whole blood or bone marrow, samples might alternatively be frozen at −20 °C or preferably at −80 °C.

It is recommended to preferentially use MNC or specific cell subpopulations (for the analysis of lineage chimerism) rather than whole blood or bone marrow for chimerism analysis. Detailed information on clinical significance of chimerism, including that of lineage specific chimerism is presented in Chap. 15.

Cell sample processing includes:

1. The isolation of mononuclear cells by density gradient centrifugation, according to a standard protocol (see Chap. 19).
2. The isolation of particular cell subset with the use of flow cytometry or immunomagnetic method (this step is optional).
3. DNA isolation with the use of column-based DNA isolation kit, according to the manufacturer's instructions. Alternatively, DNA might be isolated using salting-out method, which generates DNA of sufficient quality for STR-PCR-based chimerism analysis; however, this is not recommended for RQ-PCR-based approach. The remaining MNCs should be stored for later use, preferably in liquid nitrogen or at −80 °C.
4. The concentration of DNA optimal for chimerism analysis via STR-PCR-based approach is 20 ng/μl. In case of DNA samples of graft recipient collected at consecutive time points of chimerism monitoring one should obtain at least 10 μl DNA in this concentration (20 ng/μl). In case of DNA samples of graft donor and of the recipient before transplantation, it is recommended to obtain greater yield of DNA isolation since these DNA samples need to be amplified in line with DNA samples obtained in every consecutive time point of chimerism monitoring. The optimal DNA amount for RQ-PCR-based chimerism analysis is 5 ng/μl in a 100 μl volume.

5. The assessment of DNA quantity and quality by optical density measurement at 260 and 280 nm, preferably using a microvolume spectrophotometer (e.g., Nanodrop or a comparable equipment). In case of RQ-PCR-based approach it is additionally recommended to assess the quantity and amplifiability of DNA via RQ-PCR amplification and quantitative assessment of a suitable control gene using a relevant standard curve.
6. The preparation of working dilutions of DNA for STR-PCR or RQ-PCR.

22.3 Schedule of Material Collection and Chimerism Monitoring

In order to determine the genotypes of analyzed individuals, used as reference for the analysis of post-transplant samples, it is necessary to obtain at least 200–400 ul of blood or bone marrow from:

- the graft recipient (before transplantation),
- the graft donor (any time).

For the purpose of the identification of STR markers informative for the analyzed donor-recipient pair, DNA should be isolated using whole blood/bone marrow; it is not necessary to perform MNC/cell subset isolation. In the STR-PCR approach, the remaining blood/bone marrow should be stored for any subsequent DNA isolation, since chimerism monitoring requires the amplification of the donor and recipient DNA (obtained before transplantation) in line with DNA of the recipient obtained in every consecutive time point of chimerism monitoring.

In order to monitor chimerism throughout post-transplant period it is necessary to obtain 3–10 ml of blood or bone marrow from the graft recipient in the following time points (the following refers to acute lymphoblastic leukemia):

- once a week until day +100 post-transplantation and then,
- once a month until +18 month-post-transplantation.

Mononuclear cells should be used for DNA extraction in these time points.

In case of identification of mixed chimerism (at any time point throughout the post-transplant monitoring) or in case of suspicion of impending relapse or graft rejection, a more intensive schedule of chimerism monitoring is recommended; i.e., the collection of 3–10 ml of blood or bone marrow from the graft recipient.

- once a week until identification of full donor chimerism in at least two consecutive time points.

In case of intensive chimerism monitoring, MNC fraction, or preferably relevant cell subset should be used for DNA isolation. It is recommended to store a proportion of whole blood/bone marrow or MNCs for chimerism analysis in case of insufficient yield or unsuccessful isolation of the desired cell fraction.

22.4 Chimerism Analysis Using STR-PCR Approach

This approach is based on the identification of microsatellite sequences, informative for the analyzed donor and recipient pair (so-called "STR-screening"), i.e., the identification of STR markers present in different allelic forms in the donor and in the recipient before transplantation (See also Chap. 15). In the consecutive post-transplant follow-up time points, chimerism is analyzed qualitatively (identification of complete chimerism, CC; mixed chimerism, MC; autologous recovery, AR) and quantitatively (in case of MC) with the use of the selected optimal STR markers. Preferably, at least two informative STR markers should be used for chimerism assessment in each follow-up time point.

The sequential steps of chimerism analysis procedure, i.e., STR marker sequence amplification, electrophoretic detection of amplicons in a sequencer and data analysis are the same in case of the identification of informative STR markers (STR-screening) and chimerism analysis during post-transplant follow-up. The only difference lies in the type of chimerism analysis, i.e., solely qualitative analysis in case of STR-screening and in case of chimerism monitoring–qualitative analysis for the identification of the type of chimerism (CC/MC/AR) followed by quantitative analysis in case of MC detection. The identification and quantification of chimerism is performed with the use of the appropriate software, dependent on the sequencer used for detection and automated quantification of the amplified STR sequences.

22.4.1 Identification of Informative STR Markers

Microsatellite sequences to be used for chimerism analysis might be selected using one of the available databases, e.g., *Short Tandem Repeat DNA Internet Database*; *STRBase* (*National Institute of Standards and Technology*) (Ruitberg et al. 2001), available at: http://www.cstl.nist.gov/strbase/.

Recommended STR markers for chimerism analysis, including sequences of oligonucleotide primers, are presented in Table 22.1 (http://www.cstl.nist.gov/strbase/). One of the primers of each primer pair should be labeled with an appropriate fluorescent dye (e.g., Cy-5), dependent on the settings of the sequencer to be used for chimerism analysis.

In case of each analyzed donor and recipient pair, STR-screening includes the amplification of all STR sequences, for which oligonucleotide primers are available in a particular laboratory, in order to select at least two, most optimal, informative markers for chimerism monitoring.

The identification of informative markers includes:

1. The PCR amplification of DNA sample of the donor and of the recipient before transplantation (in independent parallel reactions) with the use of oligonucleotide primers specific for selected STR sequences.

Table 22.1 Sequences of primers used for STR-PCR chimerism analysis

Locus	Sequence 5′ → 3′
FGA	GCCCCATAGGTTTTGAACTCA
	TGATTTGTCTGTAATTGCCAGC
F13A1	GAGGTTGCACTCCAGCCTTT
	ATGCCATGCAGATTAGAAA
D21S11	ATATGTGAGTCAATTCCCCAAG
	TGTATTAGTCAATGTTCTCCAG
TH01	GTGGGCTGAAAAGCTCCCGATTAT
	GTGATTCCCATTGGCCTGTTCCTC
VWA	CCCTAGTGGATGATAAGAATAATCAGTATG
	GGACAGATGATAAATACATAGGATGGATGG
FES	GGGATTTCCCTATGGATTGG
	GCGAAAGAATGAGACTACAT
D12S391	AACAGGATCAATGGATGCAT
	TGGCTTTTAGACCTGGACTG
D8S1179	TTTTTGTATTTCATGTGTACATTCG
	CGTAGCTATAATTAGTTCATTTTCA

FGA (*FIBRA*), STR marker located within alpha fibrinogen gene; *F13A1*, STR marker located in coagulation factor XIII A subunit gene; *D21S11*, STR marker located in *D21S11* locus in chromosome 21; *TH01*, STR marker located within tyrosine hydroxylase gene; *VWA* (*vWF*) STR marker located within von Willebrand Factor gene; *FES*, STR marker located within feline sarcoma viral oncogene human homolog; *D12S391*, STR marker located in *D12S391* locus in chromosome 12; *D8S1179*, STR marker located in *D8S1179* locus in chromosome 8
References for primers' sequences are available at: http://www.cstl.nist.gov/strbase/

2. The composition of PCR reaction mix is presented in Table 22.2.
3. Recommended PCR conditions are as follows:

94 °C	5 min	
94 °C	45 s	26x
55 °C	1 min	26x
72 °C	1 min	26x
72 °C	5 min	

4. The preparation of PCR products for electrophoresis in a sequencer: 2 μl of PCR product should be mixed with 7 μl of loading buffer containing 100 bp and 300 bp fluorescently labeled size markers (so-called 'internal markers').
5. The denaturation of PCR products via incubation in 95 °C for 5 min, followed by transfer onto ice to prevent renaturation.
6. PCR products should be immediately loaded into 6 % polyacrylamide gel containing 7 M urea (denaturating conditions) and run in 0.6x TBE buffer, applying 1,500 V, and using fluorescently labeled 50–500 bp fragments sizer as an external marker.

Table 22.2 Composition of STR-PCR reaction mix

Reagent	Starting	Volume/1 reaction [μl]	Final
Water (nanopure)		4.9	
PCR buffer with 15 mM $MgCl_2$	10x	1	1x
dNTP	1.25 mM	1.6	200 μM
F primer	12.5 μM	0.2	0.25 μM
R primer	12.5 μM	0.2	0.25 μM
Taq polymerase	5 U/μl	0.08	0.4 U
DNA	20 ng/μl	2	40 ng
Reaction volume		10	

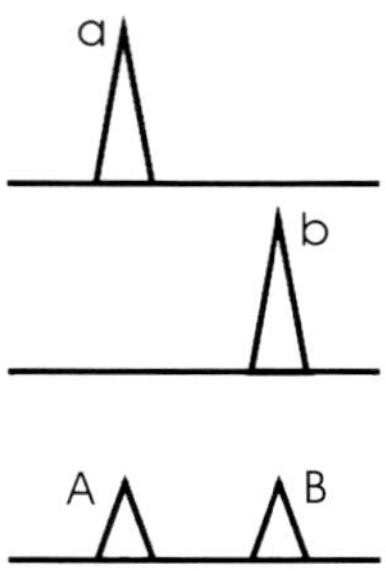

Fig. 22.1 The donor and the recipient do not share a common allele in the analyzed STR locus; both, the donor and the recipient are homozygotes

22.4.1.1 Interpretation of STR-Screening Results

STR-screening is aimed at selection of at least two optimal STR markers informative for the analyzed donor and recipient pair, i.e., enabling unequivocal discrimination between the genotypes of the donor and of the recipient. This implies that at least one allele in the analyzed STR locus must be specific exclusively for the donor or for the recipient. Possible configurations of STR alleles of the donor and of the recipient are presented in Figs. 22.1, 22.2, 22.3, 22.4, 22.5, 22.6, 22.7. In all figures, the same sample order is applied: (1) peaks specific for the recipient before transplantation in the upper panel, (2) donor-specific peaks in the middle panel, and (3) peaks detected in the recipient in the analyzed time point after transplantation in the lower panel. The upper and the middle panel reflect STR-screening. All three panels reflect post-transplant chimerism analysis, in which case the samples in the upper and in the middle panel are used as the reference, while the sample in the lower panel is subjected to qualitative and possibly to quantitative analysis.

Possible informative alleles configurations of the donor and of the recipient:

- The donor and the recipient do not share a common allele in the analyzed STR locus:

  (a) both the donor and the recipient are homozygotes (Fig. 22.1)
  (b) the recipient is a heterozygote, the donor is a homozygote (Fig. 22.2)
  (c) the recipient is a homozygote, the donor is a heterozygote (Fig. 22.3)
  (d) both, the donor and the recipient are heterozygotes (Fig. 22.4)

Fig. 22.2 The donor and the recipient do not share a common allele in the analyzed STR locus; the recipient is a heterozygote, the donor is a homozygote

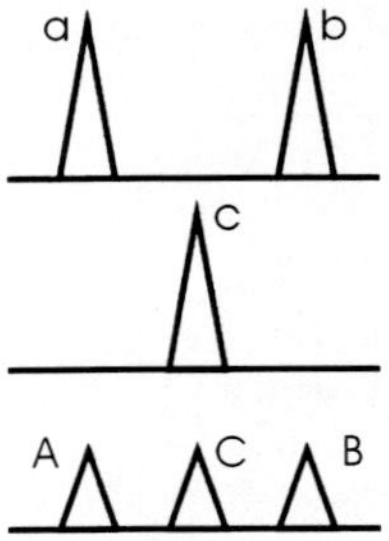

Fig. 22.3 The donor and the recipient do not share a common allele in the analyzed STR locus; the recipient is a homozygote, the donor is a heterozygote

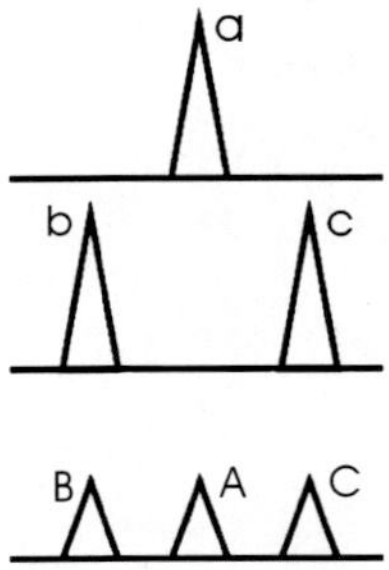

Fig. 22.4 The donor and the recipient do not share a common allele in the analyzed STR locus; both, the donor and the recipient are heterozygotes

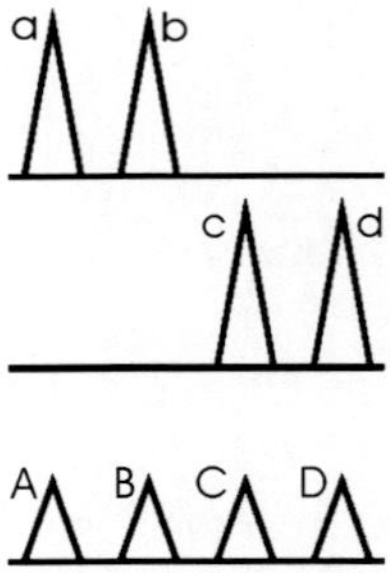

Fig. 22.5 The donor and the recipient share a common allele in the analyzed STR locus; both, the donor and the recipient are heterozygotes. The peak common for the donor and the recipient (representing the common allele) is not used for the calculation (the *crossed out peak*)

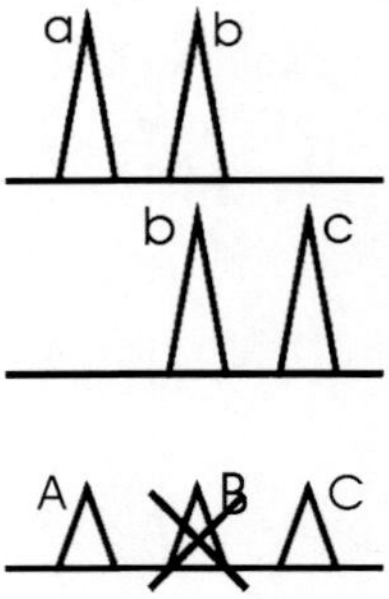

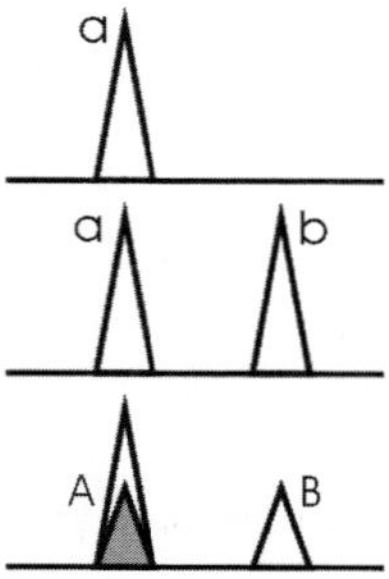

Fig. 22.6 The donor and the recipient share a common allele in the analyzed STR locus; the recipient is a homozygote, the donor is a heterozygote. The fusion peak is generated, including the component of the donor origin, which area is equal to the area of the second heterozygous allele of the donor (illustrated as the *shaded part of the peak*) and the component of the recipient origin

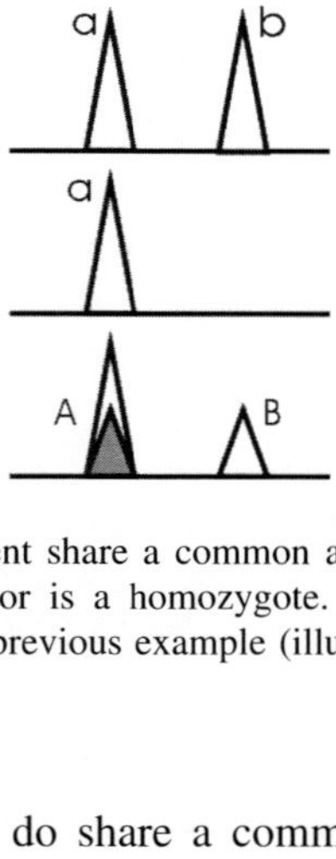

Fig. 22.7 The donor and the recipient share a common allele in the analyzed STR locus; the recipient is a heterozygote, the donor is a homozygote. For the calculation of chimerism a modification of the formula used in previous example (illustrated in Fig. 22.6) is used

- The donor and the recipient do share a common allele in the analyzed STR locus:

  (e) both, the donor and the recipient are heterozygotes (Fig. 22.5)
  (f) the recipient is a homozygote, the donor is a heterozygote (Fig. 22.6)
  (g) the recipient is a heterozygote, the donor is a homozygote (Fig. 22.7)

The power of discrimination between the genotypes of the analyzed donor and recipient, with the use of the given STR marker is dependent on:

- The above-mentioned configurations of alleles specific for the donor and the recipient (the configurations presented in Figs. 22.6 and 22.7 are characterized by the lowest power of discrimination).
- The length of the amplified fragments dependent on the number of STR repeats (it is recommended to choose STR markers, which generate amplicons differing considerably in length in the donor and in the recipient).

- The presence of nonspecific peaks representing: nonspecific amplicons resulting from the slippage of polymerase (so-called "polymerase slippage products" also referred to as "stutter peaks"), from template-independent nucleotide addition by terminal transferase activity of Taq polymerase (double peaks), or from the nonspecific fluorescence of the applied fluorochromes (so called "dye-associated fluorescence peaks").

It is recommended to choose at least two optimal STR markers for chimerism analysis; though in case of doubts, one might decide to monitor chimerism with the use of more than two available STR markers to increase the reliability of the analysis.

If the configuration of alleles in the analyzed STR locus is the same in the donor and in the recipient, such STR marker is not informative for the given donor and recipient pair and might not be used for chimerism analysis.

22.4.2 Post-Transplant Chimerism Analysis with STR-PCR Approach

Post-transplant monitoring of chimerism in whole or fractionated blood or bone marrow, obtained at consecutive time points during post-transplant follow-up is performed with the use of at least two informative STR markers. The composition of PCR reaction mix, PCR thermal cycling conditions, the preparation of PCR products for electrophoresis and conditions of electrophoresis in a sequencer are exactly the same as those applied for the identification of informative STR markers, therefore one should follow the steps described in Sect. 22.4.1. Remarks concerning these steps performed for chimerism analysis are briefly described below.

- The amplification of selected optimal informative STR markers is performed in three parallel reactions using (1) the DNA of the recipient obtained before transplantation, (2) the DNA of the donor and (3) that of the recipient obtained in the analyzed time point during post-transplant monitoring, preferably according to the schedule previously described in Sect. 22.3.
- While performing electrophoresis of PCR products in a plate sequencer it is recommended to load the samples onto the gel in the following order:

1. PCR products amplified using the DNA of the recipient before transplantation
2. PCR products amplified using the DNA of the donor
3. PCR products amplified using the DNA of the recipient in the analyzed time point.

This sample order prevents false positive results. Potentially, accidental leakage of PCR products between the neighboring wells of the gel might falsely be interpreted as mixed chimerism, if sample of the recipient before transplantation is run adjacent to the sample of the recipient post-transplantation.

22.4.2.1 Interpretation of Chimerism Analysis Results

The analysis of chimerism in consecutive time points during post-transplant follow-up is aimed at the identification of the type of chimerism through qualitative analysis, i.e., discrimination between CC, MC, and no chimerism (AR). In case of detection of MC, additional quantitative analysis is performed for the assessment of the percentage of donor-derived and recipient-derived cells in the analyzed material.

Qualitative Analysis

The following guidelines should be applied for the identification of the type of chimerism:

- Complete chimerism (also termed "complete donor chimerism")
  The configuration of alleles detected in the recipient post-transplantation is exactly the same as that identified in the donor. This implies the detection of the cells of the donor genotype exclusively.
- No chimerism (also termed "autologous recovery")
  The configuration of alleles detected in the recipient post-transplantation is exactly the same as that identified in the recipient before transplantation. This implies the detection of the cells of the recipient genotype exclusively.
- Mixed chimerism
  The configuration of alleles detected in the recipient post-transplantation is a combination of alleles specific for the donor and for the recipient before transplantation. This implies co-existence of the cells of the donor and of the recipient genotype.

Quantitative Analysis

Quantitative chimerism analysis is based on the following assumptions:

- The amount of DNA (of the donor/recipient) is proportional to the number of cells used for DNA isolation, and thus reflects the percentage share between donor-derived and recipient-derived cells.
- Theoretically, the alleles specific for the donor and for the recipient amplify with equal efficiency (though, in practice, the efficiency of amplification is dependent on the sequence length and the nucleotide composition of the analyzed STR markers).
- The intensity of fluorescence emitted by the amplicons generated with the use of fluorescently labeled primers is proportional to the amount of these PCR products.

The amplified STR sequences are automatically detected in a sequencer, which is presented graphically as specific peaks. The length of each sequence is determined relative to 100 bp, 300 bp and 50–500 bp markers, based on the time of migration of PCR products through a laser beam. The amount of each amplicon is determined based on the intensity of emitted fluorescence excited by the laser beam, which is reflected as the area beneath each peak. The sizes of detected alleles and their configuration are used for the identification of the genotype of the analyzed cells and thus, the type of chimerism. The areas of the peaks are applied for the calculation of percentage share between donor-derived and recipient-derived cells, with the use of specific mathematical formulas.

The general mathematical formula used for chimerism calculations is presented below (Kreyenberg et al. 2003):

$$\%\,\text{DNA donor} = 100 \cdot \frac{\sum D}{\sum D + \sum R}$$

where

$\sum$D cumulative area of the peaks specific for the donor
$\sum$R cumulative area of the peaks specific for the recipient

The following modifications of the above basic formula are used for chimerism quantification, dependent on the configuration of the alleles of the donor, and of the recipient (according to Figs. 22.1, 22.2, 22.3, 22.4, 22.5, 22.6, 22.7) (Fernandez-Aviles et al. 2003):

- The donor and the recipient do not share a common allele in the analyzed STR locus:

  (a) both, the donor and the recipient are homozygotes (Fig. 22.1)

$$\%D = 100 \cdot \frac{B}{A + B}$$

  (b) the recipient is a heterozygote, the donor is a homozygote (Fig. 22.2)

$$\%D = 100 \cdot \frac{C}{A + B + C}$$

  (c) the recipient is a homozygote, the donor is a heterozygote (Fig. 22.3)

$$\%D = 100 \cdot \frac{(B + C)}{A + B + C}$$

  (d) both, the donor and the recipient are heterozygotes (Fig. 22.4)

$$\%D = 100 \cdot \frac{(C + D)}{A + B + C + D}$$

- The donor and the recipient do share a common allele in the analyzed STR locus:

  (e) both, the donor and the recipient are heterozygotes (Fig. 22.5)

$$\%D = 100 \cdot \frac{C}{A + C}$$

The peak common for the donor and the recipient (representing the common allele) is not used for the calculation (illustrated in Fig. 22.5 as the *crossed out peak*)

(f) the recipient is a homozygote, the donor is a heterozygote (Fig. 22.6)

$$\%D = 100 \cdot \frac{2B}{A + B}$$

The fusion peak is generated, including the component of the donor origin, which area is equal to the area of the second heterozygous allele of the donor (illustrated in Fig. 22.6 as the *shaded part of the peak*) and the component of the recipient origin.

(g) the recipient is a heterozygote, the donor is a homozygote (Fig. 22.7)

$$\%D = 100 - \frac{2B}{A + B} \cdot 100$$

This formula is a modification of that used in the previous example.

22.4.3 Standardization of STR-PCR Approach

In order to verify the accuracy and reliability of chimerism quantification, it is recommended to perform an experimental assessment of chimerism using standard curves, representing the reconstruction of mixed chimerism (Thiede et al. 1999). All the steps of this experiment should be performed using the same conditions and guidelines for data interpretation as those used for the analysis of patients' samples.

This experiment includes:

- The preparation of a standard curve by diluting DNA of two individuals, representing the theoretical donor and recipient before transplantation, in different proportions, e.g.,:0:100 5:95 10:20 20:80 30:70 40:60 50:50 60:40 70:30 80:20 90:10 95:5 100:0
- The amplification of the standard curve with the use of primers specific for selected STR markers informative for the analyzed donor and recipient pair.
- The detection and quantification of amplicons via electrophoresis in a sequencer.
- The quantitative analysis of mixed chimerism with the use of the appropriate mathematical formula, dependent on the configuration of donor and recipient alleles.

- Plotting the curves presenting the proportion of DNA of the donor and of the recipient:
  - in the analyzed samples of the standard curve (known proportion in each sample amplified)
  - calculated with the use of mathematical formula (based on the areas of the peaks representing the alleles of the donor and of the recipient).

One might decide to prepare the standard curve by mixing the MNCs of the donor and of the recipient, which should better reflect the actual condition of mixed cellular chimerism than the standard curve prepared by mixing the DNA of the analyzed individuals (Thiede et al. 1999).

It is not necessary to perform amplification of the standard curve for each analyzed donor and recipient pair, and for all the analyzed STR markers. It is recommended to prepare standard curves for several donor and recipient pairs and to amplify them in replicates with the use of primers specific for all available STR markers, in order to test chimerism quantification for different configurations of donor and recipient alleles. The quantitative assessment of artificial mixed chimerism generated via the construction of the standard curves enables experimental determination of the accuracy, sensitivity, and reproducibility of the STR-PCR approach in the given laboratory.

22.4.4 Informativeness, Sensitivity, Reproducibility of STR-PCR Approach

- Informativeness nearly 100 %
  Discrimination between the genotype of the donor and of the recipient is possible in nearly all analyzed donor and recipient pairs (Alizadeh et al. 2002; Thiede et al. 1999).
- Reproducible sensitivity approximately 5×10^{-2}
  It is possible to detect less abundant cell population at the level of 5 %. It is often possible to detect cell population even below this level, dependent on the configuration of the donor-specific and the recipient-specific alleles; however, results are usually not reproducible, and should not be used for clinical decision making (Thiede et al. 1999; Kreyenberg et al. 2003).
- Reproducibility
  Results obtained via the amplification of the analyzed sample with the use of different STR markers usually differ within the range of 5–10 %. In some cases, this also applies to replicates analyzed with the same STR marker in independent reactions. Therefore, for greater reliability of the results it is recommended to analyze each post-transplant sample simultaneously with previously analyzed sample of this patient (as a reference) and comparison of the results obtained in the given analysis with those obtained in a previous analysis (Kreyenberg et al. 2003).

Alternatively, one might analyze post-transplant samples without such reference, but present the results in a suitable percentage range, e.g., 45 % (40–50 %).

22.5 Chimerism Analysis Using RQ-PCR Approach

Chimerism analysis with the use of RQ-PCR approach is based on the identification of unique genetic markers: one specific for the donor, another for the recipient. In the proposed protocol markers are selected from 25 polymorphisms of 15 loci (Brojer et al. 2005; Guz et al. 2010): 10 bi-allelic insertion/deletion (*indel*) polymorphisms (*S01*, *S04-5*, *S07-11*, *ACE*, *RHCE*C/c*) and 5 null (gene deletion) alleles (*SRY*, *RHD*, *GSTM1*, *S03*, *S06*) (Alizadeh et al. 2002; Lo et al. 2000; Lo et al. 1998; Legler et al. 2002; Zhang et al. 2000). The *CCR5* gene was chosen as a control for relative quantification of chimerism after allo-HSCT. Sequences of primers and probes used for RQ-PCR analysis of *indel* and null alleles, as well as the names of the genes are presented in Tables 22.3 and 22.4.

The analysis of chimerism with the use of RQ-PCR consists of three steps:

- RQ-PCR optimization,
- the selection of donor and recipient-specific markers,
- the evaluation of post-transplant chimerism based on quantitative analysis of selected markers.

In these study phases the amplification conditions for all markers are identical, although several standardization tests for optimization of PCR conditions are necessary prior to chimerism determination by RQ-PCR. Sensitivity curves for individual markers must be performed for subsequent quantitative analysis.

22.5.1 Standardization of RQ-PCR Approach

22.5.1.1 RQ-PCR Optimization

The *indel* and null markers amplification is performed with primers and a probe specific for particular polymorphism in independent RQ-PCR (Tables 22.3 and 22.4). The reaction volume depends on the RQ-PCR equipment used. Amplification is usually performed in 25 μl if 0.2 ml amplification tubes and "standard block" are used, and in 5–10 μl in case of smaller 'formats/fast' blocks. With a wide variety of commercially available reagents and equipment for RQ-PCR analysis, the choice of appropriate RQ-PCR buffer is necessary (usually 2x concentrated Master Mix with the optimal concentration of Mg^{2+} ions, dNTP, Taq

Table 22.3 Sequences of primers and probes used for RQ-PCR chimerism analysis based on *indel* markers

Marker		Sequence 5′ → 3′	
SO1	a	primer F	GGT ACC GGG TCT CCA CAT GA
		probe*	FAM-CTG GGC CAG AAT CTT GGT CCT CAC A-TAMRA
		primer R*	GGG AAA GTC ACT CAC CCA AGG
	b	primer F	GTA CCG GGT CTC CAC CAG G
SO4	a	primer R	AAG GAT GCG TGA CTG CTA TGG
		probe*	FAM-TCC TGG CAG TGT GGT CCC TTC AGA A-TAMRA
		primer F*	CTG GTG CCC ACA GTT ACG CT
	b	primer R	AGG ATG CGT GAC TGC TCC TC
SO5	a	primer F	AAA GTA GAC ACG GCC AGA CTT AGG
		probe*	FAM-CCC TGG ACA CTG AAA ACA GGC AAT CCT-TAMRA
		primer R*	AGT TAA AGT AGA CAC GGC CTC CC
	b	primer F	AGT TAA AGT AGA CAC GGC CTC CC
SO7	a	primer F	TGG TAT TGG CTT TAA AAT ACT GGG
		probe*	FAM-TCC TCA CTT CTC CAC CCC TAG TTA AAC AG-TAMRA
		primer R*	CAG CTG CAA CAG TTA TCA ACG TT
	b	primer F	CTG GAT GCC TCA CTG ATC CA
SO8	a	primer F	CTG GAT GCC TCA CTG ATC CA
		probe*	FAM-CTC CCA ACC CCC ATT TCT GCC TG-TAMRA
		primer R*	TGG GAA GGA TGC ATA TGA TCT G
	b	primer F	GCT GGA TGC CTC ACT GAT GTT
SO9	a	primer R	TCA GCT TGT CTG CTT TCT GGA A
		probe*	FAM-TGG AGG ATT TCT CCC CTG CTT CAG ACA G-TAMRA
		primer F*	GGG CAC CCG TGT GAG TTT T
	b	primer R	CAG CTT GTC TGC TTT CTG CTG
S10	a	primer F	GCC ACA AGA GAC TCA G
		probe*	FAM-CAG TGT CCC ACT CAA GTA CTC CTT TGG A-TAMRA
		primer R*	TGG CTT CCT TGA GGT GGA AT
	b	primer F	TTA GAG CCA CAA GAG ACA ACC AG
S11	a	primer F	TAG GAT TCA ACC CTG GAA GC
		probe*	FAM-CAA GGC TTC CTC AAT TCT CCA CCC TTC C-TAMRA
		primer R*	CCA GCA TGC ACC TGA CTA ACA
	b	primer F	CCC TGG ATC GCC GTG AA
ACE	ins	primer F	GCT GGG ATT ACA GGC GTG ATA
		probe*	FAM-TCA CTT TTA TGT GGT TTC GCC AAT TTT ATT CCA-TAMRA
		primer R*	GCC CTT AGC TCA CCT CTG CTT
	del	primer F	CCA TTT CTC TAG ACC TGC TGC C

(continued)

Table 22.3 (continued)

Marker		Sequence 5′ → 3′	
RHCE	C	primer F	CAT TGC TAT AGC TTA AGG ACT CA
		probe	FAM-CAA CAC CAA ACC AGG GCC ACC-TAMRA
		primer R	ATG ATT GTA CCA CTG GGA AG
	c	primer F	TCG GCC AAG ATC TGA CCG
		probe	FAM-CTT CCT CAC CTC AAA TTT CCG GAG A-TAMRA
		primer R	ATG ACC ACC TTC CCA GG

* common primer/probe
short insertion/deletion polymorphic markers located on seven different chromosomes: *SO1* (chromosome 17), *SO4* (chromosome 9), *SO5* (chromosmome 20), *SO7* (chromosome X), *SO8* (chromosome 1), *SO9* (chromosome 17), *SO10* (chromosome 18), *SO11* (chromosome 11); *ACE*, angiotensin I converting enzyme (peptidyl-dipeptidase A) 1; *RHCE*, Rh blood group, CcEe antigens
References for primers' sequences: *SO1*, *SO4*, *SO5*, *SO7*, *SO8*, *SO9*, *SO10*, *SO11*(Alizadeh et al. 2002); *ACE* (Lo et al. 1998); *RHCE* (Legler et al. 2002)

Table 22.4 Sequences of primers and probes used for RQ-PCR chimerism analysis based on null markers

Marker	Sequence 5′ → 3′	
SO3	primer F	CTT TTG CTT TCT GTT TCT TAA GGG C
	probe	FAM-CAT ACG TGC ACA GGG TCC CCG AGT-TAMRA
	primer R	TCA ATC TTT GGG CAG GTT GAA
SO6	primer F	CAG TCA CCC CGT GAA GTC CT
	probe	FAM-CCC ATC CAT CTT CCC TAC CAG ACC AGG-TAMRA
	primer R	TTT CCC CCA TCT GCC TAT TG
SRY	primer F	TGG CGA TTA AGT CAA ATT CGC
	probe	FAM-AGC AGT AGA GCA GTC AGG GAG GCA GA-TAMRA
	primer R	CCC CCT AGT ACC CTG ACA ATG TAT T
GSTM1	primer F	GGA GAA GAT TCG TGT GGA CA
	probe	FAM-TTT GGA GAA CCA GAC CAT GGA CAA C-TAMRA
	primer R	CTG GAT TGT AGC AGA TCA TAC
RHD exon 7	primer F	CCC CAC AGC TCC ATC ATG
	probe	FAM-AGC TTG CTG GGT CTG CTT GGA GAG ATC-TAMRA
	primer R	CCA CAT GCC ATT GCC GGC T
CCR5	primer F	TAC CTG CTC AAC CTG GCC AT
	probe	VIC-TTT CCT TCT TAC TGT CCC CTT CTG GGC TC-TAMRA
	primer R	TTC CAA AGT CCC ACT GGG C

null polymorphic markers located on two different chromosomes: *SO3* (chromosome 6), *SO6* (chromosome 1); *SRY*, sex determining region Y; *GSTM1*, glutathione S-transferase mu 1; *RHD*, Rh blood group, D antigen; *CCR5*, chemokine (C–C motif) receptor 5. References for primers' sequences: *SO3, SO6* (Alizadeh et al. 2002); *SRY* (Lo et al. 1998); *GSTM1* (Lo et al. 2000); *RHD* exon 7 (Zhang et al. 2000); *CCR5* (Legler et al. 2002)

polymerase, with, or without ROX used as to get the following: ROX used as a passive reference dye a passive reference dye). The temperature profile depends on the heating block parameters, the type of Taq polymerase, and the absence or presence of Uracil N-glycosylase (UNG) enzyme in the Master Mix. The optimum annealing and elongation temperature for all primer and probe sets is 60 °C, applied for 45 cycles. Each RQ-PCR should be preceded by the selection of optimum primer concentrations (the combination of 50, 300, 900 nM) followed by effective probe concentration (every 25 nM from 50 to 225 nM). Standardization, even though costly and laborious, is necessary for each new PCR apparatus and reagent. It is recommended, therefore, to perform chimerism analyses using exclusively dedicated thermocycler and reagents for which standardization has been performed.

22.5.1.2 Standard Curves

Each marker analysis requires a separate standard curve prepared via the serial dilution of DNA positive for the analyzed marker (preferably obtained from a heterozygous individual) in negative DNA (obtained from individual without target allele). The proposed protocol includes:

- The preparation of a standard curve by five-fold DNA dilutions from 12,500 copies (100 % chimerism) to four copies (0.05 % chimerism) in a constant final amount of 50 ng DNA per reaction, assuming that one cell corresponds to 6.6 pg of DNA.
- The amplification of the standard curve with the use of primers/probe set specific for the selected marker.
- Each dilution should be tested in three replicates (intra-assay variability) and the entire procedure should be repeated on three different days (inter-assay variability).
- RQ-PCR sensitivity and efficiency is deduced from three standard curves; for the assessment of post-transplant chimerism the mean value of curve slope is used in the calculation formula (see Sect. 22.5.3.2).

For standard curves preparation and chimerism analysis, it is necessary to establish a panel of DNA samples from healthy individuals (e.g., blood donors) representing all genotype combinations in each marker locus (homozygotes, heterozygotes, and male hemizygotes in the *S07* locus on X chromosome).

22.5.1.3 Informativeness, Sensitivity, Reproducibility of RQ-PCR Approach

- Informativeness 100 % for unrelated donor/recipient pairs

Over 90 % for related donor-recipient pairs. In the study by Guz et al. (2010) informativeness was 100 and 91.08 % for unrelated and related donor-recipient pairs, respectively (Guz et al. 2010). The differentiation of donor and recipient genotype is not always possible; therefore, the panel of markers used in the given laboratory usually has to be constantly expanded.

- Sensitivity 5×10^{-4}

According to Guz et al. (2010) the RQ-PCR experimental sensitivity for all described markers is four genome equivalents (geq), which represents 0.05 % of chimerism. The detection of 1–3 geq is possible but not with 100 % repeatability (Guz et al. 2010).

- Reproducibility

CV (coefficient of variation) range of RQ-PCR for assays performed on the same day (intra-assay variability) and on three different days (inter-assay variability) is 0.24–1.42 and 1.00–3.26, respectively (Guz et al. 2010).

22.5.2 Identification of Informative Markers for RQ-PCR Analysis

The selection of markers specific for the donor and for the recipient (specific for the recipient before transplantation) begins with the analysis of phenotypic characteristics of the analyzed individuals, i.e., gender, RhD (Rhesus blood group, D, antigen), and RhCE (Rhesus blood group, CcEe, antigens) phenotype. This provides information if *SRY*, *RHD* genes, or *RHCE*C/c* alleles might be used for chimerism analysis. If not, donor and recipient DNA is investigated for the presence/absence of other *indel*/null markers. This is usually performed in 1–3 subsequent tests until unique markers differentiating the donor and the recipient are found. If more than one such marker is found for either of them, markers characterized by convergent PCR efficiency are selected. It is recommended to choose different heterozygous polymorphisms in the donor and recipient (i.e., the recipient is heterozygous for the target allele, the donor is homozygous for the opposite allele, and vice versa in case of the other locus specific for the donor). If the homozygous marker has to be analyzed, the PCR standard curve must be prepared with serial dilutions of DNA homozygous for this marker.

In case of null markers analysis, the first step is the determination of zygosity of the analyzed individual (with the exception of *SRY* gene). The gene dose analysis is based on the gene-quantity and *CCR5* ratio. This requires a separate experiment in which the target gene is co-amplified with *CCR5* control gene in a multiplex RQ-PCR and the results obtained for the tested DNA are compared to those for the DNA of at least two homozygous and heterozygous individuals used as the reference for the marker/*CCR5* ratio (range of ΔCt; Ct, threshold cycle).

For the sufficient reliability of chimerism analysis by RQ-PCR approach it is desirable to analyze both donor and recipient markers. If no donor-specific marker is found, chimerism monitoring might be based solely on the recipient-specific marker analysis. This is not the case in a reverse situation (the identification of donor-specific marker exclusively). Chimerism monitoring with the use of donor-specific marker as the only target sequence is not recommended due to low

RQ-PCR precision in case of large proportions of the target sequence (donor-specific). Decrease in the percentage of donor cells might be overlooked unless the donor marker is analyzed in parallel with that of the recipient.

22.5.3 Post-Transplant Chimerism Analysis with RQ-PCR Approach

Monitoring chimerism with the use of RQ-PCR method is based on the detection of the recipient/donor-specific markers. The recommended schedule of sample collection as well as the procedures of cell sample processing have been described in Sects. 22.2 and 22.3. Guidelines for RQ-PCR amplification of target sequences and the interpretation of quantitative results are described below.

22.5.3.1 Amplification of Informative Markers

The quantitative analysis of each post-transplant sample includes:

1. Three separate RQ-PCR reactions (each performed in duplicates, each containing 50 ng DNA) with the use of appropriate primers/probe sets for the selected recipient-specific marker, donor-specific marker, and *CCR5* control gene.
2. The composition of RQ-PCR reaction mix as well as thermal cycling conditions has to be determined experimentally at the stage of RQ-PCR optimization (see Sect. 22.5.1.1).
3. The DNA of healthy volunteers of the same genotype as the donor/the recipient (prior to transplantation) is simultaneously examined to serve as a positive control and a reference ("calibrator" DNA) for the relative quantification of post-transplantation chimerism with the use of mathematical formulas (see Sect. 22.5.3.2).
4. In very rare cases, when the donor and the recipient are opposite homozygotes for the same locus, two calibrators should be tested from donors with the respective genotypes.

22.5.3.2 Analysis and Interpretation of Results

The identification of CC, MC and AR (no chimerism) is based on the determination of the presence/absence of recipient-derived and donor-derived cells, analogously as in STR-PCR approach.

In case of mixed chimerism, quantitative assessment of the proportion (%) of recipient-derived and donor-derived cells is performed using Pfaffl's formula presented below (Alizadeh et al. 2002). Calculations are done separately for the donor-specific and the recipient-specific marker. The Ct values obtained for the target sequence of the analyzed patient, and in case of the calibrator DNA—for the control *CCR5* gene, as well as mean values of the slope of the respective standard curves are used for calculations with the use of following mathematical formula:

$$\%\text{DNAdonor/recipient} = 100 \cdot \frac{(E_{\text{target}})^{\Delta\text{Ct target}(C-U)}}{(E_{\text{ref}})^{\Delta\text{Ctref}(C-U)}}$$

where

E^{target} $10^{(-1/\text{slope of PCR for the target sequence})}$; the PCR efficiency for the target sequence (donor-specific or recipient-specific marker)

E^{ref} $10^{(-1/\text{slope of PCR for the control gene})}$; the PCR efficiency for the *CCR5* control gene

C Ct value of the recipient/donor-specific marker or Ct value of the *CCR5* control gene for the calibrator DNA

U Ct value of the recipient/donor-specific marker or Ct value of the *CCR5* control gene for patient DNA

If the proportion of the donor or the recipient genotype is ≤10 %, calculation is performed by subtracting the obtained value from 100 %. If proportions of both genotypes are >10 %, both values should be added and treated as 100 %; percentage share between the donor and recipient genotype is then calculated with the use of proportion method.

22.6 Conclusions

Quantitative evaluation of chimerism has become a part of routine molecular analyses performed after allo-HSCT for the documentation of engraftment, the assessment of the risk of graft rejection, graft-versus host disease, and relapse of the malignancy. The assessment of dynamic chimerism changes during post-transplant follow-up allows early therapeutic interventions and optimal modification of treatment as well as the monitoring of its effectiveness. The STR-PCR approach using microsatellite polymorphism and RQ-PCR method based on *indel* and null polymorphism are well recognized tools for chimerism monitoring. They offer different sensitivities of chimerism analyses, but are also characterized by different levels of time-consumption, complexity of the procedures, and labour-intensity. The protocols presented in this chapter enable implementation of chimerism monitoring with the use of these two most widely applied approaches, depending on the needs and the possibilities of a given hemato-oncology unit.

Acknowledgment This chapter was partly supported by the Ministry of Science and Higher Education, grant N N407 311 839.

References

Alizadeh M, Bernard M, Danic B, Dauriac C, Birebent B, Lapart C, Lamy T, Le Prise PY, Beauplet A, Bories D, Semana G, Quelvennec E (2002) Quantitative assessment of hematopoietic chimerism after bone marrow transplantation by real-time quantitative polymerase chain reaction. Blood 99(12):4618–4625

Brojer E, Zupanska B, Guz K, Orzinska A, Kalinska A (2005) Noninvasive determination of fetal RHD status by examination of cell-free DNA in maternal plasma. Transfusion 45(9):1473–1480. doi:TRF00559.10.1111/j.1537-2995.2005.00559.x

Fernandez-Aviles F, Urbano-Ispizua A, Aymerich M, Colomer D, Rovira M, Martinez C, Nadal E, Talarn C, Carreras E, Montserrat E (2003) Serial quantification of lymphoid and myeloid mixed chimerism using multiplex PCR amplification of short tandem repeat-markers predicts graft rejection and relapse, respectively, after allogeneic transplantation of CD34+ selected cells from peripheral blood. Leukemia 17(3):613–620

Guz K, Smolarczyk-Wodzyńska J, Dawidowska M, Jółkowska-Baraniak J, Orzinska A, Skulimowska J, Sawecka J, Kraszewska M, Tomaszewska A, Nasiłowska-Adamska B, Mariańska B, Wachowiak J, Witt M, Brojer E (2010) Evaluation of chimerism after allogeneic hematopoietic stem cell transplantation using the RQ-PCR method—its standardization and comparison with the STR-PCR method. Acta Haematol Pol 41(4):535–544

Kreyenberg H, Holle W, Mohrle S, Niethammer D, Bader P (2003) Quantitative analysis of chimerism after allogeneic stem cell transplantation by PCR amplification of microsatellite markers and capillary electrophoresis with fluorescence detection: the Tuebingen experience. Leukemia 17(1):237–240

Legler TJ, Lynen R, Maas JH, Pindur G, Kulenkampff D, Suren A, Osmers R, Kohler M (2002) Prediction of fetal Rh D and Rh CcEe phenotype from maternal plasma with real-time polymerase chain reaction. Transfus Apher Sci 27(3):217–223, S1473-0502(02)00068-X

Lo YM, Lau TK, Chan LY, Leung TN, Chang AM (2000) Quantitative analysis of the bidirectional fetomaternal transfer of nucleated cells and plasma DNA. Clin Chem 46(9):1301–1309

Lo YM, Tein MS, Lau TK, Haines CJ, Leung TN, Poon PM, Wainscoat JS, Johnson PJ, Chang AM, Hjelm NM (1998) Quantitative analysis of fetal DNA in maternal plasma and serum: implications for noninvasive prenatal diagnosis. Am J Hum Genet 62 (4):768–775, S0002-9297(07)60967-7.10.1086/301800

Masmas TN, Madsen HO, Petersen SL, Ryder LP, Svejgaard A, Alizadeh M, Vindelov LL (2005) Evaluation and automation of hematopoietic chimerism analysis based on real-time quantitative polymerase chain reaction. Biol Blood Marrow Transplant 11 (7):558–566. doi:10.1016/j.bbmt.2005.04.004, S1083879105002600

Ruitberg CM, Reeder DJ, Butler JM (2001) STRBase: a short tandem repeat DNA database for the human identity testing community. Nucleic Acids Res 29(1):320–322

Thiede C, Bornhauser M, Ehninger G (2004) Strategies and clinical implications of chimerism diagnostics after allogeneic hematopoietic stem cell transplantation. Acta Haematol 112 (1–2):16–23. doi:10.1159/000077555, AHA20041121_2016

Thiede C, Florek M, Bornhauser M, Ritter M, Mohr B, Brendel C, Ehninger G, Neubauer A (1999) Rapid quantification of mixed chimerism using multiplex amplification of short tandem repeat markers and fluorescence detection. Bone Marrow Transplant 23(10):1055–1060. doi:10.1038/sj.bmt.1701779

Zhang J, Fidler C, Murphy MF, Chamberlain PF, Sargent IL, Redman CW, Hjelm NM, Wainscoat JS, Lo YM (2000) Determination of fetal RhD status by maternal plasma DNA analysis. Ann N Y Acad Sci 906:153–155

Chapter 23
Analysis of Minimal Residual Disease with the Use of Rearrangements of Ig/TCR Genes Through RQ-PCR

Małgorzata Dawidowska, Vincent H. J. van der Velden, Michał Witt and Tomasz Szczepański

Abstract The quantitative analysis of minimal residual disease (MRD) with the use of junctional regions of rearranged immunoglobulin (Ig) and T-cell (TCR) receptor genes as MRD target sequences is a complex, multi-step procedure. It includes: the processing of biological material, the detection, clonality assessment, identification, and selection of optimal MRD target sequences, and MRD analysis with the use of real-time quantitative polymerase chain reaction (RQ-PCR), which includes: probe and primer selection, standard curve preparation, testing the sensitivity of primers, DNA quality and quantity testing, quantitative MRD analysis, and data interpretation. Although this approach is laborious, it requires experienced and qualified personnel, and extensive standardization, it is applicable in more than 95 % of acute lymphoblastic leukemia (ALL) patients and enables

M. Dawidowska (✉) · M. Witt
Department of Molecular and Clinical Genetics, Institute of Human Genetics,
Polish Academy of Sciences, Strzeszyńska 32, 60-479 Poznań, Poland
e-mail: ma.dawidowska@wp.pl

M. Witt
e-mail: wittmich@man.poznan.pl

V. H. J. van der Velden
Department of Immunology, Erasmus MC, University Medical Center Rotterdam,
Dr. Molewaterplein 50, 3015 GE, Rotterdam, The Netherlands
e-mail: v.h.j.vandervelden@erasmusmc.nl

M. Witt
International Institute of Molecular and Cell Biology,
Trojdena 4, 02-109 Warsaw, Poland

T. Szczepański
Department of Pediatric Hematology and Oncology, Medical University of Silesia,
3 Maja 13/15, 41-800 Zabrze, Poland
e-mail: szczep57@poczta.onet.pl

M. Witt et al. (eds.), *Molecular Aspects of Hematologic Malignancies*,
Principles and Practice, DOI: 10.1007/978-3-642-29467-9_23,

MRD assessment with high sensitivity (10^{-4} – 10^{-5}), which makes it a valuable tool for the management of ALL treatment.

23.1 Introduction

Several studies have shown that detection of minimal residual disease (MRD) in childhood acute lymphoblastic leukemia (ALL) is clinically relevant, both in de novo ALL and relapsed ALL as well as in ALL patients undergoing stem cell transplantation (See also Chaps. 11 and 16) (van Dongen et al. 1998; Cave et al. 1998; Coustan-Smith et al. 2000; Panzer-Grumayer et al. 2000; Goulden et al. 2003; Conter et al. 2010; Bader et al. 2009; Paganin et al. 2008). Based on these results, MRD diagnostics are now implemented in many front-line ALL treatment protocols, in which patients are stratified according to MRD levels in bone marrow (BM) samples obtained during and after induction therapy (Schrappe 2002).

The quantitative assessment of MRD is mostly performed using RQ-PCR (real-time quantitative polymerase chain reaction) analysis of immunoglobulin (Ig) and T-cell receptor (TCR) gene rearrangements, as this method is applicable in the vast majority of childhood ALL patients and generally reaches the sensitivities of 10^{-4}, required for the identification of low-risk patients (Willemse et al. 2002; van Dongen et al. 1998; Szczepanski et al. 2002) (See also Chap. 11). Immunoglobulin and T-cell receptor gene rearrangements occur during early B- and T-cell differentiation, when each lymphocyte obtains a specific combination of V-(D-)J gene segments that codes for the variable domains of Ig or TCR molecules; V (variable), D (diversity), J (joining). The random insertion and deletion of nucleotides at the junction sites of V, (D), and J gene segments make the junctional regions of Ig and TCR genes into'fingerprint-like'sequences, which are most probably different in each lymphocyte and thus lymphocyte clone, also in each lymphoid malignancy. Therefore, these junctional regions can be used as patient-specific targets for RQ-PCR-MRD analysis. Such targets can be detected (e.g., by PCR heteroduplex analysis or GeneScan analysis) at initial diagnosis in >98 % of lymphoid malignancies (Szczepanski et al. 2002). Subsequently, the precise nucleotide sequence of the junctional regions can be determined by sequencing. This sequence information allows the design of junctional region-specific oligonucleotides (either probes or primers), which can be used for sensitive detection of even low levels of malignant cells, down to one malignant cell in 10^4 – 10^5 normal cells (sensitivity of 10^{-4} – 10^{-5}) (See also Chap. 11).

RQ-PCR-based detection of MRD with the use of rearranged Ig/TCR genes is, however, a complex process, involving many steps. In order to achieve consistency of MRD results between different laboratories, all steps of MRD diagnostics, including the detection and identification of Ig/TCR gene rearrangements, MRD analysis of follow-up samples, and reproducibility of RQ-PCR analysis (both experimental and data interpretation) should, at least in part, be standardized (van der Velden et al. 2007a, b; Bruggemann et al. 2008). These various steps are presented in detail in this chapter.

23.2 Cell Sample Processing at Diagnosis and During Follow-up

At the time of diagnosis (before the start of treatment) a bone marrow (BM) sample should be collected. If this is not possible, a peripheral blood (PB) sample might be used at diagnosis, if the blast count in the blood is >30 %. During follow-up the recommended type of biological material to be used for MRD assessment is generally BM, since MRD levels in PB do not accurately reflect MRD levels in BM. To prevent an admixture of blood in the BM sample, the first aspirate should be used. Samples should be collected into EDTA (ethylenediamine tetra acetic acid) or heparin containing tubes (3–5 ml of BM, 10 ml of PB), transported or stored at room temperature, and subjected to further procedures within 24 h.

Cell sample processing (both at the time of diagnosis and during follow up) includes:

1. The isolation of mononuclear cells (MNCs) by density gradient centrifugation, according to a standard protocol (see Chap. 19).
2. The assessment of blast count in the obtained MNC fraction, by cytomorphology or flow cytometry, for correction for the tumor load in the diagnostic sample performed during the preparation of a standard curve (see Sect. 23.4.2). This step refers only to the samples collected at diagnosis.
3. DNA isolation with the use of column-based DNA isolation kit, according to the manufacturer's instructions. It is recommended to perform DNA isolation using 10×10^6 freshly separated MNCs (approximately 80 % DNA isolation efficiency compared to approximately 55 % for frozen material). The remaining MNCs should be stored for later use, preferably in liquid nitrogen or at –80 °C.
4. The assessment of DNA quantity and quality by optical density measurement at 260 and 280 nm, preferably using a microvolume spectrophotometer (e.g. Nanodrop or a comparable equipment). Each sample should be measured in duplicates.
5. The amount of DNA necessary for MRD analyses is approximately 5 μg in case of a diagnostic sample and 5–8 μg, in case of the follow-up sample.
6. The preparation of working dilutions of DNA for PCR (diagnostic sample) and RQ-PCR (diagnostic and follow-up samples).

23.3 MRD Target Selection

23.3.1 PCR for Detection of Ig/TCR Gene Rearrangements in Diagnostic Sample

The detection of rearranged Ig and TCR genes is performed in a series of PCR reactions with the use of an appropriate set of standard primers, enabling the identification of target sequences for MRD analysis in more than 95 % of ALL patients (Kuppers et al. 1993; Szczepański et al. 1999; Willems et al. 2000; Szczepański et al. 2001, 2004; Pongers-Willemse et al. 1999; van Dongen et al. 2003). It is recommended to apply a stepwise strategy for the detection and identification of Ig/TCR gene rearrangements, according to the frequency of the most common rearrangements found in BCP-ALL, and T-ALL. The frequencies of Ig/TCR gene rearrangements are presented in Table 23.1. It should be noted that the age of the patient and the presence of fusion genes both influence the pattern of frequency of Ig/TCR gene rearrangements (van der Velden et al. 2003). The primer combinations applied for the basic and complementary Ig/TCR gene rearrangements screening (the latter performed if no satisfactory results—at least two MRD targets, with a suitable sensitivity are detected in the basic screening) are presented in Tables 23.2, 23.3, 23.4. In Table 23.5 appropriate PCR protocols are presented. Alternatively, one might decide to apply a different approach for the stepwise Ig/TCR gene rearrangements identification, e.g. based on singleplex, and multiplex PCR reactions (Dawidowska et al. 2008; Kraszewska et al. 2012). The chosen approach is dependent on the amount of DNA obtained at the time of diagnosis, as well as financial and human resources available for MRD diagnostics.

The detection of rearranged Ig/TCR genes includes:

1. PCR amplification of DNA sample obtained at diagnosis with the use of a set of standard primers for the detection of the most common rearrangements, in line with the amplification of DNA extracted from normal MNCs (polyclonal control), appropriate control DNA (positive control, see Tables 23.2, 23.3, 23.4) and Milli-Q water as nontemplate control.
2. PCR conditions are as follows:

95 °C	7 min	}
94 °C	30 s	} 35x
60 °C	45 s	}
72 °C	90 s	
72 °C	10 min	
15 °C	hold	

3. Electrophoresis in 1 % agarose gel for the selection of PCR products containing positive amplicons for further analysis. One might decide to omit this step and proceed directly to heteroduplex analysis. However, it is recommended to perform an agarose gel electrophoresis at least for positive and negative control.

Table 23.1 Frequency of Ig/TCR gene rearrangements in childhood ALL, detected in PCR-HD approach (van der Velden and van Dongen 2009, modified)

Gene	Type of rearrangement	Precursor-B-ALL (%)	T-ALL (%)
IGH	V_H–J_H	75–90	<10
	D_H–J_H	25–30	15–25
	Total *IGH*	80–95	20–25
IGK	Vκ–Kde	40–45	0
	Intron-Kde	15–25	0
	Total *IGK*-Kde	40–70	0
	Vκ–Jκ	30	NT
	Total *IGK*	60–75	0
IGL	Vλ-Jλ	15–20	NT
TCRD	Vδ2–Dδ3	40–50	<10
	Dδ2–Dδ3	15–25	<5
	Vδ–Jδ1	<1	30–40
	Dδ2–Jδ1	<1	10–20
	Total *TCRD*	45–55	40–50
TCRD/A	Vδ2–Jα	35–45	NT
TCRG	Vγ–Jγ	50–60	85–95
TCRB	Vβ–Jβ	20–30	70–80
	Dβ–Jβ	15–20	45–55
	Total *TCRB*	30–40	70–90

IGH immunoglobulin heavy chain genes, *IGK* immunoglobulin light chain kappa genes, *IGL* immunoglobulin light chain lambda genes, *TCRD* T-cell receptor delta chain genes, *TCRD/A* T-cell receptor delta/alpha chain genes, *TCRG* T-cell receptot gamma chain genes, *TCRB* T-cell receptor beta chain genes, *NT* not tested

23.3.2 Heteroduplex Analysis for Clonality Assessment

Clonality assessment is aimed at discrimination among monoclonal, biclonal, and oligoclonal PCR products, derived from clonal leukemic cells, and polyclonal PCR products from normal lymphocytes (See also Chap. 11). Heteroduplex analysis includes (Langerak et al. 1997):

1. The denaturation of PCR products for 5 min at 94 °C using a thermocycler.
2. The renaturation of the PCR products, enabling formation of duplexes, by cooling at 4 °C for 60 min.
3. Electrophoresis in 6 % polyacrylamide gel (PAA) (49:1 acrylamid:bisacryl-amid) in 1x TBE (Tris/Borate/EDTA) buffer, if 300 V for 75 min with a water cooling system is applied, or in 0.5x TBE if 100 V for 1 h followed by 150 V for 3 h is applied. The exact time of electrophoresis is dependent on the product sizes. One might also use commercially available ready-to-use PAA gels.
4. The incubation of the PAA gel in 1 % ethidium bromide solution (5–10 min.), washing the gel in distilled water.
5. The analysis and photodocumentation of the gel using UV light.

Table 23.2 Primer combinations for detection of Ig and TCR gene rearrangements in precursor-B-ALL (van der Velden and van Dongen 2009)

Tube	Forward primer	Reverse primer	Positive control	Product size (bp)	Protocol[a]	Reference
1	VγI	Jγ1.1/2.1	Molt-3/Molt-4	329	A	Pongers-Willemse (1999)
2	VγI	Jγ1.3/2.3	ALL-1	533	A	
3	VγII	Jγ1.1/2.1	Patient	318	A	
4	VγII	Jγ1.3/2.3	HSB2	522	A	
5	VγIV	Jγ1.1/2.1	Patient	353	A	
6	VγIV	Jγ1.3/2.3	Jurkat	557	A	
7	Vδ2	Dδ3	REH	501	A	
8	Dδ2	Dδ3	Nalm16	608	A	
9	VκI	Kde	ROS15	433	A	
10	VκII	Kde	380	443	A	
11	VκIII	Kde	REH	429	A	
12	VκIV	Kde	ROS5	445	A	
13	Intron-F1-B1	Kde	Nalm1	511	A	
14	VH1/7	JH	Nalm6	300–400	A	Kuppers et al. (1993)
15	VH2	JH	Patient	300–400	A	
16	VH3	JH	REH	300–400	A	
17	VH4/6	JH	ROS16	300–400	A	
18	VH5	JH	VH5-TL	300–400	A	
19	23xVβ: 2, 4, 5, 6a, 6b, 6c, 7a, 8a, 9, 10, 11, 13a, 13b, 14, 16, 17, 18, 19, 20, 21, 22, 23, 24	Jβ: 1.1, 1.2, 1.3, 1.4, 1.5, 1.6, 2.2, 2.6, 2.7	Jurkat/ALL-1	240–280	B	van Dongen et al. (2003)
20	23xVβ: 2, 4, 5, 6a, 6b, 6c, 7a, 8a, 9, 10, 11, 13a, 13b, 14, 16, 17, 18, 19, 20, 21, 22, 23, 24	Jβ: 2.1, 2.3, 2.4, 2.5	Peer/CMLT1	240–280	C	
21	Dβ1 + Dβ2	Jβ: 1.1, 1.2, 1.3, 1.4, 1.5, 1.6, 2.1, 2.2, 2.3, 2.4, 2.5, 2.6, 2.7	Jurkat	170–200 (Dβ2) 290–310 (Dβ1)	D	

(continued)

Table 23.2 (continued)

Tube	Forward primer	Reverse primer	Positive control	Product size (bp)	Protocol[a]	Reference
22	Vδ2	Jα29	Patient	200–350	E	Szczepański et al. (2004)
23	Vδ2	Jα9, 30, 48, 49, 52, 54, 55, 56, 57,58, 59, 61	Patient	200–350	F	
24	DH1	JH	Patient	130	A	Szczepański et al. (1999)
25	DH2	JH	Patient	240	A	
26	DH3	JH	Patient	160	A	
27	DH4	JH	Patient	180	A	
28	DH5	JH	Patient	300	A	
29	DH6	JH	Patient	200	A	
30	DH7	JH	Patient	230	A	

[a] See Table 23.5 for detailed information about PCR mixture per protocol

Table 23.3 Primer combinations for detection of TCR and D_H–J_H rearrangements in T-ALL (van der Velden and van Dongen 2009)

Tube	Forward primer	Reverse primer	Positive control	Product size (bp)	Protocol[a]	Reference
1	Vγ I	Jγ1.1/2.1-R1-B1	Molt-3/Molt-4	329	A	Pongers-Willemse et al. (1999)
2	Vγ I	Jγ1.3/2.3-R1-B1	ALL-1	533	A	
3	Vγ II	Jγ1.3/2.3-R1-B1	HSB2	522	A	
4	Vγ III	Jγ1.3/2.3-R1-B1	ALL-1	522	A	
5	Vγ IV	Jγ1.3/2.3-R1-B1	Jurkat	557	A	
6	Vδ1	Jδ1-R1-B1	Peer	452	A	
7	Vδ2	Dδ3-R1-B1	REH	501	A	
8	Vδ2	Jδ1-R1-B1	Patient	443	A	
9	Vδ3	Jδ1-R1-B1	Patient	440	A	
10	Dδ2	Dδ3-R1-B1	Nalm 16	608	A	
11	Dδ2	Jδ1-R1-B1	Loucy	550	A	
12	Sil	Tal1db1-R1-B1	ALL-1	300	A	
13	23xVβ: 2, 4, 5, 6a, 6b, 6c, 7a, 8a, 9, 10, 11, 13a, 13b, 14, 16, 17, 18, 19, 20, 21, 22, 23, 24	Jβ-R1-B2: 1.1, 1.2, 1.3, 1.4, 1.5, 1.6, 2.2, 2.6, 2.7	Jurkat/ALL1	240–280	B	van Dongen et al. (2003)
14	23xVβ2: 2, 4, 5, 6a, 6b, 6c, 7a, 8a, 9, 10, 11, 13a, 13b, 14, 16, 17, 18, 19, 20, 21, 22, 23, 24	Jβ-R1-B2: 2.1, 2.3, 2.4, 2.5	Peer/CMLT1	240–280	C	
15	Dβ1 + Dβ2	Jβ-R1-B2: 1.1, 1.2, 1.3, 1.4, 1.5, 1.6, 2.1, 2.2, 2.3, 2.4, 2.5, 2.6, 2.7	Jurkat	170–200 (Dβ2) 290–310 (Dβ1)	D	
16	DH1	JH	Patient	130	A	Szczepański et al. (1999)
17	DH2	JH	Patient	240	A	
18	DH3	JH	Patient	160	A	
19	DH4	JH	Patient	180	A	
20	DH5	JH	Patient	300	A	
21	DH6	JH	Patient	200	A	
22	DH7	JH	Patient	230	A	

[a] See Table 23.5 for detailed information about PCR mixture per protocol

Table 23.4 Additional (second phase) PCR reactions for precursor-B-ALL (van der Velden and van Dongen 2009)

Forward primer	Reverse primer	Positive control	Product size (bp)	Protocol[a]	References
Vδ2	Jα1,6,7,22,26,40,54,57	Patient	200–400	G	Szczepański et al. (2004)
Vδ2	Jα2,3,5,8,11,12,13,19	Patient	200–400	G	
Vδ2	Jα4,10,14,20,23, 29,42,48	Patient	200–400	G	
Vδ2	Jα9,16,35,37,38,41,49,51,56,60	Patient	250–400	G	
Vδ2	Jα15,18,28,34,36,43,44,45,46	Patient	200–400	G	
Vδ2	Jα17,21,24,25,27,31,32,33,39	Patient	200–400	G	
Vδ2	Jα30,47,50,52,53,55,58,59,61	Patient	200–400	G	
Vκ1/6,2,3,4,5,7	Jκ1-4,5	ROS 15	200–650	H	van Dongen et al. (2003)
Vλ1/2,3	Jλ1,2,3	ROS 5	140–165	H	

[a] See Table 23.5 for detailed information about PCR mixture per protocol

6. The interpretation of heteroduplex analysis results according to the following criteria: monoclonal rearrangement—one band, biclonal or biallelic rearrangements—two homoduplex and two heteroduplex bands (possibly comigrating), oligoclonal rearrangements—more than four bands (ladder), polyclonal rearrangements—multiple bands (smear). Schematic illustration of the idea of heteroduplex analysis is presented in Fig. 23.1. Typical results of heteroduplex analysis are represented in Fig. 23.2.

23.3.3 Sequencing for Identification of Clonal Rearrangements

The identification of Ig/TCR gene rearrangements (the identification of V, (D), J genes and of precise sequence of junctional regions, i.e. 5′ and 3′ deletions and insertion in the junction) is performed based on the results of fluorescent sequencing of clonal amplicons. Monoclonal PCR products obtained in singleplex reactions are sequenced directly using the PCR product. In case of biclonal PCR products, it is recommended to repeat amplification using a larger reaction volume (e.g. 2 × 100 μl), perform electrophoresis in PAA gel (heteroduplex analysis), resolving each PCR product in three lanes, and excise relevant bands from the gel. Both homoduplex bands should be separately excised form the gel (in case of their comigration, both heteroduplex bands should be separated) followed by DNA elution and precipitation. Fluorescent sequencing should be performed in both directions, with the use of the same primers as those used for PCR amplification (see Tables 23.2, 23.3, 23.4).

Obtained sequences are than compared, for homology analysis, with human germline V, D, J gene sequences available online in databases and against hard-copies containing germline sequences (available upon request: v.h.j.vandervelden@erasmusmc.nl).

Table 23.5 Composition of PCR mixture per protocol (van der Velden and van Dongen 2009)

Reaction mix per 50 μl reaction		Protocol							
		A	B	C	D	E	F	G	H
Reagent	Starting	Volume/1 reaction [ul]							
PCR buffer	10x	5	5	5	5	5	5	5	5
$MgCl_2$	25 mM	3	6	6	3	4	4	4	3
Milli-Q water		34	16.1	18.6	27.8	33.4	27.7	29.7/29.2/28.7	31.3/33.8
dNTP	20 mM	0.5	0.5	0.5	0.5	0.5	0.5	0.5	0.5
BSA	20 mg/ml	1	1	1	1	1	1	1	1
Forward primer	10 pmol/μl	0.7							
Reverse primer	10 pmol/μl	0.7							
Primer mix *TCRB* tube 1 (23x Vβ + 9x Jβ)	20 pmol/μl, each		16						
Primer mix *TCRB* tube 2 (23x Vβ + 4x Jβ)	20 pmol/μl, each			13.5					
Primer mix *TCRB* tube 3 (2x Dβ + 13x Jβ)	20 pmol/μl, each				7.5				
Forward primer	20 pmol/μl					0.5			
Reverse primer	20 pmol/μl					0.5			
Forward primer	20 pmol/μl						0.5		
Reverse primers	20 pmol/μl, each						6		
Forward primer	20 pmol/μl							0.5	
Reverse primer	20 pmol/μl, each							4/4.5/5	
Primer mix	20 pmol/μl, each								4 (Vκ–Jκ) 1.5 (Vλ–Jλ)
HotStart Taq Polymerase	5 U/μl	0.1	0.4	0.4	0.2	0.1	0.3	0.3	0.2
DNA	10 ng/μl	5	5	5	5	5	5	5	5

The recommended databases are:

VBASE	http://vbase.mrc-cpe.cam.ac.uk/	DNAPLOT tool	For Ig genes
IMGT	http://www.imgt.org/	IMGT/V-QEST tool	For Ig and TCR genes

The alignment of patients' sequences with germline sequences can be confirmed with the use BLAST tool (http://www/ncbi.nlm.nih.gov/BLAST) or an alternative software.

The following guidelines for the interpretation of sequencing data have been developed:

1. The identification of V, D, J genes, and precise junction sequence (5′ deletion, 3′ deletion and *N*-insertion) is performed based on homology analysis with germline sequences available in databases/in hard copies.

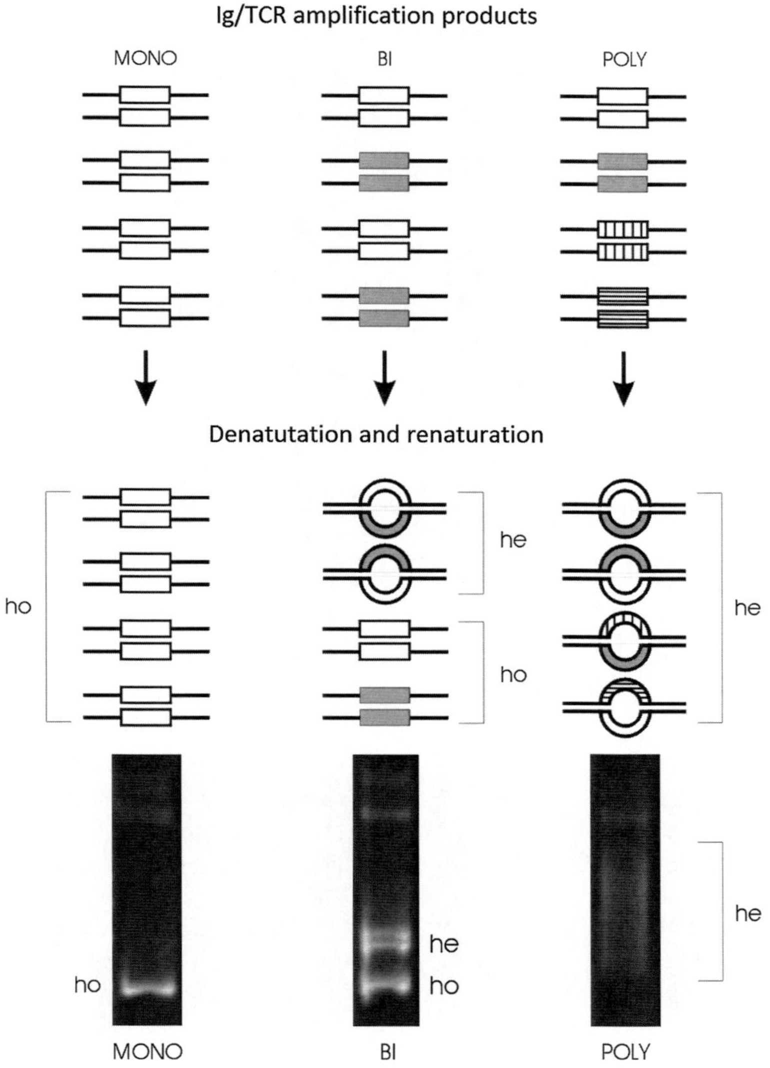

Fig. 23.1 Schematic illustration of the idea of heteroduplex analysis. *Mono* monoclonal PCR product, *bi* biclonal PCR product, *poly* polyclonal PCR product, *ho* homoduplexes, *he* heteroduplexes. For details see the text and Chap. 11

2. The identification of D genes is possible if a minimum length of one-third of germline sequence is found in the analyzed sequence (generally at least 5 nucleotides; in case of Dδ2: 4 nucleotides).
3. If the junction region is >10 nucleotides, the second D gene in this region should be searched for using the hard copies or alternatively by blasting the sequence around the junction against the databases.

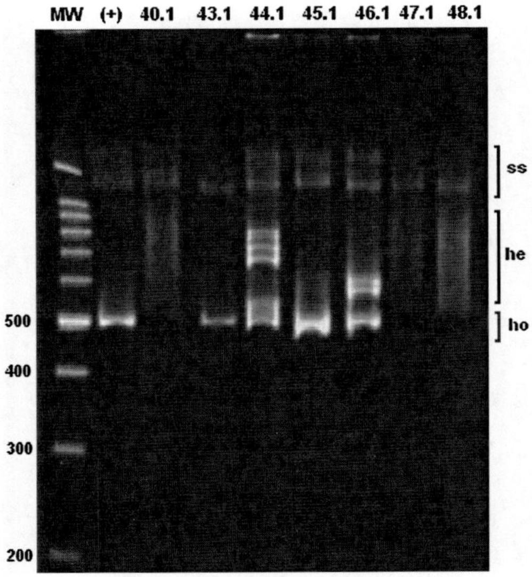

Fig. 23.2 Typical results of heteroduplex analysis. Rearrangements of *Vδ2–Dδ3* genes detected in seven BCP-ALL patients. Numbers coding for each sample are depicted over each lane: *MW* molecular weight marker 100 bp; (+) positive monoclonal control; patients' samples: 40.1, 47.1 and 48.1, containing polyclonal amplicons; 43.1 and 45.1, containing monoclonal amplicons; 44.1, containing oligoclonal amplicons; 46.1, containing biclonal amplicons; *ss* single stranded fragments, *he* heteroduplexes, *ho* homoduplexes

4. The identification of Vβ and Jβ genes is performed based on IMGT database with the use of nomenclature for *TCRB* genes used in this database (by Rowen; note that standard BIOMED primers are named using the Arden nomenclature) (Rowen et al. 1996; Arden et al. 1995).
5. The identification of 5′ and 3′ deletions and insertions in the rearranged *TCRB* genes is performed with the use of germline *TCRB* sequences published by Rowen
   (GenBank accession number: L36092.2 formerly U66059, U66060, U66061; http://www.ncbi.nlm.nih.gov/nuccore/L36092.2).

23.3.4 Selection of MRD Targets

It is strongly recommended to analyze MRD using two Ig/TCR gene rearrangements as targets in order to avoid false negative results, due to target loss (as a consequence of secondary or ongoing rearrangements) or loss of a subclone with the target sequence (Szczepański et al. 2003). Optimal MRD targets should be chosen among all rearrangements identified in a patient, based on information on target stability and target sensitivity that might be reached in RQ-PCR with the use of the MRD target sequence.

The following guidelines for target selection have been developed:

1. Monoclonal rearrangements should preferably be chosen over oligoclonal rearrangements (in BCP-ALL monoclonal rearrangements are characterized by 80–90 % stability compared to 40–50 % for oligoclonal rearrangements; in T-ALL oligoclonality at diagnosis and thus instability of rearrangements is rarely encountered) (Szczepański et al. 2003).
2. So-called 'end-stage' Ig/TCR gene rearrangements (e.g. *IGK*-Kde rearrangements) should be chosen, if available, to decrease the risk of target loss due to ongoing and secondary rearrangements (van der Velden et al. 2002b).
3. Rearrangements involving V, D, and J genes should preferably be chosen over rearrangements of V–J and V–D genes only, in order to increase the chance for higher sensitivity of RQ-PCR assay.
4. Selected MRD targets should enable RQ-PCR assay sensitivity of at least 10^{-4}.
5. Rearrangements in *TCRG* locus should be selected if no other optimal rearrangements are available, since these rearrangements are usually characterized by suboptimal sensitivity due to the generation of substantial background from similar *TCRG* gene rearrangements present in normal lymphocytes.
6. Preferred strategy for optimal target selection includes the following order:

   In BCP-ALL

   IGK-Kde → *IGH* or *TCRB* or Vδ2-Jα → *TCRD* → Vκ-Jκ *or* Vλ-Jλ → *TCRG*

   In T-ALL

   SIL–TAL1 → *TCRD* or *TCRB* → *IGH* → *TCRG*

For the names of gene loci see Table 23.1.

7. Regardless of the above priority order of rearrangements selection, nucleotide composition of the junction, influencing the design of patient-specific primer, should always be considered during MRD target selection.

23.4 RQ-PCR-MRD Analysis

23.4.1 Design of Patient-Specific Primers

In most RQ-PCR MRD assays, a germline TaqMan probe and a germline primer, complementary to a sequence downstream of the junction region, are used in combination with a patient specific, allele-specific oligonucleotide (ASO) primer, complementary to the junction region (so called ASO primer approach). The standard sets of germline primers and probes for RQ-PCR detection of rearrangements in *IGH*, *IGK*, *IGL*, *TCRG*, *TCRD*, and *TCRB* loci have been developed (Verhagen et al. 2000; van der Velden et al. 2002a, b, 2006; Szczepański et al. 2004; Bruggemann et al. 2004).

The following guidelines apply for the design of patient-specific ASO primers:

1. The design of primers should be performed with the use of an appropriate primer design software.
2. Patient-specific ASO primer should be positioned in the way that its 3′ end is complementary to a sequence within the junction or just over the junction.
3. The 3′ end of the ASO primer should encompass no more than 2–6 nucleotides of the germline sequence.
4. The melting temperature (Tm) of the ASO primer should be within the range of 57–60 °C.
5. The GC content should be within the range of 20–80 %.
6. If possible, there should be no more than 2 G/Cs within the last 5 nucleotides of the 3′ end of the primer.
7. Based on internal stability graph, generated by the software, the primer should exhibits strong binding in the middle of the primer and lower binding at the 3′ end ($\Delta G > -10$ kcal/mol).
8. Primer-dimers formation should be checked for:

3′-dimers of ASO–ASO primers	($\Delta G > -5$ kcal/mol)
3′-dimers of ASO primer-germline primer	($\Delta G > -5$ kcal/mol)
overall dimers of ASO–ASO primers	(if possible $\Delta G > -10$ kcal/mol)
overall dimers of ASO primer–germline primer	(if possible $\Delta G > -10$ kcal/mol)

9. Hairpin structures formation should be checked for. If possible, 3′ end hairpins with Tm within 10 °C from Tm of the primer should be avoided.
10. The length of the primer should be as short as possible, with the above criteria fulfilled.

23.4.2 Standard Curve and Sensitivity Testing

The sensitivity of the RQ-PCR assay, that can be reached with the use of a particular set of a patient-specific ASO primer with an appropriate germline primer and probe, is tested with the use of a standard curve (van der Velden et al. 2007a). The standard curve is obtained via serial dilution of DNA of the patient (obtained at the time of diagnosis) in control DNA (a mixture of DNA obtained from MNCs of at least 5–10 healthy donors).

Sensitivity testing includes:

1. The preparation of 60 ng/μl of patient's DNA and of the control DNA (alternative amounts can be used, but for reaching a theoretical sensitivity of 10^{-5} each reaction should contain 600 ng, equivalent to 10^5 cells).
2. The confirmation of the obtained DNA concentration by spectrophotometry and adjustment to 60 ng/μl, if necessary.

3. The dilution of the patient's DNA into the control DNA to reach a 10^{-1} dilution. At this step information on the blast percentage, determined cytomorphologically or by flow cytometry in the MNC fraction obtained at diagnosis, should be used for correction for the tumor load. One might alternatively skip the 10^{-1} dilution, if limited amount of diagnostic DNA sample is available (10^{-2} dilution should be prepared with correction for tumor load).
4. The preparation of the following standard curve dilutions, starting from 10^{-1} dilution (alternatively 10^{-2} dilution) by serial dilution of patient's DNA in control DNA:

10^{-1} 10^{-2} 10^{-3} 5×10^{-4} 10^{-4} 10^{-5}

5. The amplification of a standard curve (each dilution amplified in duplicates), in line with amplification of the control DNA (a mixture of DNA obtained from MNC of at least 5–10 healthy donors; amplified in 6 wells to check for 'background' amplification) and with Milli-Q water (nontemplate control in 2 wells) using 600 ng of DNA per well (equivalent of approximately 10^5 cells).
6. The preparation of RQ-PCR reaction mixture according to Table 23.6. The addition of BSA (bovine serum albumin) prevents inhibition of RQ-PCR, which might be a problem in case of some DNA samples.
7. Amplification using the following thermal cycling conditions:
8. The analysis of RQ-PCR data using appropriate software.

50 °C	2 min	
95 °C	10 min	
95 °C	15 s	} 50x
60 °C	1 min	

9. The determination of quantitative range and sensitivity for the tested ASO primer in combination with germline primer and probe, using the following guidelines developed by EuroMRD (formerly the European Study Group on MRD in ALL; ESG-MRD-ALL) (van der Velden et al. 2007a).

23.4.2.1 Criteria for Quantitative Range Determination

'Quantitative range' (also called 'reproducible sensitivity') is defined as the range of RQ-PCR (the range of the standard curve) in which the MRD level can be quantitatively assessed in an accurate and reproducible way. Quantitative range is determined by the lowest dilution step of the standard curve for which the following criteria are fulfilled:

- optimal shape of amplification curves of both replicates, reflecting specific amplification
- ΔCt of all replicates $\leq$1.5, reflecting reproducible amplification
- Ct values of all replicates $\geq$3.0 lower than the lowest Ct value of the background (amplification of the control DNA)

Table 23.6 RQ-PCR reaction mixtures (van der Velden and van Dongen 2009)

Reagent	Starting	Volume/reaction [μl]	Final
Milli-Q water		1	
Universal Master mix	2x	12.5	1x
Forward primer	30 μM	0.25	300 nM
Reverse primer	30 μM	0.25	300 nM
TaqMan probe	5 μM	0.5	100 nM
BSA	2 % (w/v)	0.5	0.04 %
DNA	60 ng/μl	10	600 ng
Reaction volume		25	

- mean Ct value within a defined range from the mean Ct value of the previous dilution point:
  2.6–4.0 Cts between tenfold dilutions (e.g. 10^{-3}–10^{-4})
  0.5–1.5 Cts between twofold dilutions (e.g. 10^{-3}–5×10^{-4})

23.4.2.2 Criteria for Standard Curve

After the determination of quantitative range the standard curve can be constructed. It should include only the dilution points within the quantitative range (at least 3 dilutions, 2 logs), the remaining dilution points should be treated as unknown samples. The standard curve should be characterized by:

- slope of –3.1 to –3.9
- squared correlation coefficient (coefficient of determination) (R2) ≥0.98.

If the standard curve does not fulfill these criteria RQ-PCR should be optimized and repeated (e.g. the increase of the annealing temperature, the design of an alternative ASO primer should be performed).

23.4.2.3 Criteria for Sensitivity Determination

'Sensitivity' is defined as the range of RQ-PCR (the range of the standard curve) in which the MRD level can still be detected, but not quantified in a reproducible and accurate way. Sensitivity is determined by the lowest dilution step of the standard curve for which the following criteria are fulfilled:

- amplification of at least one replicate; ΔCt of the replicates is not relevant
- optimal shape of amplification curve(s), reflecting specific amplification
- the lowest Ct value ≥1.0 lower than the lowest Ct value of the background (amplification of the control DNA)
- the lowest Ct value <20 cycles away from the intercept of the standard curve (representing the undiluted sample)

The optimal ASO primer should enable MRD RQ-PCR analysis with a quantitative range of $\leq 10^{-4}$ and a sensitivity of 10^{-4}–10^{-5}. If these criteria are not reached one can decide to increase the annealing temperature for a greater specificity of RQ-PCR. In case this approach is unsuccessful, an alternative ASO primer should be designed. It is also possible to use for MRD analysis an ASO primer with the quantitative range of 5×10^{-4} and a sensitivity of $\leq 10^{-4}$, provided that the second MRD target sequence will be detected with the use of an ASO primer of quantitative range of $\leq 10^{-4}$ and sensitivity of 10^{-4}–10^{-5}. The exact criteria depend on the clinical protocol.

23.4.3 DNA Quality and Quantity Testing

Quantity and quality of each DNA sample (obtained at the time of diagnosis and in consecutive time points during followup) should be analyzed via RQ-PCR amplification of a control, albumin gene (*ALB*) with the use of *ALB*-specific primers, and TaqMan probe (Pongers-Willemse et al. 1998). The amplification of a control gene and that of a target MRD sequence should be performed in exactly the same conditions (reaction volume, DNA content, RQ-PCR mixture components, thermal cycling conditions).

Quality and quantity test (so-called 'albumin test') includes:

1. The preparation of a standard curve (so-called albumin standard curve) by diluting control DNA (a mixture of DNA obtained from MNC of at least 5–10 healthy donors) in water.
2. The standard curve should include the following dilutions points:

   100 ng/μl   50 ng/μl   10 ng/μl   1 ng/μl

3. The amplification of the standard curve. Each dilution point should be amplified at least in duplicates (10 μl DNA per well) in line with the amplification of all DNA samples to be tested (in concentration of 60 ng/μl based on the spectrophotometry) at least in duplicates (10 μl DNA per well = 600 ng DNA per well) and with Milli-Q water as the nontemplate control amplified in 2 wells.
4. The preparation of RQ-PCR reaction mixture according to Table 23.6.
5. Amplification using thermal cycling conditions described in Sect. 23.4.2.
6. The determination of DNA content in each sample using their Ct values and a standard curve. Each sample should contain between 250 and 1,000 ng DNA. If DNA content, based on the albumin test results, is >1,000 ng, the sample should be diluted, since too high DNA concentration might inhibit RQ-PCR. If DNA quantity is <250 ng, reliable interpretation of quantitative data is generally not possible, unless high MRD levels (within the QR) are detected.

23.4.4 Quantitative MRD Analysis and Data Interpretation

Quantitative MRD analysis should preferably be performed with the use of two optimal target sequences selected from identified Ig/TCR gene rearrangements based on the criteria described in Sect. 23.3.4. In case discordant results are obtained for both MRD-targets, a higher MRD level should be considered reliable and used for clinical decision making, since the lower MRD level might represent a subclone.

Analysis of MRD level in follow-up samples includes:

1. The amplification of each follow-up DNA sample in triplicates, in line with the amplification of the standard curve (each dilution point at least in duplicates), and of control DNA (at least in 6 wells) using 600 ng DNA per well and Milli-Q water as nontemplate control (at least in 3 wells).
2. The preparation of RQ-PCR reaction mixture according to Table 23.6.
3. Amplification using thermal cycling conditions described in Sect. 23.4.2.
4. The analysis and interpretation of the quantitative data according to the following guidelines developed by EuroMRD:

   - For each RQ-PCR MRD assay quantitative range, sensitivity and standard curve should be determined according to the guidelines described in Sect. 23.4.2. If criteria for quantitative range and sensitivity are not fulfilled, one might try to reanalyze quantitative data using manual threshold (threshold should always be set within the region of exponential amplification, i.e. in the linear part of the amplification plot).
   - After determination of the quantitative range the standard curve should be corrected (it should include only the dilution points within the quantitative range (at least 3 dilutions, 2 logs), the remaining dilution points should be treated as unknown samples. The standard curve should be characterized by a slope of –3.1 to –3.9, and a squared correlation coefficient (R2) $\geq$0.98. If the standard curve does not fulfill these criteria quantitation of MRD might not be performed, due to insufficient quality of RQ-PCR data; RQ-PCR should be optimized (e.g. the increase of annealing temperature, the design of an alternative ASO primer) and repeated.
   - Nonspecific amplification (‘background amplification’ obtained from control DNA amplified in 6 wells) should always be checked for. In case of follow-up samples any amplification with Ct value >24 cycles from the intercept of the standard curve should be interpreted as ‘background amplification.’
   - The quantitative analysis of MRD level in the follow-up samples is performed if the following criteria are fulfilled:

– the mean Ct of all replicates of the analyzed follow-up sample is $\leq$ the highest Ct of quantitative range (MRD level is within quantitative range)
– ΔCt between replicates is $\leq$1.5

- The quantitation of MRD level is performed using mean Ct of the replicates and a standard curve (see Fig 23.3). It is necessary to make correction of MRD level based on quantitative data from albumin test, i.e. DNA quantity in the sample obtained at diagnosis and during follow-up tested via amplification of a control gene—*ALB*.
- If the mean Ct of the replicates is > the highest Ct of quantitative range (MRD level is beyond the quantitative range) the MRD level might not be quantified. Such MRD results are interpreted as 'positive' or 'not negative,' dependent on the clinical protocol. The results of albumin test should be checked for, although not used for the correction of the MRD level; if DNA content is beyond the range defined in Sect. 23.4.3. MRD data might not be reliably interpreted.
- The MRD results are interpreted as 'positive' if the following criteria are fulfilled:

- (in case of no background amplification) Ct of at least one of the replicates is within 4 Cts of the highest Ct for dilution point determining the sensitivity
- (in case of background amplification) Ct of at least one of the replicates is within 4 Cts of the highest Ct for dilution point determining the sensitivity and
- Is $\geq$3.0 lower than the lowest Ct of the background (in order to avoid false positive results in clinical protocols aimed at therapy intensification) or
- is $\geq$1.0 lower than the lowest Ct of the background (in order to avoid false negative results in clinical protocols aimed at therapy deintensification)

- The MRD results are interpreted as 'negative' if the following criteria are fulfilled:

- (in case of no background amplification) Ct of all of the replicates are $\geq$4 Cts away from the highest Ct for dilution point determining the sensitivity
- (in case of background amplification) Ct of all of the replicates are within one Ct of the background
- The results of albumin test should be checked for negative samples, although not used for the correction of MRD level; if DNA content is beyond the range defined in Sect. 23.4.3. MRD data might not be reliably interpreted.

23.5 Conclusions

The move from a laboratory research tool, used for a retrospective evaluation of clinical trials, to a diagnostic tool used for stratification of patients in daily clinical practise, requires uniformity in MRD data not only within single treatment protocols, but also between different protocols. Therefore, the standardization of multiple steps of this complex process, as described in this chapter, is necessary. In addition, regular quality control rounds (e.g., twice a year) should be performed to evaluate the performance of the participating laboratories. These quality control

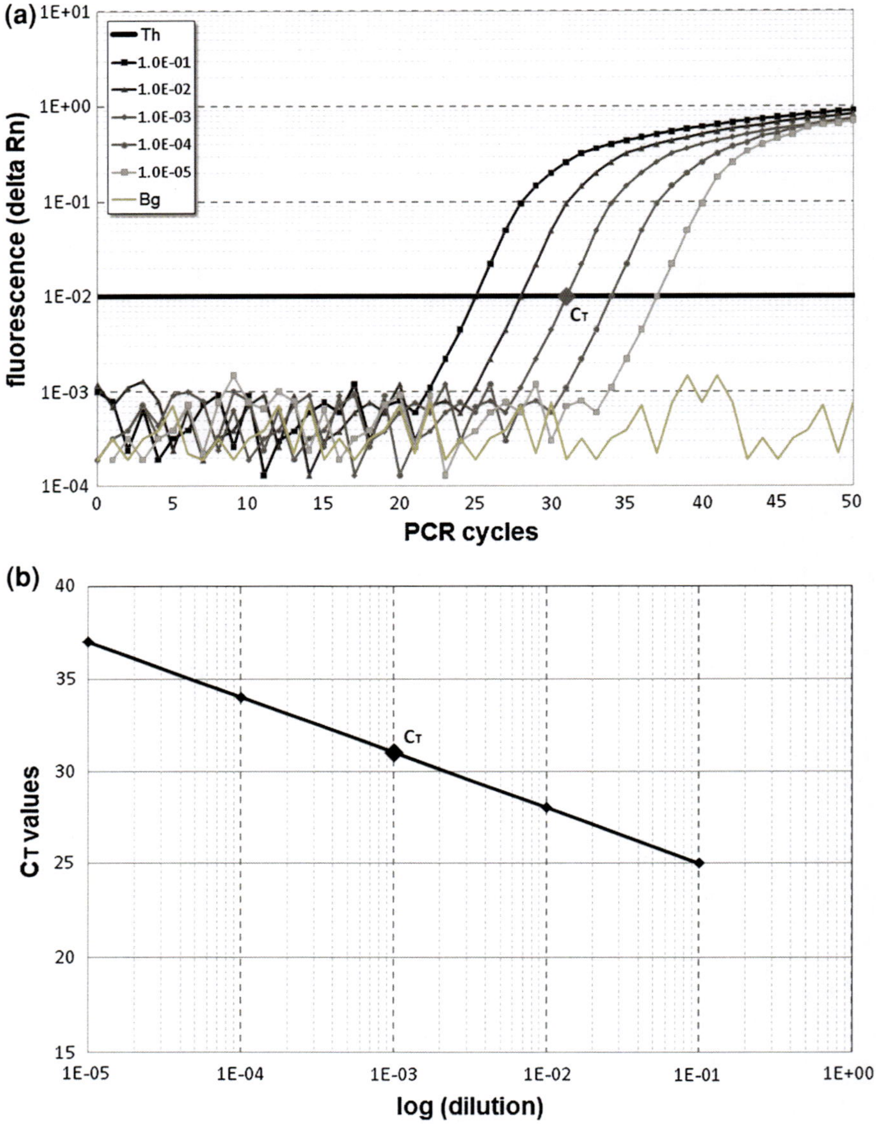

Fig. 23.3 Schematic illustration of RQ-PCR assay used for MRD analysis. **a.** Amplification plot of RQ-PCR assay. *Th* threshold, *Bg* background, C_T threshold cycle, delta Rn, the increase in normalized intensity of fluorescence. For details of RQ-PCR assay see the text and Chaps. 11 and 20. **b.** Standard curve constructed based on RQ-PCR assay. The standard curve is used for the determination of MRD levels in follow-up samples based on mean C_T values of the follow-up samples, each amplified in triplicate

programs should also include regular meetings creating the opportunity to discuss MRD results, to present new developments in the field of MRD diagnostics, and to carry out educational sessions. The EuroMRD network (formerly the European Study Group on MRD detection in ALL), including over 40 laboratories in Europe, Australia, and Asia, has organized such quality control programs since the beginning of this millennium.

This chapter is based on guidelines developed by Department of Immunology, Erasmus MC, University Medical Center Rotterdam and guidelines of the European Study Group on MRD in ALL (ESG-MRD-ALL) (van der Velden et al. 2007a).

This chapter was partly supported by the Ministry of Science and Higher Education, grant N N407 311 839.

References

Arden B, Clark SP, Kabelitz D, Mak TW (1995) Human T-cell receptor variable gene segment families. Immunogenetics 42(6):455–500

Bader P, Kreyenberg H, Henze GH, Eckert C, Reising M, Willasch A, Barth A, Borkhardt A, Peters C, Handgretinger R, Sykora KW, Holter W, Kabisch H, Klingebiel T, von Stackelberg A (2009) Prognostic value of minimal residual disease quantification before allogeneic stem-cell transplantation in relapsed childhood acute lymphoblastic leukemia: the ALL-REZ BFM Study Group. J Clin Oncol 27(3):377–384. doi:JCO.2008.17.606510.1200/JCO.2008.17.6065

Bruggemann M, van der Velden VH, Raff T, Droese J, Ritgen M, Pott C, Wijkhuijs AJ, Gokbuget N, Hoelzer D, van Wering ER, van Dongen JJ, Kneba M (2004) Rearranged T-cell receptor beta genes represent powerful targets for quantification of minimal residual disease in childhood and adult T-cell acute lymphoblastic leukemia. Leukemia 18(4):709–719. doi:10.1038/sj.leu.24032632403263

Bruggemann M, Schrauder A, Raff T, Pfeifer H, Dworzak M, Ottmann OG, Asnafi V, Baruchel A, Bassan R, Benoit Y, Biondi A, Cave H, Dombret H, Fielding AK, Foa R, Gokbuget N, Goldstone AH, Goulden N, Henze G, Hoelzer D, Janka-Schaub GE, Macintyre EA, Pieters R, Rambaldi A, Ribera JM, Schmiegelow K, Spinelli O, Stary J, von Stackelberg A, Kneba M, Schrappe M, van Dongen JJ (2008) Standardized MRD quantification in European ALL trials: proceedings of the second international symposium on MRD assessment in Kiel, Germany, 18–20 Sept 2008. Leukemia 24(3):521–535. doi:leu200926810.1038/leu.2009.268

Cave H, van der Werfften Bosch J, Suciu S, Guidal C, Waterkeyn C, Otten J, Bakkus M, Thielemans K, Grandchamp B, Vilmer E (1998) Clinical significance of minimal residual disease in childhood acute lymphoblastic leukemia. European organization for research and treatment of cancer–childhood leukemia cooperative group. N Engl J Med 339(9):591–598

Conter V, Bartram CR, Valsecchi MG, Schrauder A, Panzer-Grumayer R, Moricke A, Arico M, Zimmermann M, Mann G, De Rossi G, Stanulla M, Locatelli F, Basso G, Niggli F, Barisone E, Henze G, Ludwig WD, Haas OA, Cazzaniga G, Koehler R, Silvestri D, Bradtke J, Parasole R, Beier R, van Dongen JJ, Biondi A, Schrappe M (2010) Molecular response to treatment redefines all prognostic factors in children and adolescents with B-cell precursor acute lymphoblastic leukemia: results in 3184 patients of the AIEOP-BFM ALL 2000 study. Blood 115(16):3206–3214. doi:blood-2009-10-24814610.1182/blood-2009-10-248146

Coustan-Smith E, Sancho J, Hancock ML, Boyett JM, Behm FG, Raimondi SC, Sandlund JT, Rivera GK, Rubnitz JE, Ribeiro RC, Pui CH, Campana D (2000) Clinical importance of minimal residual disease in childhood acute lymphoblastic leukemia. Blood 96(8):2691–2696

Dawidowska M, Jolkowska J, Szczepanski T, Derwich K, Wachowiak J, Witt M (2008) Implementation of the standard strategy for identification of Ig/TCR targets for minimal residual disease diagnostics in B-cell precursor ALL pediatric patients: Polish experience. Arch Immunol Ther Exp (Warsz) 56(6):409–418. doi:10.1007/s00005-008-0045-y

Goulden N, Bader P, Van Der Velden V, Moppett J, Schilham M, Masden HO, Krejci O, Kreyenberg H, Lankester A, Revesz T, Klingebiel T, Van Dongen J (2003) Minimal residual disease prior to stem cell transplant for childhood acute lymphoblastic leukaemia. Br J Haematol 122(1):24–29

Kraszewska MD, Dawidowska M, Kosmalska M, Sedek L, Grzeszczak W, Szczepanski T, Witt M (2012) Immunoglobulin/T-cell receptor gene rearrangements in the diagnostic paradigm of pediatric T-cell acute lymphoblastic leukemia patients. Leuk Lymphoma. doi:10.3109/10428194.2011.654338

Kuppers R, Zhao M, Rajewsky K, Hansmann ML (1993) Detection of clonal B cell populations in paraffin-embedded tissues by polymerase chain reaction. Am J Pathol 143(1):230–239

Langerak AW, Szczepanski T, van der Burg M, Wolvers-Tettero IL, van Dongen JJ (1997) Heteroduplex PCR analysis of rearranged T cell receptor genes for clonality assessment in suspect T cell proliferations. Leukemia 11(12):2192–2199

Paganin M, Zecca M, Fabbri G, Polato K, Biondi A, Rizzari C, Locatelli F, Basso G (2008) Minimal residual disease is an important predictive factor of outcome in children with relapsed 'high-risk' acute lymphoblastic leukemia. Leukemia 22(12):2193–2200. doi:-leu200822710.1038/leu.2008.227

Panzer-Grumayer ER, Schneider M, Panzer S, Fasching K, Gadner H (2000) Rapid molecular response during early induction chemotherapy predicts a good outcome in childhood acute lymphoblastic leukemia. Blood 95(3):790–794

Pongers-Willemse MJ, Verhagen OJ, Tibbe GJ, Wijkhuijs AJ, de Haas V, Roovers E, van der Schoot CE, van Dongen JJ (1998) Real-time quantitative PCR for the detection of minimal residual disease in acute lymphoblastic leukemia using junctional region specific TaqMan probes. Leukemia 12(12):2006–2014

Pongers-Willemse MJ, Seriu T, Stolz F, d'Aniello E, Gameiro P, Pisa P, Gonzalez M, Bartram CR, Panzer-Grumayer ER, Biondi A, San Miguel JF, van Dongen JJM (1999) Primers and protocols for standardized detection of minimal residual disease in acute lymphoblastic leukemia using immunoglobulin and T cell receptor gene rearrangements and TAL1 deletions as PCR targets: report of the BIOMED-1 CONCERTED ACTION: investigation of minimal residual disease in acute leukemia. Leukemia 13(1):110–118

Rowen L, Koop BF, Hood L (1996) The complete 685-kilobase DNA sequence of the human beta T cell receptor locus. Science 272(5269):1755–1762

Schrappe M (2002) Risk-adapted therapy: lessons from childhood acute lymphoblastic leukemia. Hematol J 3(Supplement 2):127–132

Szczepanski T, Flohr T, van der Velden VHJ, Bartram CR, van Dongen JJM (2002) Molecular monitoring of residual disease using antigen receptor genes in childhood acute lymphoblastic leukaemia. Best Pract Res Clin Haematol 15(1):37–57

Szczepański T, Pongers-Willemse MJ, Langerak AW, Harts WA, Wijkhuijs AJ, van Wering ER, van Dongen JJ (1999) Ig heavy chain gene rearrangements in T-cell acute lymphoblastic leukemia exhibit predominant DH6-19 and DH7-27 gene usage, can result in complete V-D-J rearrangements, and are rare in T-cell receptor alpha beta lineage. Blood 93(12):4079–4085

Szczepański T, Willemse MJ, van Wering ER, van Weerden JF, Kamps WA, van Dongen JJ (2001) Precursor-B-ALL with D(H)-J(H) gene rearrangements have an immature immunogenotype with a high frequency of oligoclonality and hyperdiploidy of chromosome 14. Leukemia 15(9):1415–1423

Szczepański T, van der Velden VH, Raff T, Jacobs DC, van Wering ER, Bruggemann M, Kneba M, van Dongen JJ (2003) Comparative analysis of T-cell receptor gene rearrangements at diagnosis and relapse of T-cell acute lymphoblastic leukemia (T-ALL) shows high stability of clonal markers for monitoring of minimal residual disease and reveals the occurrence of second T-ALL. Leukemia 17(11):2149–2156

Szczepański T, van der Velden VH, Hoogeveen PG, de Bie M, Jacobs DC, van Wering ER, van Dongen JJ (2004) Vdelta2-Jalpha rearrangements are frequent in precursor-B-acute lymphoblastic leukemia but rare in normal lymphoid cells. Blood 103(10):3798–3804

van der Velden VH, van Dongen JJ (2009) MRD detection in acute lymphoblastic leukemia patients using Ig/TCR gene rearrangements as targets for real-time quantitative PCR. Methods Mol Biol 538:115–150. doi:10.1007/978-1-59745-418-6_7

van der Velden VH, Wijkhuijs JM, Jacobs DC, van Wering ER, van Dongen JJ (2002a) T cell receptor gamma gene rearrangements as targets for detection of minimal residual disease in acute lymphoblastic leukemia by real-time quantitative PCR analysis. Leukemia 16(7):1372–1380

van der Velden VH, Willemse MJ, van der Schoot CE, Hahlen K, van Wering ER, van Dongen JJ (2002b) Immunoglobulin kappa deleting element rearrangements in precursor-B acute lymphoblastic leukemia are stable targets for detection of minimal residual disease by real-time quantitative PCR. Leukemia 16(5):928–936

van der Velden VH, Szczepanski T, Wijkhuijs JM, Hart PG, Hoogeveen PG, Hop WC, van Wering ER, van Dongen JJ (2003) Age-related patterns of immunoglobulin and T-cell receptor gene rearrangements in precursor-B-ALL: implications for detection of minimal residual disease. Leukemia 17(9):1834–1844

van der Velden VH, de Bie M, van Wering ER, van Dongen JJ (2006) Immunoglobulin light chain gene rearrangements in precursor-B-acute lymphoblastic leukemia: characteristics and applicability for the detection of minimal residual disease. Haematologica 91(5):679–682

van der Velden VH, Cazzaniga G, Schrauder A, Hancock J, Bader P, Panzer-Grumayer ER, Flohr T, Sutton R, Cave H, Madsen HO, Cayuela JM, Trka J, Eckert C, Foroni L, Zur Stadt U, Beldjord K, Raff T, van der Schoot CE, van Dongen JJ (2007a) Analysis of minimal residual disease by Ig/TCR gene rearrangements: guidelines for interpretation of real-time quantitative PCR data. Leukemia 21(4):604–611

van der Velden VH, Panzer-Grumayer ER, Cazzaniga G, Flohr T, Sutton R, Schrauder A, Basso G, Schrappe M, Wijkhuijs JM, Konrad M, Bartram CR, Masera G, Biondi A, van Dongen JJ (2007b) Optimization of PCR-based minimal residual disease diagnostics for childhood acute lymphoblastic leukemia in a multi-center setting. Leukemia 21(4):706–713

van Dongen JJM, Seriu T, Panzer-Grumayer ER, Biondi A, Pongers-Willemse MJ, Corral L, Stolz F, Schrappe M, Masera G, Kamps WA, Gadner H, van Wering ER, Ludwig WD, Basso G, de Bruijn MA, Cazzaniga G, Hettinger K, van der Does-van den Berg A, Hop WC, Riehm H, Bartram CR (1998) Prognostic value of minimal residual disease in acute lymphoblastic leukaemia in childhood. Lancet 352(9142):1731–1738

van Dongen JJ, Langerak AW, Bruggemann M, Evans PA, Hummel M, Lavender FL, Delabesse E, Davi F, Schuuring E, Garcia-Sanz R, van Krieken JH, Droese J, Gonzalez D, Bastard C, White HE, Spaargaren M, Gonzalez M, Parreira A, Smith JL, Morgan GJ, Kneba M, Macintyre EA (2003) Design and standardization of PCR primers and protocols for detection of clonal immunoglobulin and T-cell receptor gene recombinations in suspect lymphoproliferations: report of the BIOMED-2 Concerted Action BMH4-CT98-3936. Leukemia 17(12):2257–2317

Verhagen OJ, Willemse MJ, Breunis WB, Wijkhuijs AJ, Jacobs DC, Joosten SA, van Wering ER, van Dongen JJ, van der Schoot CE (2000) Application of germline IGH probes in real-time quantitative PCR for the detection of minimal residual disease in acute lymphoblastic leukemia. Leukemia 14(8):1426–1435

Willems P, Verhagen O, Segeren C, Veenhuizen P, Guikema J, Wiemer E, Groothuis L, Jong TB, Kok H, Bloem A, Bos N, Vellenga E, Mensink E, Sonneveld P, Lokhorst H, van Der Schoot E, Raymakers R (2000) Consensus strategy to quantitate malignant cells in myeloma patients is validated in a multicenter study. Belgium-Dutch hematology-oncology group. Blood 96(1):63–70

Willemse MJ, Seriu T, Hettinger K, d'Aniello E, Hop WC, Panzer-Grumayer ER, Biondi A, Schrappe M, Kamps WA, Masera G, Gadner H, Riehm H, Bartram CR, van Dongen JJ (2002) Detection of minimal residual disease identifies differences in treatment response between T-ALL and precursor B-ALL. Blood 99(12):4386–4393

Chapter 24
Molecular Diagnostics of Acute Myeloblastic Leukemia

Marta Libura, Agata A. Filip and Olga Haus

Abstract Acute myeloblastic leukemia (AML) is a genetically heterogeneous disorder. In approximately 60 % of cases specific recurrent chromosomal aberrations can be identified by modern cytogenetic methods, which enable risk stratification. In these AML subgroups, molecular diagnostics serve as an additional tool to confirm and complement cytogenetic data. In the remaining 40 % of AML cases, with normal karyotype (NK), as well as in core binding factor leukemias (CBF-AMLs), molecular techniques enable the identification of intragenic aberrations and gene expression markers, which further differentiate prognosis of AML. In addition to molecular risk stratification established at the moment of diagnosis, minimal residual disease (MRD) assessment by means of highly sensitive real-time quantitative polymerase chain reaction (RQ-PCR) provides a basis for therapeutic decisions in the course of disease.

M. Libura (✉)
Department of Hematology, Oncology and Internal Medicine,
Medical University of Warsaw, Banacha 1a, 02-097 Warsaw, Poland
e-mail: marta.libura@gmail.com

A. A. Filip
Department of Cancer Genetics, Medical University of Lublin,
Radziwiłłowska 11, 20-950 Lublin, Poland
e-mail: a.filip@umlub.pl

O. Haus
Department of Clinical Genetics, Ludwik Rydygier Collegium Medicum in Bydgoszcz
Nicolaus Copernicus University in Toruń, Skłodowska-Curie 9, 85-094 Bydgoszcz, Poland
e-mail: haus@cm.umk.pl

O. Haus
Department of Hematology, Wrocław Medical University,
Pasteura 4, 50-367 Wrocław, Poland

M. Witt et al. (eds.), *Molecular Aspects of Hematologic Malignancies*,
Principles and Practice, DOI: 10.1007/978-3-642-29467-9_24,

24.1 Introduction

The identification of molecular markers at the moment of initial diagnosis as well as the monitoring of minimal residual disease (MRD) became standard procedures in the diagnosis and management of acute myeloid leukemia (AML) patients. They are used to characterize AML cases and stratify them into relevant risk groups. Molecular diagnostics of AML includes analyses performed for all AML patients, as well as those performed in AML patients assigned to specific AML subtypes, based on the results of prior cytogenetic and/or other molecular tests. Because of the genetic heterogeneity of AML, it is rational to prioritize diagnostic procedures according to clinical significance of molecular markers, economic aspects, as well as technological feasibility. The proposal of such strategy is shown in Table 24.1. It represents modified version of the international expert panel recommendations on behalf of the European LeukemiaNet (ELN) (Dohner et al. 2010) as well as recent data from the integrated mutational profiling in AML (Patel et al. 2012).

The markers studied in molecular diagnostics are divided into two categories: structural DNA aberrations and quantitative alterations of gene expression. Molecular techniques provide tools for robust and high-throughput identification of whole panel of gene aberrations with the resolution at a single base pair level. Application of different techniques for the identification of specific aberrations in AML is presented in Table 24.2.

Real-time quantitative polymerase chain reaction (RQ-PCR) preceded by reverse transcription (RT) remains a standard technique for the quantification of aberrant gene expression in the diagnostic material, as well as for MRD monitoring in the follow-up samples. Fusion gene transcripts resulting from gross structural DNA aberrations such as chromosomal translocations may be detected by means of reverse transcription PCR (RT-PCR). More complex and sophisticated techniques are required for the identification of small intragenic aberrations which include microinsertions/duplications/deletions as well as single base-pair substitutions. Detection of these mutations is of special prognostic value in the intermediate risk group (cytogenetically normal AML, CN-AML), as well as in patients with low risk rearrangements like *AML1-ETO (RUNX1-RUNX1T1)* and *CBFB-MYH11* (core binding factor leukemias, CBF-AMLs). Unless included in the text, the names of the genes are given in the legend to Table 24.1 or 24.2. This refers to the whole chapter.

24.2 Cell Processing of Diagnostic and Follow-up AML Samples

Bone marrow (BM) aspirates (3–5 ml) should be collected at the time of diagnosis/during follow-up into EDTA containing tubes, transported to the diagnostic laboratory at room temperature, and processed within next 24 h. The cell sample processing procedures include the following steps:

Table 24.1 Proposal of guidelines for the initial genetic work-up of a patient with AML—according to the international expert panel recommendations on behalf of European LeukemiaNet (Dohner et al. 2010) as well as recent data from integrated mutational analysis in AML (Patel et al. 2012)

Test/procedure	Reference laboratories	Clinical trials
Genetic tests to establish the diagnosis for all patients:		
1. Cytogenetics (CG) or FISH analysis (if CG failed) for: t(15;17)(q22;q21)/*PML-RARA*, inv(16)(p13q22) or t(16;16)(p13;q22)/*CBFB-MYH11*, and t(8;21)(q22;q22)/*AML1-ETO*	Yes	Yes
2. FISH screening for 11q23.3	Optional	Yes
3. Molecular analyses: *AML1-ETO (RUNX1-RUNX1T1), CBFB-MYH11*	Yes	Yes
4. *FLT3*-ITD	Yes	Yes
Genetic tests performed for selected groups of patients:		
1. Group of patients with normal karyotype:		
a. Intragenic aberrations: *NPM1, CEBPA, IDH1/2* mutations, *MLL*-PTD	Yes	Yes
b. Intragenic aberrations: *WT1* mutations	Optional	Yes
c. Intragenic aberrations: *RUNX1, TET2, ASXL1, DNMT3A, BCOR*	No	Investigational
d. Gene expression: *BAALC, ERG, MN1, EVI1*	Optional	Yes
2. Group of patients with CBF leukemias:		
a. exon 8 and 17 *C-KIT* mutations	Optional	Yes
b. *FLT3* D835 mutations	Optional	Yes
c. *K-* and *N-RAS* mutations	No	Investigational
3. Group of patients with 11q23 aberrations in the FISH screening:		
Confirmation of *MLL* rearrangement and verification of *MLL* partner gene using RT-PCR (e.g. *MLL-AF6, MLL-AF9, MLL-AF10, MLL-ENL, MLL-EEN, MLL-ELL)*	Optional	Yes

(continued)

Table 24.1 (continued)

Test/procedure	Reference laboratories	Clinical trials
4. Group of patients with characteristic cytomorphology and immunophenotype abnormalities or positive CG result:		
RT-PCR for *PML-RARA*	Yes	Yes
RT-PCR for *DEK-CAN*	Optional	Yes

RT-PCR reverse transcriptase polymerase chain reaction, *CG* classical cytogenetics, *FISH* fluorescence in situ hybridization

Official gene names/other designations according to National Center for Biotechnology Information gene database (NCBI; http://www.ncbi.nlm.nih.gov/, cited December 22, 2011); gene order in the list according to the succession of genes presented both in the table and in the text: *PML* promyelocytic leukemia, *RARA* retinoic acid receptor, alpha, *CBFB* core-binding factor, beta subunit, *MYH11* myosin, heavy chain 11, *AML1* (*RUNX1*), acute myeloid leukemia 1, runt-related transcription factor 1, *CBFA2* core-binding factor alfa 2 subunit, *ETO* (*RUNX1T1*) eight twenty one, runt-related transcription factor 1, translocated to, 1; *FLT3* fms-related tyrosine kinase 3, *NPM1* nucleophosmin, *CEBPA* CCAAT/enhancer binding protein (C/EBP), alpha, *MLL* myeloid/lymphoid or mixed-lineage leukemia gene, *IDH1* isocitrate dehydrogenase 1 (NADP+), soluble, *IDH2* isocitrate dehydrogenase 2 (NADP+), mitochondrial, *WT1* Wilms tumor 1, *IDH1* isocitrate dehydrogenase 1 (NADP+), soluble, *IDH2* isocitrate dehydrogenase 2 (NADP+), mitochondrial, *TET2* tet methylcytosine dioxygenase 2, *ASXL1* additional sex combs like 1, *DNMT3A* DNA (cytosine-5-)-methyltransferase 3 alpha, *BCOR* B-cell CLL/lymphoma 6 (BCL6) corepressor, *BAALC* brain and acute leukemia, cytoplasmic factor, *ERG* v-ets erythroblastosis virus E26 oncogene homolog (avian), ets-related transcriptional regulator, *MN1* meningioma (disrupted in balanced translocation) 1, probable tumor suppressor protein MN1, *EVI1*(*MECOM*), *MDS1* and *EVI1* complex locus, *KIT* v-kit Hardy-Zuckerman 4 feline sarcoma viral oncogene homolog, *C-KIT* proto-oncogene tyrosine-protein kinase Kit, *K-RAS* v-Ki-ras2 Kirsten rat sarcoma viral oncogene homolog, GTPase KRas, *N-RAS* neuroblastoma RAS viral (v-ras) oncogene homolog, transforming protein N-Ras, *AF6 ALL1*—fused gene from chromosome 6 also named *MLLT4,* myeloid/lymphoid translocated to, 4, *AF9 ALL1*–fused gene from chromosome 9 also named *MLLT3*, myeloid/lymphoid translocated to, 3, *AF10 ALL1*—fused gene from chromosome 10 also named *MLLT10*, myeloid/lymphoid translocated to, 10, *ENL* translocation gene partner of *MLL*(*ALL1*) also named *MLLT1*, myeloid/lymphoid translocated to, 1, *EEN* extra 11—19 leukemia fusion gene, *ELL* elongation factor RNA polymerase II

1. Isolation of mononuclear cells (MNCs) by density gradient centrifugation, according to the standard protocol (see also Chap. 19).
2. Isolation of RNA and DNA followed by assessment of their quantity and quality at 260 and 280 nm with microvolume spectrophotometer. 10×10^6 fresh MNCs should be used both in case of diagnostic and follow-up samples (for MRD up to 20×10^6 cells). RNA and DNA isolation procedures according to Chomczyński and Sacchi protocol are recommended (see also Chap. 20). This protocol yields the highest amounts of stable RNA/DNA, which can be safely stored for further applications. The remaining MNCs should be stored for later use in DMSO, preferably in liquid nitrogen, and as dry pellets in –80 °C.

In general, the molecular analyses performed in AML diagnostics include:

1. Reverse transcription for mRNA transcript analyses (see also Chap. 20).
2. Polymerase chain reaction (PCR)-based analyses for evaluation of DNA structural aberrations (see also Chap. 20).
3. Assessment of gene expression markers and MRD using RQ-PCR approach (see also Chap. 20).

24.3 Molecular Analyses Performed for All AML Patients

Each AML patient should be screened for the following markers:

- *AML1-ETO* and *CBFB-MYH11* according to BIOMED-1 guidelines (van Dongen et al. 1999),
- *FLT3*-ITD (Dohner et al. 2010).

Along with these molecular analyses, classical cytogenetic examination supplemented with fluorescence in situ hybridization (FISH) with molecular probes specific for particular aberrations, like *AML1-ETO, CBFB-MYH11* and *MLL* rearrangements (assessed with *MLL* break-apart probe), should be performed for each AML patient—see Table 24.1. Beside the presented above markers, recent data on integrated mutational analysis suggest that screening for *MLL*-PTD, as well as *IDH2* R140Q mutation might be introduced into panel of molecular analyses performed for all AML patients, due to the strong clinical impact of both aberrations in the entire AML population (Patel et al. 2012).

24.3.1 Fusion Gene Analyses Standardized According to BIOMED-1 Guidelines

Each diagnostic sample from AML patients should be screened by RT-PCR for the presence of fusion gene transcripts: *AML1-ETO* and *CBFB-MYH11*. Some laboratories examine also *PML-RARA*. As protocol for the detection of *PML-RARA* was standardized together with *AML1-ETO* and *CBFB-MYH11*, it is presented within this section. RT-PCR protocol and primers were designed according to the consensus of The European BIOMED-1 Concerted Action for standardization of MRD detection in acute leukemias, which also introduced the appropriate primer nomenclature for basic fusion gene analyses (van Dongen et al. 1999). It presents as follows:

A primer—an external forward primer
B primer—an external reverse primer
C primer—an internal forward primer
D primer—an internal reverse primer

Although, starting from this paragraph the nomenclature of the primers is quoted after original papers.

Detection of fusion genes according to BIOMED-1 guidelines includes:

1. PCR amplification of cDNA sample obtained at diagnosis with the use of a set of standard primers presented below, along with the amplification of appropriate control cDNA (positive control, see below) and water as nontemplate control. The composition of PCR mix according to BIOMED-1 is shown in Table 24.3. As both genes, *PML-RARA* and *CBFB-MYH11*, exist in the form of different transcript variants, their detection is held in two separate PCR tubes for each fusion gene. In case of *CBFB-MYH11*, first reaction mix is designed to detect transcript A, occurring with the incidence of 88 % in adult *CBFB-MYH*11(+) AML patients, while the second mix allows for the detection of alternative transcripts like E and D, both found in 5 % of *CBFB-MYH*11(+) cases, as well as other rare variants. Classical transcript of *PML-RARA* fusion gene described as bcr1 is found in 60 % of APL, and is identified separately from alternative variants: bcr2 and bcr3 (found in 5 and 40 % of cases, respectively; see Table 24.4 for further details). Detection of the only *AML1-ETO* transcript is performed in a single PCR tube.

   The following primers are used for PCR amplification:

   AML1-A: CTACCGCAGCCATGAAGAACC
   ETO-B: AGAGGAAGGCCCATTGCTGAA
   AML1-C: ATGACCTCAGGTTTGTCGGTCG
   ETO-D: TGAACTGGTTCTTGGAGCTCC
   CBFB-A: GCAGGCAAGGTATATTTGAAGG
   MYH11-B1: TGAAGCAACTCCTGGGTGTC
   MYH11-B2: TCCTCTTCTCCTCATTCTGCTC
   CBFB-C: GGGCTGTCTGGAGTTTGATG
   MYH11-D1: TCCCTGTGACGCTCTCAACT
   MYH11-D2: CTTGAGCGCCTGCATGTT
   PML-A1: CAGTGTACGCCTTCTCCATCA
   PML- A2: CTGCTGGAGGCTGTGGAC
   RARA-B: GCTTGTAGATGCGGGGTAGA
   PML- C1: TCAAGATGGAGTCTGAGGAGG

Table 24.2 Summary of diagnostic procedures for AML-associated gene aberrations

Type of genetic aberration	Method used in genetic diagnostics
A. Chromosomal translocations/ fusion genes	– classic CG, FISH – RT-PCR, PCR (van Dongen et al. 1999) – Southern blotting
B. Losses, duplications/amplifications of larger DNA fragments	– classic CG, FISH (> 2Mbp) – aCGH, aSNP (> 5Kbp) – Southern blotting
C. Small intragenic aberrations:	
1. *FLT3*-ITD	PCR or RT-PCR followed by the analysis of PCR products: Screening analyses – agarose gel electrophoresis (Thiede et al. 2002) – GS analysis (Thiede et al. 2002) – HRM analysis (Tan et al. 2008) Determination of *FLT3* ITD mutant : wt ratio – GS analysis (Thiede et al. 2002) – LOH analysis within the locus relative to *FLT3* (Whitman et al. 2001)
2. *NPM1* mutations	PCR or RT-PCR followed by the analysis of PCR product using: – Direct sequencing (Dohner et al. 2005) – PAGE gel electrophoresis (Calvo et al. 2009) – dHPLC (Ammatuna et al. 2005; Roti et al. 2006) – GS analysis (Thiede et al. 2006) – HRM analysis (Tan et al. 2008)
3. *CEBPA* mutations	PCR or RT-PCR followed by the analysis of PCR product using: – Direct sequencing of the whole coding region (Pabst et al. 2001) – GS analysis (Benthaus et al. 2008) – dHPLC (Wouters et al. 2009)
4. *MLL* duplication (*MLL*-PTD)	RT-PCR followed by the analysis of PCR product using: – Agarose gel electrophoresis (Poirel et al. 1996) – Southern blotting (Poirel et al. 1996)
5. *WT1* mutations	– Direct sequencing of exon 7 and 9 (Hou et al. 2010) – dHPLC of exon 7 and 9 (Paschka et al. 2008)
6. *IDH1/IDH2* mutations	– Direct sequencing (Marcucci et al. 2010) – dHPLC (Abbas et al. 2010) – HRM analysis (Tefferi et al. 2010) – RFLP analysis for *IDH1* (Green et al. 2010)
7. *TET2* mutations	– Direct sequencing of the whole coding region (Abdel-Wahab et al. 2009)
8. *RUNX1* mutations	– Direct sequencing of the whole coding region (Gaidzik et al. 2011) – dHPLC (Steensma et al. 2005)
9. *ASXL1* mutations	– Direct sequencing of the whole coding region (Gelsi-Boyer et al. 2009)
10. *DNMT3A* mutations	– Direct sequencing of the whole coding region (Ley et al. 2010)

(continued)

Table 24.2 (continued)

Type of genetic aberration	Method used in genetic diagnostics
11. *C-KIT* mutations	– dHPLC screening followed by confirmation of mutations by direct sequencing (Paschka et al. 2006)
	– HRM analysis (Fuster et al. 2009)
12. *FLT3* D835 mutations	– Screening by RFLP analysis followed by confirmation of mutations by direct sequencing (Libura et al. 2003)
	– dHPLC (Mead et al. 2007)
13. *N-RAS* and *K-RAS* mutations	– dHPLC (for *N-RAS*), SSCP for exon 12, 13, and 61 of *K-RAS* (Neubauer et al. 2008)
	– dHPLC (for *N-RAS*), RFLP for exon 12, 13, and 61 of *K-RAS* (Bowen et al. 2005)
D. Aberrant mRNA expression	– RT-RQ-PCR (Beillard et al. 2003; Gabert et al. 2003)

RT-RQ-PCR real-time quantitative polymerase chain reaction, based on reverse transcription, *aCGH* array-comparative genomic hybridization, *aSNP* array-single nucleotide polymorphism, *dHPLC* denaturing high performance liquid chromatography, *HRM* high resolution melting analysis, *LOH* loss of heterozygosity, *PAGE* polyacrylamide gel electrophoresis, *NGS* targeted next-generation sequencing, *GS* GeneScan analysis, *RFLP* restriction fragment length polymorphism, *SSCP* single strand conformation polymorphism, *wt* wild-type. The remaining abbreviations have been explained in the text

Table 24.3 Composition of PCR reaction mix according to BIOMED-1 (van Dongen et al. 1999)

Reagent	Stock concentration	Volume used for 1 reaction	Final concentration
PCR buffer	10x	2.5 μl	1x
$MgCl_2$	25 mM	2.5 μl	2.5 mM
dNTP	2 mM	2.5 μl	0.2 mM
Forward primer	10 μM	1 μl	0.4 μM
Reverse primer	10 μM	1 μl	0.4 μM
Hot-start polymerase	5 U/μl	0.2 μl	1 U
cDNA	10–15 % of RT mix volume	2–3 μl	corresponds to 100–150 ng of RNA
H_2O		up to 25 μl	
Final volume		25 μl	

PML-C2: AGCGCGACTACGAGGAGAT
RARA-D: CTGCTGCTCTGGGTCTCAAT

- PCR conditions are as follows:

94°C	8 min (with hot start polymerase)	
94°C	30 s	35 cycles
65°C	1 min	35 cycles
72°C	1 min	35 cycles
72°C	10 min	

Table 24.4 PCR products length for *AML1-ETO* (*RUNX1-RUNX1T1*), *CBFB-MYH11* and *PML-RARA* fusion genes depending on primers used for external and internal PCR (after van Dongen et al. 1999, modified)

Type of fusion gene transcript	Product length (bp) for specified primers			
AML1-ETO	A–B	–	C–D	–
Type A	395	–	260	–
CBFB-MYH11	A–B1	A–B2	C–D1	C–D2
Type A (88 %)	–	418	–	271
Type B	–	630	–	483
Type C	–	811	–	664
Type D (5 %)	338	(1,138)[a]	155	(991)
Type E (5 %)	545	(1,345)	362	(1,198)
Type F	–	322	–	175
Type G	242	(1,042)	59	(895)
Type H	344	(1,144)	161	(997)
Type I	–[b]	–[b]	–[b]	–[b]
Type J	–	1,033	–	886
PML-RARA	A1–B	A2–B	C1–D	C2–D
bcr1 (55 %)	381	(1,329)	214	(688)
bcr2 (5 %)	±345	(±819)	±178	(652)
bcr3 (40 %)	–	376	–	289

[a] PCR products presented in brackets are too long to be amplified using BIOMED-1 PCR protocol (too short elongation time)

[b] Rare transcript variant, not amplified with presented primer set

2. PCR products are assayed for positive amplicons by 2 % agarose gel electrophoresis.

The length of the PCR product is precisely determined for each transcript, depending on the primers used. The expected lengths of amplification products are shown in Table 24.4.

- Positive control cell lines for predominant fusion transcripts:
  for *AML1-ETO*—KASUMI cell line,
  for *CBFB-MYH11* type A—ME1 cell line,
  for *PML-RARA* bcr1—NB4 cell line (van Dongen et al. 1999).
  In case of rare fusion genes RNA of a verified fusion-positive patient may be used as positive control.

24.3.2 Internal Tandem Duplication of FLT3 Gene (FLT3-ITD)

All AML patients should be screened for *FLT3*-ITD, as it stratifies the prognosis in each cytogenetic subgroup.

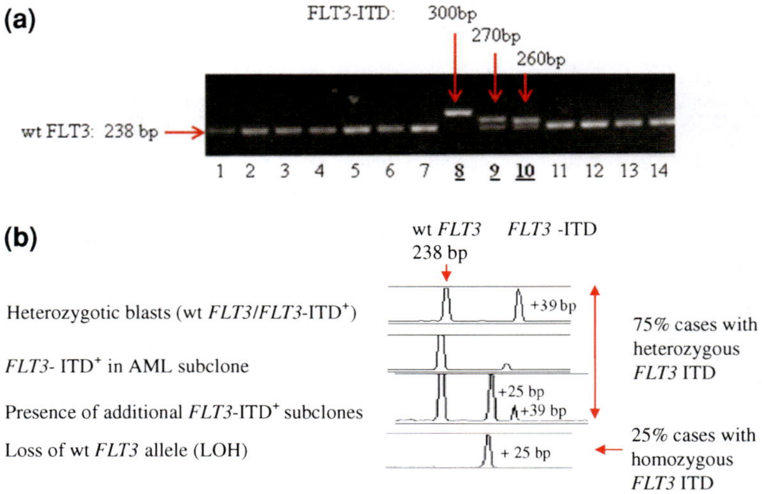

Fig. 24.1 Typical results of agarose (**a**) polyacrylamide (**b**) gel electrophoresis (PAGE) of *FLT3* amplification products. **a** Agarose gel electrophoretic analysis of *FLT*3-ITD$^+$. Samples 8, 9, 10 represent *FLT*3-ITD$^+$ cases. In sample 8 internal tandem duplication is present in two alleles (corresponding to one band of 300 bp) (loss of heterozygosity; LOH), in samples 9 and 10 both wild-type and mutant alleles are present corresponding to bands of 270 and 260 bp, respectively. Samples 1–7, and 11–14 represent cases with wild-type (wt) *FLT3* (238 bp band). **b**. PAGE analysis of *FLT3*-ITD$^+$ cases. Semi-quantitative assessment of wt/mutant allele ratio can be performed using fragment length analysis; additionally, the presence of small *FLT3*-ITD$^+$ subclones may be identified by means of PAGE. 75 % of *FLT3*-ITD (+) AML population present heterozygous pattern of mutation, while only 25 % cases with *FLT3*-ITD present loss of wt *FLT3* allele (LOH)

*FLT*3-ITD analysis includes:

1. PCR amplification of exons 13–15 of the *FLT3* gene using primers listed below (Libura et al. 2003). DNA (100 ng) or RNA (0.2 μg RNA equivalent) samples are used as a template.
   *FLT3*E: TGGTGTTTGTCTCCTCTTCATTGT
   *FLT3*Q: GTTGCGTTCATCACTTTTCCAA
   *FLT3*Q primer may be labeled with 5′HEX fluorochrome for GeneScan (GS) analysis. RT-PCR seems to be more sensitive than PCR (0.1–0.5 % vs. 10 % of cells *FLT3*-ITD- positive within the whole population of analyzed cells) and potentially enables the detection of small leukemic clones present in the examined samples (see Fig. 24.1b).The composition of PCR mix is similar to protocol proposed by BIOMED-1 (Table 24.3), it differs by final concentration of $MgCl_2$ (5 mM) and dNTPs (0.75 mM) (Libura et al. 2003).

- PCR conditions are as follows:

94°C	8 min (with hot start polymerase)	
94°C	30 s	35 cycles
60°C	1 min	
72°C	1 min	
72°C	10 min	

2. Agarose gel (2 %) electrophoresis or GS fragment length analysis by polyacrylamide gel electrophoresis (PAGE) is performed for selection of PCR products containing positive amplicons (Fig. 24.1).
3. Since it was proved that *FLT3* mutant to wild-type ratio might influence AML prognosis, it is clinically relevant to assess quantitatively the allele ratio of *FLT3*-ITD(+)/wt (Kottaridis et al. 2001; Thiede et al. 2002). This can be performed using GS analysis (see Fig. 24.1) or by determining LOH (loss of heterozygosity) at chromosome 13q12 (Whitman et al. 2001).

24.4 Molecular Analyses Performed for Selected Groups of AML Patients

More precise molecular characteristics enables prognostic stratification within the cytogenetically and/or molecularly defined subgroups (CN-AMLs and CBF-leukemias) or may be performed for the detection of rare gene rearrangements for their later application as targets in MRD monitoring, e.g. *MLL* fusions, *DEK-CAN* (*DEK* oncogene, *CAN* also named *NUP214*, nucleoporin 214 kDa). Thus, protocols presented in this section should be carried out after obtaining results of conventional cytogenetics, FISH, and/or other preliminary molecular tests.

24.4.1 Extended Molecular Diagnostics in CN-AML

24.4.1.1 Intragenic Alterations in CN-AML

Intragenic aberrations, which are particular features of CN-AML, may be clustered within specific region of the relevant gene (e.g. duplications within exon 14 of *FLT3*, mutations within exon 12 of *NPM1*, mutations within exon 4 of *IDH1* and *IDH2*), or can be scattered along the whole gene (e.g. *CEBPA, TET2* and *N-RAS* mutations) (Dohner et al. 2005; Metzeler et al. 2011b). This influences the choice of a diagnostic method used for further characterization of CN-AML cases.

Direct sequencing remains the gold standard for the detection of intragenic aberrations; however, it is neither time-efficient nor economically justified option of screening. Thus, other screening methods have been proposed. The rapid and highly sensitive techniques, e.g. denaturing high performance liquid chromatography (dHPLC), high resolution melting (HRM) analysis and targeted next-generation sequencing (NGS) enable the detection of all types of small DNA alterations (length aberrations and nucleotide changes) with the sensitivity of 99–100 % (Fuster et al. 2009; Wouters et al. 2009; Grossmann et al. 2011a). GeneScan analysis offers reliable option for screening of short length fragment aberrations, but excludes the possibility of nucleotide substitution detection. Other techniques used for the detection of intragenic alterations include restriction fragment length polymorphism (RFLP) and single strand conformation polymorphism (SSCP). The results indicated as positive by any screening technique should always be confirmed by direct sequencing. Screening methods used for the detection of different aberrations in AML patients, with relevant references, have been summarized in Table 24.2.

NPM1 Gene Mutations

NPM1 mutations (see Chap. 2) include small insertions and deletions, resulting in frame shift or premature transcription inhibition. Thus, beside sequencing, GS analysis may be also successfully used as a screening method (Thiede et al. 2006). Depending on the localization of primers, both DNA and cDNA may serve as a template for PCR.

NPM1 mutational analysis includes:

1. PCR amplification of *NPM1* exon 12 using exemplary primers (Dohner et al. 2005):
   NPM1 F: TTAACTCTCTGGTGGTAGAATGAA
   NPM1 R: CAAGACTATTTGCCATTCCTAAC
   NPM1 R2 (sequencing): GGCATTTTGGACAACACA.
   - The composition of PCR mix has been proposed by BIOMED-1 (Table 24.3).
   - PCR conditions are as follows:

94°C	8 min (with hot start polymerase)	
94°C	30 s	35 cycles
55°C	1 min	
72°C	1 min	
72°C	10 min	

2. Purification of PCR products using Exonuclease I–Shrimp Alkaline Phosphatase reagent or by means of a commercially available column-based kit.
3. Direct sequencing using commercial sequencing kit and additional primer (NPM1 R2).

CEBPA Gene Mutations

CEBPA gene is composed of a single exon of 1 kb. Mutations in *CEBPA* are very heterogeneous both at the structural and at functional level (see Chap. 2). Many groups suggest sequencing as the only approach in *CEBPA* screening (Pabst et al. 2001; Frohling et al. 2004), although dHPLC and GS analysis has also been recommended (see Table 24.2).

Table 24.5 PCR mix composition for *CEBPA* mutations and *MLL-AF6* fusion analysis (after van Dongen et al. 1999, modified)

Reagent	Stock concentration	Volume used for 1 reaction (μl)	Final concentration
PCR buffer	10x	2.5	1x
$MgCl_2$	25 mM	2.5	2.5 mM
dNTP	2 mM	2.5	0.2 mM
DMSO	100 %	1.25	5 %
Forward primer	10 μM	1	0.4 μM
Reverse primer	10 μM	1	0.4 μM
Hot-start polymerase	5 U/μl	0.1	0.5 U
cDNA	10–20 % of RT mix volume	2–5	corresponds to 100–200 ng of RNA
H_2O		up to 25	
Final volume		25	

CEBPA mutational analysis includes:

1. PCR amplification of *CEBPA* exon 1: reaction is performed using either cDNA or DNA as the template. Exemplary sequences of primers that may be used to amplify DNA (50–100 ng) or cDNA for direct sequencing are presented below (Pabst et al. 2001):
   PP1F: TCGCCATGCCGGGAGAACTCTAAC
   PP1R: CTGGTAAGGGAAGAGGCCGGCCAG
   PP2F: CCGCTGGTGATCAAGCAGGA
   PP2R: CACGGTCTGGGCAAGCCTCGAGAT.

   - The composition of PCR mix is similar to that in BIOMED-1 protocol; it includes enhancing agent (e.g. 5 % DMSO, Table 24.5) to improve the specificity and/or the yield of the amplification.
   - PCR conditions are as follows:

94°C	8 min (with hot start polymerase)	
94°C	30 s	35 cycles
62°C	1 min	35 cycles
72°C	1 min	35 cycles
72°C	10 min	

2. Purification of PCR products using Exonuclease I–Shrimp Alkaline Phosphatase reagent or one of commercially available column sets.
3. Direct sequencing with the use of commercial sequencing kit.

MLL Gene Duplications (*MLL*-PTD)

MLL partial tandem duplications (*MLL*-PTD) analysis can be performed by nested RT-PCR or by Southern blotting (Poirel et al. 1996).

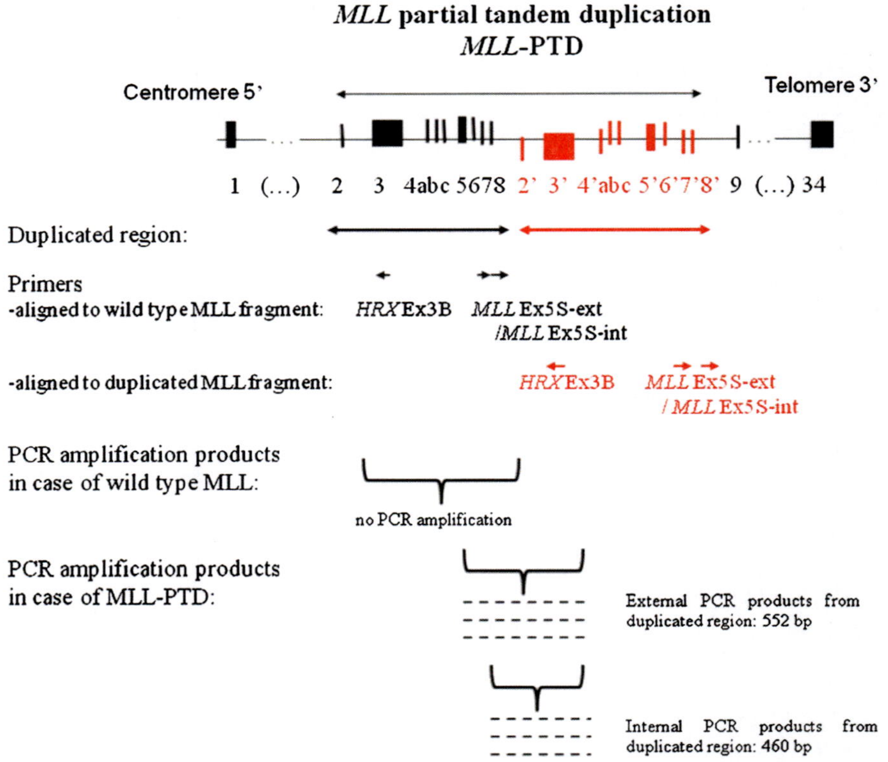

Fig. 24.2 Localization of primers for nested PCR in wild-type and mutated *MLL* gene. Partial duplication of *MLL* encompasses fragment from exon 2–8. External primers are: *MLL* Ex5S-ext and *HRX* Ex3B, while internal ones are *MLL* Ex5S-int and *HRX* Ex3B. In case of the wild-type sequence there is no amplification of the template because primers are localized in the opposite directions. *MLL* duplication positively changes amplification results, as forward primer *MLL* Ex5S-ext, specific for exon 5 is localized in the proper orientation towards reverse primer *MLL* Ex3B, specific to exon 3 of the duplicated region

Nested RT-PCR analysis includes the following steps:

1. PCR amplification of cDNA using external primers flanking longer fragment of the gene, followed by internal PCR round with internal primers, which flank smaller fragment within this gene. Primer design does not allow reaction to proceed in case of the wild-type *MLL* gene sequence (see Fig. 24.2).
   External PCR primer sequences (for external round of nested PCR):

   MLL Ex5S—ext: GAGGATCCTGCCCCAAAGAAAAG
   HRX Ex3B: AGAATCTTTCTTCTTGATCTTA
   Internal PCR primer sequences (for internal round of nested PCR):
   MLL Ex5S—int: GCCTGAATCCAAACAGGCCACCACT
   HRX Ex3B: AGAATCTTTCTTCTTGATCTTA.

- A sample from the verified *MLL*-PTD positive patient may serve as a positive control.
- The composition of PCR mix has been proposed by BIOMED-1 (Table 24.3).
- PCR conditions are as follows:

94°C	8 min (with hot start polymerase)	
94°C	30 s	35 cycles
57°C	1 min	
72°C	1 min	
72°C	10 min	

2. PCR products are assayed by 2 % agarose gel electrophoresis. The length of external PCR product of typical *MLL*-PTD encompassing fragments from either exon 2 to 6 is 552 base pairs, while internal PCR product is 460 base pairs.
3. The interpretation of results: since *MLL*-PTD might be present in a small percentage of cells both in healthy controls and in AML patients, the problem with the interpretation may arise (Marcucci et al. 1998). Thus, the experience in interpretation is necessary, as false positive results should be distinguished from true positive ones which include also the presence of subclones. Differentiation is possible after electrophoretic separation of internal PCR products: false positive samples show weak bands intensity as compared to strong bands of the true positive ones.

24.4.1.2 Other Intragenic Aberrations in CN-AML

In the last decade several new AML-associated mutations were described, involving genes like *WT1*, *IDH1*/*IDH2*, *RUNX1*, *TET2*, *ASXL1*, *DNMT3A*, *BCOR* (Hou et al. 2010; Ley et al. 2010; Rocquain et al. 2010; Metzeler et al. 2011a, b; Grossmann et al. 2011b). According to recent data (Patel et al. 2012) *IDH1/2* mutations might be considered as obligatory analysis in the initial work-up of CN-AML patients as they radically improve prognosis when co-occuring with *NPM1* mutations. Although some of these mutations are found also in other AML subtypes, they are of special prognostic value in CN-AML (Gaidzik et al. 2011; Metzeler et al. 2011b).

24.4.1.3 Gene Expression Analysis

The expression of *EVI1*, *BAALC*, *ERG* and *MN1* genes is assessed by RT-RQ-PCR, and includes the following steps:

1. The choice of specific probe and primers: the sets of oligonucleotides for the analysis of these genes are commercially available.

Table 24.6 PCR mix composition for RQ-PCR

Reagent	Stock concentration	Volume used for 1 reaction (μl)	Final concentration
RQ-PCR master mix[a]	10x	2.5	1x
Forward primer	30 μM	0.25	0.3 μM
Reverse primer	30 μM	0.25	0.3 μM
Probe	20 μM	0.25	0.2 μM
cDNA	10 % of RT mix volume	5	corresponds to 100 ng of RNA
H_2O		up to 25	
Final volume		25	

[a] RQ-PCR master mix includes polymerase buffer, dNTPs, magnesium ions, and hot start polymerase

2. Assessment of tested RNA quality by parallel analysis of the reference gene expression (e.g. *C-ABL*). According to the criteria of Europe Against Cancer program, only the samples with Ct (crossover threshold) values of less than 32 for *ABL* gene are considered appropriate (Gabert et al. 2003).

   - The composition of RQ-PCR mix is presented in Table 24.6.
   - RQ-PCR conditions are as follows:

50°C	2 min	
95°C	10 min	
95°C	15 s	50 cycles
60°C	1 min	

3. The analysis of RT-RQ-PCR results using the formula of relative quantification. The level of expression of the examined gene (*X*) is normalized in comparison to the reference gene expression level by setting the difference between Ct values of the two genes [e.g. Ct *ABL*—Ct *X* = delta Ct (dCt)]. The dCt presenting negative values are observed when mRNA copy number of *X* gene is lower (corresponding to higher Ct) than *ABL* mRNA copy number (lower Ct) in the cell, and vice versa: dCt with positive values reflect higher *X* mRNA copy number (lower Ct) in regard to *ABL* mRNA (higher Ct). The definition of the positive and negative samples in regard to gene expression is assessed by referring the analyzed samples to control samples with normal expression of the examined gene, or to empirically determined expression threshold (e.g. median gene expression for *BAALC, ERG,* and *MN1* genes).

24.4.2 Genetic Rearrangements in CBF-Leukemias

In CBF-leukemias, activating mutations of *C-KIT, RAS,* and *FLT3* cooperate with aberrations affecting CBF complex to cause overt AML (Chou et al. 2011; Wang et al. 2011). Screening for *RAS* mutations is not important in practical terms, as *RAS*(+) CBF-leukemias preserve their profile of favorable risk AML (see Tables 24.1 and 24.2). *C-KIT* and *FLT3* mutations (both *FLT3*-ITD and *FLT3* D835) are indicators of poor prognosis; mutations of *C-KIT* worsens the prognosis, especially in *CBFB-MYH11*(+) AML, although recent study presents reduced overall survival among AML1-ETO(+) patients (Patel et al. 2012). Thus, the analysis of these markers is sufficient to stratify prognosis of CBF-AML (Boissel et al. 2006).

24.4.2.1 *C-KIT* Mutations

C-KIT mutation screening approaches are presented in Table 24.2. The following primers may be applied both for dHPLC and direct sequencing, using cDNA as a template (Paschka et al. 2006):

*KIT*8 F: ATTCTGACGTCAATGCTGCC
*KIT*8 R: GGCAGTACAGAAGCAGAGCAT
*KIT*17 F: CATAGAAAGAGATGTGACTCCCG
*KIT*17 R: GCCATCCACTTCACAGGTA.

24.4.2.2 Point mutation of *FLT3* gene (D835Y)

The *FLT3* gene point mutation in the D835 locus or in its proximity was found in about 5–10 % of all AMLs, and more frequently (24 %) in the *CBFB-MYH11*(+) AMLs (Libura et al. 2003; Mead et al. 2007). Mutational analysis is performed by standard PCR or RT-PCR with subsequent RFLP analysis by PAGE. The following primers might be used (Abu-Duhier et al. 2001):

FLT3 D835 F: CCGCCAGGAACGTGCTT
FLT3 D835 R: CAGGCAGACGGGCATTG.

24.4.3 Rare Fusion Genes

The analyses of rare molecular markers, present in 1–5 % of AML patients, are performed in selected cytomorphologic or cytogenetic subgroups, and include:

– *DEK-CAN* gene analysis performed in patients with M2 subtype accompanied by myelodysplasia and basophilia; alternatively, as a confirmation of the presence of t(6; 9) detected by conventional cytogenetics (about 1 % of patients);

– molecular characteristics of *MLL* fusion partners in patients with 11q23 aberrations, detected by conventional cytogenetics or by FISH (3–7 % of AML patients).

24.4.3.1 *DEK-CAN* Fusion Gene

DEK-CAN fusion analysis includes:

1. RT-PCR reaction using primers presented below:
   DEK-CAN C: GCCAAAAGAGAAAAACCTAAA
   DEK-CAN B: GCAAGGATTTGGTGTGAGAT

   - The composition of PCR mix is the same as shown in Table 24.3, although some optimization may be necessary.
   - PCR conditions are as follows:

94°C	8 min (with hot start polymerase)	
94°C	30 s	35 cycles
60°C	1 min	
72°C	1 min	
72°C	10 min	

2. Agarose gel (2 %) electrophoresis for selection of positive cases.
3. In patients with confirmed *DEK-CAN* fusion, monitoring of MRD by RT-RQ-PCR is possible with primers and probe as follows (Garçon et al. 2005).:
   DEK S (RQ): AAAGTTGAAGAAACCCCCTACAGA
   CAN AS (RQ): CATCATTCACATCTTGGACAGCA
   DEK-CAN probe (RQ): FAM5′–CATACTGATGAAGGCGCCGAATTTCCT – 3′TAMRA.

24.4.3.2 *MLL* Gene Aberrations

After preliminary identification of *MLL* aberrations by FISH, the results may be confirmed by RT-PCR with the primers corresponding to the most typical *MLL* gene partners in AML, such as: *AF6, AF9, AF10, ENL, EEN*, *ELL* (Poirel et al. 1996). In case of positive FISH and negative PCR result, the unknown partner gene can be identified by long-distance inverse PCR (LDI-PCR) (Libura et al. 2005). The identification of *MLL* partner gene is necessary to set up the MRD assay, but is not required for prognostic stratification, as all *MLL* fusions, except *MLL-AF9*, are associated with poor prognosis.

The protocol for identification of *MLL-AF*6 fusion, one of the most common arrangements in adult AML, includes (Poirel et al. 1996):

1. RT-PCR reaction with the following primers:
   MLL-Ex5S-ext: GAGGATCCTGCCCCAAAGAAAAG
   AF6-AS-ext: CTCCGCTGACATGCACTTCATAG.
   ML2 and MM2 cell lines may serve as positive control for the fusion gene

- The composition of PCR mix is similar to that in BIOMED-1 protocol; it includes enhancing agent (e.g., 5 % DMSO; Table 24.5) to improve the specificity and/or the yield of the PCR.
- PCR conditions are as follows:

94°C	8 min (with hot start polymerase)	
94°C	30 s	35 cycles
60°C	1 min	
72°C	1 min	
72°C	10 min	

2. Agarose gel (2 %) electrophoresis for selection of positive cases.
3. Visualization and interpretation of the results.

Fusions of *MLL* with other gene partners are detected using similar protocols (Poirel et al. 1996).

24.5 MRD detection by RT-RQ-PCR

The routine MRD assessment in AML is restricted to patients carrying the aforementioned fusion genes, identified at diagnosis.

Intragenic aberrations may also serve as MRD markers, particularly *NPM1* mutations due to their genetic stability in the course of the disease (Krönke et al. 2011). A standard protocol for MRD quantification includes the following steps:

1. RT-RQ-PCR with the use of standardized primers and probes for typical fusion genes like: *AML–ETO, CBFB–MYH11, PML–RARA* (bcr1 and bcr 3 transcript variants), designed within the Europe Against Cancer (EAC) program (Gabert et al. 2003).
2. Parallel amplification of the control *ABL* gene using the same cDNA template. Primer and probe sequences used for RT-RQ–PCR of *ABL* reference gene are shown below (Beillard et al. 2003):
   ENF1003: TGGAGATAACACTCTAAGCATAACTAAAGGT
   ENR1063: GATGTAGTTGCTTGGGACCCA
   ENP1043: FAM5′—CCATTTTTGGTTTGGGCTTCACACCATT—3′TAMRA.

- The composition of RQ-PCR mix is presented in Table 24.6.
- PCR conditions are as follows:

50°C	2 min	
95°C	10 min	
95°C	15 s	50 cycles
60°C	1 min	

3. Interpretation of the results. The calculation of the absolute number of fusion gene copies and reference *ABL* gene copies is done with the use of a standard curve prepared by the amplification of consecutive dilutions of plasmids, containing the examined transcripts. The final result is expressed as the ratio of marker gene to control gene copy numbers.

24.6 Conclusions

Risk stratification by means of molecular examination of prognostic markers identified at the time of initial diagnosis, as well as the monitoring of minimal residual disease (MRD) became standard procedures in the modern work-up of AML patients. Molecular diagnostics focuses on the detection of those markers which represent already proven prognostic value. However, as it tends to follow fundamental research, this area develops very quickly, and thus presents a challenge for clinical practice. It is possible that in the near future, detailed molecular characterization of individual leukemia cases with regard to prognostic molecular markers will underlie the design of personalized therapy. Because of an extensive genetic heterogeneity of AML, continuous update and standardization of molecular diagnostics is necessary.

References

Abbas S, Lugthart S, Kavelaars FG, Schelen A, Koenders JE, Zeilemaker A, van Putten WJ, Rijneveld AW, Lowenberg B, Valk PJ (2010) Acquired mutations in the genes encoding IDH1 and IDH2 both are recurrent aberrations in acute myeloid leukemia: prevalence and prognostic value. Blood 116:2122–2126

Abdel-Wahab O, Mullally A, Hedvat C, Garcia-Manero G, Patel J, Wadleigh M, Malinge S, Yao J, Kilpivaara O, Bhat R, Huberman K, Thomas S, Dolgalev I, Heguy A, Paietta E, Le Beau MM, Beran M, Tallman MS, Ebert BL, Kantarjian HM, Stone RM, Gilliland DG, Crispino JD, Levine RL (2009) Genetic characterization of TET1, TET2, and TET3 alterations in myeloid malignancies. Blood 114:144–147

Abu-Duhier FM, Goodeve AC, Wilson GA, Care RS, Peake IR, Reilly JT (2001) Identification of novel FLT-3 Asp835 mutations in adult acute myeloid leukaemia. Br J Haematol 113:983–988

Ammatuna E, Noguera NI, Zangrilli D, Curzi P, Panetta P, Bencivenga P, Amadori S, Federici G, Lo-Coco F (2005) Rapid detection of nucleophosmin (NPM1) mutations in acute myeloid leukemia by denaturing HPLC. Clin Chem 51:2165–2167

Beillard E, Pallisgaard N, van der Velden VH, Bi W, Dee R, van der Schoot E, Delabesse E, Macintyre E, Gottardi E, Saglio G, Watzinger F, Lion T, van Dongen JJ, Hokland P, Gabert J (2003) Evaluation of candidate control genes for diagnosis and residual disease detection in leukemic patients using 'real-time' quantitative reverse-transcriptase polymerase chain reaction (RQ-PCR)—a Europe against cancer program. Leukemia 17:2474–2486

Benthaus T, Schneider F, Mellert G, Zellmeier E, Schneider S, Kakadia PM, Hiddemann W, Bohlander SK, Feuring-Buske M, Braess J, Spiekermann K, Dufour A (2008) Rapid and sensitive screening for CEBPA mutations in acute myeloid leukaemia. Br J Haematol 143:230–239

Boissel N, Leroy H, Brethon B, Philippe N, de Botton S, Auvrignon A, Raffoux E, Leblanc T, Thomas X, Hermine O, Quesnel B, Baruchel A, Leverger G, Dombret H, Preudhomme C (2006) Incidence and prognostic impact of c-Kit, FLT3, and Ras gene mutations in core binding factor acute myeloid leukemia (CBF-AML). Leukemia 20:965–970

Bowen DT, Frew ME, Hills R, Gale RE, Wheatley K, Groves MJ, Langabeer SE, Kottaridis PD, Moorman AV, Burnett AK, Linch DC (2005) RAS mutation in acute myeloid leukemia is associated with distinct cytogenetic subgroups but does not influence outcome in patients younger than 60 years. Blood 106:2113–2119

Calvo KL, Ojeda MJ, Ammatuna E, Lavorgna S, Ottone T, Targovnik HM, Lo-Coco F, Noguera NI (2009) Detection of the nucleophosmin gene mutations in acute myelogenous leukemia through RT-PCR and polyacrylamide gel electrophoresis. Eur J Haematol 82:69–72

Chou FS, Wunderlich M, Griesinger A, Mulloy JC (2011) N-Ras(G12D) induces features of stepwise transformation in preleukemic human umbilical cord blood cultures expressing the AML1-ETO fusion gene. Blood 117:2237–2240

Dohner K, Schlenk RF, Habdank M, Scholl C, Rucker FG, Corbacioglu A, Bullinger L, Frohling S, Dohner H (2005) Mutant nucleophosmin (NPM1) predicts favorable prognosis in younger adults with acute myeloid leukemia and normal cytogenetics: interaction with other gene mutations. Blood 106:3740–3746

Dohner H, Estey EH, Amadori S, Appelbaum FR, Buchner T, Burnett AK, Dombret H, Fenaux P, Grimwade D, Larson RA, Lo-Coco F, Naoe T, Niederwieser D, Ossenkoppele GJ, Sanz MA, Sierra J, Tallman MS, Lowenberg B, Bloomfield CD (2010) Diagnosis and management of acute myeloid leukemia in adults: recommendations from an international expert panel, on behalf of the European LeukemiaNet. Blood 115:453–474

Frohling S, Schlenk RF, Stolze I, Bihlmayr J, Benner A, Kreitmeier S, Tobis K, Dohner H, Dohner K (2004) CEBPA mutations in younger adults with acute myeloid leukemia and normal cytogenetics: prognostic relevance and analysis of cooperating mutations. J Clin Oncol 22:624–633

Fuster O, Barragan E, Bolufer P, Cervera J, Larrayoz MJ, Jimenez-Velasco A, Martinez-Lopez J, Valencia A, Moscardo F, Sanz MA (2009) Rapid detection of KIT mutations in core-binding factor acute myeloid leukemia using high-resolution melting analysis. J Mol Diagn 11:458–463

Gabert J, Beillard E, van der Velden VH, Bi W, Grimwade D, Pallisgaard N, Barbany G, Cazzaniga G, Cayuela JM, Cave H, Pane F, Aerts JL, De Micheli D, Thirion X, Pradel V, Gonzalez M, Viehmann S, Malec M, Saglio G, van Dongen JJ (2003) Standardization and quality control studies of 'real-time' quantitative reverse transcriptase polymerase chain reaction of fusion gene transcripts for residual disease detection in leukemia—a Europe against cancer program. Leukemia 17:2318–2357

Gaidzik VI, Bullinger L, Schlenk RF, Zimmermann AS, Rock J, Paschka P, Corbacioglu A, Krauter J, Schlegelberger B, Ganser A, Spath D, Kundgen A, Schmidt-Wolf IG, Gotze K, Nachbaur D, Pfreundschuh M, Horst HA, Dohner H, Dohner K (2011) RUNX1 mutations in acute myeloid leukemia: results from a comprehensive genetic and clinical analysis from the AML study group. J Clin Oncol 29:1364–1372

Garçon L, Libura M, Delabesse E, Valensi F, Asnafi V, Berger C, Schmitt C, Leblanc T, Buzyn A, Macintyre E (2005) DEK-CAN molecular monitoring of myeloid malignancies could aid therapeutic stratification. Leukemia 19:1338–1344

Gelsi-Boyer V, Trouplin V, Adelaide J, Bonansea J, Cervera N, Carbuccia N, Lagarde A, Prebet T, Nezri M, Sainty D, Olschwang S, Xerri L, Chaffanet M, Mozziconacci MJ, Vey N, Birnbaum D (2009) Mutations of polycomb-associated gene ASXL1 in myelodysplastic syndromes and chronic myelomonocytic leukaemia. Br J Haematol 145:788–800

Green CL, Evans CM, Hills RK, Burnett AK, Linch DC, Gale RE (2010) The prognostic significance of IDH1 mutations in younger adult patients with acute myeloid leukemia is dependent on FLT3/ITD status. Blood 116:2779–2782

Grossmann V, Kohlmann A, Klein HU, Schindela S, Schnittger S, Dicker F, Dugas M, Kern W, Haferlach T, Haferlach C (2011a) Targeted next-generation sequencing detects point mutations, insertions, deletions and balanced chromosomal rearrangements as well as identifies novel leukemia-specific fusion genes in a single procedure. Leukemia 25:671

Grossmann V, Tiacci E, Holmes AB, Kohlmann A, Martelli MP, Kern W, Spanhol-Rosseto A, Klein HU, Dugas M, Schindela S, Trifonov V, Schnittger S, Haferlach C, Bassan R, Wells VA, Spinelli O, Chan J, Rossi R, Baldoni S, De Carolis L, Goetze K, Serve H, Peceny R, Kreuzer KA, Oruzio D, Specchia G, Di Raimondo F, Fabbiano F, Sborgia M, Liso A, Farinelli L, Rambaldi A, Pasqualucci L, Rabadan R, Haferlach T, Falini B (2011b) Whole-exome sequencing identifies somatic mutations of BCOR in acute myeloid leukemia with normal karyotype. Blood 118:6153–6163

Hou HA, Huang TC, Lin LI, Liu CY, Chen CY, Chou WC, Tang JL, Tseng MH, Huang CF, Chiang YC, Lee FY, Liu MC, Yao M, Huang SY, Ko BS, Hsu SC, Wu SJ, Tsay W, Chen YC, Tien HF (2010) WT1 mutation in 470 adult patients with acute myeloid leukemia: stability during disease evolution and implication of its incorporation into a survival scoring system. Blood 115:5222–5231

Kottaridis PD, Gale RE, Frew ME, Harrison G, Langabeer SE, Belton AA, Walker H, Wheatley K, Bowen DT, Burnett AK, Goldstone AH, Linch DC (2001) The presence of a FLT3 internal tandem duplication in patients with acute myeloid leukemia (AML) adds important prognostic information to cytogenetic risk group and response to the first cycle of chemotherapy: analysis of 854 patients from the United Kingdom Medical Research Council AML 10 and 12 trials. Blood 98:1752–1759

Krönke J, Schlenk RF, Jensen KO, Tschürtz F, Corbacioglu A, Gaidzik VI, Paschka P, Onken S, Eiwen K, Habdank M, Späth D, Lübbert M, Wattad M, Kindler T, Salih HR, Held G, Nachbaur D, von Lilienfeld-Toal M, Germing U, Haase D, Mergenthaler HG, Krauter J, Ganser A, Göhring G, Schlegelberger B, Döhner H, Döhner K (2011) Monitoring of minimal residual disease in NPM1-mutated acute myeloid leukemia: a study from the German-Austrian acute myeloid leukemia study group. J Clin Oncol 29:2709–2716

Ley TJ, Ding L, Walter MJ, McLellan MD, Lamprecht T, Larson DE, Kandoth C, Payton JE, Baty J, Welch J, Harris CC, Lichti CF, Townsend RR, Fulton RS, Dooling DJ, Koboldt DC, Schmidt H, Zhang Q, Osborne JR, Lin L, O'Laughlin M, McMichael JF, Delehaunty KD, McGrath SD, Fulton LA, Magrini VJ, Vickery TL, Hundal J, Cook LL, Conyers JJ, Swift GW, Reed JP, Alldredge PA, Wylie T, Walker J, Kalicki J, Watson MA, Heath S, Shannon WD, Varghese N, Nagarajan R, Westervelt P, Tomasson MH, Link DC, Graubert TA, DiPersio JF, Mardis ER, Wilson RK (2010) DNMT3A mutations in acute myeloid leukemia. N Engl J Med 363:2424–2433

Libura M, Asnafi V, Tu A, Delabesse E, Tigaud I, Cymbalista F, Bennaceur-Griscelli A, Villarese P, Solbu G, Hagemeijer A, Beldjord K, Hermine O, Macintyre E (2003) FLT3 and MLL intragenic abnormalities in AML reflect a common category of genotoxic stress. Blood 102:2198–2204

Libura J, Slater DJ, Felix CA, Richardson C (2005) Therapy-related acute myeloid leukemia-like MLL rearrangements are induced by etoposide in primary human CD34+ cells and remain stable after clonal expansion. Blood 105:2124–2131

Marcucci G, Strout MP, Bloomfield CD, Caligiuri MA (1998) Detection of unique ALL1 (MLL) fusion transcripts in normal human bone marrow and blood: distinct origin of normal versus leukemic ALL1 fusion transcripts. Cancer Res 58:790–793

Marcucci G, Maharry K, Wu YZ, Radmacher MD, Mrózek K, Margeson D, Holland KB, Whitman SP, Becker H, Schwind S, Metzeler KH, Powell BL, Carter TH, Kolitz JE, Wetzler M, Carroll AJ, Baer MR, Caligiuri MA, Larson RA, Bloomfield CD (2010) IDH1 and IDH2 gene mutations identify novel molecular subsets within de novo cytogenetically normal acute myeloid leukemia: a cancer and leukemia group B study. J Clin Oncol 28:2348–2355

Mead AJ, Linch DC, Hills RK, Wheatley K, Burnett AK, Gale RE (2007) FLT3 tyrosine kinase domain mutations are biologically distinct from and have a significantly more favorable prognosis than FLT3 internal tandem duplications in patients with acute myeloid leukemia. Blood 110:1262–1270

Metzeler KH, Becker H, Maharry K, Radmacher MD, Kohlschmidt J, Mrózek K, Nicolet D, Whitman SP, Wu YZ, Schwind S, Powell BL, Carter TH, Wetzler M, Moore JO, Kolitz JE, Baer MR, Carroll AJ, Larson RA, Caligiuri MA, Marcucci G, Bloomfield CD (2011a) ASXL1 mutations identify a high-risk subgroup of older patients with primary cytogenetically normal AML within the ELN Favorable genetic category. Blood 118:6920–6929

Metzeler KH, Maharry K, Radmacher MD, Mrózek K, Margeson D, Becker H, Curfman J, Holland KB, Schwind S, Whitman SP, Wu YZ, Blum W, Powell BL, Carter TH, Wetzler M, Moore JO, Kolitz JE, Baer MR, Carroll AJ, Larson RA, Caligiuri MA, Marcucci G, Bloomfield CD (2011b) TET2 mutations improve the new European LeukemiaNet risk classification of acute myeloid leukemia: A Cancer and Leukemia Group B Study. J Clin Oncol 29:1373–1381

Neubauer A, Maharry K, Mrózek K, Thiede C, Marcucci G, Paschka P, Mayer RJ, Larson RA, Liu ET, Bloomfield CD (2008) Patients with acute myeloid leukemia and RAS mutations benefit most from postremission high-dose cytarabine: a cancer and leukemia group B study. J Clin Oncol 26:4603–4609

Pabst T, Mueller BU, Zhang P, Radomska HS, Narravula S, Schnittger S, Behre G, Hiddemann W, Tenen DG (2001) Dominant-negative mutations of CEBPA, encoding CCAAT/enhancer binding protein-alpha (C/EBPalpha), in acute myeloid leukemia. Nature Genet 27:263–270

Paschka P, Marcucci G, Ruppert AS, Mrózek K, Chen H, Kittles RA, Vukosavljevic T, Perrotti D, Vardiman JW, Carroll AJ, Kolitz JE, Larson RA, Bloomfield CD (2006) Adverse prognostic significance of KIT mutations in adult acute myeloid leukemia with inv(16) and t(8;21): a cancer and leukemia group B study. J Clin Oncol 24:3904–3911

Paschka P, Marcucci G, Ruppert AS, Whitman SP, Mrózek K, Maharry K, Langer C, Baldus CD, Zhao W, Powell BL, Baer MR, Carroll AJ, Caligiuri MA, Kolitz JE, Larson RA, Bloomfield CD (2008) Wilms' tumor 1 gene mutations independently predict poor outcome in adults with cytogenetically normal acute myeloid leukemia: a cancer and leukemia group B study. J Clin Oncol 26:4595–4602

Patel JP, Gönen M, Figueroa ME, Fernandez H, Sun Z, Racevskis J, Van Vlierberghe P, Dolgalev I, Thomas S, Aminova O, Huberman K, Cheng J, Viale A, Socci ND, Heguy A, Cherry A, Vance G, Higgins RR, Ketterling RP, Gallagher RE, Litzow M, van den Brink MR, Lazarus HM, Rowe JM, Luger S, Ferrando A, Paietta E, Tallman MS, Melnick A, Abdel-Wahab O, Levine RL (2012) Prognostic relevance of integrated genetic profiling in acute myeloid leukemia. N Engl J Med 366:1079–1089

Poirel H, Rack K, Delabesse E, Radford-Weiss I, Troussard X, Debert C, Leboeuf D, Bastard C, Picard F, Veil-Buzyn A, Flandrin G, Bernard O, Macintyre E (1996) Incidence and characterization of MLL gene (11q23) rearrangements in acute myeloid leukemia M1 and M5. Blood 87:2496–2505

Rocquain J, Carbuccia N, Trouplin V, Raynaud S, Murati A, Nezri M, Tadrist Z, Olschwang S, Vey N, Birnbaum D, Gelsi-Boyer V, Mozziconacci MJ (2010) Combined mutations of ASXL1, CBL, FLT3, IDH1, IDH2, JAK2, KRAS, NPM1, NRAS, RUNX1, TET2 and WT1 genes in myelodysplastic syndromes and acute myeloid leukemias. BMC Cancer 10:401–407

Roti G, Rosati R, Bonasso R, Gorello P, Diverio D, Martelli MF, Falini B, Mecucci C (2006) Denaturing high-performance liquid chromatography: a valid approach for identifying NPM1 mutations in acute myeloid leukemia. J Mol Diagn 8:254–259

Steensma DP, Gibbons RJ, Mesa RA, Tefferi A, Higgs DR (2005) Somatic point mutations in RUNX1/CBFA2/AML1 are common in high-risk myelodysplastic syndrome, but not in myelofibrosis with myeloid metaplasia. Eur J Haematol 74:47–53

Tan AY, Westerman DA, Carney DA, Seymour JF, Juneja S, Dobrovic A (2008) Detection of NPM1 exon 12 mutations and FLT3—internal tandem duplications by high resolution melting analysis in normal karyotype acute myeloid leukemia. J Hematol Oncol 1:10

Tefferi A, Lasho TL, Abdel-Wahab O, Guglielmelli P, Patel J, Caramazza D, Pieri L, Finke CM, Kilpivaara O, Wadleigh M, Mai M, McClure RF, Gilliland DG, Levine RL, Pardanani A, Vannucchi AM (2010) IDH1 and IDH2 mutation studies in 1473 patients with chronic-, fibrotic- or blast-phase essential thrombocythemia, polycythemia vera or myelofibrosis. Leukemia 24:1302–1309

Thiede C, Steudel C, Mohr B, Schaich M, Schakel U, Platzbecker U, Wermke M, Bornhauser M, Ritter M, Neubauer A, Ehninger G, Illmer T (2002) Analysis of FLT3-activating mutations in 979 patients with acute myelogenous leukemia: association with FAB subtypes and identification of subgroups with poor prognosis. Blood 99:4326–4335

Thiede C, Koch S, Creutzig E, Steudel C, Illmer T, Schaich M, Ehninger G (2006) Prevalence and prognostic impact of NPM1 mutations in 1485 adult patients with acute myeloid leukemia (AML). Blood 107:4011–4020

van Dongen JJ, Macintyre EA, Gabert JA, Delabesse E, Rossi V, Saglio G, Gottardi E, Rambaldi A, Dotti G, Griesinger F, Parreira A, Gameiro P, Diaz MG, Malec M, Langerak AW, San Miguel JF, Biondi A (1999) Standardized RT-PCR analysis of fusion gene transcripts from chromosome aberrations in acute leukemia for detection of minimal residual disease. Report of the BIOMED-1 Concerted Action: investigation of minimal residual disease in acute leukemia. Leukemia 13:1901–1928

Wang YY, Zhao LJ, Wu CF, Liu P, Shi L, Liang Y, Xiong SM, Mi JQ, Chen Z, Ren R, Chen SJ (2011) C-KIT mutation cooperates with full-length AML1-ETO to induce acute myeloid leukemia in mice. Proc Nat Acad Sci USA 108:2450–2455

Whitman SP, Archer KJ, Feng L, Baldus C, Becknell B, Carlson BD, Carroll AJ, Mrózek K, Vardiman JW, George SL, Kolitz JE, Larson RA, Bloomfield CD, Caligiuri MA (2001) Absence of the wild-type allele predicts poor prognosis in adult de novo acute myeloid leukemia with normal cytogenetics and the internal tandem duplication of FLT3: a cancer and leukemia group B study. Cancer Res 61:7233–7239

Wouters BJ, Lowenberg B, Erpelinck-Verschueren CA, van Putten WL, Valk PJ, Delwel R (2009) Double CEBPA mutations, but not single CEBPA mutations, define a subgroup of acute myeloid leukemia with a distinctive gene expression profile that is uniquely associated with a favorable outcome. Blood 113:3088–3091

Chapter 25
Assessment of the Presence and the Level of *BCR-ABL* Fusion Gene Expression and Mutational Status in *ABL* Kinase Domain

Sylwia Czekalska, Magdalena Zawada and Izabela Florek

Abstract In this chapter, selected molecular methods currently widely applied for the diagnostics and assessment of minimal residual disease (MRD) in patients with chronic myelogenous leukemia (CML) are presented. At the time of diagnosis, the qualitative RT-PCR method is employed. It allows for the identification of the type of *BCR-ABL* fusion gene. During follow-up, the quantitative RQ-PCR analysis is used for monitoring the kinetics of changes in the *BCR-ABL* fusion gene expression level. The results of these analyses might indicate the need for therapy modification. In case of undetectable *BCR-ABL* fusion gene levels in RQ-PCR, a more sensitive approach, nested RT-PCR, might be performed. In case of lack or loss of molecular response, the assessment of mutational status of *ABL* kinase domain is required.

25.1 Introduction

In patients with suspected chronic myelogenous leukemia (CML), RT-PCR method (reverse transcription and qualitative polymerase chain reaction) is employed at the moment of diagnosis. Multiplex RT-PCR, with primer pairs specific for typical and rare transcripts of the *BCR-ABL* allows for identification of the type of the fusion gene. During follow-up, the quantitative real-time PCR technique (RQ-PCR) is the best method for monitoring the response to treatment with tyrosine kinase inhibitors (TKI) in patients with CML. The quantitative

S. Czekalska (✉) · M. Zawada · I. Florek
Department of Hematology, Jagiellonian University Medical College, Kopernika 17, 31-501 Kraków, Poland
e-mail: diagmol@cm-uj.krakow.pl

M. Witt et al. (eds.), *Molecular Aspects of Hematologic Malignancies*, Principles and Practice, DOI: 10.1007/978-3-642-29467-9_25,

analysis is performed every 3 months at the beginning of TKI therapy, but it might be performed more frequently in case of suboptimal response or lack of response (e.g., every month). After fourfold to fivefold logarithmic reduction of the *BCR-ABL* transcript level or negativity in the RQ-PCR results, further monitoring of treatment results should optimally be performed by using a nested RT-PCR, characterized by higher sensitivity than RQ-PCR. When the PCR product of the *BCR-ABL* fusion gene is detected in the nested RT-PCR, the RQ-PCR analysis is performed again. In situations when the level of the *BCR-ABL* fusion gene in the logarithmic scale is doubled or higher, based on the last RQ-PCR result combined with concomitant resistance to imatinib treatment, ABL kinase domain (ABL KD) should be sequenced.

25.2 Biological Material

Peripheral blood is the best biological material used both at the time of diagnosis (the presence and the type of the *BCR-ABL* fusion gene) and during follow-up, when minimal residual disease is monitored (the level of the *BCR-ABL* expression). Peripheral blood is collected into tubes with EDTA (anticoagulant). Heparin should not be used as an anticoagulant due to its PCR-inhibiting properties.

Nuclear cells are isolated from the peripheral blood sample. The minimal volume of blood is 10 ml, but the most important factor is the number of white blood cells (WBC)—the optimal 2×10^7 per sample.

The recommended volume of blood used for isolation is no more than 12 ml; otherwise, the procedure can require additional steps with a lysis buffer, which may influence the quality of the nuclear cells and consequently RNA. Moreover, the isolation of mononuclear cells by density gradient centrifugation method is not recommended, as it may result in a lower sensitivity of the RT-PCR, RQ-PCR, and ABL KD mutation status analysis, due to the depletion of granulocytes during MNC isolation. According to current standards, the time lapse between blood collection and preservation of isolated cells should be no longer than 24 h (Branford et al. 2006).

25.2.1 White Blood Cells Isolation Protocol

1. An appropriate volume of peripheral blood, containing approximately 2×10^7 nuclear cells, is put into a 50 ml tube and filled up to 40 ml with ammonium chloride.
2. The original tube with collected blood is rinsed with an additional 10 ml of ammonium chloride and this volume is used to filling the tube (from point 1) up to 50 ml.
3. The lysis of erythrocytes is performed by keeping the sample on ice (10 min). During incubation, the sample is mixed by inverting the tube several times.

4. The sample is centrifuged (400×*g*, 10 min).
5. The supernatant is discarded.
6. About 25–30 ml of PBS buffer (without Ca^{2+} and Mg^{2+}) is added. Then the sample is mixed to suspend the pellet of cells in the PBS buffer.
7. The sample is centrifuged (400×*g*, 10 min).
8. The supernatant is discarded and the pellet is dried.
9. The pellet is suspended in reagent for RNA isolation based on a modified Chomczyński–Sacchi method. Suspending of the pellet is performed with a needle (0.9 × 40 mm) and syringe (2 or 5 ml). The shearing is performed until the mixture becomes liquid and the sample is transferred to a 2 ml tube.
10. The mixture is frozen in −20 °C or in −80 °C if the sample is to be stored for longer than 1 week.

25.2.2 RNA Isolation Protocol

Each step of isolation is performed on ice. Centrifugation is performed in 2–8 °C.

1. The frozen nuclear cell homogenate is allowed to thaw on ice, vortexed, and incubated in a thermoblock (37 °C, 10 min, 1,400 rpm). It is then placed on ice for 10 min.
2. At least 0.2 ml of chloroform (temp. 4 °C) is added and the sample is vortexed for 15 min. The sample is centrifuged (12,000×*g*, 10 min).
3. After centrifuging, the mixture is separated into two phases:

   - Lower—red—phenol:chloroform phase
   - upper—colorless—water phase—for RNA isolation.

4. The water phase is transferred to a new 1.5 ml tube and 0.2 ml of chloroform is added. The sample is vortexed for a short time—until the mixture becomes milky (very important: the mixture must be homogeneous).
5. The sample is centrifuged (12,000×*g*, 10 min). The upper water phase is transferred to a new 1.5 ml tube; 0.5 ml of cold (4 °C) absolute ethanol (EtOH) is added and the sample is incubated in −20 °C for at least 30 min or overnight (recommended).
6. The sample is centrifuged (12,000×*g*, 10 min).
7. The supernatant is discarded and at least 1 ml of ice cold 70 % EtOH (−20 °C) is added.
8. The mixture is vortexed and the sample is centrifuged (7,500×*g*, 5 min).
9. The supernatant is discarded (using a 1,000 μl tip), the pellet is dried using a 10 μl tip or a glass capillary.
10. The pellet is finally dried in a thermomixer (37 °C, 2–5 min, 300 rpm) in an open tube. The pellet is suspended in approximately 24 μl nuclease-free water.
11. RNA suspended in water is incubated in the thermomixer (65 °C, 5 min, 0 rpm)
12. RNA is stored in −80 °C.

25.2.3 Spectrophotometric Assessment of RNA Concentration and Quality

The concentration and quality of isolated RNA is assessed by the spectrophotometric measurement by using: 260 nm wave length (for RNA concentration), 280 nm (for proteins concentration), and 320 nm (phenol contamination). The ratio A_{260nm}/A_{280nm} should be ideally 2.0. The lower value means that the sample is contaminated by proteins. The absorbance measured at 320 nm should equal 0.

25.3 Reverse Transcription Reaction

During reverse transcription reaction (RT), cDNA is obtained, which is then used as a template for RT-PCR, RQ-PCR, and *ABL* mutation analysis. The guidelines for the RT-based analyses in CML patients have been developed by the European standardization program (*BIOMED 1 Concerted Action* within the confines of *European Leukemia Net*) (Branford et al. 2006; van Dongen et al. 1999).

25.3.1 Reverse Transcription Protocol

1. A volume of RNA containing 2 μg is used and water is added up to 5 μl.
2. The sample is subjected to denaturation in a thermocycler (70 °C, 10 min), then it is immediately placed on ice and incubated for 2–3 min.
3. The reaction mixture is prepared as described in Table 25.1. Then it is added to RNA with water and the sample is amplified according to the temperature profile described below:

70 °C	10 min
Incubation on ice	2–3 min
20 °C	10 min
42 °C	45 min
99 °C	3 min
4 °C	∞

4. cDNA is resuspended with nuclease-free water in a ratio: 2 parts of cDNA : 3 parts of water. cDNA should be stored at −20 °C.

The quality and efficiency of the RT reaction is checked by amplification of one of the reference genes: *ABL* (v-abl Abelson murine leukemia viral oncogene homolog 1), *BCR* (breakpoint cluster region), or *GUS* (*β*-glucuronidase). The detailed protocols of this analysis are shown in Sect. 25.7 of this chapter.

Table 25.1 Contents of reverse transcription reaction mixture (van Dongen et al. 1999)

Reagent	Initial concentration	Volume [μl]	Final concentration
Reverse transcriptase	200 U/μl	1.0	200 U
Buffer FSB (First Strand Buffer; 250 mM TrisHCl pH 8.3, 375 mM KCl, 15 mM $MgCl_2$)	5x	4.0	1x
Random hexamers	100 mM	5.0	25 mM
dNTP	25 mM	0.8	1 mM
RNase inhibitor	20 U/μl	0.5	10 U
DTT (Ditiotreitol)	100 mM	2.0	10 mM
RNase free water	–	1.7	–
Template (RNA)	–	5 (RNA + water)	2 μg
Final volume	–	20	–

Table 25.2 Sequences of primers for multiplex RT-PCR

Primer	Sequence 5′—3′
ABL a3 B	GTT TGG GCT TCA CAC CAT TCC
BCR b1 A	GAA GTG TTT CAG AAG CTT CTC C
BCR e1 A	GAC TGC AGC TCC AAT GAG AAC
BCR e6 S2	GAC TTA CCT GAG CCA CCT GGA G
BCR c3 A	ACG GCG AGA GCA CGG ACA

25.4 Multiplex RT-PCR

At the moment of diagnosis, the detection of the *BCR-ABL* fusion gene is performed by using the multiplex RT-PCR technique that allows for the identification of several transcripts of this fusion gene, resulting from different breakpoints. The mixture of reagents contains five primers: four specific for different types of transcripts (complementary to different parts of the *BCR* gene) and 1 common primer (specific for *ABL*) (Table 25.2). The contents of a reaction mixture are presented in Table 25.3.

25.4.1 Multiplex RT-PCR protocol

1. The reaction mixture is prepared as shown in Table 25.3.
2. The amplification is performed with the use of the following controls:
   - Positive controls—cDNA with known type of *BCR-ABL* transcript (*b2a2*, *b3a2*, *e1a2*).
   - Non-amplified control—cDNA without the *BCR-ABL* transcript, isolated in the same RNA batch and transcribed in the same RT reaction—the purity of the RNA isolation and RT reaction control.

Table 25.3 Contents of multiplex RT-PCR reaction mixture

Reagent	Initial concentration	Volume [μl]	Final concentration
RNase free water	–	7.7	–
PCR buffer without $MgCl_2$	10x	2.5	1x
dNTP	2.5 mM	1.2	120 μM
GC-rich solution	5x	1.2	0.24x
$MgCl_2$	25 mM	2.0	2 mM
ABL a3 B	10 μM	1.0	0.4 μM
BCR b1 A	10 μM	1.0	0.4 μM
BCR e1 A	10 μM	1.0	0.4 μM
BCR e6 S2	10 μM	1.0	0.4 μM
BCR c3 A	10 μM	1.0	0.4 μM
Polymerase (hot start type)	5 U/μl	0.4	2 U
Template (cDNA)	–	5.0	–
Final volume	–	25	–

- Negative control—non-template control—water instead of cDNA—reagents purity control.

3. 5 μl of cDNA is added to 20 μl of the PCR mixture and amplified at the temperature profile mentioned below:

95 °C	4 min	
95 °C	30 s	35 cycles
62 °C	1 min	35 cycles
72 °C	1 min	35 cycles
72 °C	7 min	
4 °C	∞	

25.5 Nested RT-PCR

A more sensitive RT-PCR method for *BCR-ABL* identification is nested RT-PCR. It is composed of external and internal PCR steps. The sensitivity of this reaction is about 10^{-6}. Nested PCR is performed for 3 typical transcripts types of the *BCR-ABL* fusion gene: *b2a2, b3a2,* and *e1a2*. According to recommendations, quantitative RQ-PCR reaction is the gold standard for monitoring the minimal residual disease (MRD). Although, when *BCR-ABL* is undetermined, nested RT-PCR reaction is performed.

25.5.1 Nested RT-PCR Protocol: External Step

Sequences of primers for the external reaction of nested RT-PCR are shown in Table 25.4.

Table 25.4 Sequences of primers for the external reaction of nested RT-PCR

Primer	Sequence 5′—3′	Transcript type
NB1+	GAG CGT GCA GAG TGG AGG GAG AAC A	*b2a2, b3a2*
ABL3 −	GGT ACC AGG AGT GTT TCT CCA GAC TG	*b2a2, b3a2, e1a2*
BCR1+	GAA CTC GCA ACA GTC CTT CGA	*e1a2*

1. The reaction mixture is prepared as shown in Table 25.5 (for transcripts *b2a2, b3a2*) or in Table 25.6 (for transcript *e1a2*).
2. Control amplification is required (see Sect. 25.4.1).
3. 5 μl of cDNA is added to 20 μl of PCR mixture and amplified at the temperature profile shown below:

95°C	4 min	
95°C	30 s	35 cycles
60°C	40 s	35 cycles
72°C	50 s	35 cycles
72°C	7 min	
4°C	∞	

25.5.2 *Nested RT-PCR Protocol: Internal Step*

Sequences of primers for the internal reaction of nested RT-PCR are shown in Table 25.7.

1. The reaction mixture is prepared as shown in Table 25.8 (for transcripts *b2a2, b3a2*) or in Table 25.9 (for transcript *e1a2*).
2. 2 μl of the external PCR product is added to 23 μl of the PCR mixture and amplified at the temperature profile shown below:

95 °C	4 min	
95 °C	30 s	35 cycles
58 °C	30 s	35 cycles
72 °C	30 s	35 cycles
72 °C	7 min	
4 °C	∞	

25.6 Agarose Gel Electrophoresis

The final step of detection of the *BCR-ABL* products is horizontal electrophoresis, in 2 % agarose gel. To prepare 100 ml of the agarose gel 2 g of agarose and 70 μl of EtBr (1 mg/ml) are added to 100 ml of TAE buffer 1x. The electrophoresis is performed at a

Table 25.5 Contents of the external RT-PCR mixture (transcripts *b2a2* and *b3a2*)

Reagent	Initial concentration	Volume [μl]	Final concentration
RNase free water	–	8.7	–
PCR buffer with $MgCl_2$	10x	2.5	1x
dNTP	2,5 mM	1.6	160 μM
GC-rich solution	5x	5.0	1x
ABL3 -	10 μM	1.0	0.4 μM
NB1 +	10 μM	1.0	0.4 μM
Polymerase (hot start type)	5U/μl	0.2	1 U
Template (cDNA)	–	5.0	–
Final volume	–	25	–

Table 25.6 Contents of the external RT-PCR reaction mixture (transcript *e1a2*)

Reagent	Initial concentration	Volume [μl]	Final concentration
RNase free water	–	7.7	–
PCR buffer with $MgCl_2$	10x	2.5	1x
dNTP	2.5 mM	1.6	160 μM
GC-rich solution	5x	5.0	1x
$MgCl_2$	25 mM	1.0	1 mM
ABL3 –	10 μM	1.0	0.4 μM
BCR1 +	10 μM	1.0	0.4 μM
Polimerase (hot start type)	5U/μl	0.2	1 U
Template (cDNA)	–	5.0	–
Final volume	–	25	–

Table 25.7 Sequences of primers for the internal reaction of nested RT-PCR

Primer	Sequence 5′—3′	Transcript type
B2A +	TTC AGA AGC TTC TCC CTG ACA T	*b2a2, b3a2*
CA3–	TGT TGA CTG GCG TGA TGT AGT TGC TTG	*b2a2, b3a2, e1a2*
E1N+	AGA TCT GGC CCA ACG ATG ACG A	*e1a2*

voltage of 5 V/cm and with a current intensity of 100 mA for about 30–40 min in the presence of the DNA molecular weight marker (50-1,000 bp). The results are analyzed in the transilluminator with the use of UV light and photo documented. The expected sizes of PCR products are shown in Tables 25.10 and 25.11.

25.7 Reverse Transcriptase Quantitative Polymerase Chain Reaction

For technical principles of this method see Chap. 20. Reverse Transcriptase Quantitative Polymerase Chain Reaction (RT-RQ-PCR) analysis of *BCR-ABL* transcript levels is performed according to the *Europe Against Cancer* program using TaqMan technology (Gabert et al. 2003) and the following guidelines:

Table 25.8 Contents of the internal RT-PCR reaction mixture (transcripts *b2a2* and *b3a2*)

Reagent	Initial concentration	Volume [μl]	Final concentration
RNase free water	–	11.7	–
PCR buffer with $MgCl_2$	10x	2.5	1x
dNTP	2.5 mM	1.6	160 μM
GC-rich solution	5x	5.0	1x
CA3–	10 μM	1.0	0.4 μM
B2A+	10 μM	1.0	0.4 μM
Polymerase (hot start type)	5U/μl	0.2	1U
Template (external PCR product)	–	2.0	–
Final volume	–	25	–

Table 25.9 Contents of internal RT-PCR reaction mixture (transcript *e1a2*)

Reagent	Initial concentration	Volume [μl]	Final concentration
RNase free water	–	10.7	–
PCR buffer with $MgCl_2$	10x	2.5	1x
dNTP	2.5 mM	1.6	160 μM
GC-rich solution	5x	5.0	1x
$MgCl_2$	25 mM	1.0	1 mM
CA3–	10 μM	1.0	0.4 μM
E1N+	10 μM	1.0	0.4 μM
Polymerase (hot start type)	5U/μl	0.2	1U
Template (external PCR product)	–	2.0	–
Final volume	–	25	–

Table 25.10 Multiplex RT-PCR products [bp]

BCR-ABL transcript type		
	a2	*a3*
b2	342	168
b3	417	243
e1	521	347
e6	621	447
c3	586	412

Table 25.11 Nested RT-PCR products [bp]

	External RT-PCR	Internal RT-PCR
b2a2	455	383
b3a2	530	458
e1a2	468	325

1. Amplification of all samples and negative controls (NTC–no template control) is performed at least in duplicates using a 96-well plate format. The contents of the reaction mix, primers, and molecular probes sequences are presented in Tables 25.12 and 25.13.

Table 25.12 RT-RQ-PCR reaction mix (Gabert et al. 2003)

Reagent	Initial concentration	Volume [μl]	Final concentration
Reaction mix (commercially available)	2x	12.5	1x
Forward primer	30 μM	0.25	300 nM
Reverse primer	30 μM	0.25	300 nM
TaqMan probe	20 μM	0.25	200 nM
RNase free water	–	6.75	–
Template (cDNA)	–	5.0	–
Final volume	–	25.0	–

Table 25.13 Sequences of primers and TaqMan probes used in RQ-PCR analysis (Gabert et al. 2003)

Analyzed gene	Name of oligonucleotide	Sequence 5′—3′
ABL	Primer ENF1003	TGG AGA TAA CAC TCT AAG CAT AAC TAA AGG T
	Primer ENR1063	GAT GTA GTT CTT GGG ACC CA
	Molecular probe ENP1043	FAM[a]-CCA TTT TTG GTT TGG GCT TCA CAC CAT T-TAMRA[b]
BCR-ABL	Primer ENF501	TCC GCT GAC CAT CAA Y[c]AA GGA
	Primer ENR561	CAC TCA GAC CCT GAG GCT CAA
	Molecular probe ENP541	TAMRA-CCC TTC AGC GGC CAG TAG CAT CTG A-FAM

[a] FAM—fluorescent dye, 6-fluoresceine, reporter
[b] TAMRA—fluorescent dye, 6-carboksytetramethylorodamine, quencher
[c] Y—cytosine or thymine; due to polymorphism in the *BCR* gene

2. Amplification is performed using the following temperature profile:

50 °C	2 min	
95 °C	10 min	
95 °C	15 s	50 cycles
60 °C	60 s	50 cycles

   A temperature of 50 °C is required for UNG (Uracil N-Glycosylase) enzyme activation. UNG hydrolyses uracil-glycosidic bonds in DNA containing dUTP (due to the substitution of dTTP with dUTP in commercially available PCR reaction mix) that causes dUTP-containing DNA degradation, thus preventing contamination with amplicons from previous RQ-PCR reactions. A temperature of 95 °C for 10 min is required for polymerase activation.
3. For precise assessment of cDNA amount and thus *BCR-ABL* transcript levels in the analyzed samples, the serial plasmid dilutions are amplified (Branford et al. 2006). The plasmid contains inserts of cDNA of the *BCR-ABL* and *ABL* genes. Serial dilutions correspond to known copy numbers of the analyzed genes:
   - for *BCR-ABL*: 10^6–10^1
     (1 000 000, 100 000, 1000, 100, 10 fusion gene copies/5 μl)

- for *ABL*: 10^5–10^3
  (100 000, 10 000, 1000 gene copies/5 μl).
  BCR-ABL plasmid contains two of the most frequently expressed transcripts: *b3a2* and *b2a2*.
  Based on the plasmid amplification results, the standard curves are automatically determined. The correctness of standard curves is estimated based on the following parameters:
- Correlation coefficient value—should be higher than 0.95
- Slope ideal value is −3.33 (acceptable between −3.2 and −3.6)
- Intercept value—approximately 40.
  Figure 25.1 presents exemplary results of the RQ-PCR assay. The X axis indicates the cycle numbers, while the Y axis displays fluorescence levels corresponding to each cycle. The threshold cycle (Ct) is defined as the number of the reaction cycle when a significant increase in the amount of the PCR product is observed for the first time (Fig. 25.1a). In the lower part of Fig. 25.1, the standard curve for *BCR-ABL* is presented. Points represent the plasmid dilutions (Fig. 25.1b).

4. In order to check the RNA quality and the RT reaction productivity, amplification of the control gene: *ABL*, *BCR*, or *GUS* is performed. Samples with the Ct values for the amplification of the control gene above 28 are not analyzed because of RNA degradation.
5. For each reaction, non-template control (NTC) is amplified: instead of template, nuclease-free water is used.
6. Reporting the results of the RQ-PCR assays: with the use of the standard curves, the *BCR-ABL* gene copy number is normalized to the control gene copy numbers—the ratio of *BCR-ABL* and control gene, e.g., *BCR-ABL/ABL* in the percentage scale. For the clinical practice, during the IRIS (*International Randomized IFN versus STI571*) study, the International Scale [IS] was established. IS makes results comparable between different local laboratories (Branford et al. 2006; Müller et al. 2009). This is the reason why every result is corrected by individual conversion factor (CF) (Table 25.14).
   For each result, the assay sensitivity is determined by the equation (Stentoft et al. 2001) (See Eq. 25.1):

$$x = 10^{\left(\frac{40 - {}_{ave}Ct_{CG}}{Y}\right)} \qquad (25.1)$$

where:

x	sensitivity of RQ-PCR
${}_{ave}Ct_{CG}$	average value of the control gene Ct for the analyzed sample
Y	intercept value (Ct value of 40 is a limit PCR cycle number for negativity)

Sensitivity of the single RQ-PCR test depends on the quality of isolated RNA (Ct of *ABL* gene) and standard curve parameters: slope and intercept.

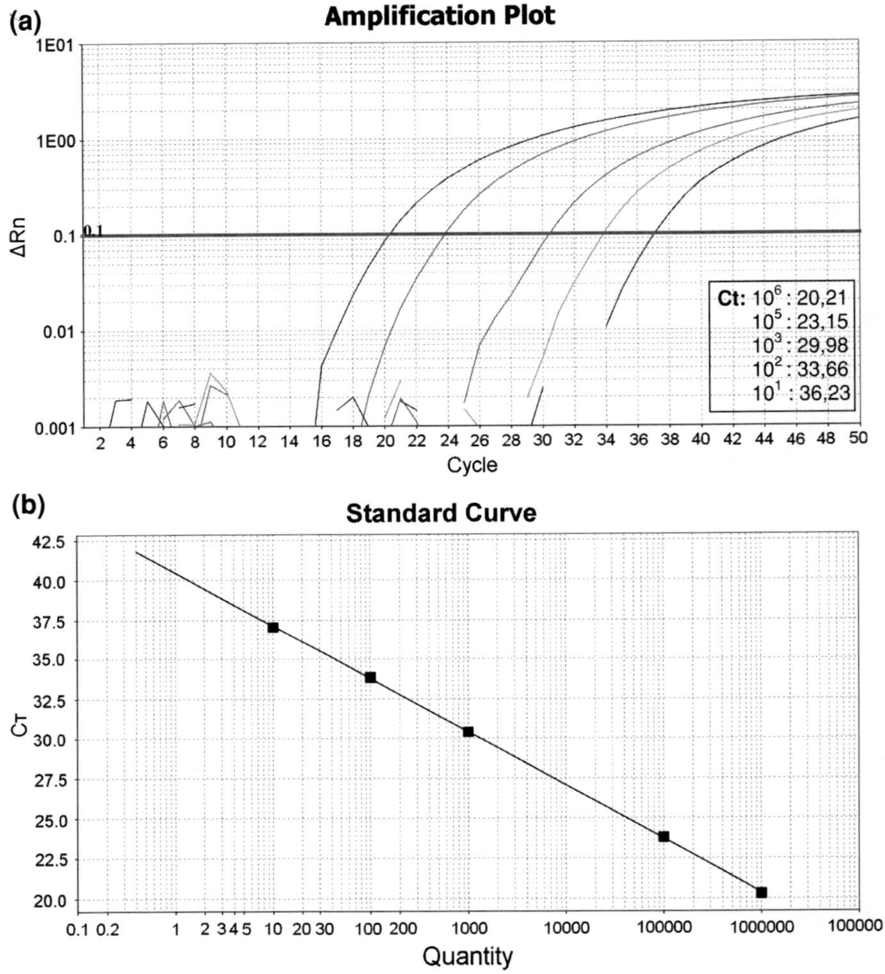

Fig. 25.1 Results of RQ-PCR amplification of serial dilution of *BCR-ABL* standard; optimal amplification plot (**a**) and standard curve (**b**) are presented

Table 25.14 The estimation of the conversion factor with example

MMR_{av} (%)	0.1 %/MMR_{av} (%) = CF	*BCR-ABL*^{L} × CF = *BCR-ABL*^{IS}
0.1	0.1/0.1 = 1	*BCR-ABL*^{L} × 1

MMR_{av}—*BCR-ABL* as MMR (*Major Molecular Response*) by IRIS
BCR-ABL^{L} —*BCR-ABL/ABL* ratio as percentage in a given laboratory
BCR-ABL^{IS} —*BCR-ABL/ABL* ratio in international scale

In Table 25.15, the suggested method for sequential reporting of results of RQ-PCR assays is shown (Hughes et al. 2006).

Table 25.15 Suggested method for sequential reporting of results of RQ-PCR assays

BCR-ABL transcripts				
Transcript type	Mean copy number of *BCR-ABL*	Mean copy number of control gene (*ABL*)	Ratio [%]	Result in IS [%]
–	–	–	–	–
BCR-ABL undetected (in all replicates)				
Total copy number of control gene (in all replicates)			–	

25.8 Analysis of Point Mutations in *ABL* Gene

One of the mechanisms of resistance to tyrosine kinase inhibitors treatment of patients suffering from CML is point mutations in *ABL* kinase domain of the *BCR-ABL* gene. To date, more than 100 point mutations have been described (Borrow 2007; Ernst et al. 2008; Shah and Sawyers 2003). Moreover, six polymorphisms, which are not reported as mutations have been described (Hughes and Branford 2009). In general, mutations may be divided into four groups depending on the affected region of the ABL domain:

- P-loop (amino acids 248–255),
- ATP-binding domain (amino acids 289–317),
- catalytic domain of oncogenic protein (amino acids 351–359),
- activation loop (amino acids 379–402) (Jones et al. 2009; Martinelli et al. 2005).

The most important point mutations are placed within the sequence coding the P-loop. Nevertheless, the entire kinase domain of *ABL* gene must be analyzed, in particular codons 240–486, with the use of the sequencing technique.

During mutation analysis, the following steps are performed: RT-PCR (external and semi-nested) to generate amplicons to be used as templates for sequencing, and PCR-based dideoxy sequencing followed by electrophoresis in high-resolution sequencing acrylamide gels or capilars. In the external RT-PCR, the whole *BCR-ABL* transcript is amplified and in semi-nested RT-PCR, only the specific *ABL* kinase domain is amplified. The sequencing reaction requires high quality of the template, determined based on the amplification of the control gene (Hughes and Branford 2006) (See Sect. 25.7).

25.8.1 Semi-Nested RT-PCR

Semi-nested RT-PCR comprises of two steps: external and semi-nested. In this type of RT-PCR only three primers are used: one common reverse for external and semi-nested steps and two forward primers, one specific for the external and the second specific for the semi-nested step. After both PCR steps, purification is required. It allows for removal of the excess of primers, nucleotides, possible unspecific PCR products, and salts (inhibition of the reaction).

Table 25.16 The contents of the external and the semi-nested PCR reaction mixture

Reagent	Initial concentration	Volume [μl]		Final concentration
		external	semi-nested	
PCR buffer for long templates	10x	2.5	2.5	1x
dNTP	2.5 mM	4	4	0.4 mM
$MgCl_2$	25 mM	0.75	0.75	0.75 mM
Forward primer	50 μM	0.2	0.2	0.4 μM
Reverse primer	50 μM	0.2	0.2	0.4 μM
Polymerase	5 U/μl	0.375	0.375	1.875 U
RNase free water	–	11.975	14.975	–
Template cDNA	–	2.5–5.0	2	–
Final volume	–	25	25	

Below are presented methods of PCR product purification:

- purifying from agarose gel,
- column-based method,
- enzymatic method,
- product dilution.

In case of obtaining single PCR product, the column-based method is recommended. When unspecific products are present it should be preceded by the excision of specific PCR product from the gel (purification from agarose gel).

25.8.1.1 The Protocol of Semi-Nested RT-PCR (Branford and Hughes 2006)

1. The external reaction is performed in the final volume of 25 μl. The components of the reaction mixture are presented in Table 25.16, primers' sequences are presented in Table 25.17. Depending on *BCR-ABL* transcript level, 2.5–5 μl of cDNA is added to the reaction mixture (see Sect. 25.3).
2. Control amplification is required (see Sect. 26.4.1).
3. The temperature profile:

94 °C	2 min	
94 °C	10 s	} 10 cycles
60 °C	30 s	
68 °C	2 min	
94 °C	10 s	} 20 cycles (external PCR)
60 °C	30 s	
68 °C	2 min plus 20 s./cycle	30 cycles (semi-nested PCR)
68 °C	7 min	

4. The obtained product is purified according to instruction enclosed in the purifying set.

Table 25.17 Sequences of primers used in the *ABL* gene mutation analysis (Branford and Hughes 2006)

Step of PCR	Primer	Sequence 5′—3′	Type of transcript
External	Forward (S1)	TGA CCA ACT CGT GTG TGA AAC TC	*b2a2 i b3a2*
	Forward (S1E)	ACC GCA TGT TCC GGG ACA AAA G	*e1a2*
External and semi-nested	Reverse (AS)	TCC ACT TCG TCT GAG ATA CTG GAT T	*b2a2, b3a2, e1a2*
semi-nested	Forward (S2)	CGC AAC AAG CCC ACT GTC T	*b2a2, b3a2, e1a2*

Table 25.18 External and semi-nested RT-PCR products [bp]

Step of PCR reaction	Type of transcript	Product size (bp)
External	*b2a2*	1,504
	b3a2	1,579
	e1a2	1,641
Semi-nested	*b2a2, b3a2 i e1a2*	863

5. Electrophoresis is performed in 2 % agarose gel (5 µl PCR product and 1 µl loading buffer is added to the well). The sizes of obtained RT-PCR products are presented in Table 25.18.
6. The semi-nested reaction is performed only when there is no band after external RT-PCR or the band is weak. If the band is clear and strong, PCR product is directly used for sequencing PCR.
7. The semi-nested reaction is performed in the final volume of 25 µl. The contents are presented in Table 25.16, primer sequences are presented in Table 25.17.
8. About 2 µl of the external PCR product is added to 23 µl of the semi-nested PCR mixture and amplified at the temperature profile shown above (with one difference: 30 cycles instead of 20 cycles).
9. After PCR, electrophoresis is performed (see point 5).
10. PCR product purification (see introduction to Sect. 26.8.1).
11. Until PCR-based dideoxy sequencing, the product should be stored at 4 °C; it should not be frozen.

25.8.2 Sequencing

The principles of sequencing technique are described in Chap. 20. The sequencing of the *BCR-ABL* fusion gene fragment encoding ABL domain is carried out in the forward and reverse direction, with the use of primers employed in the semi-nested reaction (Table 25.17). On the basis of intensity of the band obtained in the agarose electrophoresis, the amount of the purified product to be used in the

Table 25.19 The contents of the reaction mixture for the sequential PCR

Reagent	Initial concentration	Volume of reagent in μl	Final concentration
RNase free water	–	7.8	–
Buffer	5x	1	0.25x
Big Dye 3 Sequencing	–	4	–
Primer forward/Primer reverse	1 μM	3.2	0.16 μM
PCR product	–	2–4	–
Final volume	–	20	–

sequencing PCR is determined; usually it is 2 μl. There are several methods of purifying products of the sequencing PCR:

- precipitation with ethanol,
- column-based method,
- purification with the use of commercially available set—this method allows for obtaining a large amount of the highest quality product.

25.8.2.1 Dideoxy Sequencing PCR Protocol

1. The ready reaction mixture, which is a part of a commercially available set for sequencing, is thawed on ice (protected from light).
2. PCR reaction is performed as described in Table 25.19. For each primer, a separate mixture is prepared.
3. 2 μl (the maximum of 6 μl) of the purified PCR product is added to 18 μl of each reaction mixture.
4. The temperature profile of the sequencing PCR reaction:

96 °C	1 min	
96 °C	10 s	25 cycles
50 °C	30 s	
60 °C	4 min	

After the reaction and the purification, the products are separated by electrophoresis in high-resolution sequencing acrylamide gels or capilars. Until then, the samples may be stored at 4 °C (for 10 days), not exposed to light.

25.8.3 High-resolution Sequencing Electrophoresis

The electrophoresis is carried out with the use of 2–10 μl of the purified product of the sequencing PCR reaction, in accordance to the requirements of the manufacturer of the genetic analyzer applied. The obtained nucleotide sequences are compared

Table 25.20 A scheme of *ABL* gene mutation study result according to the recommendation of Hughes et al. (2006)

Replacement of amino acid	Replacement of the nucleotide	Occurrence of the P-loop	% mutant allele
–	–	–	–

with the reference sequences for the wild *ABL* gene, available in gene databases (e.g., GenBank, sequence number: M14752, X16416, U07563), with the use of a sequence analysis program. If a mutation is detected for the first time, the study must be repeated, as recommended, with the use of another blood or RNA sample taken at the same time, to guarantee that the identified nucleotide change is the result of a real mutation, and not an artifact resulting from the analysis imperfections. In Table 25.20, the *ABL* gene mutation analysis result scheme is presented.

25.9 Conclusions

Chronic Myeloid Leukemia is one of the most extensively studied malignancies. Thanks to the identification and molecular characterization of *BCR-ABL* fusion gene modern targeted therapy based on tyrosine kinase inhibitors has been implemented. CML has become a model malignancy for the application of TKI. Such sophisticated treatment needs very sensitive and specific tools for diagnosis and minimal residual disease monitoring. The methods presented in this chapter are essential molecular tools required for the proper diagnostics and monitoring of CML patients, enabling optimization of therapy and rapid clinical decision making in case of treatment failure. The methods presented in this chapter, although labor intensive and time-consuming, are characterized by high sensitivity and specificity. Standardized protocols and procedures developed in recent years enable the application of these methods for optimal management of CML treatment.

References

Borrow J (2007) Guidelines for mutation analysis of BCR/ABL kinase domain: interpreting TKI-resistance mutations in CML patients. West Midlands Regional Genetics Laboratory. Available via http://www.bwhct.nhs.uk/tki_sensitivities_final.pdf. Cited 9 Dec 2011

Branford S, Hughes T (2006) Detection of BCR-ABL mutations and resistance to imatinib mesylate. Methods Mol Med 125:93–106

Branford S, Cross NC, Hochhaus A, Radich J, Saglio G, Kaeda J, Goldman J, Hughes T (2006) Rationale for the recommendations for harmonizing current methodology for detecting BCR-ABL transcripts in patients with chronic myeloid leukaemia. Leukemia 20:1925–1930

Ernst T, Hoffmann J, Erben P, Hanfstein B, Leitner A, Hehlmann R, Hochhaus A, Müller MC (2008) ABL single nucleotide polymorphisms may masquerade as BCR-ABL mutations associated with resistance to tyrosine kinase inhibitors in patients with chronic myeloid leukemia. Haematologica 93:1389–1393

Gabert J, Beillard E, van der Velden VH, Bi W, Grimwade D, Pallisgaard N, Barbany G, Cazzaniga G, Cayuela JM, Cavé H, Pane F, Aerts JL, De Micheli D, Thirion X, Pradel V, González M, Viehmann S, Malec M, Saglio G, van Dongen JJ (2003) Standardization and quality control studies of 'real-time' quantitative reverse transcriptase polymerase chain reaction of fusion gene transcripts for residual disease detection in leukemia—a Europe Against Cancer program. Leukemia 17:2318–2357

Hughes T, Branford S (2006) Molecular monitoring of BCR-ABL as a guide to clinical management in chronic myeloid leukaemia. Blood Rev 20:29–41

Hughes T, Branford S (2009) Monitoring disease response to tyrosine kinase inhibitor therapy in CML. Hematol Am Soc Hematol Educ Program 477-87

Hughes T, Deininger M, Hochhaus A, Branford S, Radich J, Kaeda J, Baccarani M, Cortes J, Cross NC, Druker BJ, Gabert J, Grimwade D, Hehlmann R, Kamel-Reid S, Lipton JH, Longtine J, Martinelli G, Saglio G, Soverini S, Stock W, Goldman JM (2006) Monitoring CML patients responding to treatment with tyrosine kinase inhibitors: review and recommendations for harmonizing current methodology for detecting BCR-ABL transcripts and kinase domain mutations and for expressing results. Blood 108:28–37

Jones D, Kamel-Reid S, Bahler D, Dong H, Elenitoba-Johnson K, Press R, Quigley N, Rothberg P, Sabath D, Viswanatha D, Weck K, Zehnder J (2009) Laboratory practice guidelines for detecting and reporting BCR-ABL drug resistance mutations in chronic myelogenous leukemia and acute lymphoblastic leukemia: a report of the Association for Molecular Pathology. J Mol Diagn 11:4–11

Martinelli G, Soverini S, Rosti G, Cilloni D, Baccarani M (2005) New tyrosine kinase inhibitors in chronic myeloid leukemia. Haematologica 90:534–541

Müller MC, Cross NC, Erben P, Schenk T, Hanfstein B, Ernst T, Hehlmann R, Branford S, Saglio G, Hochhaus A (2009) Harmonization of molecular monitoring of CML therapy in Europe. Leukemia 23:1957–1963

Shah NP, Sawyers CL (2003) Mechanisms of resistance to STI571 in Philadelphia chromosome-associated leukemias. Oncogene 20(22):7389–7395

Stentoft J, Pallisgaard N, Kjeldsen E, Holm MS, Nielsen JL, Hokland P (2001) Kinetics of BCR-ABL fusion transcript levels in chronic myeloid leukemia patients treated with STI571 measured by quantitative real- time polymerase chain reaction. Eur J Haematol 67:302–308

van Dongen JJ, Macintyre EA, Gabert JA, Delabesse E, Rossi V, Saglio G, Gottardi E, Rambaldi A, Dotti G, Griesinger F, Parreira A, Gameiro P, Diáz MG, Malec M, Langerak AW, San Miguel JF, Biondi A (1999) Standardized RT-PCR analysis of fusion gene transcripts from chromosome aberrations in acute leukaemia for detection of minimal residual disease. Report of the BIOMED-1 Concerted Action: investigation of minimal residual disease in acute leukaemia. Leukemia 13:1901–1928

Chapter 26
Studies of Rearrangements and Somatic Hypermutation of IGHV Genes in Chronic Lymphocytic Leukemia

Anton W. Langerak, Richard Rosenquist, Paolo Ghia, Chrysoula Belessi, Kostas Stamatopoulos and Frederic Davi

Abstract In this chapter, we present protocols used for the study of several aspects of immunoglobulin heavy variable (IGHV) gene mutational status, including material collection and preparation, polymerase chain reaction amplification, clonality testing, sequencing, and also data analysis, interpretation, and reporting. This chapter is based on guidelines on technical aspects and interpretation (Ghia et al., Leukemia 21:1–3, 2007; Davi et al., Leukemia 22:212–214, 2008; Langerak et al., Leukemia 25:979–984, 2011), as developed by the

A. W. Langerak (✉)
Department of Immunology, Erasmus MC, University Medical Center,
Dr. Molewaterplein 50, 3015 GE, Rotterdam, The Netherlands
e-mail: a.langerak@erasmusmc.nl

R. Rosenquist
Rudbeck Laboratory, Department of Immunology, Genetics and Pathology,
Uppsala University, Uppsala, Sweden

P. Ghia
Laboratory of B Cell Neoplasia and Unit of Lymphoid Malignancies,
Division of Molecular Oncology and Department of Onco-Hematology,
Università Vita-Salute San Raffaele and Istituto Scientifico San Raffaele, Milan, Italy

C. Belessi
Hematology Department, Nikea General Hospital, Pireaus, Greece

K. Stamatopoulos
Center for Research and Technology Hellas, Institute of Agrobiotechnology, Thessaloniki, Greece

K. Stamatopoulos
Hematology Department and HCT Unit, G. Papanicolaou Hospital, Thessaloniki, Greece

F. Davi
Laboratory of Hematology, Hôpital Pitié-Salpètrière, Université Pierre et Marie Curie, Paris, France

M. Witt et al. (eds.), *Molecular Aspects of Hematologic Malignancies*,
Principles and Practice, DOI: 10.1007/978-3-642-29467-9_26,

European Research Initiative on chronic lymphocytic leukemia (CLL) (ERIC) (www.ericll.org). Consideration of all of these aspects in a clinical diagnostic setting is highly relevant in order to generate a reliable IGHV–IGHD–IGHJ gene rearrangement sequence and to correctly report the IGHV mutational status for individual CLL patients to the referring clinician.

26.1 Introduction

Several clinical and biological parameters have been found to be associated with prognosis and outcome in chronic lymphocytic leukemia (CLL), which is, nowadays, recognized as a clinically heterogeneous disease. Since the end of the 1990s one prognostic parameter stands out as being very informative: the somatic hypermutation status of the immunoglobulin heavy variable (IGHV) genes (Damle et al. 1999; Hamblin et al. 1999), leading to its utilization for inclusion, or stratification in many clinical protocols. Indeed, it is well established that CLL cases can be categorized into two clinical subsets using the IGHV gene mutational status; one subgroup with unmutated IGHV genes (generally showing a less favorable prognosis with short time to treatment, poorer response to therapy, and an inferior overall survival), and a second group with mutated IGHV genes (with a more favorable predicted outcome). The clinically relevant distinction between 'mutated (M)' and 'unmutated (UM)' CLL is mostly made using a cut-off value of 98 % identity of the rearranged IGHV gene to the closest germline IGHV gene. Cases with less than 98 % identity are classified as M, whereas those with equal or greater than 98 % identity as UM (Damle et al. 1999; Hamblin et al. 1999). In most cases, the prognostic implications of IGHV gene analysis can be ascertained reliably using the 98 % identity cut-off level. Nevertheless, as for any mathematical cut-off value, great caution is warranted when dealing with CLL cases of 'borderline' IGHV gene mutational status (Ghia et al. 2007; Langerak et al. 2011).

26.2 Sample Source, Collection, and Preparation

Peripheral blood (PB) is generally the source of leukemic cells for IGHV gene mutational analysis, due to the high peripheral leukocyte count in most CLL patients (Table 26.1). Alternatively, bone marrow (BM), lymph node, or any other tissue/fluid with CLL cells, can be used. As the IGHV gene mutational status is a stable feature of the leukemic clone, it can be evaluated at any time point as long as a reasonable leukemic cell population is present.

PB or BM aspirates are best collected in tubes containing EDTA (ethylenediamine tetra acetic acid) as anticoagulant or in CPT (citrate/pyridoxal 5′-phosphate/

Table 26.1 Recommendations for IGHV mutational analysis procedure

Parameter	Recommended	Alternative options
Source of cells	PB	BM, lymph node, other
Anticoagulant (PB/BM)	EDTA or CPT tubes	Heparinized tubes
Work-up of cells	Ficoll gradient (PB/BM)	Tissue biopsy or cell suspension of biopsy
Type of nucleic acid	gDNA or RNA/cDNA[a]	None
PCR primers	IGHV leader or IGHV FR1[a]	IGHV FR2 (restricted)
PCR protocol	Various existing protocols	NA
Taq polymerase	No specific enzyme	NA
Clonality analysis	GS or HD analysis[a]	PAGE (without prior HD)
Sequencing	Direct, via eluted PCR product	Cloning (with caution)

[a] See Table 26.2 for specific advantages and disadvantages of each option. *BM* bone marrow; *CPT* citrate/pyridoxal 5′-phosphate/Tris; *EDTA* ethylenediamine tetra-acetic acid; *FR* framework region; *GS* GeneScan; *HD* heteroduplex; *IGHV* immunoglobulin heavy V gene; *NA* not applicable; *PAGE* polyacrylamide gel electrophoresis; *PB* peripheral blood; *PCR* polymerase chain reaction

Tris) tubes (Table 26.1). Heparin tubes, which are regularly used for flow cytometric or cytogenetic evaluation, are also an option.

1. Isolate mononuclear cells (MNCs) by density gradient centrifugation, according to a standard protocol (e.g. Ficoll). Use of whole lysed BM/PB material is possible but has drawbacks: (i) lower CLL percentage in whole lysed material might create difficulties in detection; (ii) inhibitors of polymerase chain reaction (PCR) amplification (e.g. hemoglobin) might give complications in amplification.
2. Use either cell suspensions (also appropriate for parallel-flow cytometric analysis) or total biopsies (fresh, archival) in case of lymph node material.
3. Isolate genomic DNA (gDNA) and/or RNA using column-based genomic DNA/RNA isolation kits. Alternatively, noncolumn-based DNA isolation methods (phenol/chloroform) or RNA isolation methods (e.g. Chomczyński-based method with the use of Trizol or another commercially available reagent) can also be used. Perform DNA or RNA isolation using 5–10 × 10^6 (freshly separated) MNCs. The remaining MNCs can be stored for later use, preferably in liquid nitrogen or at −80°C.
4. Assess gDNA and/or RNA quantity and quality in duplicate by optical density measurement at 260/280 nm, preferably using a microvolume spectrophotometer (e.g. Nanodrop or comparable equipment).
5. Reverse transcribe 1–2 μg RNA into complementary DNA (cDNA) using any commercially available kit.
6. Prepare working dilutions of gDNA (e.g. 20 ng/μl) for PCR amplification.

Table 26.2 Typical advantages and disadvantages of several parameters in the IGHV gene mutational analysis procedure

Parameter	Advantage	Disadvantage
Type of nucleic acid		
gDNA	More optimal for archival material (FFPE, frozen) More stable in case of material transport over long distances (reference laboratory, sample exchange) No reverse transcription step	Unproductive or second productive rearrangement might also be amplified (~15 % of cases)
RNA/cDNA	Mostly only one productive rearrangement amplified (in ~4 % also second allele) Isotype identification	Additional reverse transcription step required
PCR primers		
IGHV leader	Accurate percentage identity based on whole IGHV gene	Detection rate slightly lower than with VH FR1 set
VH FR1	Widely used in IGH clonality analysis protocols Detection rate slightly better than with IGHV leader set	Estimated percentage identity due to lack of information on 5′ part of IGHV gene
Clonality analysis		
HD analysis	Unlabeled PCR products allow direct sequencing	Detection limit slightly lower than GS
GS analysis	Detection limit slightly better than HD Optimal visualization of clonality patterns	Labeled PCR products less optimal for direct sequencing

cDNA complementary DNA; *FFPE* formalin-fixed paraffin-embedded; *FR* framework region; *gDNA* genomic DNA; *GS* GeneScan fragment; *HD* heteroduplex; *IGHV* immunoglobulin heavy V gene; *PCR* polymerase chain reaction

26.3 PCR-Based Amplification

26.3.1 gDNA Versus cDNA

Both gDNA and cDNA (from RNA) can be used as starting material for PCR-based determination of IGHV gene mutational status (Table 26.1). From a scientific point of view there is no clear preference, as both have their advantages and disadvantages (Table 26.2). However, it is advisable to have both types of material available, as occasionally proper sequence analysis from either of the two starting materials fails. Also, for a more standardized analysis in multi-center clinical trials, it is recommended to attune starting material.

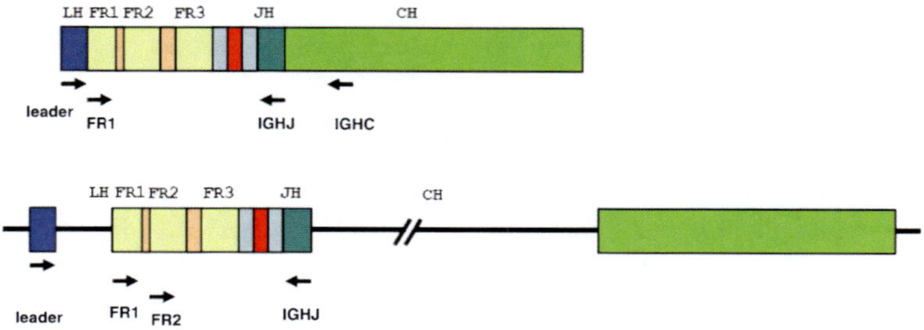

Fig. 26.1 Schematic representation of rearranged IGH transcript (*upper*) and IGH rearrangement at DNA level (*lower*), with the most relevant types of forward (IGHV leader, FR1, FR2, FR3), and reverse (IGHJ, IGHC) primers indicated

26.3.2 Primer Sets

In order to amplify IGH variable (IGHV)–IGH diversity (IGHD)–IGH joining (IGHJ) gene rearrangements, several different PCR strategies have been published (Campbell et al. 1992; Küppers et al. 1993; Aubin et al. 1995; Fais et al. 1998; Van Dongen et al. 2003). Many of these primer sets are being applied routinely in a clinical diagnostic setting, mostly for IGH clonality analysis. In principle, they can be utilized for IGHV gene mutational analysis as well. Depending on the use of gDNA or cDNA as starting material (see above), there are several options of primer sets (Fig. 26.1): (1) IGHV leader primers plus isotype-specific IGHC primer, mostly IGHM (cDNA); (2) IGHV leader primers plus consensus IGHJ primer (gDNA/cDNA); (3) VH FR1 primers plus consensus IGHJ primer (mostly gDNA). There are pros and cons with respect to the use of IGHV leader versus VH FR1 primers (Table 26.2). Most importantly, in strategies employing IGHV leader primers the whole IGHV gene is amplified, thus enabling precise calculation of the actual percentage of the identity to the germline. On the contrary, at best an estimation of the percentage identity can be obtained using VH FR1 primers. In daily practice, this estimation is virtually always accurate enough to classify the individual CLL case in a proper way, although more caution is warranted if the percentage identity is around the 98 % cut-off level (Tobin et al. 2005). In such 'borderline' cases reevaluation of the IGHV gene mutational status via a leader primer-based PCR strategy is strongly recommended. The limited IGHV gene sequence information is the reason why FR2- and FR3-based strategies are discouraged, although an FR2 strategy might occasionally be considered as an alternative if IGHV leader/FR1 PCR strategies fail or are not informative (Table 26.1). A comprehensive approach should probably include a leader-based and an FR1-based strategy. Furthermore, in multi-center clinical studies it is probably wise to standardize PCR protocols and primer sets.

26.3.3 Multiplex Versus Single PCR

For efficiency reasons, mostly a multiplex PCR protocol is employed with multiple IGHV subgroup-specific forward primers and a (consensus) reverse IGHJ or IGHM primer, rather than several single PCR reactions. However, in a fraction of cases (15 % of gDNA-based analyses, 4 % of cDNA-based analyses; Langerak et al. 2011) this will result in multiple clonal products, which pose problems for sequencing. In such cases, single PCR reactions can be employed in an attempt to generate single clonal products (see also Sect. 26.4).

26.3.4 PCR Protocol and Conditions

With respect to the detailed PCR protocol and conditions (reagents, times, temperatures), there is no preferred approach or critical parameter to be considered and/or specially optimized for the mere purpose of IGHV gene mutational analysis. Conditions of standardized protocols for IGH rearrangement analysis are in principle directly applicable (Table 26.1). Extensive experience of many laboratories has shown that the use of *Taq* polymerases with proofreading activity is not required (Table 26.1). As the rate of misincorporation during DNA amplification is low (10^{-4}–10^{-5}), this does not influence determination of the somatic mutation level on an IGHV sequence of only a few hundred nucleotides.

1. Prepare a PCR reaction mixture containing 50–100 ng of gDNA or 2 μl cDNA in a total volume of 25–50 μl.
2. Add *Taq* polymerase and forward and reverse primer(s).
3. Amplify for 35–40 cycles using a standardized PCR protocol for the employed primer sets (e.g. 7 min activation at 94°C, 30 s denaturation at 94°C, 45 s annealing at 60°C, 90 s extension at 72°C).

26.3.5 IGK and IGL Analysis

Evaluation of the mutational status is routinely performed via analysis of IGHV genes. Immunoglobulin kappa or lambda light chain variable genes (IGKV or IGLV genes, respectively) could also be tested, but mutational levels are generally lower and clinical implications have never been validated. If IGKV/IGLV genes are studied for mutations, this is usually done for specific research questions, using existing primers (Stamatopoulos et al. 2005; Belessi et al. 2005).

26.4 Clonality Testing

A key aspect of the entire IGHV gene mutational analysis procedure is post-PCR evaluation. First, it is very informative to investigate whether PCR amplicons of the correct size are present in gel electrophoresis. To this end, agarose gels or preferably polyacrylamide gels should be used, as the latter have better resolution. Second, further analysis is also required to evaluate the presence of single monoclonal (monoallelic) PCR products as opposed to patterns showing double monoclonal (biallelic) products, or even oligo/polyclonality. The latter might reflect the presence of a limited amount of leukemic cells (as might occur in small lymphocytic lymphoma, SLL or monoclonal B-cell lymphocytosis, MBL) or even the lack of a true clone in the sample (requiring reevaluation of the diagnosis). Before questioning the presence of a monoclonal B cell population, the possibility should be ruled out that no reliable sequence can be generated because the utilized primer is not annealing to the specific CLL rearrangement. Hence, in cases of unexpected lack of clonality, other primer sets should be utilized to try to amplify the true CLL clonal IGHV–IGHD–IGHJ gene rearrangement for mutational analysis.

For evaluation of monoclonal versus oligoclonal versus polyclonal patterns, two standardized methods are available: GeneScan (GS) fragment analysis (Kneba et al. 1995; Linke et al. 1997) and heteroduplex (HD) analysis (Bottaro et al. 1994; Langerak et al. 1997; González et al. 1999). Both have been proven as robust and reliable approaches in a European consortium on clonality analysis (Van Dongen et al. 2003; Evans et al. 2007). Both approaches exploit the heavy complementarity determining region 3 (VH CDR3) size heterogeneity, whereas in the HD method the differences in the actual CDR3 nucleotide sequences are also exploited. In HD analysis, PCR products are denatured and enforced to reanneal at low temperatures, resulting in smears or clear bands that reflect polyclonal or monoclonal rearrangements, respectively (Fig. 26.2). In GS analysis, fluorescently labeled PCR products are separated by high resolution gel or capillary electrophoresis, resulting in clear visualization of the level of heterogeneity of the IGHV–IGHD–IGHJ PCR products, based on CDR3 length (Fig. 26.3). In principle, GS and HD analysis serves equally to study clonality patterns (Table 26.1), although there are considerations to choose one or the other approach (Table 26.2).

1. Evaluate successful PCR amplification via gel electrophoresis. Use 5–10 μl of the PCR reaction mixture to load onto a 1 % agarose gel and visualize PCR products with e.g. ethidium bromide upon electrophoresis.
2. Evaluate the presence of clonal IGH product(s) by HD analysis. Use 25–30 μl of the PCR reaction mixture for denaturation (5 min, 95°C) and reannealing (1 h, 4°C) and load onto a 6 % polyacrylamide gel (pre-cast or hand-made gels). Following electrophoresis, visualize homo- and hetero-duplex PCR products via ethidium bromide staining or silver staining.

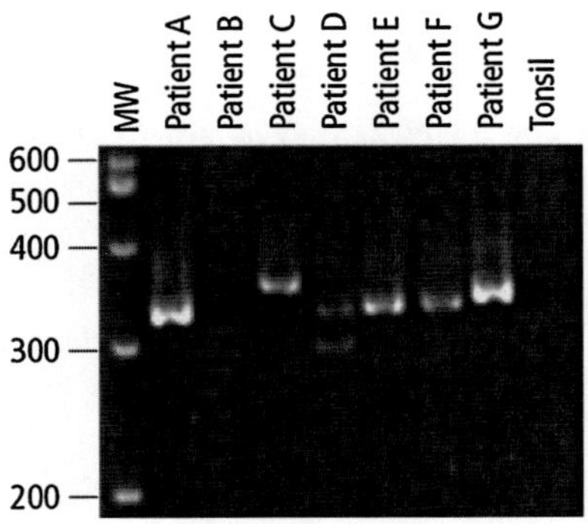

Fig. 26.2 Heteroduplex analysis of gDNA-based multiplex FR1-IGH PCR products. In patients *A, C, E–G* clear monoallelic products of the expected size are seen, which implies direct sequencing. In case *D* biallelic PCR products are found, prompting further analysis via single PCR reactions and/or gel excision of the PCR products prior to sequencing. In case *B* no clonal IGH product is found; possible explanations are (i) non-CLL lymphocytosis; (ii) small CLL clone below detection limit (e.g. follow-up sample after treatment); (iii) CLL clone that is not recognized by the primers used, prompting the use of different primer sets, and/or different starting material

3. Evaluate the presence of clonal IGH product(s) by GS fragment analysis. Load 1 μl of a 1:10 diluted PCR reaction mixture on an automated sequencer. Analyze GS profiles using commercially available software.

The results of HD- or GS-based clonality testing are decisive for determining the subsequent strategy. Several scenarios are possible, which are discussed more extensively in Figs. 26.2 and 26.3 and in Sect. 26.5: (a) single clonal (monoallelic) product; (b) >1 clonal product; (c) no clonal products.

26.5 Sequencing

In case of a monoallelic rearrangement (see Sect. 26.4), direct sequencing of the PCR product can be performed. However, in case of biallelic rearrangements, the two PCR products should be excised from the polyacrylamide gel, eluted, and sequenced in separate reactions. Alternatively, when multiplex strategies are used, it is worthwhile to perform single PCR reactions to generate single products that can subsequently be directly sequenced. In cases where both rearrangements utilize an IGHV gene of the same subgroup, the latter approach will fail and gel excision is the only option (Fig. 26.4). When all other attempts to generate a reliable IGHV–IGHD–IGHJ sequence have failed, subcloning and subsequent sequencing of individual colonies might be considered as a final option (Fig. 26.4). In practice, the only situation where cloning may be required is in the case of

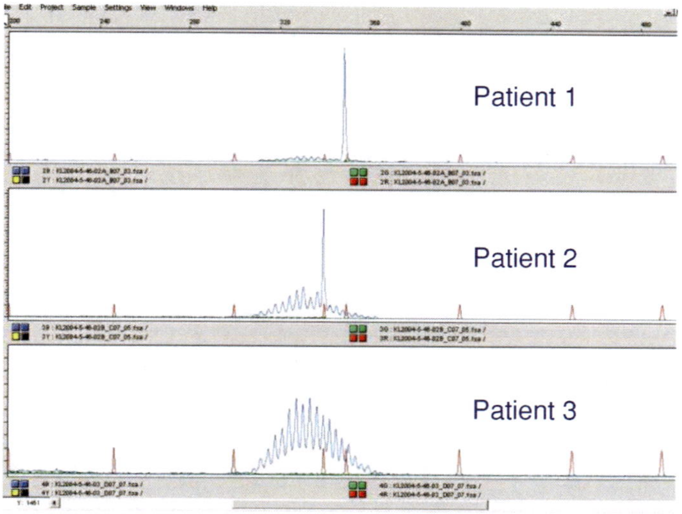

Fig. 26.3 GeneScan analysis of gDNA-based multiplex FR1-IGH PCR products. In patient *1*, a monoallelic IGH rearrangement is observed without background, making direct sequencing possible. In patient *2*, a monoallelic IGH rearrangement is observed with a more prominent background, which probably still can be sequenced directly; alternatively, the monoclonal PCR product can be excised from a gel and then sequenced, or the amplification can be performed with single IGHV subgroup primers (instead of multiplex reaction) in order to reduce background. In patient *3*, polyclonal IGH rearrangements are seen, either due to (i) lack of leukemic clone; (ii) small clone below the detection limit (e.g. follow-up sample); (iii) rearrangement that is not detectable by the employed primer set

biallelic rearrangements where the size difference of the two PCR products does not allow their physical separation by gel excision.

1. Perform direct sequencing (cycle sequencing or Sanger method), using a consensus IGHJ primer or an IGHC (mostly, though not always, IGHM) primer (Fig. 26.1), depending on the starting material and the primers used. From the resulting sequence that largely covers the IGHV gene, the IGHV subgroup (and, in most cases, the actual IGHV gene) can be identified (see Sect. 26.6). Note: primers used for sequencing can be identical to the primers used for amplification or can be nested primers.
2. Perform direct sequencing using a forward IGHV subgroup or leader primer. This can be done either in parallel to or following sequencing with the reverse (IGHJ or IGHC) primer (Fig. 26.1).
3. Evaluate the sequencing reaction by checking chromatograms via suitable software. Depending on sequence readability (no double sequences, no background), further analysis can be performed (see Sect. 26.6).
4. In case sequences are not very well readable, purification of PCR products, excision of PCR products from the polyacrylamide gel, and/or cloning of PCR

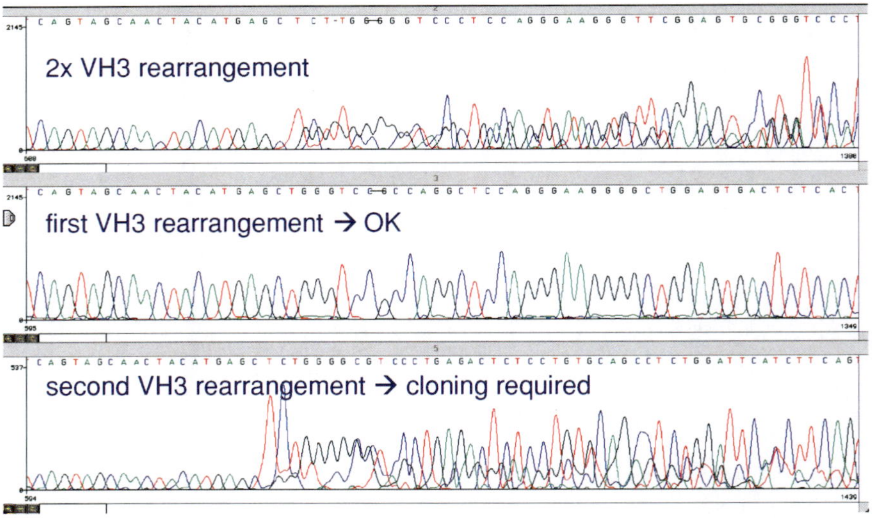

Fig. 26.4 Sequencing results in a CLL case with a double IGHV3 rearrangement. Direct sequencing of the IGH PCR product revealed a mixture of two sequences (*upper* pherogram). Following gel excision of the two IGHV3 subgroup rearrangements, one could be sequenced directly without any problem (*middle* pherogram), whereas the second still was not optimally readable (*lower* pherogram) and finally had to be cloned for proper reading of the sequence

products using a commercially cloning vector should be performed, and sequencing repeated.

In our experience there are few, if any, discrepancies that could be attributed to *Taq* polymerase errors, making it unnecessary to run two independent PCR reactions on every sample, although it is conceivable for borderline cases.

26.6 Analysis of Data and Interpretation

In case of a two-step sequencing strategy, first the IGHV subgroup (and, as already mentioned, actual IGHV gene) usage is determined by analyzing the sequence obtained with the reverse primer via IMGT/V-QUEST (www.imgt.org). Then a second sequencing reaction is performed (see above) with the use of a forward IGHV subgroup-specific primer (either leader or FR1, depending on initial amplification; Fig. 26.1). When a one-step sequencing strategy is chosen, all sequences are in parallel available to proceed with data analysis.

IMGT/V-QUEST is the best available online tool for sequence analysis and interpretation, as IMGT is more comprehensive and also more regularly updated to include polymorphic alleles (Davi et al. 2008). The latter is especially relevant for accurate calculation of the percentage identity of the involved IGHV gene/allele. For this reason, the newest IgBlast version is directly linked to IMGT database.

1. Construct a consensus sequence by aligning all available sequences from both strands (upper and lower) from 1 to 2 independent PCR reactions.
2. Analyze the consensus sequence using IMGT/V-QUEST.
3. Evaluate whether the IGH rearrangement is productive (in-frame, no pseudogene, no stop codon). NOTE: in case of an unproductive IGH rearrangement, evaluation of the mutation percentage does not have any clinical implication. In that case, PCR amplification should be repeated, using alternative primer sets, and/or another starting material.
4. Determine IGHV, IGHD, and IGHJ gene/allele usage via IMGT/V-QUEST.
5. Identify the percentage identity of the rearranged IGHV allele to closest germline IGHV allele, by calculation of the number of mutated nucleotides over the total number of nucleotides in the IGHV gene (excluding possible primer binding site when FR1 primers were used). In case of low identity percentage (e.g. below 85 %), this could be due to the presence of deletion(s) or insertion(s); the analysis should therefore be repeated including the option 'Search for insertions and deletions' in 'Advanced parameters' of IMGT/V-QUEST.
6. Interpret IGHV mutational status as M ($<$98 % identity) or UM ($\geq$98 %).

26.7 Reporting

As for any genetic test, also for reporting IGHV mutational status data, it is important to include information on all relevant test parameters in the diagnostic report next to the actual results and the overall conclusion on the data. The majority of CLL cases can be readily classified as either M or UM. However, in a small portion of cases the assignment will be less straightforward; for instance, in cases showing a single unproductive rearrangement or cases with double productive rearrangements of discordant mutational status (see below). A multi-center analysis of 'problematic cases' and guidelines how to handle such cases was recently published (Langerak et al. 2011). Furthermore, an online troubleshooting forum, launched in 2007 by ERIC, assists laboratories performing IGHV gene mutational status with advice on trouble sequences (http://www.ericll.org/projects/IGVHMutationalAnalysis.php).

1. Report the most relevant test parameters such as material, type of nucleic acid, primers used, sequencing strategy (direct, cloning, etc.).
2. Report the presence of a single or multiple rearrangements and their functionality (productive or unproductive).
3. Report the IGHV, IGHD, and IGHJ gene usage and the percentage identity of the involved IGHV gene/allele. An additional remark on cautious interpretation should be made in case of a borderline percentage identity (97–99 % identity).

4. Report the overall interpretation of mutational status as follows:
   Single rearrangement

   - Productive: interpreted as UM or M, with remark on borderline identity (if applicable)
   - unproductive: inconclusive

   Multiple rearrangements

   - concordant mutational status: interpreted as UM or M, with remark on borderline identity (if applicable)
   - discordant mutational status

- productive UM + productive M: inconclusive
- productive UM + unproductive M: (currently still) inconclusive (NOTE: in cDNA-based analysis this situation might not be encountered, and hence interpreted as UM)
- productive M + unproductive UM: interpreted as M

Note: for particular IGHV gene usage (e.g. IGHV3-21) or BCR stereotypy (see Chap. 5) the association with clinical prognosis can be remarked.

26.8 Conclusions

Since the late 1990s IGHV gene mutational analysis has become an important prognostic parameter in CLL. Using a mathematically defined cut-off of 98 % identity, CLL with unmutated IGHV genes, presenting with therapy resistance, and inferior survival can be distinguished from mutated CLL that generally show a more favorable prognosis. As the whole procedure of IGHV mutational analysis (both the analytical phase and post-analytical phase) has been standardized in much detail through the efforts of the ERIC-IgCLL group (Ghia et al. 2007; Davi et al. 2008, Langerak et al. 2011), this method is now robust enough to be used for inclusion or stratification purposes in multi-center clinical protocols.

In analyzing the percentage identity to the closest IGHV gene, much information on IGHV/IGHD/IGHJ gene usage and CDR3 stereotypy has been generated in CLL. It remains to be studied what the latter parameters reveal about the underlying CLL biology. Perhaps more importantly, the clinical implications of these features need to be disclosed in future clinical studies. If prognostically valuable, the here described molecular method can also be utilized for such analysis.

References

Aubin J, Davi F, Nguyen-Salomon F, Leboeuf D, Debert C, Taher M, Valensi F, Canioni D, Brousse N, Varet B (1995) Description of a novel FR1 IgH PCR strategy and its comparison with three other strategies for the detection of clonality in B cell malignancies. Leukemia 9:471–479

Belessi C, Stamatopoulos K, Hadzidimitriou A, Hatzi K, Smilevska T, Stavroyianni N, Marantidou F, Paterakis G, Fassas A, Anagnostopoulos A, Laoutaris N (2005) Analysis of expressed and non-expressed IGK locus rearrangements in chronic lymphocytic leukemia. Mol Med 11:52–58

Bottaro M, Berti E, Biondi A, Migone N, Crosti L (1994) Heteroduplex analysis of T-cell receptor gamma gene rearrangements for diagnosis and monitoring of cutaneous T-cell lymphomas. Blood 83:3271–3278

Campbell MJ, Zelenetz AD, Levy S, Levy R (1992) Use of family-specific leader region primer for PCR amplification of the human heavy chain variable region gene repertoire. Mol Immunol 29:193–203

Damle RN, Wasil T, Fais F, Ghiotto F, Valetto A, Allen SL, Buchbinder A, Budman D, Dittmar K, Kolitz J, Lichtman SM, Schulman P, Vinciguerra VP, Rai KR, Ferrarini M, Chiorazzi N (1999) Ig V gene mutation status and CD38 expression as novel prognostic indicators in chronic lymphocytic leukemia. Blood 94:1840–1847

Davi F, Rosenquist R, Ghia P, Belessi C, Stamatopoulos K (2008) Determination of IGHV gene mutational status in chronic lymphocytic leukemia: bioinformatics advances meet clinical needs. Leukemia 22:212–214

Evans PA, Pott Ch, Groenen PJ, Salles G, Davi F, Berger F, Garcia JF, van Krieken JH, Pals S, Kluin P, Schuuring E, Spaargaren M, Boone E, González D, Martinez B, Villuendas R, Gameiro P, Diss TC, Mills K, Morgan GJ, Carter GI, Milner BJ, Pearson D, Hummel M, Jung W, Ott M, Canioni D, Beldjord K, Bastard C, Delfau-Larue MH, van Dongen JJ, Molina TJ, Cabeçadas J (2007) Significantly improved PCR-based clonality testing in B-cell malignancies by use of multiple immunoglobulin gene targets: report of the BIOMED-2 Concerted Action BHM4-CT98-3936. Leukemia 21:207–214

Fais F, Ghiotto F, Hashimoto S, Sellars B, Valetto A, Allen SL, Schulman P, Vinciguerra VP, Rai K, Rassenti LZ, Kipps TJ, Dighiero G, Schroeder HW Jr, Ferrarini M, Chiorazzi N (1998) Chronic lymphocytic leukemia B cells express restricted sets of mutated and unmutated antigen receptors. J Clin Invest 102:1515–1525

Ghia P, Stamatopoulos K, Belessi C, Moreno C, Stilgenbauer S, Stevenson F, Davi F, Rosenquist R (2007) European Research Initiative on CLL. ERIC recommendations on IGHV gene mutational status analysis in chronic lymphocytic leukemia. Leukemia 21:1–3

González M, González D, López-Pérez R, García-Sanz R, Chillón MC, Balanzategui A, Mateos MV, Alaejos I, Langerak AW, Orfão A, Van Dongen JJ, San Miguel JF (1999) Heteroduplex analysis of VDJ amplified segments from rearranged IgH genes for clonality assessments in B-cell non-Hodgkin's lymphoma. A comparison between different strategies. Haematologica 84:779–784

Hamblin TJ, Davis Z, Gardiner A, Oscier DG, Stevenson FK (1999) Unmutated Ig V(H) genes are associated with a more aggressive form of chronic lymphocytic leukemia. Blood 94:1848–1854

Kneba M, Bolz I, Linke B, Hiddemann W (1995) Analysis of rearranged T-cell receptor beta-chain genes by polymerase chain reaction (PCR) DNA sequencing and automated high resolution PCR fragment analysis. Blood 86:3930–3937

Küppers R, Zhao M, Rajewsky K, Hansmann ML (1993) Detection of clonal B cell populations in paraffin-embedded tissues by polymerase chain reaction. Am J Pathol 143:230–239

Langerak AW, Szczepanski T, Van der Burg M, Wolvers-Tettero ILM, Van Dongen JJM (1997) Heteroduplex PCR analysis of rearranged T cell receptor genes for clonality assessment in suspect T cell proliferations. Leukemia 11:2192–2199

Langerak AW, Davi F, Ghia P, Hadzidimitriou A, Murray F, Potter KN, Rosenquist R, Stamatopoulos K, Belessi C (2011) Immunoglobulin sequence analysis and prognostication in CLL: guidelines from the ERIC Review Board for reliable interpretation of problematic cases. Leukemia 25:979–984

Linke B, Bolz I, Fayyazi A, von Hofen M, Pott C, Bertram J, Hiddemann W, Kneba M (1997) Automated high resolution PCR fragment analysis for identification of clonally rearranged immunoglobulin heavy chain genes. Leukemia 11:1055–1062

Stamatopoulos K, Belessi C, Hadzidimitriou A, Smilevska T, Kalagiakou E, Hatzi K, Stavroyianni N, Athanasiadou A, Tsompanakou A, Papadaki T, Kokkini G, Patarakis G, Saloum R, Laoutaris N, Anagnostopoulos A, Fassas A (2005) Immunoglobulin light chain repertoire in chronic lymphocytic leukemia. Blood 106:3575–3583

Tobin G, Thunberg U, Laurell A, Karlsson K, Aleskog A, Willander K, Söderberg O, Merup M, Vilpo J, Hultdin M, Sundström C, Roos G, Rosenquist R (2005) Patients with chronic lymphocytic leukemia with mutated VH genes presenting with Binet stage B or C form a subgroup with a poor outcome. Haematologica 90:465–469

Van Dongen JJM, Langerak AW, Brüggemann M, Evans PA, Hummel M, Lavender FL, Delabesse E, Davi F, Schuuring E, Garcia Sanz R, Van Krieken JH, Droese J, Gonzalez D, Bastard C, White HE, Spaargaren M, González M, Parreira A, Smith JF, Morgan G, Kneba M, Macintyre EA (2003) Design and standardization of PCR primers and protocols for detection of clonal immunoglobulin and T-cell receptor gene rearrangements in suspect lymphoproliferations. Report of the BIOMED-2 Concerted Action BMH4-CT98-3936. Leukemia 17:2257–2317

Chapter 27
Molecular Biology Methods in the Diagnosis of Multiple Myeloma

Anna Dmoszyńska and Sylwia Chocholska

Abstract The development of multiple myeloma (MM) is a multistep process including sequential series of genetic abnormalities. Failure to obtain informative metaphases from conventional cytogenetic techniques might be overcome by using molecular cytogenetic methods, which utilize DNA from interphase nuclei, thus permitting the evaluation of chromosomal regions in non-dividing cells. The advent of molecular biology methods, such as fluorescence in situ hybridization (FISH), comparative genomic hybridization (CGH) or gene expression profiling (GEP) has provided new insights into the biology of MM. These methods may help to explain clinical heterogeneity of MM and to differentiate between the disease subtypes related to good and bad prognosis.

27.1 Introduction

In contrast to other hematological neoplasms, the analysis of chromosomal abnormalities in multiple myeloma (MM) using conventional cytogenetics is informative in only 30–40 % of patients. The reason for this is a generally very low mitotic activity of tumor cells, as indicated by a median bone marrow plasma cell labeling index (PCLI, a measure of plasma cells in the S phase) of less than 1 % (Debes-Marun et al. 2003; Liebisch and Döhner 2006). In the remaining cases, no metaphases or only normal metaphases originating from myeloid bone marrow cells can be obtained.

A. Dmoszyńska · S. Chocholska (✉)
Department of Hematooncology and Bone Marrow Transplantation,
Medical University of Lublin, Staszica 11, 20-081 Lublin, Poland
e-mail: sylwia.chocholska@umlub.pl

A. Dmoszyńska
e-mail: annadmosz@wp.pl

M. Witt et al. (eds.), *Molecular Aspects of Hematologic Malignancies*, Principles and Practice, DOI: 10.1007/978-3-642-29467-9_27,

Karyotypes are usually complex and show more than 10 abnormalities in almost half of cases and even more than 20 aberrations in about 10 % of patients (Tricot et al. 1997). Numerical and large structural abnormalities can be relatively easily diagnosed, demonstrating that numerical changes are observed with hyperdiploid karyotypes and rare translocations, while nonhyperdiploid karyotype is associated with high frequency of translocations, mainly involving the 14q32 region. Another limitation of conventional cytogenetics is that small interstitial deletions or partial genomic gains as well as translocations with telomeric breakpoints, for instance t(4;14)(p16;q32) and t(14;16)(q32;q23), can easily be overlooked (Avet-Loiseau et al. 1999; Higgins and Fonseca 2005). Molecular-based techniques, such as comparative genomic hybridization (CGH) and fluorescence in situ hybridization (FISH), enable the detection of genetic aberrations in non-proliferating cells in practically all MM patients (Higgins and Fonseca 2005; Liebisch and Döhner 2006).

In order to report reliable cytogenetic results, plasma cells have to be clearly identified either using simultaneous cytoplasmic immunoglobulin staining and FISH (cIg-FISH) or immunomagnetic plasma cell separation. Performing FISH in unsorted bone marrow samples carries a high risk of low sensitivity for chromosome abnormalities detection (Ahmann et al. 1998; Fonseca et al. 2009). Moreover, bone marrow samples contain considerably fewer plasma cells than the corresponding smear used for morphological assessment. Therefore, in order to obtain good quality samples for FISH studies clinicians should send part of the first draw of the aspirate and further aspiration should involve repositioning of the needle. Since FISH is a time consuming method and the obtained results depend on plasma cells of good viability it is not recommended to perform bone marrow aspirates on Friday (Fonseca et al. 2004; Ross et al. 2007).

FISH analysis should be performed at the time of diagnosis in order to determine therapy and long-term outcome for an individual patient. However, it should be emphasized that even if chromosomal abnormalities of known predictive value are detected, the overall outcome may still be variable because of the influence of other genetic and microenvironmental factors. At present, it is recommended that FISH tests should be repeated at the time of disease relapse. Chromosomal abnormalities evolve over the disease course and it is also possible that aberrations undetected in the first analysis may become evident in the second analysis (Munshi 2008).

27.2 Identification of Chromosomal Abnormalities in Bone Marrow Plasma Cells Using Cytoplasmic Immunoglobulin Staining and FISH

27.2.1 Bone Marrow Cell Culture

cIg-FISH is performed on bone marrow plasma cells. Bone marrow samples are cultured in RPMI 1640 medium supplemented with 10 % heat-inactivated fetal bovine serum for 24 h at 37 °C in 5 % CO_2. The cells are harvested using hypotonic potassium chloride, fixed by methanol/glacial acetic acid (3:1) and stored at −20 °C for further analysis (Ahmann et al. 1998).

27.2.2 Microscopic Slide Preparation

1. Collect fixed bone marrow cells by centrifugation at 400×*g* for 10 min at room temperature.
2. Remove the supernatant, resuspend the sediment in 8 ml of 96 % ethanol and incubate 15 min at room temperature.
3. Repeat steps 1 and 2.
4. Resuspend the pellet in 96 % ethanol and place a drop of cells onto a clean microscopic slide.
5. Air-dry the slides and examine under phase contrast microscope to check cell density.

27.2.3 cIg-FISH Protocol

1. Incubate slides in 10 mM citrate buffer (1:1 mixture of citric acid—1 g/500 ml H_2O and natrium citrate—1.45 g/500 ml H_2O; pH 6,0) for 10 min at 95 °C.
2. After incubation, wash slides twice in phosphate buffered saline (PBS) solution for 2 min at room temperature.
3. Apply 20 µl of AMCA (7-amino-4-methylcoumarin-3-acetic acid)-labeled anti-human kappa chain antibody or anti-human lambda chain antibody, diluted 1:10 in PBS, onto each slide and incubate under 24 × 24 mm coverslip in a prewarmed humidified box for 60–90 min at 37 °C.
4. After incubation, wash slides twice in PBS solution for 2 min at room temperature.
5. Apply 20 µl of AMCA-labeled anti-goat IgG (H + L) antibody, diluted 1:20 in PBS, onto each slide and incubate under 24 × 24 mm coverslip in a humidified box for 60–90 min at 37 °C.
6. After incubation, wash slides twice in PBS solution for 2 min at room temperature.
7. Dehydrate slides for 2 min in 70 % ethanol, followed by 2 min in 85 % ethanol, and 2 min in 96 % ethanol.
8. View slides under fluorescent microscope to check staining of cytoplasmic immunoglobulin.
9. Apply 10 µl of FISH probe mixture to the target area of the slide and immediately apply 22 × 22 mm coverslip. Prepare probe mixture according to the manufacture's protocol.

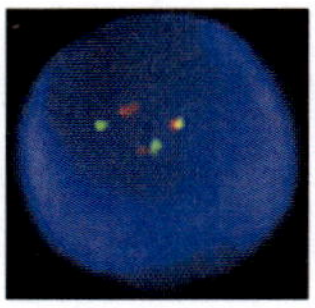

Fig. 1 FISH to interphase nuclei with LSI IGH/FGFR3 dual color, dual fusion translocation probe on plasma cells. The *FGFR3* (fibroblast growth factor receptor 3) gene is located at 4p16 and the *IGH* (immunoglobulin heavy chain) gene is located at 14q32. An abnormal nucleus, containing t(4;14)(p16;q32), shows one orange (*FGFR3*), one green (*IGH*) and two fusion signals for der(4) and der(14) chromosomes

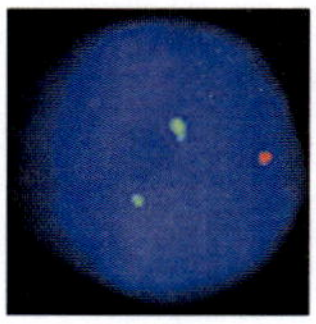

Fig. 2 FISH to interphase nuclei with LSI IGH/MAF dual color, dual fusion translocation probe on plasma cells. The *MAF* (v-maf musculoaponeurotic fibrosarcoma oncogene homolog) gene is located at 16q23 and the *IGH* gene is located at 14q32. An abnormal nucleus shows one orange (*MAF*) and two green (*IGH*) signals indicating del(16q23). No t(14;16)(q32;q23) is observed

10. Seal coverslip with rubber cement and incubate slides in a humidified box for 6–16 h at 37 °C.
11. After incubation, wash slides in 0.4× SSC (sodium chloride–sodium citrate buffer)/0.3 % Nonidet-P40 (NP-40) solution for 2 min at 73 °C and then in 2× SSC/0.1 % NP-40 for 5 s to 1 min at room temperature.
12. Air-dry slides in darkness and apply 10 μl of antifade solution (0,01 % p-phenylenediamine dissolved in glycerol/PBS buffer, pH 8.0). Apply coverslip and analyze under fluorescent microscope.
13. Wherever possible score 100 AMCA-positive plasma cells for each slide. Results are acceptable from less than 50 cells only when more than 75 % of them have the abnormality.

It is recommended that the following chromosomal abnormalities should be tested in all cases:

- t(4;14)(p16;q32);
- t(14;16)(q32;q23);
- del(17p13).

In the expended panel, hyperdiploidy, t(11;14)(q13;q32), chromosome 13 and chromosome 1 abnormalities should be analyzed. The cutoff levels should be 10 % for dual fusion and break-apart probes and 20 % for numerical abnormalities and single fusion results with dual fusion probes. (Fonseca et al. 2009; Ross et al. 2007). Examples of cIg-FISH on plasma cells are presented in Figs. 27.1, 27.2, 27.3, 27.4, 27.5, 27.6.

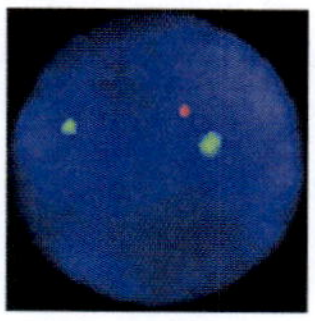

Fig. 3 FISH to interphase nuclei with LSI TP53/CEP 17 probe on plasma cells. The *TP53* (tumor protein p53) gene is located at 17p13.1 and the CEP17 probe is located at the centromere of chromosome 17. An abnormal nucleus with *TP53* gene deletion shows one orange signal for the 17p13 region. Green signals distinguish 17p13 deletion from chromosome 17 monosomy

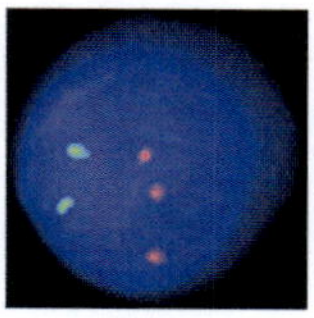

Fig. 4 FISH to interphase nuclei with LSI IGH/CCND1 dual color, dual fusion translocation probe on plasma cells. The *CCND1* (cyclin D1) gene is located at 11q13 and the *IGH* gene is located at 14q32. An abnormal nucleus with trisomy 11 shows three orange (*CCND1*) and two green (*IGH*) signals. No t(11;14)(q13;q32) is observed

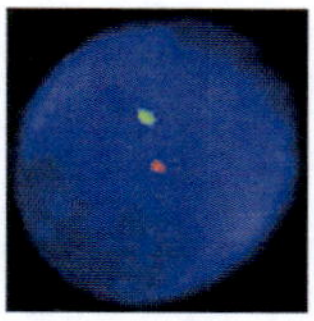

Fig. 5 FISH to interphase nuclei with LSI 13q14/13q34 probe on plasma cells. The *RB1* (retinoblastoma 1) gene is located at 13q14. An abnormal nucleus with del(13q14) shows one orange signal. Green signals differentiate between the interstitial deletions and the loss of the entire q arm

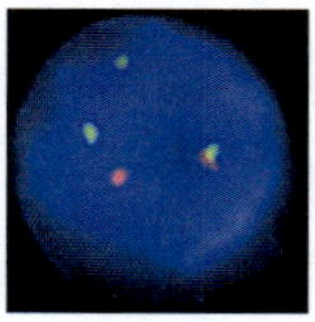

Fig. 6 FISH to interphase nuclei with LSI 1q21/1p36 probe on plasma cells. An abnormal nucleus with amp(1q21) shows three green signals. Red signals specific for the 1p36 region distinguish amp(1q21) from trisomy or tetrasomy of chromosome 1

When reporting the results of FISH analysis, the method of plasma cells identification should be stated. The proportion of affected plasma cells should be reported, though it is not clear what the cutoff level for clinical significance is. It is suggested that anomalies in less than 40 % of cells should be interpreted as low level. The results presented to the clinician should be expressed as clearly as possible with a hypothetical sample report as follows: 17p13 (*TP53*) deleted (75 %) 4p16 t(4;14) single fusion (100 %) 16q23 normal 13q14 (*RB1*) normal. Therefore, the European Myeloma Network FISH Working Party do not endorse the use of an International System for Human Cytogenetic Nomenclature (ISCN) (Fonseca et al. 2004, 2009; Ross et al. 2007).

27.3 Conclusions

The development of MM is a multistep process including series of genetic changes. MM plasma cells are characterized by a high degree of karyotypic instability resulting in a complex pattern of chromosomal abnormalities. The recent advances in molecular cytogenetic techniques have resulted in the development of innovative laboratory methods that, along with traditional tools, have improved the process of MM diagnosis and monitoring of the disease status.

References

Ahmann GJ, Jalal SM, Juneau AL, Christensen ER, Hanson CA, Dewald GW, Greipp PR (1998) A novel three-color, clone-specific fluorescence in situ hybridization procedure for monoclonal gammopathies. Cancer Genet Cytogenet 101:7–11

Avet-Loiseau H, Brigaudeau C, Morineau N, Talmant P, La JL, Daviet A, Li JY, Praloran V, Rapp MJ, Harousseau JL, Facon T, Bataille R (1999) High incidence of cryptic translocations involving the Ig heavy chain gene in multiple myeloma, as shown by fluorescence in situ hybridization. Genes Chromosomes Cancer 24:9–15

Debes-Marun C, Dewald GW, Bryant S, Picken E, Santanat-Dávila R, González-Paz N, Winkler JM, Kyle RA, Gertz MA, Witzig TE, Dispenzieri A, Lacy MQ, Rajkumar SV, Lust JA, Greipp PR, Fonseca R (2003) Chromosome abnormalities clustering and its implications for pathogenesis and prognosis in myeloma. Leukemia 17:427–436

Fonseca R, Barlogie B, Bataille R, Bastard C, Bergsagel PL, Chesi M, Davies FE, Drach J, Greipp PR, Kirsch IR, Kuehl WM, Hernandez JM, Minvielle S, Pilarski LM, Shaughnessy JD Jr, Stewart AK, Avet-Loiseau H (2004) Genetics and cytogenetics of multiple myeloma: a workshop report. Cancer Res 64:1546–1558

Fonseca R, Bergsagel PL, Drach J, Shaughnessy J, Gutierrez N, Stewart AK, Morgan G, Van Ness B, Chesi M, Minvielle S, Neri A, Barlogie B, Kuehl WM, Liebisch P, Davies F, Chen-Kiang S, Durie BG, Carrasco R, Sezer O, Reiman T, Pilarski L, Avet-Loiseau H, International Myeloma Working Group (2009) International Myeloma Working Group molecular classification of multiple myeloma: spotlight review. Leukemia 23:2210–2221

Higgins MJ, Fonseca R (2005) Genetics of multiple myeloma. Best Pract Res Clin Haematol 18:525–536

Liebisch P, Döhner H (2006) Cytogenetics and molecular cytogenetics in multiple myeloma. Eur J Cancer 42:1520–1529

Munshi NC (2008) Investigative tools for diagnosis and management. Hematology Am Soc Hematol Educ Program 298–305

Ross FM, Avet-Loiseau H, Drach J, Hernandez Rivas JM, Liebisch P, European Myeloma Network FISH Working Party (2007) European Myeloma Network recommendations for FISH in myeloma. Haematologica 92(Suppl 2):100–101

Tricot G, Sawyer JR, Jagannath S, Desikan KR, Siegel D, Naucke S, Mattox S, Bracy D, Munshi N, Barlogie B (1997) Unique role of cytogenetics in the prognosis of patients with myeloma receiving high-dose therapy and autotransplants. J Clin Oncol 15:2659–2666

Chapter 28
Molecular Methods in Myeloproliferative Neoplasms

Aleksandra Leszczyńska, Witold Prejzner, Maria Bieniaszewska and Andrzej Hellmann

Abstract In this chapter molecular methods that are clinically useful in the diagnosis of myeloproliferative neoplasms are presented. The methods described are the essential elements of contemporary hematological diagnostic procedures and allow a diagnosis to be reached more easily and precisely. Detailed protocols for the detection of mutations in *JAK2, MPL,* and *KIT* genes, as well as for the detection of the fusion gene *FIP1L1/PDGFRA*, are presented.

28.1 *JAK2* V617F Mutation

Many different protocols are available for detection of *JAK2* gene mutations: protocols based on allele-specific polymerase chain reaction (AS-PCR) with fluorescent primers, direct sequencing, melting curve assay, pyrosequencing, and many others (James et al. 2005; McClure et al. 2006; Murugesan et al. 2006; Steensma 2006). The most commonly used method in the routine laboratory setting is amplification refractory mutation system polymerase chain reaction (ARMS-PCR) (Jones et al. 2005; Chen et al. 2007). The method is highly sensitive, fast, uncomplicated, and inexpensive.

Purified granulocytes are the best clinical material for *JAK2* V617F identification. However, the total genomic DNA isolated from unfractionated whole blood or bone marrow samples is also acceptable for daily routine diagnostics.

A. Leszczyńska · W. Prejzner · M. Bieniaszewska · A. Hellmann (✉)
Department of Haematology and Transplantology, Medical
University of Gdańsk, Dębinki 7, 80-952 Gdańsk, Poland
e-mail: klhem@gumed.edu.pl

M. Witt et al. (eds.), *Molecular Aspects of Hematologic Malignancies*,
Principles and Practice, DOI: 10.1007/978-3-642-29467-9_28,

Table 28.1 Composition of PCR reaction mixture for detection of *JAK2* V617F mutation

Reaction component	Starting	Volume (μl)	Final
DNA template	20–100 ng/μl	1–5	20–100 ng
Primer FO	10 pmol/μl	2	0.8 pmol/μl
Primer RO	10 pmol/μl	2	0.8 pmol/μl
Primer Fwt	10 pmol/μl	2.5	1 pmol/μl
Primer Rmut	10 pmol/μl	2.5	1 pmol/μl
PCR buffer	10x	2.5	1x
$MgCl_2$	50 mM	1	2 mM
dNTPs mix	10 mM	0.5	0.2 mM
Hot Start *Taq* polymerase	5 U/μl	0.2	1 U
Water		To final volume 25 μl	–

28.1.1 ARMS-PCR Protocol for JAK2 *V617F Mutation Analysis*

Four primers are used in ARMS-PCR. Forward outer (FO) and reverse outer (RO) primers flank the mutation site and result in a 463 bp band. This product is generated regardless of the presence of mutation and constitutes the internal control of the PCR reaction.

The primers Fwt (wild-type-specific) and RO amplify a wild-type allele and produce a 229 bp band. The primers Rmut (mutation-specific) and FO amplify a mutant allele and generate a 279 bp PCR product.

Primer sequences:

FO	5' TCC TCA GAA CGT TGA TGG CAG 3′
RO	5' ATT GCT TTC CTT TTT CAC AAG AT 3′
Fwt	5' GCA TTT GGT TTT AAA TTA TGG AGT AT<u>A</u> **TG** 3′
Rmut	5' GTT TTA CTT ACT CTC GTC TCC ACA <u>A</u>A**A** 3′

The nucleotides highlighted in bold at the 3′ end anneal at the site of mutation.

The nucleotides underlined are intentionally introduced mismatches to the wild-type sequence to maximize allelic specificity.

The composition of a PCR reaction mixture is shown in Table 28.1.

The following PCR cycling parameters are used:

Initial denaturation	95 °C	1–5 min (depending on polymerase used)	
Denaturation	95 °C	40 s	30x
Annealing	60 °C	50 s	30x
Extension	72 °C	75 s	30x
Final extension	72 °C	5 min	

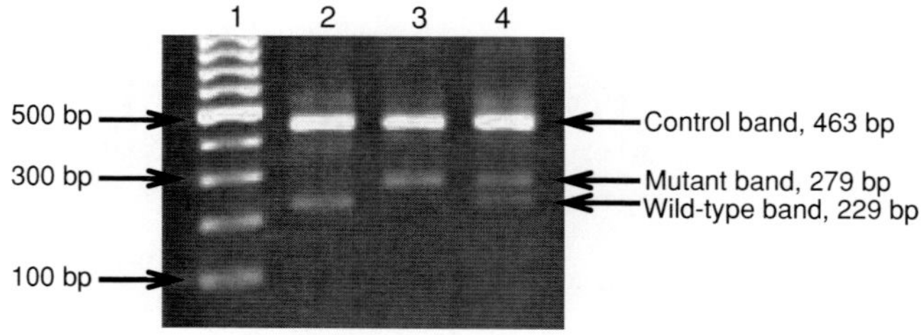

Fig. 28.1 ARMS-PCR detection of *JAK2* V617F mutation. The results of electrophoresis of ARMS-PCR products in 2 % agarose gel stained with ethidium bromide and visualized in UV light. *Line 1* Size marker 100–1000 bp. *Line 2* Wild-type sample—control and wild-type allele bands are visible. *Line 3* Mutant sample—control and mutant bands are visible, wild-type allele band is hardly visible. *Line 4* Mutant sample—control, mutant, and wild-type allele bands are visible

Three controls should be run together with the samples being examined:

- positive control: DNA from a previously confirmed *JAK2* V617F-positive patient or from a homozygous mutant HEL cell line
- negative control: DNA from any *JAK2* V617F-negative sample or a negative cell line
- no template control: water instead of DNA

28.1.1.1 PCR Product Analysis

The PCR products are separated in 2 % agarose gel, stained with ethidium bromide and visualized in UV light. The presence of the following bands should be interpreted as: 463 bp and 229 bp for wild-type alleles; 463 bp, 229 bp, and 279 bp for the presence of wild-type and mutant alleles, and 463 bp and 279 bp for mutant homozygotes (Fig. 28.1).

28.2 *JAK2* Exon 12 Mutations

About 10 different mutations in exon 12 of the *JAK2* gene have been described so far. There is no universal diagnostic technology allowing for identification of all these changes. However, techniques allowing for a rapid identification of seven different mutations in these regions have been developed. High resolution melting (HRM) method enables to distinguish each individual mutation based on characteristic melting profiles they result in. The alternative option is to use such screening methods as SSCP (single strand conformation polymorphism), DGGE (denaturing gradient gel electrophoresis), or dHPLC (denaturing high performance

Table 28.2 Composition of PCR mixture for *JAK2* exon 12 amplification

Reaction component	Starting	Volume (μl)	Final
DNA template	20–100 ng/μl	1–5	20–100 ng
Primer JAK2-ex12-F	10 pmol/μl	5	2 pmol/μl
Primer JAK2-ex12-R	10 pmol/μl	5	2 pmol/μl
PCR buffer	10x	2.5	1x
$MgCl_2$	50 mM	0.75	1.5 mM
dNTPs mix	10 mM	0.5	0.2 mM
Hot Start *Taq* polymerase	5 U/μl	0.2	1 unit
Water		To final volume 25 μl	–

liquid chromatography). The method presented here involves direct sequencing of the *JAK2* exon 12 PCR product and cloning, in cases when the sequencing chromatogram cannot be read. However, it should be emphasized that low level mutant alleles could be missed because of the limitation in sensitivity of the sequencing method.

28.2.1 Protocol for JAK2 Exon 12 Mutations Analysis

The method is based on the PCR amplification of 495 bp DNA fragment. The primers are designed to flank the complete exon 12 (Jones et al. 2008).

Primer sequences:

JAK2-ex12-F	5′ CTC CTC TTT GGA GCA ATT CA 3′
JAK2-ex12-R	5′ GAG AAC TTG GGA GTT GCG ATA 3′

The composition of a PCR mixture is given in Table 28.2

The following PCR cycling parameters are used:

Initial denaturation	95 °C	1–5 min (depending on polymerase used)	
Denaturation	95 °C	40 s	35x
Annealing	55 °C	40 s	35x
Extension	72 °C	55 s	35x
Final extension	72 °C	5 min	

28.2.1.1 PCR Product Analysis

In order to verify the specificity and homogeneity of amplification, 3 μl of PCR products are separated in 2 % agarose gel. The remaining 22 μl of PCR product is purified using any commercially available PCR product purification kit and sequenced.

The sequencing reaction is carried out using the fluorescent dye terminator variant of Sanger sequencing method. Briefly, the mixture contains 10–20 ng template, 4 μl of terminator ready reaction mix, 1x concentrated buffer, 3.2 pmol of primer, and deionized water to final volume of 20 μl. The terminator mix is used in 0.5x dilution. The following cycling conditions are used: 96 °C, 1 min; 96 °C, 10 s; 50 °C, 5 s; 60 °C, 4 min, for 25 cycles. The excess of non-incorporated nucleotide terminators and the remaining sequencing primers are removed using any commercially available purification kit.

Sequencing is performed in both directions. The products of the sequencing reaction are separated in a capillary genetic analyzer. Using appropriate software the resulting sequence is aligned with the reference sequence (wild-type sequence of exon 12) for comparison aimed at identification of mutations.

In case the sequence obtained directly from the PCR product is questionable, cloning and plasmid sequence analysis is performed. The PCR product is cloned using any of the commercially available cloning system to the DH5α Escherichia coli strain or any other strain recommended by manufacturer of the cloning kit. The plasmid is purified and sequenced with the same primers as used for PCR amplification.

It should be stressed that cloning is not a suitable method for routine laboratory use. This method is extremely labor intensive and does not always give the expected results. After cloning, a mixed sequence could still be present (the bacterial cell could take up two or more particles of the plasmid) and sometimes large numbers of clones must be sequenced until the mutant allele is found.

28.3 *MPL* Mutation

Due to a high level of variability of mutations described in the *MPL* gene, a direct sequencing method is most suitable for identification of all possible mutations. However, one should be aware of the limited sensitivity of this method, which is estimated to be about 20–30 % (Baxter et al. 2005).

28.3.1 Protocol for MPL Exon 10 Mutation Analysis

This protocol is based on PCR amplification of the 248 bp fragment, including the most frequently mutated 515 codon (exon 10), and followed by sequencing of the PCR product.

Primer sequences (Pancrazzi et al. 2008):

MPL-ex10-F	5′ TAG CCT GGA TCT CCT TGG TG 3′
MPL-ex10-R	5′ AGA GGT GAC GTG CAG GAA GT 3′

Table 28.3 Composition of PCR mixture for *MPL* exon 10 amplification

Reaction component	Starting	Volume (μl)	Final
DNA template	20–100 ng/μl	1–5	20–100 ng
Primer forward	10 pmol/μl	4	1.6 pmol/μl
Primer reverse	10 pmol/μl	4	1.6 pmol/μl
PCR buffer	10x	2.5	1x
$MgCl_2$	50 mM	0.5	1 mM
dNTPs mix	10 mM	0.5	0.2 mM
Hot Start *Taq* polymerase	5 U/μl	0.2	1 U
Water		To final volume 25 μl	–

The composition of a PCR mixture is given in Table 28.3.
The following PCR cycling parameters are used:

Initial denaturation	95 °C	1–5 min (depending on polymerase used)	
Denaturation	95 °C	30 s	35x
Annealing	55 °C	40 s	35x
Extension	72 °C	45 s	35x
Final extension	72 °C	5 min	

28.3.1.1 PCR Product Analysis

In order to verify the specificity and homogeneity of amplification, 3 μl of PCR products are separated in 2.5 % agarose gel. The remaining 22 μl of the PCR product is purified by any commercially available PCR product purification kit. It is recommended that the quantity of purified PCR product be verified spectrophotometrically or by agarose gel electrophoresis.

The sequencing reaction is carried out using the fluorescent dye terminator variant of Sanger sequencing method. The products of the sequencing reaction are separated in a capillary genetic analyzer. The sequencing results are checked using any free or commercially available software for sequence analysis.

28.4 *FIP1L1-PDGFRA* Fusion Gene Analysis

Fusion of the *FIP1L1-PDGFRA* genes is commonly detected with the use of reverse transcriptase-polymerase chain reaction (RT-PCR) method. However, a combination of fluorescence in situ hybridization (FISH) and RT-PCR is recommended for a comprehensive diagnostics. Both methods used alone are not precise enough and false negative results might occur. The FISH technique is not as sensitive as the RT-PCR method, while in PCR some of the positive results might be missed, due to the heterogeneity of breakpoints in the *FIP1-L1* gene.

28.4.1 Nested RT-PCR Protocol for *FIP1-L1-PDGFRA* Detection

For this protocol RNA is extracted from white blood cells using guanidinium thiocyanate-phenol–chloroform extraction (modified Chomczyński and Sacchi method) or a commercially available spin column purification kit. Complementary DNA (cDNA) is synthesized from 1.5 μg total RNA with random hexamers and one of the commercially available reverse transcriptase according to the manufacturer's protocol. The following primers for the first round and nested reaction are used (Cools et al. 2003).

Primer sequences:

FIP1L1_F1	5′ ACC TGG TGC TGA TCT TTC TGA T 3′
PDGFR_R1	5′ TGA GAG CTT GTT TTT CAC TGG A 3′
FIP1L1_F2 nested	5′ AAA GAG GAT ACG AAT GGG ACT TG 3′
PDGFR_R2 nested	5′ GGG ACC GGC TTA ATC CAT AG 3′

The composition of a PCR mixture is presented in Table 28.4.

The following PCR cycling parameters are used:

Initial denaturation	95 °C	1–5 min (depending on polymerase used)	
Denaturation	95 °C	30 s	30x
Annealing	58 °C	30 s	
Extension	72 °C	90 s	
Final extension	72 °C	5 min	

In the nested round, 2 μl of the PCR product from the first round is used as a template. The remaining components and PCR cycling parameters are as used in the first round.

As a routine the following controls should be used:

- positive control: cDNA from previously confirmed *FIP1L1-PDGRFA*-positive patients or from the EOL-1 cell line
- negative control: cDNA from any *FIP1L1-PDGRFA*-negative samples or a negative cell line
- no template control: water instead of cDNA

28.4.1.1 PCR Product Analysis

The PCR products are separated in 1.5 % agarose gel, stained with ethidium bromide, and visualized in UV light. Due to considerable variability of the location of *FIP1L1* breakpoints and thus the heterogeneity of the resulting *FIP1L1-PDGRFA* fusion genes, different sizes of PCR products are generated in each

Table 28.4 Composition of PCR mixture for *FIP1L1-PDGFRA* fusion gene amplification

Reaction component	Starting	Volume (μl)	Final
cDNA template	20–100 ng/μl	5	20–100 ng
FIP1L1_F1	10 pmol/μl	3	1.2 pmol/μl
PDGFR_R1	10 pmol/μl	3	1.2 pmol/μl
PCR buffer	10x	2.5	1x
$MgCl_2$	50 mM	1	2 mM
dNTPs mix	10 Mm	0.5	0.2 mM
Hot Start *Taq* polymerase	5 U/μl	0.2	1 U
Water		To final volume 25 μl	–

individual patient. In addition, due to the complexity of alternative splicing of *FIP1L1* gene, multiple bands can be obtained in each patient. In case of doubtful results, the sequencing method can be used to verify the specificity of the amplification products (Cools et al. 2003).

28.5 *KIT* Mutation

Detection of the D816V mutation is one of the minor diagnostic criteria according to the WHO classification of systemic mastocytosis (SM); it is found in more than 90 % of all patients with SM. Among several techniques developed for D816V mutation of the *KIT* gene three are recommended as being sufficiently specific and precise for diagnostic purposes: RT-PCR and RFLP (restriction fragment length polymorphism), allele-specific PCR, and peptide nucleic acid (PNA)-mediated PCR. Due to its simplicity, RFLP analysis is the method most often used (Valent et al. 2007).

Analysis of the *KIT* mutation is often performed in patients with low mast cell burden, thus requiring an assay sensitive enough to detect the nucleotide change present only in a small fraction of marrow cells. Therefore, RT-PCR-based analysis of cDNA transcribed from RNA of bone marrow cells is strongly advised since it is more sensitive than the analysis of genomic DNA. If genomic DNA is used, nested or semi-nested PCR should be performed to enhance the sensitivity. Analysis of peripheral blood for the *KIT* mutation is not recommended. In the following section, semi-nested PCR and RFLP analysis are described.

28.5.1 PCR–RFLP Protocol for the KIT D816V Mutation Analysis

This protocol is based on restriction endonuclease digestion of the PCR product obtained by the semi-nested reaction (A > T substitution creates a new restriction

Table 28.5 Composition of PCR mixture the for detection of *KIT* D816 V mutation

Reaction component	Starting	Volume (μl)	Final
DNA template	20–100 ng/μl	5	20–100 ng
Ex17_F	10 pmol/μl	2	0.8 pmol/μl
Ex17_R	10 pmol/μl	2	0.8 pmol/μl
PCR buffer	10x	2.5	1x
$MgCl_2$	50 mM	0.75	1.5 mM
dNTPs mix	10 mM	0.5	0.2 mM
Hot Start *Taq* polymerase	5U/μl	0.2	1 U
Water		to final volume 25 μl	–

site for HinfI). DNA is extracted using any commercially available DNA purification kit.

Primer sequences (Sotlar et al. 2000):

Ex17_F	5′ CAC AGA GAC TTG GCA GCC AG 3′
Ex17_R	5′ CAG GAT TTA CAT TAT GAA AGT CAC GG 3′
Ex17_Fnested	5′ ATC CTC CTT ACT CAT GGT CGG ATC 3′

The composition of a PCR mixture and cycling parameters are presented in Table 28.5.

The following PCR cycling parameters are used:

Initial denaturation	95 °C	1–5 min (depending on polymerase used)	
Denaturation	95 °C	30 s	30x
Annealing	56 °C	30 s	
Extension	72 °C	45 s	
Final extension72 °C	3 min		

In the semi-nested round 1.5 μl PCR product of the first round PCR is used as a template. The same reverse primer as used in the first round and the Ex17_F nested forward primer are used. The remaining components of the PCR mixture and PCR parameters are as used in the first round.

The semi-nested PCR product of 189 bp is cleaved with the restriction endonuclease HinfI for 1 h at 37 °C. Purification of the PCR product is recommended prior to digestion to remove the remaining PCR reaction components. The predicted sizes of the digested fragments are: 121 bp and 68 bp for the wild-type alleles; 121 bp, 68 bp, 54 bp, and 14 bp for the heterozygous sample; 121 bp, 54 bp, and 14 bp for the homozygous mutant. The cleavage products are separated in 6 % polyacrylamide gel or in 4 % agarose gel, stained with ethidium bromide and visualized in UV light.

28.6 Conclusions

Molecular techniques for the detection of mutations in *JAK2, MPL,* and *KIT* genes, as well as for the detection of the fusion gene *FIP1L1/PDGFRA* provide valuable information in the process of diagnosis of myeloproliferative neoplasms. The protocols for the molecular analyses of these genetic aberrations were outlined in this chapter, although some adjustments, due to different reagents and devices used in each laboratory, might be necessary.

References

Baxter EJ, Scott LM, Campbell PJ, East C, Fouroclas N, Swanton S, Vassiliou GS, Bench AJ, Boyd EM, Curtin N, Scott MA, Erber WN, Green AR, Cancer Genome Project (2005) Acquired mutation of the tyrosine kinase JAK2 in human myeloproliferative disorders. Lancet 365:1054–1061

Chen Q, Lu P, Jones AV, Cross NC, Silver RT, Wang YL (2007) Amplification refractory mutation system, a highly sensitive and simple polymerase chain reaction assay, for the detection of JAK2 V617F mutation in chronic myeloproliferative disorders. J Mol Diagn 9:272–276

Cools J, DeAngelo DJ, Gotlib J, Stover EH, Legare RD, Cortes J, Kutok J, Clark J, Galinsky I, Griffin JD, Cross NC, Tefferi A, Malone J, Alam R, Schrier SL, Schmid J, Rose M, Vandenberghe P, Verhoef G, Boogaerts M, Wlodarska I, Kantarjian H, Marynen P, Coutre SE, Stone R, Gilliland DG (2003) A tyrosine kinase created by fusion of the PDGFRA and FIP1L1 genes as a therapeutic target of imatinib in idiopathic hypereosinophilic syndrome. N Engl J Med 348:1201–1214

James C, Ugo V, Le Couédic JP, Staerk J, Delhommeau F, Lacout C, Garçon L, Raslova H, Berger R, Bennaceur-Griscelli A, Villeval JL, Constantinescu SN, Casadevall N, Vainchenker W (2005) A unique clonal JAK2 mutation leading to constitutive signalling causes polycythaemia vera. Nature 434:1144–1148

Jones AV, Cross NC, White HE, Green AR, Scott LM (2008) Rapid identification of JAK2 exon 12 mutations using high resolution melting analysis. Haematologica 93:1560–1564

Jones AV, Kreil S, Zoi K, Waghorn K, Curtis C, Zhang L, Score J, Seear R, Chase AJ, Grand FH, White H, Zoi C, Loukopoulos D, Terpos E, Vervessou EC, Schultheis B, Emig M, Ernst T, Lengfelder E, Hehlmann R, Hochhaus A, Oscier D, Silver RT, Reiter A, Cross NC (2005) Widespread occurrence of the JAK2 V617F mutation in chronic myeloproliferative disorders. Blood 106:2162–2168

McClure R, Mai M, Lasho T (2006) Validation of two clinically useful assays for evaluation of JAK2 V617F mutation in chronic myeloproliferative disorders. Leukemia 20:168–171

Murugesan G, Aboudola S, Szpurka H, Verbic MA, Maciejewski JP, Tubbs RR, Hsi ED (2006) Identification of the JAK2 V617F mutation in chronic myeloproliferative disorders using FRET probes and melting curve analysis. Am J Clin Pathol 125:625–633

Pancrazzi A, Guglielmelli P, Ponziani V, Bergamaschi G, Bosi A, Barosi G, Vannucchi AM (2008) A sensitive detection method for MPLW515L or MPLW515 K mutation in chronic myeloproliferative disorders with locked nucleic acid-modified probes and real-time polymerase chain reaction. J Mol Diagn 10:435–441

Sotlar K, Marafioti T, Griesser H, Theil J, Aepinus C, Jaussi R, Stein H, Valent P, Horny HP (2000) Detection of c-kit mutation Asp 816 to Val in microdissected bone marrow infiltrates in a case of systemic mastocytosis associated with chronic myelomonocytic leukaemia. Mol Pathol 53:188–193

Steensma DP (2006) JAK2 V617F in myeloid disorders: molecular diagnostic techniques and their clinical utility: a paper from the 2005 William Beaumont Hospital symposium on molecular pathology. J Mol Diagn 8:397–411

Valent P, Akin C, Escribano L, Födinger M, Hartmann K, Brockow K, Castells M, Sperr WR, Kluin-Nelemans HC, Hamdy NA, Lortholary O, Robyn J, van Doormaal J, Sotlar K, Hauswirth AW, Arock M, Hermine O, Hellmann A, Triggiani M, Niedoszytko M, Schwartz LB, Orfao A, Horny HP, Metcalfe DD (2007) Standards and standardization in mastocytosis: consensus statements on diagnostics, treatment recommendations and response criteria. Eur J Clin Invest 37:435–453

Vannucchi AM, Antonioli E, Guglielmelli P, Pancrazzi A, Guerini V, Barosi G, Ruggeri M, Specchia G, Lo-Coco F, Delaini F, Villani L, Finotto S, Ammatuna E, Alterini R, Carrai V, Capaccioli G, Di Lollo S, Liso V, Rambaldi A, Bosi A, Barbui T (2008) Characteristics and clinical correlates of MPL 515 W > L/K mutation in essential thrombocythaemia. Blood 112:844–847

Chapter 29
Informed Consent for Participation in Research Project

Małgorzata Dawidowska and Michał Witt

Abstract The participation in a research project as well as the process of obtaining informed consent for such participation are associated with many ethical, legal, and even logistical problems; therefore, they are subject to relevant laws, regulations, and policies at both national and international level. These regulations vary from country to country, and in some countries there are still no clear regulations dedicated directly for research. This chapter discusses most relevant issues of obtaining the informed consent for participation in a research project, including those concerning preservation of samples for future research. General guidelines for the construction of an informed consent form and an information sheet for participants have been outlined in this chapter. Additionally, sample forms have been included. These guidelines might be adopted with respect to current local law regulations and the nature of a particular research project.

29.1 Introduction

Informed consent is a written, dated, and signed, decision of a patient/legal guardian of the patient to take part in a medical procedure, clinical trial, or a research project. Before giving the informed consent the participant or his/her legal representative has the right to talk to a relevant member of a research team

M. Dawidowska (✉) · M. Witt
Department of Molecular and Clinical Genetics,
Institute of Human Genetics, Polish Academy of Sciences,
Strzeszyńska 32, 60-479 Poznań, Poland
e-mail: ma.dawidowska@wp.pl

M. Witt
International Institute of Molecular and Cell Biology,
Trojdena 4, 02-109 Warsaw, Poland
e-mail: witmich@man.poznan.pl

M. Witt et al. (eds.), *Molecular Aspects of Hematologic Malignancies*, Principles and Practice, DOI: 10.1007/978-3-642-29467-9_29,

(usually a physician). During the conversation, information on the purpose, the schedule, the possible advantages, risk, and inconveniences related to participation in the project/procedure is provided in a manner understandable to the participant/ legal guardian, without exerting any pressure. The patient/legal representative should be informed about voluntary participation in the research and the right to withdraw from the project at any time, without any consequences, by revoking the informed consent.

Obtaining the informed consent should be treated as a process which, in more complex cases, may and should take longer than a single conversation with a physician, enabling the patient/legal guardian/family to obtain comprehensive information and knowledge on the proposed procedures and their consequences. It should be strongly emphasized that the mere signing of the relevant form does not fulfill the actual requirements to obtain fully informed consent. As a result of this process the person should receive complete information, so that he/she alone, without the participation of third parties, aware of the consequences, would be able to decide whether to consent to participation in research.

The person leading the process of obtaining the informed consent (usually a physician) should provide information on the project/procedures and only if requested should assist in decision making, in the most possible objective manner, without exerting any pressure.

The main objective of the process of obtaining informed consent, although it is often wrongly perceived, is not legal safeguards for the institution/research team (this is undoubtedly an important side effect), but the patient's conscious acceptance of the participation in the study. The role of the legal guardians should be emphasized particularly in case of minors or people who are not able to make conscious decisions and/or are not able to verbalize them in an unambiguous way.

In addition to communicating the necessary content during the conversation, the most important information concerning the nature and the purpose of participation in research and potential risks and inconvenience for the patient (if any), should be included in the written form of information for the patient/legal guardian which is provided along with a form of conscious consent. Both the informed consent form and the information sheet should be dated and signed not only by the participant but also by the person asking for consent (usually a physician), whose contact details should be included in the form. This will enable the patient/legal guardian to obtain additional information or to withdraw the informed consent.

Despite differences in legal regulations in each country general recommendations for obtaining informed consent and the construction of informed consent form and information sheet can be formulated. These principles are presented in subsequent sections of this chapter.

29.2 Information Sheet for Patients, Parents, or Legal Representatives

The information sheet for patients, parents or legal representatives should include:

1. The title of the research project.
2. The name and contact details of persons responsible for the project realization (project manager, principal investigator).
3. The name and address of the involved institution (institution coordinating the project—in the case of multi-center projects).
4. The most relevant information for the patient/guardian on the research project and the procedures performed during its realization (the aims and the nature of research, the expected benefits of research, possible risks, and inconveniences, if any).
5. The description of patient's involvement in the research (e.g., the manner and timing of sample collection, any additional tests, and procedures that go beyond the standard therapeutic procedures).
6. Information on the type of data concerning the participant/the sample to be collected and processed during the research.
7. Information on the system of sample identification (coded, i.e., traceable or anonymized).
8. Information on the possibility of retaining biological samples obtained from the patient for future molecular studies. It is strongly advised to clarify the reason for retaining the samples in a repository of biological material and the benefits of the idea of biobanking for further research and future patients. It is also recommended to inform on the place of the deposit of biological samples (the name and address of the institution) and to indicate that any further studies with its use will be possible only after approval of a relevant Ethics Committee.
9. Information on the principle of voluntarism and the possibility of withdrawing from participation in the study at any stage, with no consequences.
10. Information on confidentiality and protection of personal data in accordance with applicable regulations.
11. Information about the possibility to obtain further details of the project/procedures and to ask questions.

29.3 The Form of Informed Consent of Patients, Parents, or Legal Representatives

The form of informed consent of patients, parents, or legal representatives should include:

1. The title of the research project.
2. The name and contact details of persons responsible for the project realization (project manager, principal investigator).
3. The name and address of the involved institution (institution coordinating the project—in the case of a multi-center projects).
4. The declaration of the patient/legal guardian to have got acquainted with the proposed project based on conversation(s) with a member of the research team (mostly physician) and the patient information sheet, a copy of which the patient received. The participant/legal guardian should state that he/she has been familiarized with the nature and the aims of the project, including details of participation, sample collection, storage, and potential use in further research.
5. The statement of the patient/legal guardian that the above information has been understood, and any doubts have been clarified during a conversation with a member of the research team.
6. The declaration that the patient/guardian is aware of a voluntary participation in the study with the possibility to withdraw from the project at any stage, with no consequences.
7. The declaration that the patient/guardian is aware of his/her rights to confidentiality and privacy, and to protection against the misuse of biological material preserved in a repository (the need for approval by the relevant Ethics Committee of any future studies with the use of the deposited material).
8. The confirmation of informed consent for participation in the research.
9. The confirmation of informed consent for preservation of the biological material for future research.

Particularly noteworthy is the inclusion in these forms the consent of the patient/guardian for retaining of biological material for further scientific projects. The acquisition and storage of biological samples is an integral part of any research, involving the analysis of biological material. Therefore, all projects should include the consent of research participants for the storage and further use of the residual biological material, so that the scientific value of the obtained samples goes beyond the frameworks of a single research project. The idea of biobanking may raise doubts of participants and/or their guardians. It is therefore recommended to clarify (in conversation and in the form of information sheet for patients/guardians) the reason for retaining the biological material and the benefits of such procedures. It is recommended to provide the name and the address of the institution responsible for the storage of biological material and to emphasize that approval of the appropriate Ethics Committee is a prerequisite for the use of the material in any further research.

The samples of biological material always remain the property of the person from whom it was collected. Therefore, the participant or his/her legal representative may at any time change the previous decision concerning the storage and the use of the samples. This information may greatly contribute to dispelling possible doubts of the patient/guardian on the idea of biobanking. The role of the member of a research team responsible for obtaining the informed consent (usually a physician) for the success of the process and the comfort of the participant should be strongly emphasized. The conversation with the patients should be focused not only on providing the basic information on the project, but it should also enable the patient to get additional explanations, including those on the idea of biobanking.

The idea of using biological samples in other research projects implicates the possibility of obtaining results which may affect the health of the participant or his/her relatives. Therefore, the participant should have the right to choose whether he/she wants to be informed on this situation, depending on the current possibilities of prevention, treatment, and genetic counseling.

29.4 Examples

A sample informed consent form and a sample information sheet for a patient/legal representative prepared for an exemplary research project are included in the Appendix.

29.5 Conclusions

Due to rapid advances in molecular studies and relevant legislative changes, whose pace varies in different countries, guidelines presented in this chapter should be treated as general rules of obtaining informed consent to participate in a research project. These will probably require modification and/or adaptation for the needs of particular research projects conducted in different countries. However, the general idea of obtaining the informed consent should be unchanged: to promote research, potentially beneficial to the society, with respect of the rights of the individual, in accordance with the internationally accepted ethical rules.

Acknowledgments This chapter was partly supported by the Ministry of Science and Higher Education, grant N N407 311 839.

Appendix

Information for Patients, Parents, or Legal Representatives

EXAMPLE

'Advanced molecular methods in hematology. Development and implementation of standards for molecular diagnostics of minimal residual disease, post-transplant hematopoietic chimerism, and chromosomal translocations in childhood acute lymphoblastic leukemia'

PROJECT MANAGER: *name, surname, institution*
PRINCIPAL INVESTIGATORS: *names, surnames, institutions*
INSTITUTION RESPONSIBLE FOR THE PROJECT REALIZATION: *name and address of the institution*

Dear Patient, Dear Parents/Guardians,

For further progress in the treatment of childhood acute lymphoblastic leukemia in our country, it is essential to implement therapeutic protocols including the adjustment of treatment intensity to the results of molecular testing. In many countries, modern molecular techniques have already been successfully used for reliable assessment of prognosis, accurate evaluation of treatment response, and early, thus giving a greater chance to cure, detection of disease recurrence. Below you will find information about a research project aimed at the implementation of molecular methods for monitoring the treatment of children with acute lymphoblastic leukemia. Consent to participation in this project might contribute to further improvement of the outcome of this malignancy in our country. It is also possible that the children participating in the project might directly benefit from the results of the performed molecular analyses, which may provide additional information helpful in clinical decision making.

1. Participation in the Project

A necessary condition for the realization of the project is to obtain your permission to collect samples of blood or bone marrow from you (to a patient)/your child/children (to parents/guardians). These samples will be subjected to molecular analyses aimed at the detection of the so-called minimal residual disease, and in case of children undergoing transplantation, these will additionally be used for the assessment of the functioning of transplanted bone marrow. Our procedures require some extra sampling which will be performed in due course. Sampling will be carried out according to the following schedule:

Patients with newly diagnosed leukemia

- additional 5–7 ml of bone marrow obtained during bone marrow collection for the diagnosis of leukemia
- additional 5–7 ml of bone marrow obtained during bone marrow sampling for routine assessment of treatment effects on 15th and 33rd day of treatment, in 12th week of therapy and at the end of treatment

Patients subjected to transplantation

- 5–7 ml of blood collected once a week until 14th week after transplantation, then once a month, until the end of 18th month after transplantation

Bone marrow or peripheral blood stem cells donors

- molecular tests will be performed with the use of a small volume (approximately 5 ml) of material collected for transplantation, without need for additional sampling

2. Potential Risk and Inconveniences

Blood/bone marrow will be collected in low volumes, i.e., 5–7 ml (equivalent to 1–1.5 teaspoons) on the occasion of blood/bone marrow sampling for routine diagnostics or treatment monitoring. In case of sick children the blood will be collected by the so-called central venous catheter or port catheter, installed at the beginning of treatment, thus avoiding the subsequent puncture of peripheral veins.

Since the research project will be performed with the use of blood/bone marrow samples that have already been taken for routine diagnostic or treatment monitoring procedure, you/your child will not be exposed to any additional physical risk.

3. Coding of Samples

Collected samples will be marked with unique codes. These codes will be used by the research team during the storage and handling of the samples, to ensure the anonymity and personal data protection according to the Confidentiality principle (see point 7). If necessary, decodification will only be made by the principal investigator (*name*) or by a person authorized by the principal investigator.

4. Sample Storage and Further Use

Due to the enormous scientific value of the obtained blood/bone marrow samples, the unused portion of the biological material, *with your permission*, will be retained and secured for further research into leukemia and related diseases. This material will be deposited in: *name and address of the institution; contact details of a person responsible for the repository.* Any study with the use of this material will only be possible after approval by the respective Ethics Committee, whose task is to protect the rights of patients. By agreeing to preserve and share the residual material for further research, you and your children may greatly contribute to medical advances in the diagnosis and treatment of leukemia, which can bring benefits to future patients.

If you consent to the use of biological samples in future research projects, it is possible that the obtained results might potentially have an impact for your health/for the health of your relatives. Participants donating their samples for future research have the right to decide whether they want to be informed about such outcomes, depending on available options for treatment, prevention, and genetic counseling. Therefore, if you wish to be informed on such results, please provide us with your contact details (point 3 of the form 'Informed consent of patients, parents or legal representatives') and communicate to us via the resource person (see point 8) any changes regarding your contact details.

5. Access to Medical Record

For the purpose of this research it will be necessary for the research team to get access to medical records of the participants. Data collection and processing will be performed according to the Confidentiality principle (see point 7).

6. Voluntariness Principle

Consent to participate in the study is entirely voluntary. Each participant has the right to withdraw their consent, at any stage, without giving reasons thereof. In order to withdraw the permission, please contact the resource person (see point 8).

7. Confidentiality Principle

This ensures the confidentiality of any data obtained from the patient, i.e., the collection, storage, and analysis will be held to rules and regulations regarding the protection of personal data of patients *(local legislation should be specified; safety systems according to local law should be described).*

8. Resource Person

Should you need additional information regarding participation in the project or wish to withdraw your consent, please contact: *name, institution, contact details of the responsible person.*

....

Name and surname of the person asking for consent

....

Signature of the person asking for consent

....

Date

Informed Consent of Patients, Parents, or Legal Representatives

EXAMPLE

'Advanced molecular methods in hematology. Development and implementation of standards for molecular diagnostics of minimal residual disease, post-transplant hematopoietic chimerism, and chromosomal translocations in childhood acute lymphoblastic leukemia'

PROJECT MANAGER: *name, surname, institution*
PRINCIPAL INVESTIGATORS: *names, surnames, institutions*
INSTITUTION RESPONSIBLE FOR THE PROJECT REALIZATION: *name and address of the institution*

....

Name and surname of the patient/donor *Date and place of birth*

I declare that I have been informed about the objectives and the manner of implementation of the project, including procedures, to which participants are subjected, and about potential related risk, inconveniences, and benefits. I have also been informed about the possibility of retaining the remains of my biological samples for future research into leukemia and related diseases. I have read and understood 'Information for patients, parents or legal representatives'. I have had the opportunity to ask questions and I have understood the answers.

I had been given enough time to make a decision to carry out molecular tests with the use of blood/bone marrow samples collected from me/my child and to use the remnants of biological material for further research. I understand that the confidentiality of my/my child's personal data will be protected, and the use of residual biological material will be placed under the control of the Ethics Committee.

I am aware that the participation in this research is voluntary, and the expressed consent can be withdrawn at any time. I have received a copy of the form 'Information for patients, parents or legal representatives', and the copy of the form 'Informed consent of patients, parents or legal representatives'.

I hereby give consent (*please mark YES/NO*):

(1) for my participation/participation of my child in the above-mentioned research project
..... YES ..... NO

(2) for the preservation of blood/bone marrow samples obtained from me/my child and their further use in future research projects (under the control of Ethics Committee)
..... YES ..... NO

(3) to be informed about scientifically validated results of research with the use of my blood/bone marrow samples that might potentially influence my/my relatives' health
..... NO
..... YES in all cases
..... YES, but only if preventive or curative treatment and/or genetic counseling is available

....
Name and surname of the patient/donor

....
Contact details (address, telephone) of the patient/donor

....
Signature of the of the patient/donor giving consent *

* Signature of patient/donor required only for children over 12 years of age

....
Name and surname of the parent/legal representative of the participant

....
Signature of the parent/legal representative of the participant

....
Name and surname of the person asking for consent

....
Signature of the person asking for consent

....
Date

Further Reading

Council of Europe (1992) Recommendation (92) 3 of the Council of Europe, on genetic testing and screening for health care purposes. Available via http://www.coe.int/t/dg3/healthbioethic/Texts_and_documents. Accessed 20 Feb 2012

Council of Europe (1997) Convention for the protection of human rights and dignity of the human being with regard to the application of biology and medicine. Available via http://conventions.coe.int/Treaty/en/Treaties/html/164.htm. Accessed 20 Feb 2012

Council of Europe (1997) Recommendation (97) 5 of the Council of Europe on the protection of medical data. Available via http://www.coe.int/t/dg3/healthbioethic/Texts_and_documents. Accessed 20 Feb 2012

Council of Europe (2005) Additional protocol to the convention on human rights and biomedicine, concerning biomedical research. Available via http://conventions.coe.int/treaty/en/treaties/html/195.htm. Accessed 20 Feb 2012

Deschênes M, Cardinal G, Knoppers BM, Glass KC (2001) Human genetic research, DNA banking and consent: a question of 'form'? Clin Genet 59:221–239

Directive 95/46/EC of the European Parliament and of the Council of 24 October 1995 on the protection of individuals with regard to the processing of personal data and on the free movement of such data (1995) Off J Eu Un L 281:31–50. Available via http://eur-lex.europa.eu/. Accessed 20 Feb 2012

Directive 2001/20/EC of the European Parliament and the Council of 4 April 2001 on the approximation of laws, regulations and administrative provisions of the Member States relating to the implementation of good clinical practice in the conduct of clinical trials on medicinal products for human use (2001) Off J Eu Un L 121:34–44. Available via http://eur-lex.europa.eu/. Accessed 20 Feb 2012

Directive 2004/23/EC of the European Parliament and of the Council of 31 March 2004 on setting standards of quality and safety for the donation, procurement, testing, processing, preservation, storage and distribution of human tissues and cells (2004) Off J Eu Un L 102: 48–58. Available via http://eur-lex.europa.eu/. Accessed 20 Feb 2012

Martín Uranga A, Martín-Arribas C, Donato J, Posada de la Paz M (2012) Outstanding legal and ethical issues on biobanks. An overview on the regulations of member states of the EuroBioBank project. Available via http://www.eurobiobank.org/en/intranet/workflow/uploadDir/PDFmarcadoresEUROBIOBANK-ING.pdf. Accessed 20 Feb 2012

Regidor E (2004) The use of personal data from medical records and biological materials: ethical perspectives and the basis for legal restrictions in health research. Soc Sci Med 59:1975–1984

UNESCO (1997) Universal declaration on the human genome and the human rights. Available via http://www.unesco.org/new/en/social-and-human-sciences/themes/bioethics/human-genome-and-human-rights/. Accessed 20 Feb 2012

UNESCO (2003) International declaration on human genetic data. Available via http://www.unesco.org/new/en/social-and-human-sciences/themes/bioethics/human-genetic-data/. Accessed 20 Feb 2012

Index

A
Aberrations, 165
Abnormal cell clone, 164
Activation of NF-jB, 77
Acute leukemias (AL), 165
Acute lymphoblastic leukemia (ALL), 184, 202
Acute myeloid leukemia, 206, 388
AID, 57
Albumin gene, 379
Albumin test, 379
Alleles, 238
Allele-specific oligonucleotides (ASO), 187
Allorecognition, 240
All-trans-retinoic acid (ATRA), 35
AML-1 ETO, 35, 388
Antibodies, 143, 146
Antigen recognition site, 238
Antigen, 143, 146
Antigen-specificity, 92
Apoptosis, 109–15
ARMS-PCR, 451, 452
Array CGH, 174
ASO primer, 375

B
BAALC, 40
Background amplification, 381
Balanced and unbalanced chromosomal rearrangements, 161
Balanced, 165
Bar coding, 287
B-cell precursor all (BCP-ALL), 4, 6, 8, 20
BCR signaling, 64, 93
BCR/ABL, 103, 109
BCR/ABL1, 7–9, 12, 14, 206
Biobank, 299
Biobanking, 299, 465
Blood, 300
Bone marrow microenvironment, 219
Bone marrow, 300

C
CBFB-MYH11, 388
CC analysis, 163
CDNA, 432
CEBPA mutations, 393
CEBPA, 38
Cell culture, 163
Chromosomal aberrations, 162
Chromosome, 23, 86
Chromosome 1 abnormalities, 76
Chromosome 12p deletions, 77
Chromosome 13 abnormalities, 75
Chromosome 16q abnormalities, 77
Chromosome 17p13 deletion, 76
Chronic lymphocytic leukemia, 85, 430
Chronic lymphoid leukemias, 153
Chronic lymphoproliferative disorders, 153
Chronic myeloid leukemia, 103, 206
C-kit, 42
Class I mutations, 30
Class II mutations, 31
Cloning, 454, 455
Clonality testing, 435
  GeneScan (GS) fragment analysis, 435
  heteroduplex (HD) analysis, 367, 435

M. Witt et al. (eds.), *Molecular Aspects of Hematologic Malignancies*, Principles and Practice, DOI: 10.1007/978-3-642-29467-9,

C (*cont.*)
C-myc, 37
Comparative genomic
hybridization (CGH), 172
Complete chimerism, 242
Complex karyotype, 177
Conditioning regimen, 222
Consent form, 286, 287
Consent, 300
Control, 379
Conventional (classical)
cytogenetics (CC), 162
Conventional cytogenetic analysis, 162, 164
Copy number alterations
(CNAS), 7, 11, 12, 44
Core binding factor leukemias, 388
CRKL, 109–112
CRLF2, 10
Cross-lineage expression, 185
Cyclin D translocation, 73
Cytogenetic analysis, 161
Cytogenetic remission, 178
Cytogenetically normal AML, 388
Cytogenetics, 161, 162, 164
Cytometers, 144

D
Deletion, 309
Density gradient
centrifugation, 305, 306
DLBCL, 59
DMSO, 293
DNA damage, 112
DNA microarrays, 174
DNMT3A, 40
Donor lymphocyte
infusion (DLI), 278
Donor, 241
DR haplotype, 239
Duplication, 309

E
Electrophoresis, 316
Epigenetic mechanisms, 44
Epigenetics, 15, 309
  CpG island, 319, 320
  DNA methylation, 309, 319, 320
  DNA hypermethylation, 319
ERG, 41
ETV6–RUNX1, 7, 9, 12
European group for the immunological
characterization of leukemias (EGIL), 6

F
FBXW7, 17
FIP1l1-PDGFRA genes, 456
FIP1l1-PDGFRA, 130, 134
Flow cytometer, 144, 145
FLT3, 37
FLT3-ITD, 391
Fluorescence in situ hybridization
(FISH), 163, 168
Fluorochrome, 145, 146
FOXO, 111, 113, 114
Freezing, 289, 301
French–American–British (FAB)
classification, 5–7

G
gDNA, 432
Gene expression profiling, 14
Genetically targeted therapeutic
approaches, 177
Genetics, 87
Genome wide association
study (GWAS), 5, 11
Germinal center, 56, 58
Graft versus leukemia effect, GVL, 276, 278
Graft-versus-leukemia reaction, 217

H
Hematopoietic chimerism, 256
  complete chimerism (CC), 256
  mixed chimerism (MC), 256
  autologous recovery (AR), 256
  transient mixed chimerism (TMC), 256
  stable mixed chimerism (SMC), 256
  progressive mixed chimerism (PMC), 256
Hematologic malignancies, 161, 164
Hematopoietic stem cell transplantation
(ALLO-HSCT), 256
  short tandem repeat (STR)
  polymorphism, 257
Hemato-oncology, 161
HLA, 238
Homologous, 90
Human HSC, 218
Hyperdiploid, 72

I
IDH1, 39
IDH2, 39
IG/TCR, 20
IGHV gene mutational status, 429

IKZF1, 5, 12, 14
Immunoglobulin and t-cell receptor gene rearrangements, 18
Inactivation of p18, 78
Information sheet, 465
Informed consent, 463–465
Insertion, 309
Insertion/deletion (indel) polymorphism, 257
Inversion, 309
Isochromosome, 106

J

JAK2 gene mutation, 130, 131, 133, 451

K

Kinase substrates, 109
KIR, 239
Kit gene mutations, 135
Kit gene, 458
K-RAS, 42

L

Lasers, 145
Leukemia, 85
Leukemia-/lymphoma, 149
Linkage disequilibrium, 239
LOH, 44
Lymph node, 301
Lymphoblastic crisis, 112
Lymphoma, 55, 59

M

MAF translocation, 73, 75
M-bcr, 107, 108
MDS, 165
Methylation of p16, 78
MHA, 240
MHC, 238
microRNAs, 43, 78
Minimal residual disease (MRD), 7, 11, 47, 276
Mismatch, 240
Mixed chimerism, 242
MLL, 7, 9, 10, 12, 14, 16, 19, 36
MLL-PTD, 39
MMSET translocation, 73
MN1, 41
Monoclonal antibodies, 158
Mononuclear cells (MNCs), 305, 365
Monoploidity, 309
Monosomal karyotype, 177
MPL gene mutations, 131
MPL gene, 455
MRD, 7, 14, 19, 20, 276
Multiple myeloma (MM), 443, 444, 448
Multiple myeloma, 164
Mutation, 309
Mutations of immunoglobulin heavy chain gene, 72
MYC abnormalities, 79
Myelo proliferative neoplasms (MPN), 174
Myelodysplastic syndromes (MDS), 163, 207
Myeloproliferative neoplasms, 130, 137

N

Non-hodgkin lymphomas (NHL), 153, 163
Non-hyperdiploid, 72
Normal karyotype, 177
NOTCH1, 17
NPM1, 38
NPM1 mutations, 393
N-RAS, 42

P

Pathophysiology, 87
PAX5, 12, 13
Phenotype, 143, 146
Philadelphia chromosome, 103
PML–RARA, 35, 391
Poliploidity, 309
Polymerase chain reaction (PCR), 309, 311, 320, 432
  component, 315, 316
  conditions, 315
  inhibition, 311, 315
  multiplex PCR, 434
  methylation specific polymerase chain reaction (MS-PCR), 319, 320
  primer design, 215, 216
  purification of products, 318
  single PCR, 434
Primary chromosome aberration, 165
Prognosis, 175
Prognostic significance, 175
Pyrosequencing, 257

Q

Quality assurance, 290
Quantitative range, 377, 378, 380
Quantity and quality of DNA, 379

R

RAS mutations, 78
RAS, 105, 109, 110, 111
Rearranged immunoglobulin (IG), 6
Reduced intensity conditioning (RIC), 262
Restriction, 240
RFLP analysis, 458
RIC transplantation, 263
Reverse transcription (RT), 309, 314, 316
  one-step, 317
  two-step, 317

S

Sample retrieval, 302
Sample storage, 469
Secondary chromosome aberrations, 166
Sensitivity, 378, 380
Sequencing, 371, 436, 454, 455
Single nucleotide polymorphism (SNP), 257
SnuPE, 257
Standard curve, 376, 380
Stereotyped BCR, 90
STR-PCR approach, 257

T

T(8;14)(q24;q32), 75
T(9;22)(q34;q11), 103
TET2, 39
T lymphoblastic leukemia/lymphoma (T-ALL), 4, 6, 7, 9, 11, 14, 16, 20
Taqman technology, 186, 187
T-cell receptor (TCR) genes, 6
TEL–AML1 (ETV6–RUNX1), 7, 14
Therapy, 177
Threshold cycle, 186
Tissue
  collection, 309, 311, 312
  preparation, 311, 313
  storage, 309, 310
Tissue establishment, 286, 288
Translocation t(11;14)(q13;q32), 74
Translocation t(14;16)(q32;q23), 75
Translocation t(4;14)(p16;q32), 74
Translocation t(6;14)(p21;q32), 75
Translocation t(14;20)(q32;q11), 75
Translocation, 104, 105, 107–109, 309
Trisomy, 103, 106
Tumor supressor p53 gene, 107
Two hits model, 30, 31
Tyrosine kinase, 108, 109, 110, 112, 113

U

UPD, 44

V

V-(D-)J gene segments, 364
VDJ recombination, 56, 57

W

World health organization (WHO), 4, 6
WT1, 40

MIX
Papier aus verantwortungsvollen Quellen
Paper from responsible sources
FSC® C105338

Printed by Books on Demand, Germany